Cardiovascular Mathematics

Luca Formaggia
Alfio Quarteroni
Alessandro Veneziani (Eds.)

Cardiovascular Mathematics

Modeling and simulation of the circulatory system

Springer

Luca Formaggia
MOX, Department of Mathematics
Politecnico di Milano, Milan, Italy

Alfio Quarteroni
MOX, Department of Mathematics
Politecnico di Milano, Milan, Italy
and
CMCS-IACS, École Polytechnique Fédérale de Lausanne
Lausanne, Switzerland

Alessandro Veneziani
MOX, Department of Mathematics
Politecnico di Milano, Milan, Italy
and
Department of Mathematics and Computer Science
Emory University, Atlanta, GA, USA

ISBN 978-88-470-5805-7 Springer Milan Berlin Heidelberg New York
e-ISBN 978-88-470-1152-6 Springer Milan Berlin Heidelberg New York
DOI 10.1007/978-88-470-1152-6

Springer is a part of Springer Science+Business Media

springer.com

Softcover re-print of the Hardcover 1st edition 2009

9 8 7 6 5 4 3 2 1

Typesetting: PTP-Berlin, Protago TEX-Production GmbH, Germany (www.ptp-berlin.eu)
Cover-Design: Francesca Tonon, Milano

Springer-Verlag Italia srl – Via Decembrio 28 –20137 Milano

Preface

This book is addressed to graduate students and researchers in the field of bioengineering, applied mathematics and medicine wishing to engage themselves in the fascinating task of modelling how the cardiovascular system works. This effort is motivated by the fact that cardiovascular diseases have a major impact in Western countries and by the widespread recognition that mathematical models and numerical simulations can aid to better understand physiological and pathological processes. It complements the information provided to medical doctors by medical imaging and other non-invasive means and opens the possibility of more in-depth surgical planning.

The expertise required by a researcher wishing to work in this field, from the bioengineering, medical or mathematical side, is vast and multidisciplinary. This book offers a mathematically sound and up-to-date foundation to the training of researchers and serves as a useful reference for the development of mathematical models and numerical simulation codes. It is structured into different chapters, written by recognised experts in the field. However, the book is not just a collection of different contributions. A careful editing process has ensured the progression of the material as well as the consistency of notation and expressions and systematic cross-referencing.

To model blood flow and the circulatory system, many fundamental issues need to be addressed. Blood flow interacts both mechanically and chemically with the vessel walls and tissue, giving rise to complex fluid-structure interactions whose mathematical analysis is complex (and in part still incomplete) and which are difficult to simulate numerically in an efficient manner. At a macroscopic level, the arterial wall is a complex multi-layer structure which deforms under the action of blood flow. Even though sophisticated constitutive equations have been proposed for the structural behaviour of the vessel wall, its elastic characteristics *in vivo* are still very difficult to determine and are usually inferred from pulse propagation data. The modelling of the interaction between blood flow and the vessel wall mechanics needs algorithms which correctly describe the energy transfer between them to accurately represent wave propagation phenomena.

Blood is in fact a suspension of cells and particles in plasma. A Newtonian constitutive equation is generally accepted as a good approximation of blood behaviour for large vessels. However, the study of circulation in smaller vessels and capillaries needs to abandon the Newtonian assumption for the fluid and account for the shear-thinning behaviour of blood. At a microscopic scale, the orientation of the endothelial cells depends on the wall shear stress induced by the blood. This can be related to possible degenerative pathologies of the vascular tissue. An accurate description of the local flow field is thus required to address this type of interaction.

Another source of alteration of biochemical exchanges is the modification of the flow field caused by, for instance, vessel stenosis (a localised narrowing), which often results in the development of fat deposits in the lumen. The modelling of this process, known as atherogenesis, requires the coupling of the flow equations with appropriate models to describe the wall absorption of the chemicals involved and their transport, diffusion and kinetics. Sound mathematical models of these phenomena are needed to develop effective numerical schemes for the solution of these coupled problems.

Realistic simulations cannot be carried out without a proper geometrical reconstruction from medical imaging data, another important subject by itself. Medical imaging has progressed enormously in the last decade and the amount of information it can provide has increased by an order of magnitude at least. Yet, how to extract data in a form useful for the simulations is not an obvious task.

The complexity of the cardiovascular system calls for the integration of different models, operating at different levels of complexity and adapting to the need of the research at hand. For instance, the study of the flow recirculation in a carotid bifurcation requires to the use of a sophisticated three-dimensional model. But this model has to be fed with boundary conditions that have to take into account the rest of the circulatory system, which has then to be modelled, even if at a lower level of detail. The coupling of different mathematical models is one of the most active aspects of the research in haemodynamics. Following a sort of "divide and conquer" strategy the cardiovascular system is subdivided into "compartments" either at the geometric or at the functional level, and each is treated with the model best suited to the problem at hand. This way sophisticated (and expensive) models are used only where necessary, while the "global" nature of the cardiovascular system is maintained.

All the aspects just described find a place in this book. A general overview of the cardiovascular system physiology is given in Chapter 1, whose aim is to introduce the most important terms and concepts to the readers less acquainted with this topic. It is complemented by Chapter 2, which illustrates the basic mathematical models for blood flow and biochemical transfer. Chapter 3 provide more details on the derivation of the equations that govern blood flow, while Chapter 4 is devoted to the treatment of medical images to obtain geometries suitable for numerical computations. The most up-to-date techniques are explained in detail, focusing on the issues relevant to the use of the geometries for numerical simulations. Chapter 5 illustrates the important relations between geometry and type of flow, pointing out also the main characteristics of the different flow regimes that may be encountered in the cardiovascular system. The issue of mathematical models for blood rheology is tackled in Chapter 6. Here, different non-Newtonian models are presented and their range of applicability discussed. Indications are given on their implementation for practical flow computations. In Chapter 7 mathematical and numerical models of biochemical transport are explained in detail, with practical examples. This is a complex topic which involves the coupling of equations of different types and acting on different domains. The mathematical analysis of such coupled models is an important and recent research topic. Its foundation and major results are illustrated in Chapter 8, while Chapter 9 focuses on the mechanical coupling between blood flow and the vessel structure. It deserves special treatment because of its practical importance and abundance of results both from the theoretical and the algorithmic side. Indeed, the compliance of blood vessels influences blood flow and gives rise to the so-called "pulse waves". Chapter 10 deals with the derivation of reduced models of the cardiovascular system, and the numerical method for their solution. Reduced models are important since they are able to provide simulations of large parts, if not the whole cardiovascular system in an affordable way, at the price of a reduced spatial resolution. One-dimensional and lumped parameter models will be considered. The former are of particular importance for the study of the pulse wave propagation along the main arterial tree. The latter represent the simplest (and historically the first) way of simulating the cardiovascular system. The intertwining of such models with more complex three-dimensional ones is the foundation of the so-called geometric multiscale approach illustrated in detail in Chapter 11. Finally, Chapter 12 provides a set of well described and reproducible test cases and applications. When necessary, geometry data will be made available through the HaeMOdel project web page. The value of the main physical parameters, the definition of the major quantities of interest as well as a glossary of the more technical terms are given in the Appendices.

This book is a follow-up of the scientific results and experience collected during the four-year activity of the VI-framework European Funded project *HaeMOdel* (contract n. HPRN-CT-2002-002670), a Research and Training Network started in 2002. The aim of the project was to develop, analyse and assess numerical models for the simulation of the human cardiovascular system.

The authors want to acknowledge also the contribution to the research from different national agencies; in particular we mention the contributions of the Italian "Istituto Nazionale di Alta Matematica" (INDAM), the project COFIN 2003 by the Italian Ministry of Research, the project CNR 2000, the Fonds Nationale Suisse (FNS), the Portuguese Fundação para a Ciência e a Tecnologia (project POCTI/MAT/41898/2001), the British Engineering and Physical Sciences Research Council, the Canadian Institutes of Health

Research (CIHR), the Heart and Stroke Foundation of Ontario and the Austrian Science Foundation, Vienna, Projects N. P11982-TEC, P1414321-TEC.

The authors A. Quarteroni, A. M. Robertson and A. Sequeira appreciate support from the National Science Foundation for the grant NSF 0104680 U.S.-Portugal-Switzerland Cooperative Research Program: "Multiscale models of blood flow in the cerebral vasculature". This grant provided support for collaborative meetings for work included in this book.

We would like to gratefully acknowledge the vital scientific contribution of all the young researchers of the *HaeMOdel* project: Jordi Alastruey, Sylvia Anicic, Santiago Badia, Tomas Bodnar, Paola Causin, Lukasz Janski, Zinedine Kathir, Nuno Niniz dos Santos, Vincent Martin, Alexandra Moura, Martin Prosi, Alessandro Radaelli, Gianluigi Rozza, Keith Smith, and Christian Vergara.

Further information on the *HaeMOdel* project can be found on the project home page `mox.polimi.it/haemodel`.

Milan, January 2009

Alfio Quarteroni
Luca Formaggia
Alessandro Veneziani

Contents

List of Contributors

Luca Antiga
Mario Negri Institute
Bergamo, Italy
antiga@marionegri.it

J. Alastruey Arimon
Aeronautics Department
Imperial College
London, UK

Rossella Balossino
Laboratory of Biological Structure Mechanics
Department of Structural Engineering
Politecnico di Milano
Italy
rossella.balossino@polimi.it

Carlo D'Angelo
MOX, Department of Mathematics
Politecnico di Milano
Italy
carlo.dangelo@polimi.it

Denis Doorly
Department of Aeronautics
Imperial College
London, UK
d.doorly@imperial.ac.uk

Gabriele Dubini
Laboratory of Biological Structure Mechanics
Department of Structural Engineering
Politecnico di Milano
Italy
gabriele.dubini@polimi.it

Miguel A. Fernández
INRIA Paris-Rocquencourt
Le Chesnay Cedex, France
miguel.fernandez@inria.fr

Luca Formaggia
MOX, Department of Mathematics
Politecnico di Milano
Italy
luca.formaggia@polimi.it

Jean-Frédéric Gerbeau
INRIA Paris-Rocquencourt
Le Chesnay Cedex, France
jean-frederic.gerbeau@inria.fr

Sergio Giordana
Work performed while the author was working at
Aeronautics Department
Imperial College
London, UK

Yvon Maday
UPMC Univ Paris 06
Laboratoire Jacques-Louis Lions
Paris, France
and
Brown University
Providence, USA
maday@ann.jussieu.fr

Francesco Migliavacca
Laboratory of Biological Structure Mechanics
Department of Structural Engineering
Politecnico di Milano
Italy
francesco.migliavacca@polimi.it

Robert Owens
Département de Mathématiques et de Statistique
Université de Montréal
Canada
owens@dms.umontreal.ca

Kim Parker
Department of Bioengineering
Imperial College
London, UK
k.parker@imperial.ac.uk

Joaquim Peiró
Department of Aeronautics
Imperial College
London, UK
j.peiro@imperial.ac.uk

Giancarlo Pennati
Laboratory of Biological Structure Mechanics
Department of Structural Engineering
Politecnico di Milano
Italy
giancarlo.pennati@polimi.it

Karl Perktold
Institute of Mathematics
Graz University of Technology
Austria
karl.perktold@tugraz.at

Martin Prosi
Work performed while the author was working at
MOX, Department of Mathematics
Politecnico di Milano
Italy
mprosi@gmx.net

Alfio Quarteroni
MOX, Department of Mathematics
Politecnico di Milano
Italy
and
CMCS-IACS, EPFL
Lausanne, Switzerland
alfio.quarteroni@epfl.ch

Anne M. Robertson
Department of Mechanical Engineering
and
Materials Science
University of Pittsburgh
Pittsburgh, PA USA
annerob@engr.pitt.edu

Adélia Sequeira
Departamento de Matemática and CEMAT
IST, Instituto Superior Técnico
Lisboa, Portugal
asequeir@math.ist.utl.pt

Spencer Sherwin
Department of Aeronautics
Imperial College
London, UK
s.sherwin@imperial.ac.uk

David A. Steinman
Mechanical and Industrial Engineering
University of Toronto
Toronto, Ontario, Canada
steinman@mie.utoronto.ca

Marc Thiriet
INRIA team REO
Laboratoire Jacques-Louis Lions
CNRS UMR 7598
University Pierre and Marie Curie
Paris, France
Marc.Thiriet@inria.fr

Alessandro Veneziani
MOX, Department of Mathematics
Politecnico di Milano
Italy
and
Department of Mathematics and Computer Science
Emory University
Atlanta, GA USA
ale@mathcs.emory.edu

Christian Vergara
Department of Information Technology and Mathematical Methods
University of Bergamo
V.le Marconi 5
Dalmine (BG), Italy
christian.vergara@unibg.it

Marina Vidrascu
INRIA-Rocquencourt
Le Chesnay Cedex, France
marina.vidrascu@inria.fr

Paolo Zunino
MOX, Department of Mathematics
Politecnico di Milano
Italy
paolo.zunino@polimi.it

1

Physiology and pathology of the cardiovascular system: a physical perspective

Marc Thiriet and Kim H. Parker

The purpose of this chapter is to introduce the reader to cardiovascular physiology and pathology. These are vast, complex subjects, each filling large tomes and severely exercising the memory of medical students. By necessity, this will be a very brief and, in places, simplistic introduction to the subject. Despite its simplicity, it can be very daunting to the newcomer who has not been trained in biology and physiology. Although we would strongly discourage it, those readers interested only in the mathematics of the modelling could skip this chapter initially, returning to it as the need arises.

Since the book primarily concerns the modelling of the mechanical and biochemical behaviour of the cardiovascular system, we have concentrated on the anatomy and physiology that bear directly upon mechanics. Living systems, however, are both complex and exquisitely adaptable and so it is impossible *a priori* to predict just how one facet of the physiology will interact with another. In the middle of the last century, it was generally assumed that blood vessels were relatively inert conduits for the blood and arterial disease was often compared to the 'furring' of water mains in the water supply system of a city. We now know that the cardiovascular system is a very active organ that both controls and adapts to its environment.

Consider, as an example, the uterine arteries. In the non-pregnant woman they have a diameter of less than 1 mm and supply a small part of the pelvic floor. In pregnancy, however, they provide the major source of blood to the placenta and thus nutrients to the fetus. The uterine arteries respond to the increasing demands of the fetus by increasing in size so that at term they are approximately 4 mm in diameter and supply about 20 times the volume flow rate of blood. After delivery, the demand decreases almost instantaneously and they respond within a few weeks, exactly how quickly is not known, to their original size and function. Our understanding of the mechanisms involved in this normal physiological reaction of the artery is rather perfunctory and good models would certainly help.

Another feature of the cardiovascular system that should not be neglected is its flexibility. The differences between rest and maximal exercise can be very

Formaggia L, Quarteroni A, Veneziani A (Eds.): Cardiovascular Mathematics. Modeling and simulation of the circulatory system

large; trained athletes, for example, can increase their heart rate and cardiac output by a factor of 5 for sustained periods. Normal individuals commonly experience increases of 2–3 times in their heart rate and cardiac output during periods of exertion or stress and such variation is important for health.

There are also enormous changes in design and size between individuals in their cardiovascular system. In this chapter we will cite a number of 'average' values for the cardiac system, but it should be remembered that these refer to the average adult, usually at rest conditions, and that there will be a very wide range of values in the population as a whole and in individuals under different conditions.

The primary motivation for cardiovascular modelling must be the prevalence of cardiovascular diseases, the single largest cause of death worldwide, which is responsible for more than half of mortality in the developed countries. Atherosclerosis is responsible for both heart attacks and stroke. It is a complex disease that generally takes decades to develop. There is widespread study of its origins, its treatment and, hopefully, its reversal. Of the many risk factors that have been identified – blood cholesterol and triglyceride levels, smoking, obesity, genetics, etc. – only haemodynamic and mechanical factors can explain the focal nature of the disease. A better understanding of these factors is essential to our understanding of the disease.

In this chapter we will introduce the basic anatomy, physiology and pathology of the cardiovascular system together with a collection of data necessary for the later chapters. Our primary interests are in the mechanical properties of the system, which will be the principal target of the models discussed in this book. While there is some discussion of the regulation and control of the cardiovascular system, we have largely ignored the enormous and medically very important subject of cardiovascular pharmacology. Drug delivery and action is undoubtedly influenced by haemodynamics but little is known about these interactions.

Because all of the material in this chapter is introductory and available in a number of standard textbooks, we will not cite individual papers. Instead, we include an annotated bibliography at the end of the chapter as a guide to further reading in cardiovascular anatomy, physiology and pathology.

1.1 Anatomy of the cardiovascular system

The cardiovascular system is composed of the heart, which pumps the blood, and the network of blood vessels that convey blood to the body and drain it from the body tissues to the heart. All parts of the system work in concert, but initially will be considered individually.

1.1.1 The heart

The heart is a muscular organ made of two synchronised pumps in parallel: the right side, which collects deoxygenated blood from the systemic veins and

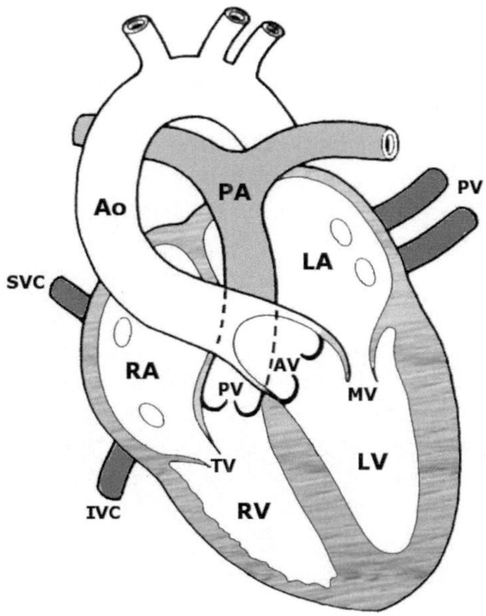

Fig. 1.1. A sketch of a cross section of the heart showing the gross anatomy. Chambers: LA left atrium, LV left-ventricle, RA right atrium, RV right ventricle. Vessels: Ao aorta, PA pulmonary artery, SVC superior vena cava, IVC inferior vena cava, PV pulmonary veins. Valves: TV tricuspid valve, AV aortic valve, PV pulmonary valve, MV mitral valve. LA is supplied by veins from the lungs and transfers blood through the mitral valve into the LV. LV ejects blood through the aortic valve into the aorta. RA collects blood from the inferior and superior venae cavae and transfers it through the tricuspid valve into RV. RV ejects blood through the pulmonary valve into the main pulmonary artery

perfuses the lungs, and the left side, which collects oxygenated blood from the pulmonary veins and perfuses the rest of the body. The heart is comprised almost entirely of myocardium, specialised muscle cells (cardiomyocytes) that differ from other muscle cells in their contractibility (lower) and their resistance to fatigue (much higher). The heart has four cavities: upper left (LA) and right (RA) atria that collect the blood from the veins and lower left (LV) and right (RV) ventricles that contract to propel the blood into the systemic and pulmonary veins (Fig. 1.1). The left ventricle, the largest chamber with the thickest walls, is located posteriorly and leftwards from the right ventricle, which can be thought of as a chamber wrapped around the right side of the left ventricle from the heart base to the apex. The two ventricles share a septum, which separates the heart into the left and right sides. The heart is surrounded by the pericardium, a serous, inelastic membrane that restricts excessive dilation of the heart and can limit ventricular filling.

There are four valves in the heart, one at the exit of each heart cavity. All of the valves are embedded in the fibrous skeleton of the heart, which divides the atria from the ventricles. The mitral valve, which prevents blood from flowing back from the LV to the LA, has two leaflets and is prevented from prolapsing by the chordae tendons and papillary muscles running from the cusps of the valve leaflets to the side of the LV. The aortic valve guards the exit of the LV into the aorta, the major systemic artery. It has three leaflets which are inserted into the walls of the sinuses of Valsalva, roughly hemispherical bulges at the root of the aorta. The aortic valve has three simple leaflets without any attachments that come together, providing mutual support when they are closed. The corresponding valves in the right heart are the tricuspid valve between the RA and RV and the pulmonary valve between the RV and the root of the main pulmonary artery.

The heart itself is perfused by the right and left coronary arteries, originating from two of the three sinuses of Valsalva just above the aortic valves. The large coronary arteries form a network that lies on the outer layer of the heart wall. The smaller arteries dive into the wall where they branch off to form the microcirculation of the myocardium. Because the myocardium lacks the ability of other muscle cells to contract anaerobically (without oxygen), the constant supply of oxygen by the coronary vessels is crucial to the regular function of the heart.

The heart is innervated by both components of the autonomic nervous system: the parasympathetic and the sympathetic nerves. Normally, the parasympathetic innervation is the dominant neural influence on the heart.

Deoxygenated blood from the head and the upper body and from the torso and lower limbs is brought to the right atrium by the superior and inferior venae cavae. While there are valves in the medium-sized veins that prevent the back-flow of blood, there are no valves between the venae cavae and the atria. This blood flows through the tricuspid valve into the RV. When the RV contracts, the tricuspid valve closes and the pulmonary valve opens, allowing the blood to flow into the main pulmonary artery. Oxygenated blood from the lungs flows into the LA through a variable number (most often 4) of pulmonary veins. There are no valves at the outlet of these veins; it is difficult, in fact, to distinguish where the veins end and the atrium begins. This blood flows through the mitral valve into the LV. When the LV contracts, the mitral valve closes and the aortic valve opens, allowing the blood to flow into the aorta and thence the systemic circulation. The detailed physiology of the cardiac cycle will be discussed in Section 1.2.1.

1.1.2 The vascular networks

Blood is ejected from the heart in discrete pulses under relatively high pressure into the main arteries (at a lower pressure in the pulmonary circulation than in the systemic circulation) where it flows through a network of branching arteries of decreasing size to the arterioles and then the capillaries where it delivers oxygen and nutrients to the tissues and removes carbon dioxide and

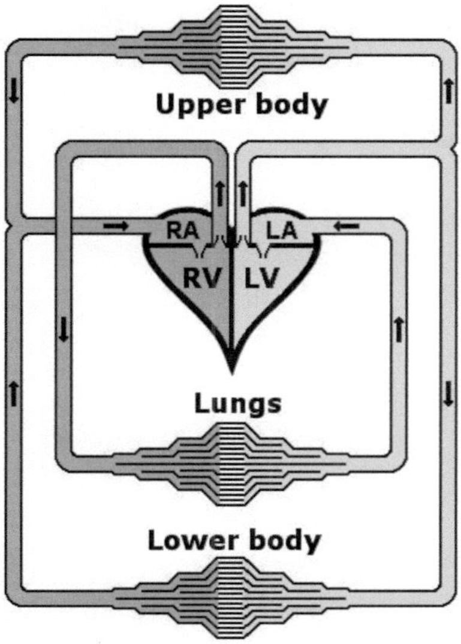

Fig. 1.2. A sketch of the cardiovascular system. LA left atrium, LV left ventricle, RA right atrium, RV right ventricle. Oxygenated blood is pumped from the LV into the aorta, which connects through the conduit arteries to the microcirculation in all parts of the body. The oxygen is transferred to the tissue and carbon dioxide is transferred to the blood. The deoxygenated blood is collected by the systemic venous system and returned to the RA. The blood is then ejected from the RV into the main pulmonary artery where it is distributed to the pulmonary microcirculation. Oxygen is transferred to the blood and carbon dioxide is transferred to the airways where it is breathed out. The newly oxygenated blood is collected by the pulmonary venous system and carried back to the LA where the cycle starts again

catabolites. Blood is collected from the capillaries through merging venules and returns to the heart at low pressure through a network of veins.

Each blood circuit, systemic and pulmonary, is thus composed of three main compartments: arteries, capillaries and veins (Fig. 1.2, Tables 1.1 and 1.2). The primary purpose of the arterial and venous vessels is to carry blood to and from the various tissues, the conduit function, while the microcirculatory compartment carries out the various exchange processes, the perfusion function. The vascular networks are closed, tortuous, multi-generation systems of branching or merging junctions of deformable vessels with widely different diameters and lengths.The arterial and venous systems are primarily bifurcating trees although there are numerous interconnections, anastomoses, at different places in the body. It is estimated that there are approximately twenty generations of bifurcations going from the heart to the most distant capillary beds in both the systemic and pulmonary circulation. The venous network roughly parallels the arterial network, except in the skull. The major arteries and their corresponding veins often run together with nerves as a neurovas-

Table 1.1. Properties of the human systemic vessels. The numbers of vessels are very crude estimates. Adapted from Caro et al. [62]

Vessel	*Diameter of lumen* (mm)	*Wall thickness* (mm)	*Number of vessels*	*Blood volume* (%)	*Mean pressure* (kPa)
Aorta	25	2	1	2	12.5
Large arteries	1–10	1	50	5	12
Small arteries	.5–1	1	10^3	5	12
Arteriole	.01–.5	0.03	10^4	5	7
Capillary	.006–.01	0.001	10^6	5	3
Venule	.01–.5	0.003	10^4	25	1.5
Vein	.5–15	0.5	10^3	50	1
Vena cava	30	1.5	2	3	0.5

Table 1.2. Properties of the human pulmonary circulation. PA: pulmonary artery. Adapted from Singhal et al. [465]

Diameter range (mm)	*Number of vessels*	*Volume* (ml)	*Mean velocity* (mm/s)
30 (main PA)	1	64	110
8–30	10	21	155
1–8	10^3	37	104
0.1–1	$.25 \times 10^6$	19	44
.02–0.1	20×10^6	5	23
.01 (capillaries)	300×10^6	5	2

cular bundle surrounded by a fascia of dense connective tissue. Veins, unlike arteries, have valves that prevent backflow of blood away from the heart.

The boundary between the large vessels and the microcirculation is defined differently by different authors, ranging from diameters of 100 to 250 µm. This boundary is somewhat artificial since the structure and composition of the smallest arteries and arterioles and of the narrowest veins and venules are very similar. Capillaries, the smallest blood vessels, are very different in their properties and connectivity. Capillaries can be as small as 5 µm in diameter, which is considerable smaller than the largest diameter of a red blood cell. In general, the topology of capillary beds is very complex with many interconnections. Most capillaries have a continuous lining of endothelial cells, like the arteries and veins. Fenestrated capillaries which have a discontinuous endothelium are found in the kidney, the gut, the choroid plexi of the brain and in many other locations where rapid exchange of water and small solutes is desirable. The common feature of flow in the microcirculation is that the Reynolds number (see Section 1.2 for the definition of the Reynolds number) is very low, generally $\ll 1$, indicating that viscous effects dominate completely.

The vasculature has many peculiar features such as vascular loops and anastomoses. Arteriovenous anastomoses are found in the skin and the gut, the interconnecting vessels often being muscular allowing for active control of the degree of anastomosis. Arterial anastomoses are found in many organs. The four arteries supplying the brain, the right and left internal carotid and vertebral arteries, are connected together through the circle of Willis at the base of the brain. The hands and the feet are each supplied by two separate arteries that are connected through the palmar and pedal arches. The arteries supplying the intestines have a large number of loops along their length. The liver has a very specialised circulation where the portal vein takes blood from the microcirculation of the gut directly to microcirculatory vessels in the liver so materials absorbed into the blood can be stored, metabolically converted or excreted immediately. While many generalisations can be made about the vascular system, it is probably safest to assume that the vasculature of every different organ has some special features.

The vasculature is characterised by three properties: complexity, diversity and variability. The complexity arises from the biological functioning, the complicated structure and sheer number of blood vessels. The diversity is the consequence of the large variability between individuals in vessel origin, shape, path and branching. The variability is due to the wide range of demands made on the circulatory system during different normal and abnormal activities. These properties place stringent demands on modelling of the circulation. On one hand it is highly desirable to find generalisations that allow us to predict the effect of various changes and interventions in the 'average' individual. On the other, the ability to generate subject-specific models will be necessary to predict detailed changes in each individual.

1.1.3 The microstructure of the heart and vessels

The cardiovascular system is made up of relatively few basic components. The endothelial cells provide a continuous interface, the endothelium, between the blood and the walls, with the exception of the fenestrated capillaries where there are gaps in the endothelium. The endothelial cells are 0.5–2 μm thick and attach tightly to each other with clefts between them approximately 10–20 nm wide. Within the intercellular clefts there are specialised tight junctions where the two cell membranes are held even closer together, particularly in the brain where they are referred to as the blood-brain barrier. It is not certain whether these tight junctions are continuous around the whole of the endothelial cell or not. The shape of the endothelial cell is dependent upon the flow over it. In regions of low flow the cells are roughly circular in aspect with a diameter of $\sim$ 50 μm. In regions where flow is high and unidirectional, the cells have an aspect ratio of $\sim$10 and the same surface area. Experiments show that endothelial cells will reorient themselves within a few hours in response to changes in the flow direction and magnitude.

The walls of the large components of the vasculature contain another cellular component, striated myocytes in the heart and smooth muscle cells in the vessels. They are also made of fibrous proteins, collagen and elastin; ground substance, proteoglycans and glycoproteins, and interstitial fluid, water containing electrolytes and small plasma proteins. Apart from their active role in pumping blood and controlling the tone of the vessels, the cells also produce the proteins and ground substance necessary for growth and maintenance of the tissue. Collagen forms relatively stiff, high-strength fibres that are normally tortuous in the relaxed tissue. Elastin forms complex, cross-linked networks that are very distensible, being able to stretch up to 100 % elastically. Thus, elastin provides the elasticity of the tissue at small strains and collagen provides tensile strength at large strains. This results in highly non-linear elastic properties. The role of the ground substance is less clear, but it is certainly involved in the visco-elastic properties of tissue and affects the permeability of the tissue to water and small solutes.

The heart

The heart achieves an efficient, co-ordinated contraction of its myofibre population in order to eject blood into both circulatory networks in each cycle. It is a highly evolved organ that combines structural and functional heterogeneity to attain its primary function as a pump. The activation phase of the myofibres matches the mechanical heterogeneity for a suitable electromechanical coupling. The heart wall is composed of three layers: (i) the internal thin endocardium (ii) the thick muscular myocardium, and (iii) the external thin epicardium. The endocardium is made up of an endothelium which is continuous with the blood vessel endothelium and elastic connective tissue that merges with the myocardium. The myocardium is composed mainly of cardiomyocytes, collagen fibres and capillaries. Its outer layer contains nodal cells. The epicardium has an external layer of flat mesothelial cells lying on a support tissue, which contains elastic fibres.

External to the heart wall is the double-layered pericardium containing a lubricating fluid ($\sim$ 25–35 ml) which separates the two pericardial layers: the outer, thick, fibrous, layer (the parietal pericardium) and the inner layer (the epicardium, or visceral pericardium). The pericardium is composed of collagenous connective tissue that can restrict overexpansion of the heart. It is attached to the diaphragm, thus anchoring the heart, and fuses with the outer wall of the blood vessels entering and leaving the heart.

The heart has a fibrous skeleton with its central fibrous body lying between the atria and the ventricles. It prevents early propagation of the action potential (Section 12.4.4). The central fibrous body provides support for the interventricular septum and the valve rings, supporting the four cardiac valves. The cardiac valves are sheets of connective tissue covered by an endothelium and are composed of intramural cells (smooth muscle cells, fibroblasts and myofibroblasts), reinforced by collagen and elastic bundles. The interstitial cells synthesise and remodel the extracellular matrix. The cusps of the atrio-ventricular valves, the mitral valve on the left and the tricuspid valve on the right, are connected via the chordae tendinae to papillary muscles attached to the ventricle walls to prevent them prolapsing into the atria during the ventricular contraction. The semilunar valves guarding the outlets of the ventricles, the aortic valve on the left and the pulmonary valve on the right, are tricuspid valves which do not require muscular support since the three cusps support each other when the valves are closed (the significant contact surface is called the coaptation zone). The aortic and pulmonary valves have smooth ventricular and wavy arterial faces. The free edge is indented, with, characterised by a high concentration of collage fibres, the Arantius nodule in its thicker middle part. The cusp is a multi-layer structure with (i) the fibrosa, (ii) the spongiosa, absent in the coaptation region, and (iii) the ventricularis.

The heart structure provides the three properties of contractibility, automatism and conduction due to two kinds of cardiac muscular cells: cardiomyocytes and nodal myocytes. The nodal cells are small (80–100×10–20 µm) muscular cells which either generate, thus acting as the pacemaker for the heart, or quickly spread the depolarisation in the myocardium. The sino-atrial node is located at the top of the right atrium. Due to its automatic self-excitation, it initiates the electrochemical signal ("natural pacemaker"), which propagates throughout the heart as a depolarisation wave (which can be measured as an electrocardiogram – ECG), the so-called action potential. Since the sino-atrial node fibres fuse with the surrounding atrial cardiomyocytes, the action potential spreads through the atria and produces the atrial contraction. However, several nodal bundles conduct action potentials with a greater speed. The action potential reaches the atrio-ventricular node, located in the right atrium near the lower part of the interatrial septum. The atrio-ventricular node imposes a delay of $\sim$ 100 ms in the transmission of the depolarisation wave to the ventricles after the atria have completed their contraction. From the atrio-ventricular node, the wave of contraction propagates rapidly along a network of conduction paths, including the His bundle (beneath the endocardium in the interventricular septum), its right and left branches (along respective sides of the interventricular septum) and the Purkinje fibres, which activate the contraction of ventricular cardiomyocytes.

Cardiomyocytes (70–150 × 20–35 µm), of given local orientation, are striated, nucleated cells which are electrically excited in order to rhythmically contract and relax. The sarcomere, the array of thick and thin myofilaments between the Z-lines, is the anatomical unit of muscular contraction (the hemi-sarcomere is the functional unit). The sarcomeres formed by packed contractile proteins (actin, myosin and multiple associated proteins) fill most of the cytosol. Cardiomyocytes have a richer supply of mitochondria, and a greater dependence on ATP (adenosine triphosphate), than skeletal muscle. They act more slowly and generate less force than skeletal muscle cells but are remarkably resistant to fatigue. Unlike skeletal muscle cells, myocardial cells rely entirely on aerobic metabolism. The microcirculation of the heart is arranged so that the capillaries run parallel to the myocardial fibres and they take up approximately half of the extracellular space in the myocardium.

Excitation of contraction requires the ion Ca^{++} and there is a complex cycle of calcium flux during the contraction/relaxation cycle of a myocyte involving active membrane transport, through special intracellular structures. The sarcolemma with its ion channels repeatedly invaginates to form transverse tubules (T-tubules) which plunge into the sarcoplasma (see Section 12.4.4), close to the sarcoplasmic reticulum. The sarcoplasmic reticulum stores calcium ions from diastolic uptake for systolic release. Owing to its speed, the action potential arrives almost simultaneously at all tubules of the T-system, ensuring that all sarcomeres have a coordinated contraction. It should be remembered that the relaxation phase of the cycle also requires metabolic energy and is not a simple mechanical relaxation. The depolarisation of the membrane which initiates the contraction cycle propagates from cell to cell as a wave. The potential changes due to this wave are detectable on the surface of the chest, the electrocardiogram (ECG), which provides an invaluable diagnostic marker of heart activity.

Cardiomyocytes are joined by intercalated discs that contain clusters of gap junctions in order to allow action potential to spread rapidly. Cardiomyocytes then act as a syncytium; stimulation of an individual cell results in the contraction of the whole myocardium. Cardiomyocytes are surrounded by a trellis of collagen and elastin, which supports the cells and limits dilation.

Structurally, the myocardium can be thought of as a left ventricle with a right ventricle added to it in a form similar to a hip pocket on a pair of trousers. The wall of the left ventricle is approximately 8 mm when relaxed and thickens to 12 mm when contracted. The wall of the right ventricle is thinner, 5 mm (range 2–7 mm). The myocardium is oriented in the wall of the left ventricle in a roughly helical manner with its direction varying with depth (Fig. 1.3). The myofibre orientation varies from the epicardial layers to the endocardial layers in a given ventricle wall slice and with the myocardium region from the base to the apex. The inner aspect of the walls of the ventricles is, contrary to most sketches, highly variegated with trabeculae carnae and papillary muscle. The role of the papillary muscles is to prevent the prolapse of the mitral valve during systole, but the role of the trabeculae is not well known. It is, however, highly likely that some of the thickening of the myocardium measured by various imaging modalities includes a component due to the coming together of the trabeculae as the volume of the ventricle decreases.

Large vessels

The walls of the large arteries have a circumferentially layered structure (Fig. 1.4). The internal, lumenal layer is the intima made up of the endothelium attached to a basement membrane and a thin layer of connective tissue (subendothelium) connected to the internal elastic lamella. The internal elastic lamella delimits the intima from the media. The media is formed by layers

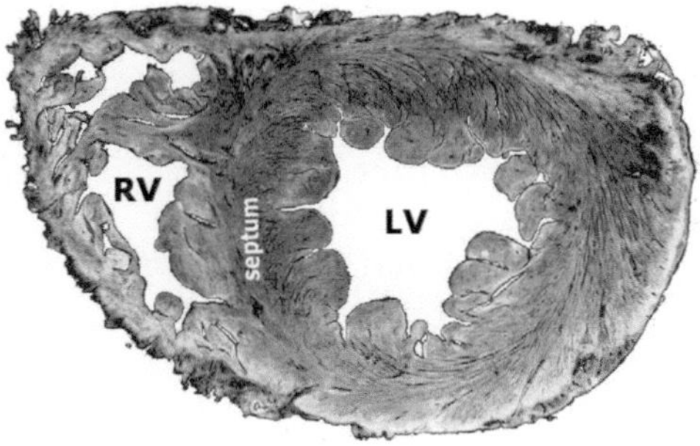

Fig. 1.3. A cross-sectional view of the human heart taken approximately halfway between the apex and the fibrous body. The orientation of the myocardial fibres is evident from the lines of staining and shows the roughly helical nature of the orientation. The septum dividing the LV and RV can be thought of as a continuation of the LV wall. Note the high degree of invagination of the internal surface of both ventricles, indicating the extent of the trabeculae carnae on the surface of the ventricles. LV: left ventricle, RV: right ventricle (adapted from [304])

of smooth muscle cells interspersed with elastic lamellae. These lamellae are about 15 μm thick and their structure is conserved across different sized arteries, larger arteries simply having more lamellae. The thickness of the media is $\sim 10\,\%$ of the internal diameter of the artery for the larger arteries. The outer limit of the media is delineated by the external elastic lamella. The outer layer of the arteries is the adventitia, consisting mainly of loose connective tissue with some smooth muscle cells. In larger vessels the adventitia contains nerves, vasa vasorum and lymphatic vessels. The adventitia is generally con-

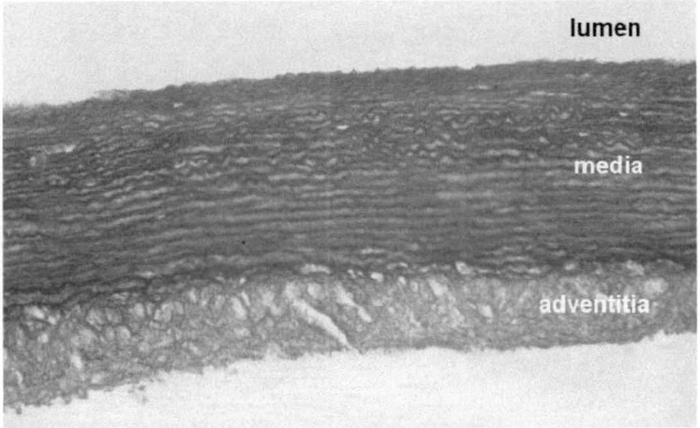

Fig. 1.4. A cross-sectional view of a part of the rabbit thoracic aorta. The artery has been fixed at physiological pressure, sectioned into thin slices and stained with orcein stain, which stains elastic tissue, collagen and basement membrane. At this magnification, the endothelium and intima are not visible. The dark lamellar structures in the media are elastic tissue with the smooth muscle cells lying between. The adventitia layer at the outside of the vessel is less organised than the media and is thought not to contribute significantly to the mechanical properties of the artery

sidered to play only a minor role in the mechanics of the vessel wall, although damage to the adventitia can lead to chronic changes in the properties of the artery wall.

There are subtle differences in the structure and properties of the large arteries at different locations in the arterial tree. Arteries proximal to the heart, particularly the ascending aorta, are known as elastic arteries. Their walls can be slightly thinner than more distal arteries with a smaller fraction of smooth muscle cells. As a result they are more distensible and provide much of the Windkessel (compliance chamber; Section 12.4.4) effect (blood systolic storage followed by diastolic restoration) whereby the starting-stopping nature of the blood flow expelled from the ventricle is smoothed out over the cardiac cycle to become pulsatile without any zero flow period (but with possible diastolic back-flow in certain territories) downstream from the main elastic arteries. The more distal muscular arteries have a larger fraction of smooth muscle, a thinner internal elastic lamella and a much more clearly delineated external elastic lamella. The smooth muscle can alter the tone of the arteries and can respond to both neural and humoral stimuli in the control of the cardiovascular system. The elastin composes a complex network of elastic tissue that forms a scaffold for the smooth muscle cells with many connections between the different lamellae. The elastic tissue can make up more than 50 % of the dry weight of the large arteries. The collagen fibres are oriented in a roughly helical form around the artery and are generally tortuous under normal conditions. As the artery is distended, the collagen fibres straighten and, because of their large tensile strength, bear more and more of the load. Because of their variability and number, very little is known about the medium-sized arteries. It is usually assumed that they resemble scaled down versions of the more distal muscular arteries which have been studied.

Cerebral arteries have distinct properties, probably because of the constant volume of the cranium in which they reside. Cerebral arteries have thinner walls without any external elastic lamella compared to similar sized arteries elsewhere in the systemic circulation. The internal elastic lamella is well developed.

Pulmonary arteries are much thinner than systemic arteries. The wall thickness is typically only 1 % of their diameter. Down to a diameter of about 1 mm they are classified as elastic arteries because they contain relatively little smooth muscle and collagen. They then transform into muscular arteries as their diameters decrease to 0.1 mm where the media is composed almost entirely of smooth muscle. This difference in structure of the pulmonary arteries is almost certainly due to the much lower blood pressure in the pulmonary circulation, generally less than one third of the systemic blood pressure. It is also interesting that pulmonary arteries are almost universally spared from atherosclerosis.

The walls of the large veins are thinner than their corresponding arteries and their bore is generally larger. The intima is very thin and the internal and external elastic lamellae are either absent or very thin. The media is thinner than the adventitia. Medium-sized veins are characterised by the presence of valves that prevent blood from flowing distally (i.e., in the direction away from the heart) during muscular compression of the veins. The largest veins of the abdomen and thorax have very thick adventitia, which contains bundles of longitudinal smooth muscle cells and vasa vasorum. Valves are absent.

The veins of the leg form a parallel system of deep veins passing through the large muscles and superficial veins lying close to the skin. They are connected by perforator veins with ostial valves allowing blood flow only from the deep to the superficial veins. This system provides a muscle pump whereby venous return of blood to the heart is facilitated against the hydrostatic pressure gradient that is present when the body is erect.

Venous valves are generally bicuspid and located in stiffer expanded segments of the vein. Venous valves are made of connective tissue with elastic fibres and few smooth muscle cells, covered by the endothelium. Veins are often elliptical in cross-section. Valve leaflets are inserted on the lower curvature faces of the vein wall while tributary veins usually enter the edges with the higher curvature.

Small vessels

Arterioles are usually defined as being less than 30 µm in diameter. They are composed of a continuous endothelium surrounded by one or two concentric layers of smooth muscle cells. Arterioles receive both sympathetic and parasympathetic innervation and are the principle regulators of local blood flow, through the action of muscular cells.

Capillaries are small exchange vessels composed of endothelium surrounded by a basement membrane with three structural types. Continuous capillaries, found in muscles, skin, lungs and the central nervous system, have a continuous basement membrane and tight intercellular clefts between endothelial cells. They, thereby, have the lowest permeability. Fenestrated capillaries, found in endocrine glands, renal glomeruli and intestinal mucosa, are characterised by perforations in the endothelium and, thus, by relatively higher permeability. Discontinuous capillaries, found in liver, spleen and bone marrow, are defined by large gaps in the endothelium and the basement membrane and, consequently, have very high permeability.

Venules are composed of a continuous endothelium surrounded by a basement membrane for the post-capillary venules and smooth muscle for the larger venules. Venules have been classified into microvenules (bore of 15–100 µm), minivenules (bore of 100–300 µm, wall with a continuous layer of smooth muscle cells) and venules (bore of 300–500 µm, wall with an adventitia).

Vascular smooth muscle cells

The smooth muscle cells found in the walls of blood vessels are capable of slower and much more sustained contraction than myocytes. Myogenic activity has been observed in all vessels except capillaries, including lymphatics. In smooth muscle, unlike striated muscle, the actin and myosin that produce the contractions are not arranged in distinct bands but are organised for the maintenance of tonic contractions. Vascular smooth muscle contraction can be initiated by mechanical, electrical and chemical stimuli. In particular, vascular smooth muscle contraction can be initiated by stretching of the muscle.

The endothelium

The endothelium constitutes the interface between the flowing blood and the deformable vessel walls (Fig. 1.5). In all vessels except the fenestrated capillaries the endothelium forms a continuous layer with very small gaps 10–20 nm wide between adjacent endothelial cells. At the microscopic level, the luminal surface of the endothelium is slightly wavy due to the thickening of the cells over the nuclei, measurements showing that the maximum height variations are $\sim$ 750 nm.

The entire surface of the endothelium and the intercellular gaps is covered with the glycocalyx, which forms the first contact between blood and the vessel wall. The glycocalyx is composed of highly negatively charged glycoproteins that are attached to the bilipid membrane of the cell wall. The glycocalyx is highly hydrated and extends up to 100 nm into the lumen of the vessel. The presence of the highly charged glycocalyx provides the first barrier to transport between the blood and the vessel wall and has a large influence on mass transport, particularly in the intercellular gaps.

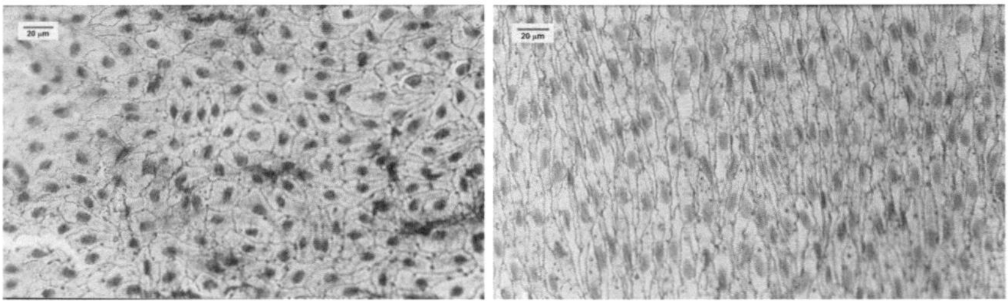

(a) ascending aorta (b) carotid artery

Fig. 1.5. An *en face* view of rabbit endothelium which lines all of the cardiovascular system. The tissue is stained to delineate the junctions between the cells (silver stain) and the cell nuclei (Weigert's iron haematoxylin) which are slightly out of focus in the centre of the cell. The mean flow direction is from the top to the bottom. a) The ascending aorta. The cells are roughly circular with no particular orientation. It may be significant that flow in the ascending aorta is highly unsteady and disorganised during some periods of the cardiac cycle. b) The carotid artery. The cells are highly elongated and aligned with the mean flow direction. Although flow in the carotid artery is also unsteady, it is much more organised and unidirectional than flow in the ascending aorta

Endothelial cells, like most cells, monitor both their internal state and the state of their environment. Endothelial cells experience normal stresses from the blood pressure, axial and circumferential tension from neighbouring cells, and shear stresses (see Chapters 2 and 3 for a precise definition) due to the friction of the flowing blood. The applied forces are unsteady with large spatial variations due to complex geometry of the vessels and the nature of the blood flow.

The endothelium is involved in the control of blood-wall exchange, in the modulation of the vasomotor tone, in the regulation of blood coagulation, in vessel wall growth and remodelling, and in the initiation and control of inflammation and immune responses through its effects on the adhesion of leukocytes. Much is known about the response of the endothelium to hydrodynamic stimuli, mainly from *in vitro* studies that can only approximate the complexity of *in vivo* behaviour. Virtually every function of the cell, from gene expression to nano- and microstructure, is affected to some extent by changes in the level or pattern of wall shear stress. Wall shear stress also affects the secretion of vasoactive substances, particularly nitric oxide (NO), and of molecules involved in coagulation and fibrinolysis. High wall shear stress also hinders leukocyte adhesion to the endothelium.

Transendothelial mass transfer

Transport across the endothelium depends on relative pressure and concentration gradients. Endothelial permeability can vary according to the state of the cytoskeleton and the size of the intercellular gaps. Molecular transport across endothelial cells is affected by the characteristics of the molecule (size, charge, shape and hydrophobicity). There are two different transport mechanisms: an intercellular transport through the intercellular gaps for small molecules and an intracellular transport for macromolecules. Intracellular transport can involve active transport across the cell membrane or transport via vesicles. Another possible mechanism for the control of endothelial permeability to macromolecules is the contraction of the cytoskeleton to induce an increase in the size of the intracellular gap. This contraction involves myosin chains interacting with actin filaments that make up the cytoskeleton. Nitric oxide induces a relaxation of the cytoskeleton and reduces endothelial permeability.

Extravasation

Flowing cells interact with each other, with the endothelium and with the subendothelial matrix in haemostasis, in thrombosis, in inflammation and in healing. These interactions involve cell-cell and cell-matrix attachments. Circulating blood cells have adhesion receptors which, once they penetrate the glycocalyx, enable them to adhere to the endothelial cell membrane. The cell-wall attachment is initially reversible but can become irreversible, tethering the cells together. Flowing cells thus undergo a sequence of steps leading to extravasation, with kinetics that are shear-dependent. The steps include rolling, tethering, activation, firm adherence, locomotion, diapedesis and finally transendothelial migration.

The endothelium can either enhance or inhibit flowing cell adhesion on its wetted surface. NO can inhibit adhesion of cells involved in inflammation or coagulation. Endothelial cells continually produce 13-hydroxyoctadecadienoic acid, which enhances the resistance to platelet or monocyte adherence. Conversely, adhesion molecules (integrins, selectins, immunoglobulin-like adhesion molecules) attract leukocytes for transmigration. Leukocyte extravasation also requires chemoattractants and cell-surface enzymatic reactions on both the leukocyte and endothelial cells. Ectoenzymes, membrane proteins that have catalytic domains outside the plasmalemma, regulate cell recruitment.

Clotting

Rapid clotting of the blood is vital in response to injury, but circulating clots can also lead to serious impairment of perfusion when they become lodged in the microcirculation of critical organs (thrombosis). We will look at the process of clotting in some detail because it is indicative of the complexity of biological reactions, a fact that should not be overlooked in modelling (Fig. 1.6).

When the endothelium is damaged, platelets aggregate and adhere to the regions where the wall matrix is exposed and initiate the coagulation cascade. The coagulation cascade is a complex process that results in a solid fibrin clot that covers the damaged region and stops haemorrhage. Primary haemostasis

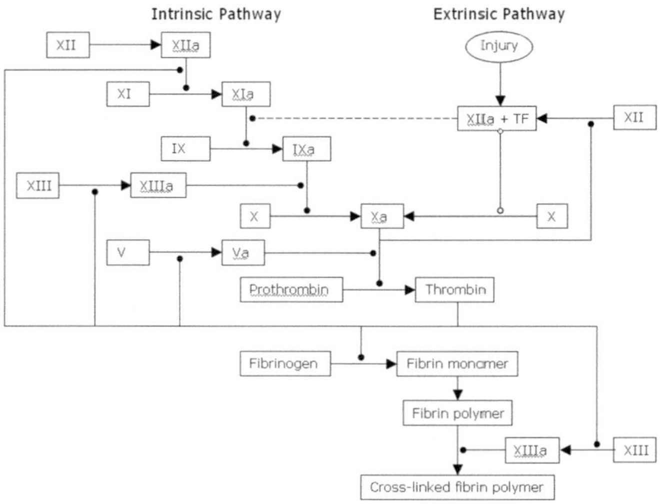

Fig. 1.6. A sketch of the pathways involved in the clotting cascade. See Table 1.3 for a definition of the different factors

Table 1.3. Coagulation factors

Coagulation factor	*Targets*
I (fibrinogen)	fibrin
II (prothrombin)	I, V, VII, XIII, protein C, platelets
III (tissue thromboplastin)	
IV (Ca^{++})	V, VIII, IX, X
V (proaccelerin)	X, II
VI (accelerin or Va)	
VII (proconvertin)	IX, X
VIII (antihaemophilic factor A)	IX, X
IX (plasma thromboplastic component)	X
X (prothrombin converting enzyme)	II
XI (plasma thromboplastin antecedent)	II, prekallikrein
XII (Hageman or contact factor)	XIa, prekallikrein, fibrin
XIII (fibrin-stabilising factor)	fibrin

refers to the plug formed by the aggregating platelets at the site of injury. Various plasma clotting factors then respond to form fibrin strands which strengthen the platelet plug. The platelets are then activated and secrete the contents of their granules into the plasma. The granules contain ADP, which is a potent inducer of platelet aggregation, which provides positive feedback for the accumulation of platelets at the site of injury. Secondary haemostasis has two pathways, intrinsic and extrinsic, which join in a common pathway leading to fibrin formation. The intrinsic pathway is characterised by the formation of the primary complex on collagen by high-molecular-weight kininogen, prekallikrein and FXII (Hegeman factor). FXII activates FXI which, in turn, becomes a protease until fibrinogen is transformed into fibrin to form the clot. In the extrinsic pathway, FVII is activated by tissue factor, which is released from cellular membranes during injury. FVIIa activates FIX and FX. The common pathway begins with activation of FX by FIXa and/or FVIIa, a process that requires FVIIIa, to produce thrombin. Thrombin not only converts fibrinogen to fibrin but also activates FVII, FV and their inhibitor PC as well as platelets.

Haemostasis involves four components: (i) the endothelium, (ii) the flowing platelets, (iii) the plasma coagulation factors and (iv) the fibrinolytic molecules. In normal conditions, the endothelium prevents clotting (thrombin inactivation and profibrinolytic activity). Endothelial cells have cell-surface substances, such as thrombomodulin, protein C, lipoprotein-associated coagulation inhibitor, tissue factor pathway inhibitor, protease-nexin and heparan sulphate. They inhibit platelet aggregation, releasing inhibitors like prostacyclins and NO. They activate fibrinolysis by binding the plasminogen activator inhibitor, which inhibits the fibrinolytic system. (Fibrinolysis occurs after coagulation during the healing process. It involves plasmin which cleaves fibrin in the clot.)

Thrombosis
The clotting process continually produces thrombi in blood vessels and cardiac chambers, probably triggered by unusual material circulating in the blood. When the blood flow is high enough, the microthrombi do not adhere strongly to the walls of the vessels and can be destroyed by the fibrinolytic system. When the blood flow is low, the competition between the self-activation and inhibition of coagulation can favour thrombis formation and the thrombus can develop to block the vessel lumen inducing ischaemia of the tissues that it irrigates. The thrombis can also detach to form an embolus, which can lodge in a smaller vessel somewhere downstream from the site of thrombosis. These blockages are called infarcts and the results can be serious when they occur in the brain (stroke), the heart (heart attack) or the lungs (pulmonary embolism).

Mechanotransduction

Blood vessel walls are constantly subjected to hydrostatic pressure, tension and shear stress. Vessels react to changes in these parameters by inducing changes that restore basal condition either by altering the conditions in the cardiovascular system as a whole acutely or by remodelling themselves chronically. The cell can change its shape and adapts to the mechanical loading. The cytoskeleton of mural cells transmits and modulates stresses within the cell via cellular junctions and cell-extracellular matrix adhesion sites. Moreover, applied forces initiate mechanotransduction cascades leading to transcription factor activation and subsequent gene expression. Cells not only sense applied forces and respond to received signals, but also evaluate the mechanical properties of their environment, in particular the stiffness of the extracellular matrix. However, the reaction depends on the cell type. For instance, mechanosensitive signalling via elastin-laminin receptors depends on the artery type and the particular region in the vessel.

There are several different mechanical stresses and various types of mechanical environments associated with flow patterns and unsteadiness. The vessel wall is sheared by the moving blood on one hand and stretched and compressed by the pressure applied by the blood. Wall shear stress has attracted much attention because of its correlation with the focal distribution of atheroma (see 1.3.1). Average wall shear stress on most arteries is $\sim 15\,\mathrm{Pa}$ but, because of the highly pulsatile nature of arterial flow, the wall shear stress vector undergoes large variations in magnitude and direction during the cardiac cycle. The normal stresses applied to the artery wall are orders of magnitude larger than the wall shear stresses; mean arterial blood pressure is $\sim 12.5\,\mathrm{kPa}$. Because of the unsteadiness of the pressure pulse, the complexity of the structure of the artery wall (particularly near branches) and the anisotropic nature of the walls, it seems likely that stress concentration could lead to large, unsteady gradients of stress locally within the wall. This, coupled with the need to displace interstitial fluid when the wall tissue is deformed, could have implications for the development of disease that, to date, remain unexplored. The stresses acting on vessel walls generate a basal tone of the smooth muscle even in the absence of neurogenic and hormonal influences. The haemodynamic stresses act on the smooth muscle via direct stress transmission or via the release of vasoactive compounds by the endothelium.

Various mechanosensors detect stresses and strains applied to the endothelial cells. Transduction elements on the cell surface include (i) mechanosensitive ion carriers, especially the stress-gated ion channels, (ii) cell-membrane receptors such as receptor tyrosine kinases and G-protein-coupled receptors and (iii) adhesion molecules. Simulation of the mechanosensors initiates different signalling pathways in order to trigger responses. Stresses can act directly on stretch-activated channels, which are sensitive to tension imposed on the cell membrane, and on shear-stress-activated channels. They convert external mechanical forces into electrochemical signals in the cell. Shear stress and luminal pressure either promote or repress gene expression in the endothelial cells. Although a small fraction of targeted genes respond to both pressure and shear stress stimulation, generally the two stimuli induce distinct gene expression. The complexity and variety of mechanical responses is hinted at in Fig. 1.7, which indicates some of the known responses of the endothelial cell and of the adjoining smooth muscle cell. Referring to the figure, initiation is done via (i) ion channels, such as stress-gated calcium ion channels (SGCC), (ii) growth factor receptors and others tyrosine kinase receptors (RTK), including the receptor type 2 of vascular endothelial growth fac-

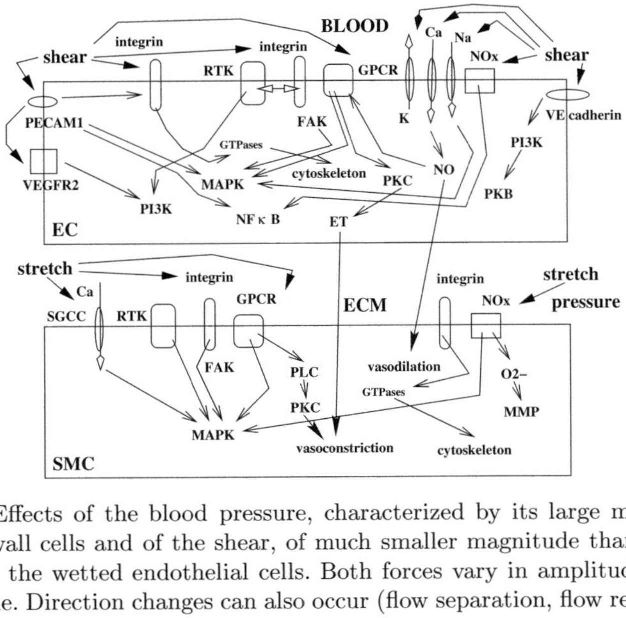

Fig. 1.7. Effects of the blood pressure, characterized by its large magnitude, on the vessel wall cells and of the shear, of much smaller magnitude than the applied pressure on the wetted endothelial cells. Both forces vary in amplitude during the cardiac cycle. Direction changes can also occur (flow separation, flow reversal during the diastole)

tor (VEGFR2), (iii) G-protein-coupled receptors (GPCR), (iv) membrane NADH/NADPH oxidase (NOx) and (v) adhesion molecules, mainly integrins, but also VE-cadherins and PECAM1. Effectors include small guanosine triphosphatases (GTPases), members of the mitogen-activated protein kinase (MAPK) family, phosphatidylinositol 3-kinase (PI3K), phospholipase PLC, protein kinases PKB and PKC, nitric oxide (NO), endothelin (ET), focal adhesion kinases (FAK) and superoxide anion O_2^-. The main targets are the transcription factors for cell and tissue remodelling (with possible degradation via matrix metalloproteinases (MMP) after long-duration pressure rise), such as NFκB, the cytoskeleton, adhesion molecules and ion channels. More details may be found in [276].

There is also cell-cell communication (i) between neighbouring endothelial cells, (ii) between adjoining smooth muscle cells and (iii) between endothelial cells and smooth muscle cells through fenestrae in the internal elastic lamella. Shear stresses imposed on monolayers of endothelial cells in culture increase the hydraulic conductivity of the endothelium by altering the state of the occludins of the tight junctions between cells.

Nitric oxide

Nitric oxide is produced by endothelial cells, smooth muscle cells, cardiomyocytes, and other cell types by the enzyme nitric oxide synthase (NOS). The continuous NO production is enhanced by many different stimuli (ATP, acetylcholine, ...). Two signalling pathways can be involved in shear-mediated changes in the NO production. The initial rapid phase of NO production is dependent upon protein G and Ca^{++} and is affected by the rate of change of shear and not on the level of shear. The subsequent slower phase of NO production does depend upon the level of shear and is involved in the sustained release of NO. NO is a potent vasodilator that acts by inhibiting vasoconstrictor influences (angiotensin-II, sympathetic vasocontriction). NO also inhibits platelet and leukocyte adhesion to the endothelium and has an antiproliferative effect on endothelial and smooth muscle cells. NO acts via cyclic guanosine monophosphate (cGMP), after binding to guanylyl cyclase.

Endothelin

Endothelin (ET) is a potent vasoconstrictor secreted by endothelial cells. The endothelin isoform ET1 is produced in endothelial cells stimulated by ischaemia or shear stress. The release of ET1 from endothelial cells in culture varies with the duration and the level of shear. It stimulates Ca^{++} influx from the sarcoplasmic reticulum of smooth muscle cells inducing vasoconstriction. ET1 also induces proliferation of endothelial and smooth muscle cells, thereby regulating the production of extracellular matrix. In human myocardium *in vitro*, endothelin exerts a positive inotropic effect (increase in myocardial contractility) via sensitisation of cardiac myofilaments to calcium and through the activation of sodium exchange. However, endothelins also induce coronary vasoconstriction and delayed negative inotropic effects, which balance and cancel the transient positive inotropic and chronotropic (increase in cardiac frequency) effects. Endothelin is also a growth factor for cardiomyocytes.

Other vasoactive substances

Several substances cause either contraction or relaxation of smooth muscle cells once they bind to specific surface receptors. Important endothelium-derived vasodilators are prostacyclin (PGI2), acetylcholine, adenosine diphosphate and adrenomedullin. Adrenomedullin also functions in many cell types including smooth muscle cells, cardiomyocytes and various blood cells. It enhances cardiac contractility, activates nitric oxide synthase, possibly induces hypotension and is involved in the regulation of fluid and electrolyte balance. Important endothelium-derived vasoconstrictors are adenosine triphosphate, superoxide anions, endoperoxides and thromboxane A2. Uridine adenosine tetraphosphate, which is stimulated by adenosine triphosphate, uridine triphosphate, acetylcholine, endothelin and mechanical stress, also produces vasoconstriction, probably via purinic receptors.

Vessel wall remodelling

Blood vessels respond to chronic changes in blood pressure and flow rate by remodelling, reduced pressure and flow lead to reduction of the lumenal diameter and media mass initiated by the up-regulation of endothelin and the down-regulation of NO. Similarly, a rapid increase in pressure or flow rate is characterised by an increase in vessel bore followed by a reactive contraction of smooth muscle cells. Prolonged increases lead to structural changes that are characterised by the proliferation of smooth muscle cells. Smooth muscle cells can also migrate into the intima, proliferate, synthesise extracellular matrix and form a neointima. Arterial wall layers thicken non-uniformly during induced hypertension. The inner wall layers thicken more in the acute phase, whereas the outer layers are thicker than the inner layers when the vessel is subjected to long-term hypertension. Medial collagen content increases quickly during the acute phase and more slowly during the chronic response. Elastin levels increase steadily but only slightly. Vascular smooth muscle tone increases rapidly but returns almost to control levels chronically.

Wall remodelling is thereby characterised by a rapid first stage of geometrical changes. Mechanical changes occur during the second stage of wall remodelling. Remodelling in response to hypertension involves the accumulation of collagens in order to counteract the increased distension of the wall, which makes the wall stiffer. However, the release of matrix metalloproteinases, which can cleave the fibrous matrix proteins, leads to progressive degradation of the extracellular matrix, increasing wall distensibility.

NO mediates the remodelling in response to increased wall shear stresses. NO released from cells exposed to excess shear stress triggers growth factor and matrix metalloproteinase activation, which contribute to the restructuring of the vessel wall. The expression of purinergic receptors in the vessel wall increases strongly in response to injury of the endothelium by balloon catheters, with a much higher level in the media, a very much higher level in the neointima and a ten-fold increase in the endothelium. It therefore seems likely that activated purinergic receptors are involved in neointimal proliferation.

1.1.4 Blood

Blood contains living cells and plasma (Table 1.4). The plasma represents $\sim 55\,\%$ of the blood volume with the remaining being the cells; the volume fraction of cells is called the haematocrit. Because erythrocytes (red blood cells) represent $97\,\%$ of the cell volume, the haematocrit is variously defined as the red blood cell volume fraction. The plasma contains $\sim 92\,\%$ water with the rest being made up of proteins, small molecules and ions. The major electrolytes in blood are the cations Na^+, K^+, Ca^{++} and Mg^{++} and the anions Cl^-, HCO_3^-, HPO_4^- and SO_4^-. Small sugars and carbohydrates are transported in the blood. Blood glucose is the most important of the small molecules and its concentration (glycaemia) depends upon the exogenous supply and the degredation of hepatic glycogen and is controlled by the hormone insulin. The circulating blood proteins include fibrinogen and other clotting factors as discussed above. Albumin is the main plasma protein, synthesised in the liver. It binds many small molecules for transport through the blood. Albumin, together with the electrolytes, is the main determinant of the osmotic pressure of the blood, which maintains the water balance between blood and the tissues. The non-protein nitrogen in the blood is contained in urea, uric acid, creatine, creatinine, ammonium salts and amino acids.

Lipids are essential for the formation and repair of cell membranes but are highly hydrophobic. They are transported in the blood in the lipoproteins, which are classified by their size and density; chylomicrons are the largest and are mainly involved in the transport of hydrophobic molecules from the small intestine to the liver where they are sequestered and processed. Very-low-density lipoproteins (VLDL) are synthesised in the liver and contain lipids, triglycerides and cholesterol esters. VLDL is converted into intermediate density lipoprotein (IDL) and low-density lipoprotein (LDL) through a complex cascade. LDL is the primary mode of transport of lipid and cholesterol through the body. Most cells have LDL receptors that are involved in the transport of lipids. High-density lipoprotein (HDL), a separate lipoprotein also synthesised in the liver, is primarily involved in the transport of excess lipids and cholesterol from the tissues to the liver for storage or excretion.

There are three main kinds of blood cells: erythrocytes, leukocytes (white blood cells) and platelets (thrombocytes). The erythrocytes are highly spe-

Table 1.4. Composition and properties of blood in the healthy human. The blood cells include erythrocytes (red blood cells), leukocytes (white blood cells) and thrombocytes (platelets). Leukocytes are divided into five classes by their morphological and histological characteristics. Neutrophils, eosinophils and basophils are known as granulocytes due to the presence of granules in their cytoplasm. Monocytes and lymphocytes are involved in scavenging and the immune defence system. Blood plasma consists of water (90 %) with the remainder being electrolytes (Na^+, 142 mmol/l; Cl^-, 102 mmol/l; and K^+, 5 mmol/l), carbohydrates, lipids, amino acids and other molecules

Erythrocytes	#/mm^3	$4.2–6.3 \times 10^6$
average haematocrit		46 % (male)
average haematocrit		42 % (female)
Leukocytes	#/mm^3	$4–10 \times 10^3$
neutrophils		40–70 %
eosinophils		1–2 %
basophils		0.5–1 %
lymphocytes		20–40 %
monocytes		2–10 %
Platelets	#/mm^3	$2–4 \times 10^5$
Ions	mEq/l	295–310
Protids	g/l	70–80
Lipids	g/l	5–7
Glucids	g/l	0.8–1.1
Density	kg/m^3	1050 (1040–1060)
Viscosity	Pa s	0.004 (.003–.04)
Haematocrit		47 % (40–50 %)
Osmotic pressure	mOsm	280–300
pH		7.39–7.41

cialised cells that contain neither a nucleus nor mitochondria. They consist of a bilipid membrane and membrane cytoskeleton surrounding a solution of haemoglobin. At rest they assume a biconcave discoid shape approximately 8 µm in diameter and 2 µm thick. Since the capillary diameters are often smaller than 6 µm, the cells must deform considerably during their passage through the microcirculation. Haemoglobin is a protein with a high affinity for oxygen and most oxygen is transported from the lungs to the tissues via this route. Erythrocytes have an average life span of ~3 months and they are constantly being generated by the bone marrow ($\sim 6 \times 10^6$ cells/s). The high cell content of the blood means that it has very complex rheological properties associated with cell deformability and agregation, which will be dealt with in Chapter 6.

Leukocytes are globular cells principally involved in the immune defence of the body and they have an average life span of only a few days. There are five types of leukocytes: neutrophils, eosinophils and basophils (collectively called granulocytes), lymphocytes and monocytes. The granulocytes are densely packed with granules and are primarily involved in the immune system. Neutrophils, 50–70 % of all leukocytes, diameter 8–15 µm, are able to phagocytise foreign cells, toxins and viruses. The eosinophils, less than 5 % of all leukocytes, diameter $\sim$ 15 µm, phagocytise antigen–antibody complexes. The basophils, less than 1 % of all leukocytes, diameter 12–15 µm, release (i) preformed granule-associated mediators, including histamine, which causes vasodilation, serotonin, bradykinin, heparin, which is an anticoagulant, and cytokines and (ii) newly generated mediators, such as prostaglandins and leukotrienes. The lymphocytes, 25–35 % of all leukocytes, diameter 8–15 µm, also play an important role in the immune response by providing antigen-specific acquired immunity (immunological memory). The monocytes, 3–9 % of all leukocytes, diameter 15–25 µm, give rise to mature macrophages that reside in the tissues and defend the body against viruses and bacteria.

The platelets, diameter 2–4 µm, are non-nucleated cells with an average life span of 10 days that are involved in coagulation. Platelets are dense in granules which contain serotonin, granulophysin, P-selectin, growth factors, clotting molecules and chemotactic compounds. Circulating platelets are kept in an inactive state particularly by prostacyclin and NO released by the endothelium. Platelet activation is affected by haemodynamic forces. At sites of injury, the platelets adhere to the exposed subendothelium, aggregate and initiate the coagulation cascade. Platelets are also active in inflammation, synthesizing proteins involved in the inflammatory pathways.

1.2 Cardiovascular physiology

The cardiovascular system is divided into the systemic circulation supplied by the left ventricle (LV) and the pulmonary circulation supplied by the right ventricle (RV). Each circulation can be divided conveniently into four parts: the corresponding heart pump, the arteries, the microcirculation and the veins. We will discuss each part separately although it should always be remembered that it is a closed system with each part interacting with every other part more or less strongly. For example, over time the same amount of blood must flow through the left and the right side of the heart. There can be transient variations which lead to the redistribution of blood within the circulatory system, but these differences cannot be sustained for long and haemostasis will soon be reestablished.

The heart is a single organ that is divided into the left and right sides. The arteries are the larger blood vessels that carry blood from the heart to the microcirculation in the tissue to be perfused and then the veins carry the blood back to the heart. In terms of mechanics, the large arteries and veins are differentiated from other vessels by their size and the predominance of inertial effects over viscous effects in the flow of blood in them. This is characterised by relatively large values of the Reynolds number,

$$Re = \frac{\rho D U}{\mu} \tag{1.1}$$

a dimensionless number that depends on the diameter of the vessel D (or radius R), the mean blood velocity U, the density ρ and viscosity μ of the blood. In Table 1.7 we report some typical values of the Reynolds number in the main blood vessels. More insight on the significance of this and other dimensionless numbers characterising fluid flow is given in Chapters 2 and 5. Here we just mention that the large difference in Re results in profoundly different fluid mechanics characteristics in the large and small vessels and so it is usual to treat them separately.

1.2.1 The cardiac cycle

The heart beat is a two stage pumping action over a period of about 1 s. Systole is defined as the period during which the myocardium contracts and blood is ejected from the ventricle. Cardiologists tend to define systole by the activity of the myocardium, usually through the electrocardiograph (ECG). Vascular doctors tend to define systole as the period between the closing of the mitral valve and the subsequent closing of the aortic valve. Functionally, the two definitions are very similar. Diastole is defined either as the period when the myocardium is relaxing or the period between the closing of the aortic valve and the closing of the mitral valve. At rest diastole occupies approximately two thirds of the cardiac period. As the heart rate increases, diastole is shortened while systole remains approximately the same duration. At maximal heart rate systole is also shortened.

Because of it predominance, we will focus our attention on the left ventricle in the discussion of the cardiac cycle. The right side of the heart is obviously just as important as the left, but it tends to follow the patterns established by the left. Also, because it is a cycle, the choice of the starting point is arbitrary. The wave of contraction over the ventricular surface gives rise to the QRS-complex in the ECG. This is a very singular event in the ECG and is often taken as the 'start' of the cardiac cycle. We will start the description of the cardiac cycle with the closure of the mitral valve (Fig. 1.8).

The four main phases of the ventricular activity can be defined by the state of the inlet and outlet valves. When the ventricular myocardium begins to contract, the pressure in the LV increases rapidly, exceeding the LA pressure and causing retrograde flow through the mitral valve. This flow causes the valve to close, initiating the *isovolumic contraction phase* when both the mitral and aortic valves are closed and the myocardium is contracting. Because blood is incompressible, the volume of the LV remains constant, but it undergoes a significant change in its shape as the myocardium continues to contract and the pressure in the ventricle increases rapidly. The mitral valve is prevented

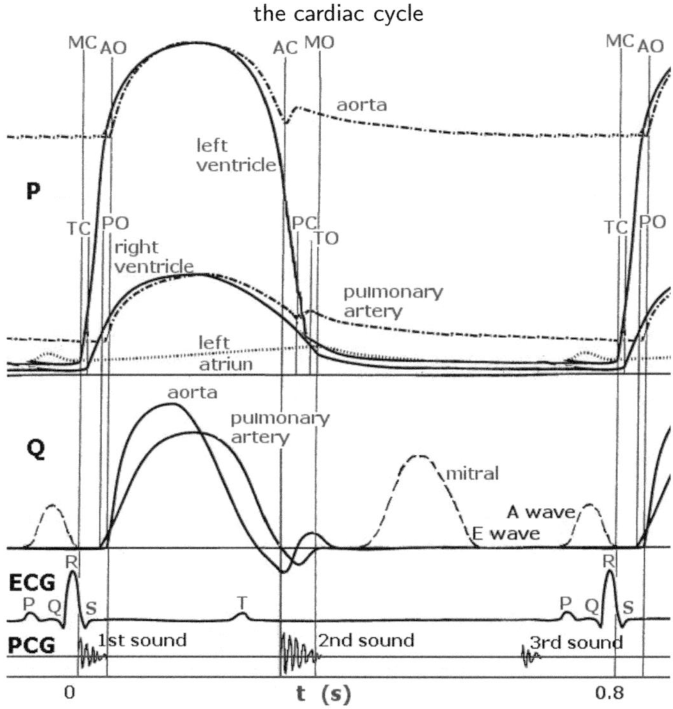

Fig. 1.8. A sketch of the events occurring during the cardiac cycle. P: pressure, Q: volume flow rate, ECG: electrocardiogram, PCG: phonocardiogram, t: time. MO: mitral valve open, MC: mitral valve close, AO: aortic valve open, AC: aortic valve close, TO: tricuspic valve open, TC: tricuspic valve close, PO: pulmonary valve open, PC: pulmonary valve close, PQRST: PQRST waves of the ECG. In the left ventricle, the isovolumic contraction phase is between MC and AO, the ventricular ejection phase is between AO and AC, the isovolumic relaxation phase is between AC and MO and the ventricular filling phase between MO and MC. Systole is the period between MC and AC, diastole the period between AC and MC

from prolapsing into the LA by the chordae tendinae and papillary muscles connecting the cusps of the valve to the wall of the ventricle.

When pressure in the LV exceeds the pressure in the aorta, the aortic valve opens, beginning the *ventricular ejection* phase of the cardiac cycle. The aortic pressure begins to rise because of the expansion of the vessels by the blood ejected from the heart, but as long as the myocardium is contracting quickly enough, the pressure difference between the LV and aorta remains negative[1] and flow into the aorta continues to accelerate up to peak flow.

[1] By convention, distance along the circulatory system is measured in the direction of mean blood flow, i.e. away from the heart in the arteries and towards the heart in the veins.

After a short time, the rate of contraction of the myocardium begins to slow and eventually it ceases to contract and begins to relax. At the time during this process when the rate of contraction of the ventricle becomes less than the volume flow rate in the root of the aorta, the pressure difference between the LV and the aorta becomes practically zero. This time coincides with the time of maximum flow rate into the aorta. Because of inertial effects, this time does not necessarily correspond to the start of relaxation of the myocardium as is frequently stated. Once the peak flow is reached, the aortic valve starts to close down to complete closure at the end of the decelerating phase of the flow across the aortic valve.

When the myocardium begins to relax, there is a spontaneous repolarisation of the cardiomyocytes that gives rise to the T-wave of the ECG. It should be remembered that myocardial relaxation is a metabolically active process (in particular, calcium sequestration in the cell stores, the sarcoplasmic reticulum).

As ventricular relaxation continues, the pressure difference between the left ventricle (LV) and the aorta reverses, becoming positive. This positive pressure gradient decelerates the flow into the aorta. After a period, this deceleration causes the flow in the ascending aorta to reverse so that blood starts to flow back into the aorta. The aortic valves closes, however, stopping this reversal of flow. Because the pressure in the LV is still much larger than the pressure in the left atrium (LA), the mitral valve is also closed and so the closing of the aortic valve marks the start of the *isovolumic relaxation phase*. During this period, the myocardium continues to relax and the pressure in the LV to fall.

When the LV pressure decreases below the pressure in the LA, the mitral valve opens, beginning the phase of *ventricular filling* when the mitral valve is open and the aortic valve closed. Filling initially occurs passively, the E-wave of mitral flow driven by the pressure in the atrium. There is considerable debate about the role of the ventricle during the passive filling, some cardiologists believing that the ventricle generates suction during this period due to the over-contraction of the ventricle past its equilibrium configuration. There is no debate about the second phase of filling, the A-wave, which is generated by the contraction of the left atrium as evidenced by the P-wave on the ECG. In healthy young adults at rest, about one third of the filling of the ventricle is contributed by the A-wave. This fraction increases with exercise and with age. At fast heart rates, the E and A-wave overlap to become a summation wave. There is a delay between the contraction of the LA and the contraction of the LV due to delays of the conduction wave through the atrio-ventricular node. Typical timings for the different phases of the cardiac cycle in a healthy adult at rest are given in Table 1.5.

The stroke volume can be modified by changes in ventricular contraction (the rate of development of tension in the myocardium; Table 1.6). Two of the major influences are the degree of filling, the rate of contraction of a myofibril depending upon the amount that it is stretched (the *Frank-Starling effect*), and the velocity of contraction (the magnitude of tension produced in a myofibril

Table 1.5. Typical duration of the four phases of the cardiac cycle (left ventricle) in a healthy young adult at rest, with a heart rate of $HR = 75$ beats/min

Phase	*Duration* (ms)	*Starting event*
Isovolumic relaxation	100	aortic valve closure
Ventricular filling	400	mitral valve opening
Isovolumic contraction	50	mitral valve closure
Ventricular ejection	250	aortic valve opening

Table 1.6. Typical properties of the heart functioning for a young adult

Property		*Units*	*Typical*	*Range*
Mass		g	300	250–350
Volume (LV)		ml		
	end diastolic		120	70–150
	end systolic		40	20–50
	stroke volume		80	50–100
	ejection fraction	%	67	60–80
Flow rate		ml/s	100	70–120
Heart rate		Hz	1.25	0.6–4.0
Duration		ms		
	isovolumic contraction		50	40–60
	systolic ejection		300	230–400
	isovolumic relaxation		80	70–90
	diastolic filling		370	250–400

depends upon its rate of shortening). The coupling of the dynamics of the heart to the vascular system, venous return and aortic dynamics makes control of the cardiovascular system very complex. It is observed that a premature depolarisation results in a weaker systole than usual, but that the following heart beat is stronger (*potentiation*). Similarly, a delayed depolarisation causes a more energetic contraction. The mechanical effects on cardiac contraction are dominated, however, by neural and humoral effects.

The variety of control mechanisms working simultaneously in the cardiovascular system results in a rather irregular behaviour of the heart rate. This is probably desirable in a pump that must react quickly to changes in the environment of the body. In fact, a very stable heart beat is associated with diseases such as congestive heart failure. This feature, however, is a handicap in cardiovascular signal and image processing. Ensemble averaging over a certain number of beats is, indeed, often used to improve the signal-to-noise ratio.

In order to supply adequate oxygenation to itself, the heart requires an average blood flow rate of 60–80 ml/min per kg of tissue. Approximately 80 % of the oxygen consumption is related to its mechanical work and 20 % to its basal metabolism. The myocardium also requires different substrates for its energy production, primarily fatty acids, which supply $\sim 70\,\%$ of the energy requirement, and glucids.

The cardiac output (CO) is the average volume of blood that is pumped by each ventricle per unit of time. In a healthy person at rest, CO is $\sim$ 5–6 l/min. Because the cardiac cycle is roughly periodic, the CO is equal to the stroke volume (SV) $\times$ the heart rate (HR), SV being the difference in volume of the ventricle at the end of the filling phase (diastole, EDV) and the end of the contraction phase (systole, ESV), hence[2], CO = (EDV − ESV) $\times$ HR.

Various factors determine the cardiac output. The force of contraction of myocardium depends upon the degree to which it is stretched and therefore the degree of filling of the ventricle prior to contraction. Cardiologists refer to anything that influences this as the preload. The rate of contraction of myocardium depends upon the load that it experiences and therefore upon the forces which resist ejection. Cardiologists refer to this as the afterload.[3] Moreover, the contractility of the heart is also affected by different molecules that originate either humorally or neurologically. Body size affects cardiac demand and studies have shown that CO varies not with body mass but with body area; so clinicians use the cardiac index (CI), which is the ratio of CO to the surface area of the body. For healthy people, $2.8 < \mathrm{CI} < 4.2\,\mathrm{l/min/m^2}$. Clinicians also refer to the cardiac reserve as a measure of the ability of the heart to quickly adjust to immediate demand, as measured by various standard tests. In healthy young adults, the cardiac reserve is 300–400 %.

The mechanical work done by the heart

The mechanical work done by the heart during one beat can be measured from the PV loop, a plot of LV pressure *vs.* LV volume (Fig. 1.9):

$$W = \oint P dV.$$

During the isovolumic relaxation and contraction phases, the ventricular volume is constant while the pressure falls or rises. Thus the integral over the loop is simply the difference between the ventricular pressure during the ejection phase and the filling phase. The work done by the LV is $\sim 1\,J$ under resting conditions, which corresponds to a mechanical power of $\sim 1.25\,W$. The latter is obtained by multiplying W by the heart rate and increases to $\sim 8\,W$ during heavy exercise, primarily due to the increase in heart rate.

[2] Clinicians are fond of using acronyms as variable names. This is very convenient for the medical student cramming for examinations, but very inconvenient for modellers writing equations.

[3] These terms derive historically from measurements on muscle fibres where they are well defined and measured in units of force. Their current use by cardiologists is less well defined, even to the extent that the units of measurement of preload and afterload are no longer clear.

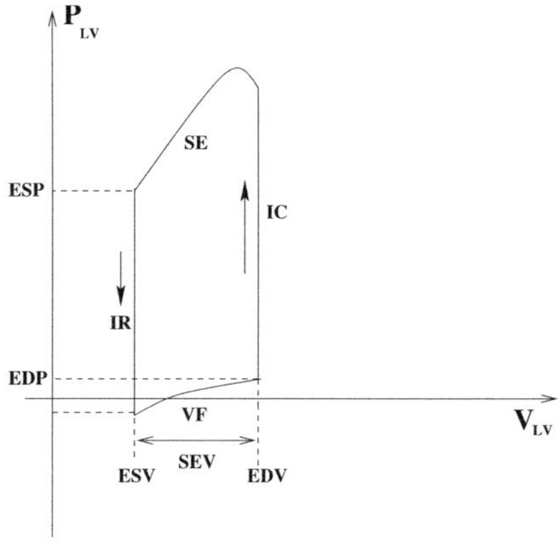

Fig. 1.9. Pressure (P)–volume (V) curve of the left ventricle (LV). SE: systolic ejection, IR: isovolumetric relaxation, VF: ventricular filling, IC: isovolumetric contraction, EDV, EDP: end diastolic volume and pressure, ESV, ESP: end systolic volume and pressure, SEV: systolic ejection volume

The mechanical state of the contracting myocardium is frequently expressed in terms of its elastance. Elastance is defined as the ratio

$$E(t) = \frac{P(t)}{V(t) - V_0},$$

where V_0 is the volume of the ventricle at zero transmural pressure. If myocardium were a simple elastic tissue, this would be the elastic modulus of the passive tissue. Because it is contractile, E varies with time during the cardiac cycle.

The use of the elastance to describe the state of the heart is supported by the work of Suga et al. [487, 489] in isolated heart preparations. They showed that the elastance at the end of systole (the end systolic pressure–volume relationship) was nearly constant for all kinds of interventions that altered heart function (pacing, volume loading, pharmacological interventions, etc.). In terms of the PV loop, this means the line from the end systolic shoulder of the loop to the intercept $V = V_0$ is almost invariant with the operating conditions of the heart. Furthermore, they found empirically that the metabolic energy consumed by the heart was related to the mechanical work (i.e. the area under the PV loop). This observation has limited clinical application despite its success in isolated hearts because of the difficulty of measuring V, particularly V_0. Nevertheless, it is at the base of the lumped parameter models for heart action presented in Chapter 10.

1.2.2 The large blood vessels

Because of the pulsatile nature of cardiac output, the arterial pressure varies between the diastolic pressure p_d (minimum) and systolic pressure p_s (maximum). The pulse pressure $\Delta P \equiv p_s - p_d$. Cardiologists are taught that p_s reflects the cardiac output and the distensibility of the arteries, p_d depends upon the state of the peripheral vessels and Δp is proportional to the stroke volume and inversely proportional to arterial compliance. In fact, the interrelations are much more complex than this. Cardiologists often calculate the mean arterial pressure from the formula $mAP = p_d + \Delta p/3$, which is a crude approximation of the time-average arterial pressure assuming that the pressure waveform is triangular.

Most arteries experience biphasic flow waveforms with a small amount of backward flow occurring in late systole and early diastole. Despite the common belief that arterial flow can be approximated by steady flow, this is a serious misrepresentation of the nature of blood flow in the arteries. In fact, the stroke volume ejected by the heart occupies less than 20 cm of the ascending aorta. The values of two major dimensionless parameters which govern the blood flow, the Reynolds number and the Womersley number (the frequency parameter), are given in Table 1.7. Both parameters become much lower than unity in the microcirculation. We have already given the definition of the Reynolds number and we postpone that of the Womersley number to Chapter 5.

Flow in the arteries is effectively wave-like. Elastic tubes, like the arteries, support one-dimensional waves in which the energy is transferred between the

Table 1.7. Properties of typical systemic vessels for an adult (LAD = left anterior descending). The numbers for the named arteries are based on measurements. The numbers for the representative vessels at the bottom of the table should only be considered as approximate, as there are very many of these vessels and a wide range of properties for individual vessels should be expected. The wave speed for veins is based on measurements of the distensibility of veins. As far as we know, the wave speed in veins has never been measured

	Bore (mm)	*Length* (cm)	*Peak velocity* (cm/s)	*Wave speed* (m/s)	*Reynolds number*	*Womersley number*
Ascending aorta	15	4	1.0	5	4000	10.5
Thoracic aorta	11	15	0.8	6	2500	7.7
Iliac artery	5	20	0.8	6	1000	3.5
Femoral artery	4	45	0.8	7	800	2.8
Brachial artery	5	40	0.8	7	1000	3.5
Common carotid artery	4	20	0.8	7	800	2.8
LAD coronary artery	3	12	0.5	12	400	2.1
Small artery	2	10	0.2	20	100	1.4
Arteriole	.02	.4	0.01	-	0.5	0.014
Capillary	.01	.2	0.001	-	0.003	0.007
Venule	.02	.4	0.01	-	0.5	0.014
Small vein	2	10	0.6	2	100	1.4
Large vein	8	50	0.8	1	1700	5.6

elastic potential energy of the distensible walls and the kinetic energy of the blood. The wave speed c depends upon the *distensibility* (sometimes also called *compliance*) of the vessel C and the density of blood ρ, $c \sim (\rho C)^{-1/2}$. More details will be found in Chapter 10. Under normal conditions, a wave generated by the contraction of the heart propagates throughout the arterial system. These waves will give rise to reflections whenever there is a discontinuity in the geometrical or elastic properties of the arteries. Bifurcations and high resistance regions can give rise to reflections that propagate back towards the heart. These backward waves are also reflected by the bifurcations giving rise to a very complex pattern of reflected and re-reflected waves that determine the local pressure and velocity waveforms in the arteries. This process will be discussed in detail in later chapters.

The pressure in veins is very much less than the pressure in arteries. When lying down, venous pressure is generally in the range of 1–2 kPa. Because of hydrostatic effects, the venous pressure is very dependent upon posture and pressure in the veins of the foot can rise to 15 kPa when standing. Of course, hydrostatic pressure also effects the arteries, but because their mean pressure is much higher, the fractional changes are much less. Mean flow in veins must be equivalent to the flow in arteries and so they have very similar values of *Re*. Flow in veins is also very pulsatile but in a much less regular way than the arteries. Venous flow is very dependent upon muscle contractions, particularly in the arms and legs, respiratory effects in the thorax and atrial contractions nearer the heart. Because of its irregularity and complexity, venous flow has not been studied seriously either experimentally or theoretically. It is a subject waiting to be explored.

1.2.3 The microcirculation

The microcirculation is made up of three parts; the arterioles, the capillaries and the venules. These vessels are very small (5–30 μm in diameter) but very numerous so that local velocities are very small ($\sim$ 1 mm/s). This means that the characteristic values of *Re* are very small so that viscous forces completely dominate any inertial forces in the flow. As a result, virtually all of the resistance to flow is found in the microcirculation. This is not to say that viscous effects are not important in the large vessels, the no-slip condition at the vessel walls ensures that viscosity is important in determining the detailed distribution of flow in the large vessels. However, it does mean that almost all of the pressure head losses in the circulation occur in the microcirculation.

Most of the pressure head losses actually occur in the arterioles. The arterioles have very thick muscular and highly ennervated walls; the ratio of wall thickness to lumen diameter is $\sim$1. The distribution of blood flow to different tissues is determined largely by these vessels whose resistance is highly dependent upon their diameter, which is controlled by contraction or relaxation of the smooth muscle in the wall.

The capillaries are the smallest vessels in the circulatory system and they are responsible for the bulk of exchange between the blood and the various tissues. Capillaries range from 5–8 µm in diameter and 200–400 µm in length. The bore of most capillaries is smaller than the largest dimension of the red blood cells, which means that the cells pass through the capillaries in single file and they must deform during their passage. In the capillaries, therefore, blood can no longer be thought of as a homogeneous fluid and it is necessary to treat it as a multi-phase fluid composed of plasma and cells (particle flow).

There is a reduction in the effective viscosity of blood in the microcirculation (the *Fahraeus-Lindquist effect*) due to the steric exclusion of the blood cells from the wall regions of the vessels (the *Fahraeus effect*). As the red blood cells pass through the microvessels, there is a very small lubrication layer between the red blood cell membrane and the microvessel wall that promotes mass transfer between them. It is unclear how the larger leukocytes pass through capillaries, probably relying upon larger anastomoses within the capillary network. Because of these effects, the blood cells circulate more slowly through the circulatory system than does the plasma.

Capillary density varies greatly between different tissues depending upon their metabolic requirements. In skeletal muscle there are 300–1000 capillaries per cm^3 of tissue, which corresponds to a total surface area of $\sim 20\,cm^{-1}$. In the highly metabolically active myocardium or the brain, the surface area per volume of tissue is $\sim 500\,cm^{-1}$. In lungs where there is little tissue except for airways and capillaries, the capillary surface area is $\sim 3500\,cm^2$ per g of tissue.

The capillary circulation, characterised by a low flow velocity and a short distance between the capillary lumen and the tissue that it perfuses, is well adapted to molecular exchange. In addition, fluid and the smaller solutes in the plasma can move from the capillary to the extravascular space, composed of the cellular, interstitial and lymphatic subcompartments. The flux of water between the capillary and the surrounding tissue depends upon the transmural difference between hydrostatic pressure p and plasma osmotic pressure Π, $J = L_P(\Delta p - \Delta\Pi)$, where L_P is the hydraulic permeability of the wall (*Starling's law*). The pressure drop along the capillary is 1–2 Pa, which means that the lumenal pressure is considerably higher at the arteriole end of the capillary than at the venule end (Table 1.8). Therefore, even under homeostatic conditions of water exchange, there is a net flux out of the arteriole end of the capillaries into the tissues and back into the capillaries at the venule end. This flux of water is very important in the exchange of small solutes carried in the blood.

In microvessels with continuous endothelium, the main route for water and small solutes is the endothelial cleft. Macromolecules can cross the endothelium between the cells (paracellular transport) or through endothelial cells (transcytosis), using receptors, specific or not, and vesicles. Microvascular transport has been modelled using pore theory for small and intermediate-sized molecules and transendothelial channels for macromolecules.

Table 1.8. Main features of the capillary circulation

	Units	*Value*
Length	µm	200–400
Diameter	µm	6–8
Distance between capillaries	µm	10–30
Capillary density	$\#/cm^3$	300–6000 (myocardium)
Total surface density	cm^2/cm^3	20–500 (myocardium)
Hydrostatic pressure	kPa	3–4 (arteriole end)
		1.5–3 (venule end)
Plasma osmotic pressure	kPa	2.5–4.0
Mean velocity	mm/s	< 1
Cell transit time	s	0.5–3
Haematocrit	%	30
Viscosity	Pa s	0.001 (plasma)
Total capillary volume	ml	~ 300 ($\sim 5\,\%$ total blood volume)

1.2.4 Regulation of the circulation

In order to meet the body's changing needs, the cardiac output changes through changes in the cardiac frequency and/or the ejection volume (see also Section 10.2.4). The cardiovascular system is controlled by a complex set of regulation mechanisms, which mainly involve the central nervous system (neural) and the release of hormones from the endocrine organs (humoral).

Nervous signals are integrated in the cardiovascular centre, located in the brainstem. Efferent nerves connect to the sino-atrial node and the myocardium in the heart, controlling the heart rate and the rate and strength of the myocardial contraction. Efferent nerves to the smooth muscles in the blood vessel walls control arterial tone, resistance in the microcirculation and blood volume in the large veins. The brain gets signals from various sensors distributed around the body.

The nervous system primarily regulates the cardiac frequency in order to adapt to the changing needs of the body. However, the increase in frequency is bounded by the rate of diastolic filling, which is determined by the venous return and the diastolic perfusion of the coronary arteries. The cardiac frequency is also influenced by other factors such as body temperature and the circulatory hormones. The main flowing hormones are the catecholamines (adrenaline and noradrenaline – also known as epinephrine and norepinephrine), secreted by the adrenal gland, vasopressin (or antidiuretic hormone ADH), secreted by the hypothalamus, angiotensin-II, secreted by the kidney, and natriuretic peptides, such as the atrial natriuretic peptide (ANP), secreted by atrial myocytes.

Blood pressure is regulated by short-term and long-term mechanisms. Short-term adjustments are made by neural mechanisms involving the control of the cardiac output and peripheral resistances in response to signals from the cardiovascular baroreceptors. Long-term control of the blood pressure involves indirect monitoring of blood volume. Hormonal mechanisms, including (i) the renin-angiotensin system, (ii) ANP and (iii) the antidiuretic hormone, regulate blood volume and indirectly the blood pressure.

Cardiovascular sensors

Mechano- and chemoreceptors are widely distributed throughout the cardiovascular system: in the heart, the coronary arteries, the carotid sinuses, the large intrathoracic blood vessels (particularly along the inner aortic arch and at the bases of both venae cavae) and the cervical vessels. These receptors continuously monitor the state of the circulation and feed their signals to the corresponding afferent neurons.

The chemoreceptors transduce reduced O_2 concentration and increased CO_2 and H^+ concentrations into an action potential. The impulses are transmitted via the vagus into the vasomotor centres, as well as the respiratory centres. The baroreceptors are sensitive to both mean pressure and the rate of change of pressure. An increase in mean pressure or pulse pressure increases the firing rate of the baroreceptor nerves, which not only inhibits sympathetic tonic activity to the heart and blood vessels, but also increases vagal tone to the heart. Conversely, a fall in arterial pressure reduces afferent signals, which relieves inhibition of sympathetic tone and increases the peripheral resistances, thereby restoring the blood pressure. The stretch receptors are located in the ventricular walls and the lower pressure parts of the cardiovascular system: the pulmonary artery and venae cavae. They are activated by long-term stretch of the tissue and are primarily involved in the regulation of blood volume.

Delayed control of the circulation

Blood volume is controlled by the kidneys, which control Na^+ and water reabsorption via the renin-angiotensin-aldosterone system. Renin cleaves angiotensinogen into angiotensin-I. Angiotensin-converting enzyme produces angiotensin-II, which constricts the arterioles. Angiotensin-II acts on the adrenal cortex to release aldosterone, which increases Na^+ and water retention by the kidneys and stimulates the release of vasopressin from the posterior pituitary, which also increases water retention. Angiotensin-II favours noradrenaline release from sympathetic nerve endings and inhibits its re-uptake, hence enhancing the sympathetic function.

The heart also has an endocrine function. Atrial natriuretic peptide (ANP) and brain natriuretic peptide (BNP) are synthesised by cardiomyocytes as preprohormones, which are processed to yield prohormones and, ultimately, hormones. They are released into the circulation at a basal rate. Augmented secretion follows haemodynamical or neuroendocrine stimuli. They relax vascular smooth muscle cells and regulate their proliferation. They decrease the baroreflex activity and have direct and indirect renal actions. ANP increases the renal blood flow, inhibits renin release by the kidneys, increases the rate of glomerular filtration, decreases the tubular Na^+ reabsorption, and inhibits aldosterone synthesis and release by the adrenal cortex. C-type natriuretic peptide (CNP) released by the endothelial cells reduces local vascular tone and growth. The diuretic and natriuretic effects of CNP are much weaker than those of ANP and BNP.

1.3 Cardiovascular diseases

Cardiovascular diseases are the leading cause of death in developed countries. Heart failure is a progressive disease in which the myocardium loses the ability to adequately perfuse the body. It has many causes including failure of the myocardium itself, chronic valve disease and chronic arterial disease. Direct disease of the heart is relatively rare. It can occur through bacterial or viral infection (endocarditis or rheumatic disease), parasitical infestation (Chagas disease) or the accumulation of protein complexes (cardiac amyloid). The two major vascular diseases, atherosclerosis and aneurysms, account for the vast majority of cardiovascular disease and have received the bulk of attention from modellers.

Another type of cardiovascular problem are genetic disorders.[4] The development of the cardiovascular system can lead to a large number of congenital disorders, many of which lead to problems that must be corrected by surgery. The most common congenital diseases of the heart are septal defects (holes in the septum) in either the atria or ventricles. Also relatively common is the Tetralogy of Fallot where there is a ventricular septal defect, pulmonary stenosis, aortic dislocation and thickening of the right ventricle. Another problem that has received considerable attention is the Fontan procedure for the amelioration of pulmonary atresia (an absent or disfunctional right ventricle) by connecting the pulmonary artery directly to the venae cavae so that the left ventricle supplies both the systemic and the pulmonary circulation in series. Perhaps the most severe, non-lethal disorder is the transposition of the great arteries where the systemic vessels are connected to the right side of the heart and the pulmonary to the left. All of these disorders and the surgical procedures that have been devised to treat them result in alterations of the haemodynamics that would benefit greatly from modelling.

[4] It has been said that adult cardiologists deal with man's mistakes while paediatric cardiologists deal with nature's mistakes.

1.3.1 Atherosclerosis

Atherosclerosis is defined by the accumulation of fatty materials, fibrous elements and calcium in the intima of arteries (Fig. 1.10). The development of the disease is very complex and there are conflicting theories about how it is initiated and progresses. There are four main stages in the progression of the disease: (i) the appearance of fatty streaks, (ii) the appearance of macrophages (foam cells), (iii) the development of fibrous plaque and (iv) calcification and the development of complicated plaques. It is a progressive disease that can take decades for the development of symptoms. The early stages are completely benign but as the lesion develops it can intrude into the lumen of the vessel creating a stenosis that obstructs blood flow leading to clinical complications. More dangerous, clinically, is the development of thrombi or the rupture of the plaque leading to emboli that get lodged in downstream vessels causing infarctions. Blockages in the heart are called heart attacks while blockages in the brain are called strokes; together they comprise approximately half of all deaths in developed countries.

Atherosclerosis is distributed throughout the systemic arteries, but is virtually unknown in the pulmonary arteries or the venous system. It is not distributed uniformly throughout the arteries but shows a strong predilection for particular sites in the arteries. Lesions are commonly found on the inside of bends in tortuous arteries and on the outer walls of bifurcations (they are rare on the flow divider or inner walls of bifurcations). This focal nature of the lesions has focused attention on mechanical effects on the development of the disease since most of the other risk factors, such as the concentration

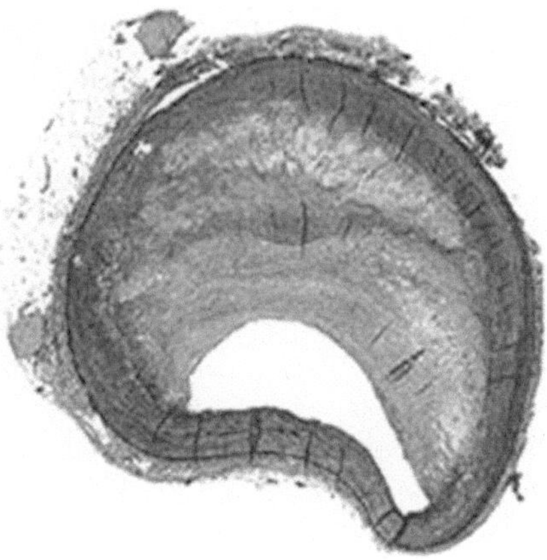

Fig. 1.10. A cross-sectional view of a very advanced atherosclerotic plaque in a human coronary artery. The plaque involves approximately three-quarters of the circumference of the arterial wall and occludes most of the original lumen of the vessel. Note that the arterial wall at the bottom of the section appears to be normal. This image was obtained by optical coherence tomography (Adapted from [301])

of lipids in the blood, obesity, cigarette smoking, etc., affect the arteries uniformly. Mechanical effects are also important in the classification of stable and unstable lesions, unstable lesions being prone to rupture and the formation of emboli.

1.3.2 Aneurysms

An aneurysm is a gradual dilation of an arterial segment over a period of years (Fig. 1.11). The aneurysm wall stretches and becomes thinner and weaker than normal arterial walls. Consequently, untreated aneurysms can rupture causing massive haemorrhage, except in the brain where rupture leads to possibly lethal vasospasm. The plastic deformation of the arterial wall is associated with structural changes in the connective tissue.

There are two types of aneurysms: *fusiform aneurysms*, cylindrical dilations where the entire circumference of the artery is weakened (Fig. 1.12), and *saccular aneurysms*, balloon-like bulges resulting from a weakening of one side of the artery wall. Fusiform aneurysms are often complications of atherosclerosis, local stenoses leading to the release of vasoactive drugs that cause the artery to remodel. They can be located in any artery but are most commonly seen in the ascending and abdominal aortae. Saccular aneurysms can be caused by trauma or certain infections of the blood. Congenital aneurysms are located at branching sites in the cerebral circulation, most often at the

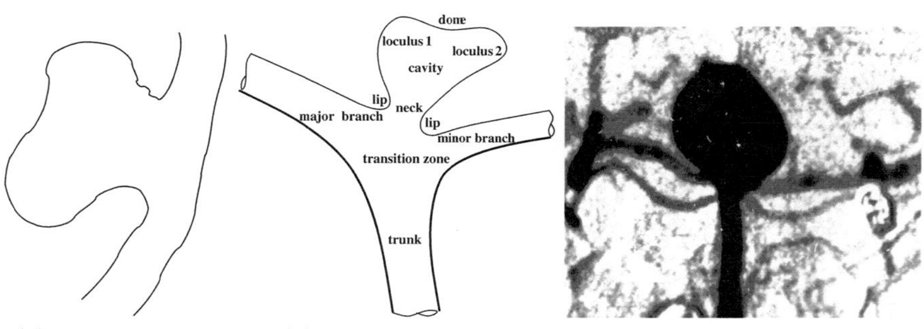

(a) side aneurysm (b) lateral aneurysm (c) terminal aneurysm

Fig. 1.11. Saccular aneurysms are located either on the vessel edge (side aneurysm; left panel), or at a branching region, and called lateral (mid panel; medical observations – traumatism of the artery wall) or terminal (right panel, aneurysm of the basilar artery; courtesy of A Gaston) whether the vessel trunk (or stem) gives birth to a lateral branch or divides into two main daughter vessels. Centre: Schematic drawing with geometry definitions of a saccular aneurysm at the apex of a branching segment of an artery. The neck is defined as the channel between the artery and the wall dilation. The main region is called the cavity (or pouch or sac). Opposite to the neck is the dome (or fundus). The cavity can be biloculated with a large projecting end part. Saccular aneurysms are classified into three categories according to the largest width (small, large – $12 \leq w_a \leq 25$ mm – and giant)

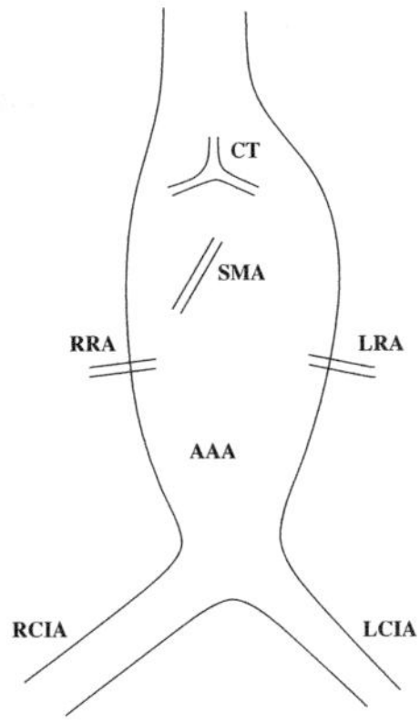

Fig. 1.12. Schematic drawing of a large fusiform aneurysm of the abdominal aorta (AAA; CT: coeliac trunk, SMA: superior mesenteric artery, RRA and LRA: right and left renal arteries, RCIA and LCIA: right and left common iliac arteries)

branches of vessels leading to or away from the Circle of Willis, although they can also be found on the sides of vessels.

1.3.3 Treatment of cardiovascular diseases

Modelling and simulations of blood flow through arterial grafts, through reconstructed vascular segments and through vessels with implanted medical devices, have been carried out by many groups in order to provide knowledge of flow behaviour and the applied stress fields. Such investigations are useful to optimise surgical procedures or the design of medical devices. Most of the studies have been performed in idealised geometries but there is a growing interest in computations carried out in realistic geometries determined from medical imaging.

Heart surgery

Heart surgery deals with repair of congenital heart defects, with valve repair and replacement, with pacemaker placement, with normal rhythm and/or conduction restoration (arrhythmia surgery, such as the Maze procedure for atrial fibrillation), with coronary revascularisation and, if all else fails, with heart transplantation. Surgery now makes extensive use of imaging systems for surgical planning and, increasingly, robotic assist during operation. Because the donor pool for cardiac transplantation is insufficient, ventricular assist devices (VAD) have been designed to unload the heart and to provide adequate perfusion of the body organs both as a bridge to transplantation, and, recently, as long-term treatment.

Malfunctioning valves can be removed and replaced with prosthetic heart valves. There are two main types of heart valves: mechanical valves, and bioprosthetic tissue valves, both stentless and stented. There are three main designs of mechanical valves: the caged ball valve (e.g., Starr-Edwards valve), the tilting disc valve (e.g., Medtronic Hall and Bjork-Shiley valves) and the bileaflet valve (e.g., St Jude, CarboMedics and ATS valves). Valved grafts have also been proposed (e.g., St Jude aortic valved graft, ATS aortic valve graft prosthesis). Bioprosthetic (xenograft) valves are made from porcine valves (e.g., Carpentier-Edwards and Hancock valves) or bovine pericardium (e.g., Ionescu-Shiley and Carpentier-Edwards valves). In order to be successful, the prosthetic valve must mimic the static and dynamic characteristics of the natural human valve and the mechanics of flow through it. It should not produce turbulence, flow stagnation or excessive shear stress (the latter can cause haemolysis, i.e., the damaging of blood cells).

Grafting

Two surgical procedures can be applied to severely stenosed arteries: endarterectomy, which removes the plaque and preserves the artery, and grafting. There are two types of grafts: (i) vessel replacement and (ii) bypass. Replacement, or end-to-end anastomosis, involves removing the diseased artery and replacing it with another vessel sutured end-to-end with the remaining arteries. Bypass, or side-to-side anastomosis, provides an alternative route for blood to bypass the stenoses which are left in place.

Vascular grafts can be divided into three types: (i) grafts using arteries or veins from the patient (autologous) or a donor (homologous), (ii) xenografts using vessels from other species (usually bovine or porcine) and (iii) artificial grafts (usually either woven or knitted dacron or expanded polytetrafluoroethylene PTFE). Autologous grafts have the advantage that they do not elicit any immune responses and are probably the preferred method of replacement despite the problem caused by removing the replacement vessel. With proper typing, homologous vessels can also be incorporated into the body with few or no problems. Xenografts have the advantage that they are biological material, but they must be treated so that they are not rejected by the immune system and this treatment limits their lifetime. Artificial grafts have the advantage that they can be very durable, but there is always the problem of incorporation of the material into the body so that it is not thrombogenic. There is very active research into the development of new materials for grafts and for drug treatments of the grafts that will promote acceptance of the graft by the immune system and suppress hyperplasia.

All grafts suffer from complications; 50 % close within 10 years after surgery. The most common modes of failure are thrombus formation, restenosis of the vessel due to intimal hyperplasia at the artery-graft junction, aneurysms at the graft junction, dilation, kinking and deterioration of the graft material. Some of these problems result from an incomplete covering by the endothelium (endothelialisation) of the graft lumen leading to the formation of thrombus: inflammation of the graft junction leading to the excess proliferation of cells (hyperplasia), and long-term degeneration of the graft material.

As in the natural arteries, haemodynamics are thought to play a role in the development of lesions in grafts. Better understanding of the flow and stresses present in grafts and graft junctions will aid in surgical planning of grafting and may improve the lifetime of grafts. As well as predicting the effects of graft geometry on flow patterns, it is also important to consider the solid mechanical interaction between the graft and the native arteries. This can affect local wall stresses through stress concentration and the transmission of the arterial pressure and velocity waves.

Stenting

The number of vascular graft operations has declined during the past decade because of the development of stenting. Stenting is a minimally invasive procedure where a catheter is advanced from a peripheral artery to the site of stenosis. The stenosis is generally disrupted by dilating it with a balloon (angioplasty) used to expand a wire mesh stent which supports the vessel walls. Nowadays, shape memory alloys are also used. The stent is left in place permanently (Fig. 1.13).

The most common problem with stents is restenosis, which occurs at a significant rate (see also Chapter 12). Consequently coated metallic stents and biodegradable stents have been developed. Several types of drug-eluting stents have been tested in clinical trials to limit cell migration and proliferation into the intima in the region of the stent. Mathematical modelling of the effect of stents on the artery and the process of intimal remodelling will certainly play an important role in the development of more successful stents.

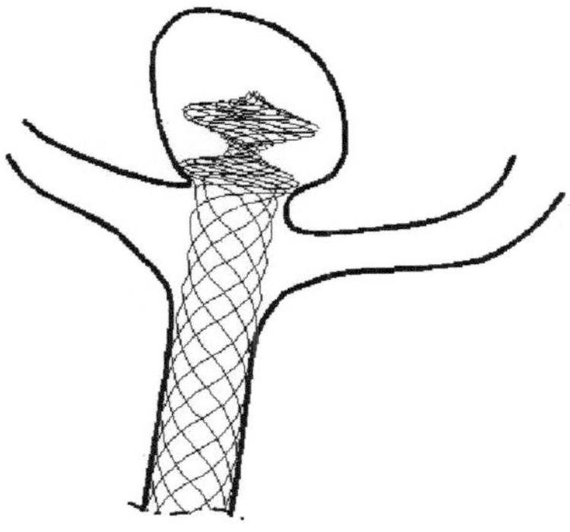

Fig. 1.13. Stent for saccular branching aneurysms (courtesy of Cardiatis). The part within the trunk serves as support. In an arterial segment (more or less curved), a uniform mesh is used to dilate a stenosis

Aneurysm clipping

The surgical treatment of saccular aneurysm consists in placing a small metallic clip around the base of the aneurysms to establish normal flow in the affected artery. Aneurysm surgery is performed on both ruptured aneurysms and to prevent rupture in aneurysms at risk. The presence of the clip and the isolated aneurysm will certainly affect the behaviour of the artery after operation, but little is known about these effects. Postoperative complications of this procedure include infection and damage to neighbouring blood vessels.

Coils and external stents

Fusiform aneurysms are treated by grafting, or external or internal stenting. Both grafting and external stenting are surgical procedures while internal stents are inserted by catheter-based methods. External stents are a recent development that rely upon the custom fabrication of the external stent using computer-aided prototyping based upon accurate medical images from magnetic resonance (MR), computed tomography (CT) or positron emission tomography (PET). Because it is so new, there is little information about the long-term outcome of external stenting.

In coiling, a catheter is advanced from a peripheral artery to the neck of a targeted saccular aneurysm under image guidance. Very thin metallic coils are then advanced into the aneurysm cavity, avoiding both rupture of the wall and the formation of emboli. Once the coils are released, the blood external to the coils compacted by the blood flow clots while the free space forms the new lumen of the artery, comprising a more or less large area of the aneurysmal cavity (the greater this area, the higher the recanalisation risk; Fig. 1.14). There are a number of problems with coiling that could benefit from suitable mathematical modelling. Therapeutic results are often unsatisfactory when the volume of the aneurysm is large, when the neck of the aneurysm is broad, or when there is a small angle between the inflow and the axis of the aneurysmal cavity.

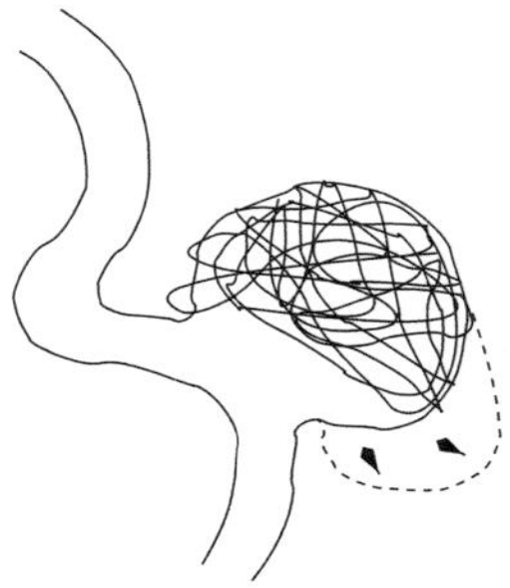

Fig. 1.14. Coiled side aneurysm. Coil compaction by blood flow leads to a residual cavity of significant volume with possible recanalisation (arrows: schematic drawing from a clinical observation)

Embolisation

Catheter-based transarterial chemoembolisation (TACE) is a a relatively new technique used in the treatment of some cancers. TACE is similar to intra-arterial infusion of chemotherapy but small emboli are included in the infusion to block small blood vessels downstream from the site of infusion, thereby increasing the residence time of the chemotherapeutic agents. This treatment commonly induces regional side effects if the emboli are not injected close enough to the target tissue.

Vein devices

The two most common problems in the veins are deep vein thrombosis and varicose veins. Therapy to prevent deep vein thrombosis includes advice about posture and exercise and the use of elastic stockings. The problem of post-operative deep vein thrombosis is usually dealt with by the use of anticlotting drugs such as heparin, although intermittent external compression by means of an inflatable boot has also been used as a prophylactic measure. Varicose veins are usually treated by surgical removal of the affected veins or by injection sclerotherapy. A number of endovascular devices have been developed that can be implanted in the veins. A venae cavae filter is a device inserted into a major vein to prevent multiple pulmonary embolisms. When veins become dilated, they lose their elliptical shape, which reduces the efficiency of the venous valves. V-shaped clips can be put into varicose veins to restore the usual configuration of their lumen in order to restore valve function.

Ventricular assist devices (VAD)

Ventricular assist devices (VAD) have been developed to assist the failing heart initially as a bridge to transplantation but more recently as a bridge to recovery. The oldest and most common devices consist of intra-aortic balloons which are inflated and deflated in phase with the cardiac cycle. The balloon is inflated during diastole to increase the aortic pressure, which increases the perfusion through the coronary arteries. The balloon is deflated just before systole, which decreases the pressure in the aorta and unloads the left ventricle. Similar effects can be obtained by external compression of the arteries, either directly invasively or indirectly non-invasively. The timing of the VAD interventions is critical to the success of the intervention; being out of phase with the cardiac cycle is highly detrimental to the functioning of the heart.

A number of implanted VADs have been developed which actively pump blood from the ventricle to the aorta. These pumps can be classed as positive displacement devices that mimic the functioning of the LV and turbine pumps, which act predominantly as pressure generators. The turbine pumps are the most recent development, primarily because it was wrongly believed that red blood cells could not survive passage through a high-speed turbine. All types of VADs would benefit from modelling of their effects and efficiency in the cardiovascular system.

Drawbacks of vascular medical devices

Any device implanted into a blood vessel can induce several biological and mechanical disturbances when it is made from inappropriate material and its rheology does not match the properties of the vessel wall. Devices inserted into regions of high blood velocity can cause the breakup of red blood cells (haemolysis), which is particularly dangerous. In any case, an implanted device provides a matrix for the formation of thrombus, especially when the endothelium is removed or damaged during implantation. Vessel wall damage also generates an intimal proliferation response, which can lead to rapid restenosis. Finally, any device implanted in a blood vessel will disturb the blood flow to some degree and the long-term effects of these disturbances can be serious. Mathematical modelling, together with new biomaterials, can and should help us to overcome all of these problems.

1.4 Conclusions and annotated bibliography

This chapter is intended as an introduction to the anatomy, physiology and pathology of the cardiovascular system for haemodynamic modellers. It is, by necessity, a very superficial look at three very broad subjects. We hope that it covers the basic topics in a way that will be accessible to engineers and physical scientists who would like to apply their expertise to the study of the cardiovascular system. At the same time we are aware that many of the 'facts' that we have presented will be contested by anatomists, physiologists and clinicians who are experts in the subjects that we have covered. We hope that it conveys some of the complexity of the subject, something that should never be forgotten in the process of modelling.

This chapter has been condensed from a book to be published by one of the authors, M. Thiriet, *Biology and Mechanics of Blood Flows* [497]. The book was originally written as a long version of an invited contribution text on "Biochemical and Biomechanical Aspects of Blood Flows", for the survey article collection "Modelling of Biological Materials" and as notes for a lecture series on the cardiovascular system for the CRM–INRIA Spring School held in Montréal, Canada. It contains many more details and references on specific topics, which have has been omitted from this brief introduction.

The anatomy of the cardiovascular system is covered in any good text on anatomy. We have made extensive use of M.F. Martini, *Fundamentals of Anatomy & Physiology* [315] in the preparation of this chapter. The combination of anatomy and physiology makes this book particularly useful.

The physiology of the heart is covered in detail in A.C. Guyton, *Medical Physiology* [213], which has become one of the standard medical physiology texts. An early work by the same author, A.C. Guyton, *Circulatory Physiology: Cardiac Output and Its Regulation* [212], is an excellent introduction to cardiac control, although there have been a number of advances in our understanding since its publication. It is, however, still a good introduction to the subject.

The physiology of the cardiovascular system is the subject of two excellent textbooks, J.R. Levick, *An Introduction to Cardiovascular Physiology* [279], and M.N. Levy and R.M. Berne, *Cardiovascular Physiology* [282]. Both books are intended as textbooks for medical students and their success is indicated by the number of editions that have been published. They are both highly recommended.

The standard textbooks on blood flow in the arteries are W.W. Nichols and M.F. O'Rourke, *McDonald's Blood Flow in Arteries* [350], a thoroughly rewritten edition of D.A. McDonald, *Blood Flow in Arteries* [317] containing a wealth of information that was not available to McDonald, who died shortly after the publication of the 2nd edition of his book, and W.R. Milnor, *Hemodynamics* [334]. Probably the best book on the pulmonary circulation, with particular emphasis on the pulmonary microcirculation, is J.M.B. Hughes and N.W. Morrell, *Pulmonary Circulation: Basic Mechanisms to Clinical Practice* [237].

The Mechanics of the Circulation, written by C.G. Caro, T.J. Pedley, R.C. Schroter and W.A. Seed [62], is a relatively old book, written before technological advances in ultrasound and magnetic resonance imaging opened new windows into the circulatory system. However, it is an excellent introduction to the cardiovascular system and the basic mechanical principles that are needed to study it. It is currently out of print, but well worth the search for anyone new to the subject.

Cardiac electrophysiology, an extremely important facet of cardiological function, which has only been touched upon in this chapter, is covered in detail in D.P. Zipes, *Cardiac Electrophysiology: from Cell to Bedside* [560].

All of the biochemistry contained in this chapter is dealt with in detail in A.L. Lehninger, *Principles of Biochemistry* [347]. In the tradition of medical textbooks, this book has outlived its original author and is almost continuously updated and revised to keep pace with developments in biochemistry.

Finally, cardiovascular pathology is the subject of a plethora of books, including *Heart Disease for Dummies* [427]. One of the standard textbooks is E. Braunwald, *Braunwald's Heart Disease: A Textbook of Cardiovascular Medicine* [50], which strives to encompass the whole of the subject.

2

Basic mathematical models and motivations

Luca Formaggia, Karl Perktold, and Alfio Quarteroni

As explained in Chapter 1, the cardiovascular system is the main responsible of the transport of various chemicals to and from the various organs, enabling their correct functioning and, in fact, life.

The desire to model this system is longstanding. Indeed, the well known Euler equations (nowadays standing at the ground of gas dynamics models) were infact developed by Euler in 1775 with the intent of describing blood flow in the human arteries [139]. We mention also the works by Bernoulli, Poiseuille and Young on this subject.

However, it is only in the past few decades that the application of mathematical models of the cardiovascular system have become widespread within the bioengineering and medical research community. The main reasons are the advancements in the power of modern computers, the progress in imaging and geometry extraction techniques (see Chapter 4) as well as the development of better numerical algorithms (like the ones described in the later chapters of this book).

Nowadays, computer simulations can provide researchers with an invaluable tool for the interpretation and analysis of the circulatory system functionality, in both physiological and pathological situations.

Clearly a main impulse to develop this field of study is the increasing demand from the medical community for scientifically rigorous and quantitative investigations of cardiovascular diseases, which are unfortunately responsible for a large percentage of early mortality in industrialised societies, see for instance [229]. The ageing of the population and the consequent increase of health care costs also call for more effective treatments.

Besides their employment in medical research, numerical models of vascular flows can also provide a virtual experimental platform to be used as training system for new vascular surgeons [494] or anaesthesiologists [91,357]. In perspective, they can give specific design indications for the realisation of surgical operations [331,494] or for the design of better prosthetic devices. For instance, numerical studies have shown how shape optimisation techniques may be used for minimising the downstream vorticity in coronary by-pass

Formaggia L, Quarteroni A, Veneziani A (Eds.): Cardiovascular Mathematics. Modeling and simulation of the circulatory system

grafts [1, 434]. Investigations of this type can help the surgeon in understanding how different surgical solutions may affect blood circulation and guide the choice of the most appropriate procedure for a specific patient or type of patients. Another interesting application of computational haemodynamics to surgical planning is found in [329].

The mathematical modelling of the various functions of the cardiovascular system is, however, still an incredibly challenging problem. The difference in space and time scale of the processes involved, highlighted in the previous chapter, makes the treatment of the system as a whole unfeasible. It is then useful to identify a hierarchy of models, each suited for a different type of investigation or to different parts of the system, see Chapter 10, and possibly devise strategies to couple them, using for instance the multiscale framework that will be illustrated in Chapter 11.

In the following we will focus our attention on models for the main systemic cardiovascular tree, providing for each of them a justification from a physical and computational point of view. A more formal derivation of the equations is postponed to other chapters of the book, in particular Chapters 3 and 7.

Numerical simulations are of course less invasive than *in vivo* investigation, and potentially more accurate and flexible than *in vitro* experiments. Numerical models require patients data: the value of the parameters characterising the properties of blood and possibly the vessel wall, the initial and boundary conditions for the partial differential equations to be solved as well as geometrical data that defines the shape of the computational domain. The latter can be obtained by radiological acquisition through, e.g., computer tomography, magnetic resonance, Doppler anemometry, etc., as will be addressed in Chapter 4.

2.1 Mathematical models for local blood flow dynamics

The mathematical equations of fluid dynamics are the key components of haemodynamics modelling. Rigorously speaking blood is not a fluid but a suspension of particles in the *plasma*, the latter being mainly made of water. As discussed in Chapter 1, the most important blood particles are red cells (erythrocytes), white cells (leukocytes), and platelets (thrombocytes). Being the most numerous, red cells are the main responsible for the special mechanical properties of blood. The prominent macroscopic effect of their presence is that blood is a *shear-thinning*, or thixotropic fluid. A precise definition will be given in Chapter 6, here we just say that a shear-thinning fluid the more it stirs the more it fluidifies (just think to the behaviour of tomato ketchup, another shear-thinning fluid). In other words, its (apparent) viscosity decreases with the increase of the rate of deformation. This effect is stronger in smaller vessels, like the arterioles, venules and the capillaries. Viscoelastic effects can be very important at the fine spatial scale (micro-circulation). Below a critical vessel calibre (about 1 mm), blood viscosity becomes dependent on the vessel radius and decreases very sharply. This is known as Fahraeus-Lindquist effect (see Chapter 1): red blood cells move to the central part of the capillary, whereas the plasma stays in contact with the vessel wall. This layer of plasma facilitates the movement of the red cells, thus causing a decrease of the apparent viscosity. High shear rate and increased blood cell deformation are further important factors that explain viscoelastic behaviour.

Things get even more complex in the smallest capillaries, since here the size of a red blood cell becomes comparable to that of the vessel and the continuum hypothesis may become questionable.

Therefore, a first separation line between models for blood flow may be drawn: on one side the *Newtonian model* which neglects shear thinning and viscoelastic effects and is suitable in larger vessels or when we are not interested in the finer details of the flow, as non-Newtonian behaviour may affect, for instance, the size of the recirculation area behind a severe stenosis [382]. On the other side, in vessels of diameter, say, less than 1 mm the use of Newtonian models is hardly justifiable. The small velocities and shear stress here involved call for the use of one of the non-Newtonian models described in Chapter 6, see also [348]. Computationwise, non-Newtonian models which just modify the expression for the viscosity by making it dependent on the shear rate would increase the cost of computations of approximately 10 % [382], because of the extra calculations and the increased non-linearity of the problem. Full visco-elastic models may instead be much more costly in terms of computing time.

In the sequel of this section we will focus our investigation on flow in *large and medium sized vessels*. The flow is here governed by the Navier-Stokes equations. If we take $t = 0$ as the initial time of our analysis, we are required to solve for $t > 0$ the following system of partial differential equations,

$$\frac{\partial \boldsymbol{u}}{\partial t} + \rho(\boldsymbol{u} \cdot \boldsymbol{\nabla})\boldsymbol{u} + \boldsymbol{\nabla} P - \mathbf{div}(\mu \boldsymbol{D}(\boldsymbol{u})) = \boldsymbol{f}, \mathbf{div}\boldsymbol{u} = 0, \tag{2.1}$$

in a domain $\Omega \subset \mathbb{R}^3$ representing the lumen of the vessel, or system of vessels, under investigation.

The first equation expresses the conservation of linear momentum. It is a vector equation formed by three differential equations, one for each component of the velocity. The second equation is the continuity equation. The domain Ω is here fixed with time, in Chapter 3 we will discuss the modifications needed for the case of moving computational domain. The viscosity μ is in non-Newtonian models a function of the *strain rate*

$$\boldsymbol{D}(\boldsymbol{u}) = \frac{\boldsymbol{\nabla u} + \boldsymbol{\nabla u}^T}{2}, \tag{2.2}$$

while is kept constant when adopting the hypothesis of a Newtonian behaviour. The principal unknowns are the velocity $\boldsymbol{u}$ and the pressure P, while the density ρ is here constant. The term $\boldsymbol{f}$ in the right hand side accounts for the possible action of external forces, like gravity, and is often taken equal to zero in haemodynamics. We will derive and discuss this system of equations in

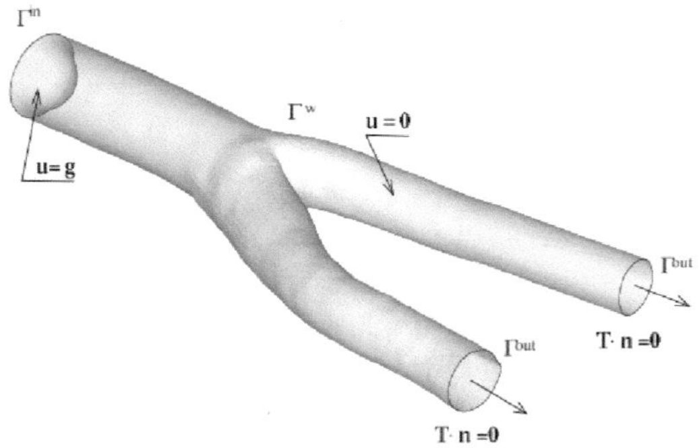

Fig. 2.1. A typical computational domain. Here we have a model of a carotid bifurcation developed by K. Perktold and his research group at Graz University of Technology on the basis of an experimental lumen cast prepared and digitised by D. Liepsch, FH Munich

detail in the next chapter, here we wish only to point out their main characteristics.

The equations have to be supplemented with boundary conditions on $\partial\Omega$. Referring to Fig. 2.1 describing a carotid bifurcation we typically prescribe a velocity profile at the *proximal* boundary Γ_{in}, that is the section closest to the heart along the direction of the mean blood flow, which we will also denote as "inflow" boundary, even if the term "inflow" in not completely correct since in some major vessels we can have flow reversals. We then prescribe zero velocity at the fixed walls and the normal stresses $\mathbf{T} \cdot \mathbf{n}$ at the *distal* boundaries Γ_{out} (also called "outflow" boundaries). Again, the term distal is meant with respect to the heart.

Proximal and distal boundaries are often indicated as *artificial boundaries* since they do not correspond to a physical interface between the fluid and the exterior, but to sections that have been artificially created to separate the region of interest for our investigation from the remaining part of the circulatory system. The set up of boundary conditions on artificial boundaries is an important issue for fluid dynamic computations. Treatments of the boundary data specially suited for haemodynamics will be discussed in Chapter 11.

We need also to prescribe the initial status of the fluid velocity, for instance

$$\boldsymbol{u}(\boldsymbol{x}, 0) = \boldsymbol{u}_0(\boldsymbol{x}) \qquad \boldsymbol{x} \in \Omega,$$

being $\boldsymbol{u}_0$ a given quantity. We recall that $\boldsymbol{u}_0$ cannot be arbitrary, since it has to satisfy $\mathbf{div}\boldsymbol{u}_0 = 0$ to be admissible.

Unfortunately, in haemodynamics computations usually we do not know a physically relevant "initial condition". Therefore $\boldsymbol{u}_0$ is usually chosen rather arbitrarily, often just equal to zero everywhere. It means that numerical computations may suffer a "false transient" linked to the incorrect initial data. If the boundary conditions are correct, however, it will decay quite rapidly and after two or three heart beats we may consider that the solution is not anymore influenced by the incorrect initial data. A possibility to get a better guess of the initial data is to solve a stationary Stokes problem for $\boldsymbol{u}_0$ in Ω, that is

$$-\mathbf{div}(\mu \boldsymbol{D}(\boldsymbol{u}_0)) + \boldsymbol{\nabla} P = \boldsymbol{f},$$

$$\mathbf{div}\boldsymbol{u}_0 = 0.$$

where the forcing and boundary terms are those of the original problem at $t = 0$. In this way, $\boldsymbol{u}_0$ is certainly compatible and accounts already of part of the physics of the problem, the only missing terms being those related to fluid inertia. With this choice the "false transient" effect is greatly reduced and in practise one may assume that it has faded away completely after just a few time steps of the solution procedure.

The situation is worsened when the compliance of the wall is taken into account. The continuous exchange of energy between fluid and wall effectively makes the decay slower. In calculations of flow in compliant vessels it is normal practise to wait for at least three cardiac cycles before considering the influence of the initial data negligible.

The solution of the Navier-Stokes equations may develop instabilities, which are normally called *turbulence*. The responsible is the dynamics induced by the non-linear convection term $\rho(\boldsymbol{u} \cdot \boldsymbol{\nabla})\boldsymbol{u}$. It is therefore natural to measure the importance of this term compared with the diffusive part given by $\mathbf{div}(\mu \boldsymbol{D}(\boldsymbol{u}))$. This information is provided by the Reynolds number, defined in (1.1). Typical values of the Reynolds number along the arterial tree are given in Table 1.7. If the Reynolds number is small, say at most of the order of 1000, the flow remains stable, and is called *laminar*. In normal physiological situations, then, the values of the Reynolds number reached in the cardiovascular system do not allow the formation of full scale turbulence. Some flow instabilities may occur only at the exit of the aortic valve and limited to the systolic phase. In this region the Reynolds number may reach the value of few thousands only for the portion of the cardiac cycle corresponding to the peak systolic velocity, however, there is not enough time for a full turbulent flow to develop. When departing from physiological conditions, there are several factors that may induce transition from laminar to turbulent flows. For instance, the increase of flow velocity because of physical exercise, or due to the presence of a stenotic artery or a prosthetic implant such as a shunt, may produce an increase of the Reynolds number and lead to localised turbulence. Smaller values of blood viscosity also raise the Reynolds number; this may happen in the presence of severe anaemia, when the hematocrit drops sharply (and so does the viscosity). More details on the relations among domain geometry, flow characteristics and type of flow regime will be given in Chapter 5, where the definition of other adimensional numbers that characterise blood flow will be given as well.

Knowing the velocity and the pressure fields allows the computation of the *stresses*, in particular the shear stresses to which an arterial wall is subjected due to the blood movement. Wall shear stresses, whose precise mathematical definition will be given in Chapter 3, are the force per unit area exerted by the fluid tangentially to the wall. We have already mentioned their importance in relation with some vascular diseases, since endothelium cells react to shear stresses. Irregular, and in particular small or "oscillating" [1] shear stresses may cause an alteration in the endothelium covering and induce inflammatory processes. Their calculation require a "point-wise" knowledge of the velocity and pressure field.

To account for the compliance of the vessel wall we need to introduce another unknown, namely the wall displacement $\boldsymbol{\eta}$. The mechanical interaction between the flowing blood and the vessel structure is rather complex. Its general mathematical description will be given in Chapter 3, while more details on the numerical techniques that can be adopted for fluid structure interaction problems are found in Chapter 9. Yet, even with the most advanced techniques available today, accurate computations of fluid structure interaction models of haemodynamics are rather costly. One reason is that the two dynamics (fluid and structure) are here strongly coupled and most of the simplest and cheapest techniques often used in other fields (like aeronautics) simply don't work. Consequently, one of the factors that may affect the choice of a fixed geometry model versus a fluid-structure interaction one is computation time: the latter may be one order of magnitude as expensive as the former.

It is therefore important to appreciate when the approximation of a fixed geometry could be reasonable. It depends on the type of vessels, the type of answers we are seeking and, finally, the type of data available. Smaller vessels experience a smaller relative movement than larger ones, where the change of radius during the heart beat may be of the order of 15 %, like in the aorta. Therefore, the flow in the peripheral vessels, lets say more than two branching levels down from the aorta, can be reasonably modelled using a fixed geometry. An exception being the coronaries, whose movement is however dominated by the heart movement more than the fluid-structure interaction in the vessel. In [396] the effect of heart movement in the shear stress distribution in a coronary artery has been investigated. It has been found that it can be relevant, particularly in vessels with high curvature.

Even in the larger vessels, at least in physiological situations, the main characteristic of the flow are already captured by a fixed geometry model. However, if more details are needed, such as a precise computation of shear stresses or the size of a recirculation region, then compliant models are better suited [250,481]. Furthermore, if it is necessary to have an accurate description of pulse waves, for instance if one wants to investigate altered pressure pattern

[1] Wall shear stress is considered to be oscillating when its component along the main flow direction changes sign during the heart beat. In normal situations the component of wall shear stress along the main flow is always negative. Oscillating shear stresses are usually found in recirculation regions.

possibly caused by anomalous pulse wave reflections, like in the study of aortic aneurysms [285], then compliant models are mandatory. The reason is that fixed geometry models simply cannot describe pulse waves: the propagation speed is here infinite because of the incompressible fluid. It is indeed the mechanical interaction between blood flow and vessel wall deformation that generates the pulse waves.

Lack of sufficient data on the mechanical parameters of the vessel wall may in some cases make compliant models less interesting. This is an important issue in cardiovascular simulations. It is often difficult to obtain accurate values for those parameters for a specific subject. They have often to be inferred from literature data obtained from experiments on animal or human cadaver tissues. More recently, a novel technique called elastography allows to infer some elastic properties from images of the vessel wall movement taken non-invasively. It may then be used to characterise a specific subject. Yet, this technique is still not well widespread. Therefore, sometimes the choice of using a fixed geometry model may be driven by the fact that no data is available to characterise the mechanical property of the vessel under investigation. It must be understood, however, that in large vessels these type of computations may provide qualitative information on the general flow but they may lack precision.

From the mathematical point of view, the analysis of fluid-structure interaction problems is still subject of open research. At the best of our knowledge, a complete mathematical analysis of the coupled fluid-structure problem is not available yet. In the steady case, for small enough applied forces, existence of regular solutions is proved in [201]. In the unsteady case, local solvability in time is proved in the simple case where the structure is a collection of rigid moving bodies in [202]. See also [73, 120]. Formulations based on optimal control on simpler models have been investigated, e.g., in [107, 292, 292, 345, 346, 361]. A overview on the most recent results on the analysis of this type of problems may be found also in Chapter 8.

As for the structural model for the vessel wall, several level of approximation can be considered, depending on the objective of the study and the data available. As we have described in detail in Section 4.2 of Chapter 1, the internal structure of the wall of a blood vessel is rather complex and varies largely with the type of vessel under consideration. The computation of the displacements (and thus the stress) field inside the vessel wall requires to solve the three dimensional equations of elastodynamics which are presented in all generality in the next chapter. Their solution requires to have precise data about the mechanical characteristics of the different layers forming the vessel wall. A piece of information difficult to obtain even by *in vitro* experiments, let alone *in vivo*. Published results like those in [222, 562] may help in the set-up of a proper structural models, yet also in this case we are still far from having the possibility of extracting routinely such type of information for a given person by non invasive techniques. However, technology in this field is progressing fast. As already mentioned, elastographic measurements will probably become common in the near future, and this will be of great help to the set up of patient-specific models also for the structural part.

Whenever there is little interest in a detailed description of the stress and displacement fields inside the vessel wall while the focus is more on their action on the flow field, it is a common practise to resort to simplified (or reduced) structural models. A first simplification is of course to use uniform "space averaged" parameters to describe the mechanical characteristics of the vessel wall, thus ignoring its internal structure. A further step is to use the so called *shell models*, where the displacement field is defined on the surface described by the lumen-wall interface, as indicated in Fig. 2.2. Shell theory, whose mathematical derivation will be sketched in Chapter 3, is in fact based on the assumption of a thin structure. In the case of a vessel it means that the ratio h/R between the wall thickness and vessel radius should be small. Indeed this assumption is questionable, particularly in arteries, which have normally quite a thick wall (see Chapter 1). Yet, the approximation can still be justified by two empirical observations. The first is that the main responsible of the mechanical strength of the vessel wall (at least in physiological situations) is the elastin, which is mainly present in the media. Thus the "effective" thickness is smaller. The other is that, despite its use beyond the fundamental hypothesis, a shell model has proved to be capable of representing the dynamics of the fluid-wall interface with a sufficient level of accuracy, provided that appropriate averaged values of the mechanical characteristics are given. From the computational point of view, shell models are usually cheaper than three dimensional models, as one has to discretise a surface and not a three dimensional domain, with a reduction of the degrees of freedom required. For this reason they are often used in haemodynamic simulations involving fluid-structure interactions, also on realistic geometries, see for instance [187].

Further down in the hierarchy of structural models one may find one dimensional models (see Fig. 2.2). These models assume a cylindrical type geometry and therefore are suited only to study a single artery without bifur-

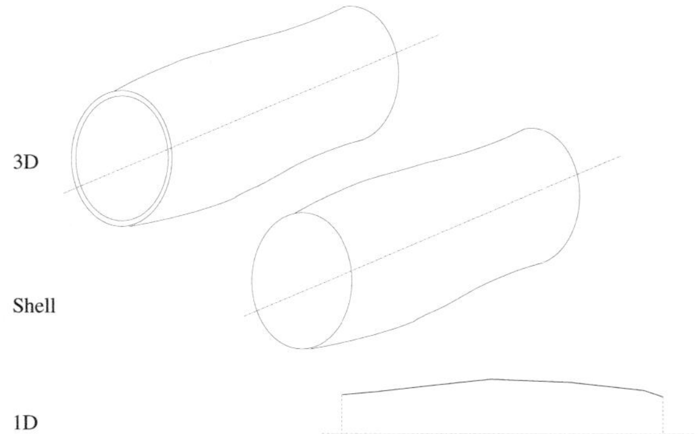

Fig. 2.2. A hierarchy of structural models

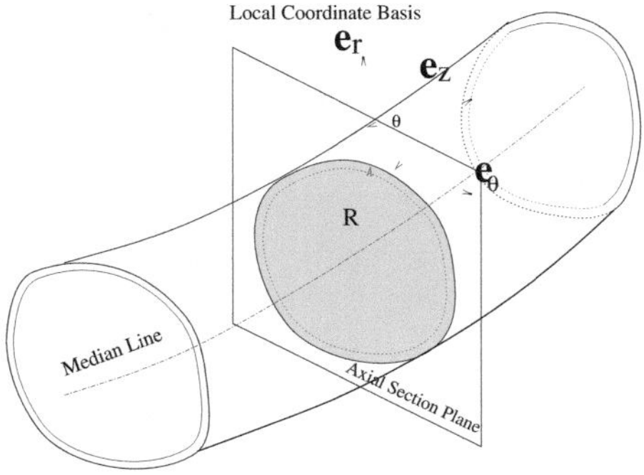

Fig. 2.3. The local coordinate system on the wall surface of a single vessel

cations. They are based on the fact that one can identify on each point of the fluid-structure interface a local system of coordinates $\mathbf{e}_r$, $\mathbf{e}_\theta$, $\mathbf{e}_z$, with $\mathbf{e}_z$ aligned along the vessel axis and $\mathbf{e}_r$ normal to the surface. The corresponding cylindrical coordinates are (r, θ, z), where the z coordinate axis is made to coincide with the centerline of the vessel (see Fig. 2.3).

If one assumes that the circumferential component of the shear stresses at the wall is negligible (this is true for an axial-symmetric geometry and axial-symmetrical deformations) it is possible to write a differential equation in the z variable and time. Often, the additional assumption of only radial displacements, i.e. $\boldsymbol{\eta} = \eta\mathbf{e}_r$ is made as well. No derivatives depending on the circumferential coordinate θ appear in the equations and we may consider each plane θ = const. independently. The resulting displacement field will depend only parametrically on θ. If, in addition, we assume that the problem has an axial symmetry (which implies the further assumption of a straight axis) the dependence on θ is completely neglected. In this case, also the fluid would be described by a 2D axi-symmetric model (see [117]).

Some more details on the derivation of models of this type are given in the Chapter 3. Clearly, we have here quite an important simplification also from the computational point of view, and this explains why these models are widely used to develop and test fluid-structure interaction algorithms. Another reason is that they lend naturally to axi-symmetric formulations [117]. However, their validity in practical computations is limited due to the geometrical restrictions.

Yet, this is not the end of the story. Even simpler structural models may be devised where the normal component of the stress on the fluid-wall interface is directly linked to the normal displacements at the same point by an algebraic relation (or possibly an ordinary differential equation in the time variable). Here the wall mechanics is greatly oversimplified, and these models are indeed used mainly to derive reduced models for blood flow in arteries, like the ones discussed in Chapter 10, even if they have also been used in some early studies of blood flow in simple or 2D geometries [481].

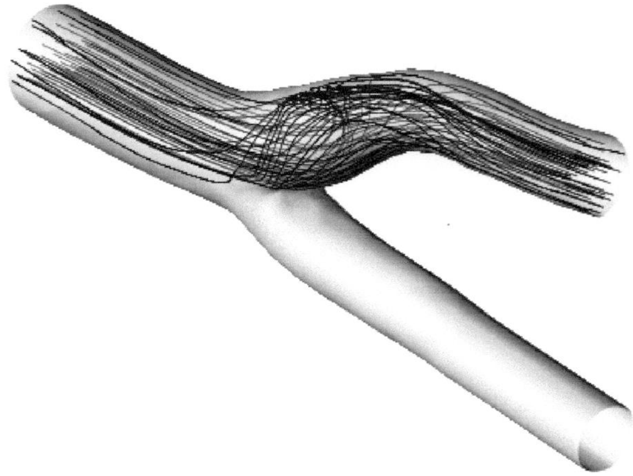

Fig. 2.4. Recirculation in a model of the carotid bifurcation[3]. We show the path of the particles entering the bifurcation. The presence of a recirculation region is evident

A clear major feature of blood flow is its pulsatility. It may induce flow reversal and recirculations near the arterial wall, a phenomenon that can have negative effects on the endothelium and stimulate the deposit of lipids and atherosclerosis. The latter effect is more likely to occur in specific vascular districts, like the carotid bifurcation, see Fig. 2.4.

With some approximation one may think that blood flow is periodic in time. Yet, this can be considered true only for relatively short periods, since the various human activities require to change the amount of blood sent to the various organs. Also the elastic properties of arteries (especially the arterioles) may vary depending on the request of blood by the peripheral organs. Indeed one of the aspects of current research in computational haemodynamics is the interaction between blood flow and the metabolic regulation [108]. It presents several challenges from the mathematical modelling and numerical side. For the sake of space and because only partial results are available so far this aspect has not been extensively covered in this book (see Chapter 10).

In several early studies, however, blood computations were made using steady flow. This can be considered acceptable in peripheral arteries, the capillary bed and in the veins,where the pulsatility of the flow is reduced thanks to the regularising effect of the compliance of the major arteries. In particular, micro-circulation is practically (but not completely) steady. The use of steady computations in larger vessels may again by justified by the lower computational cost. If we eliminate the time derivative in (2.1) we still have a non-linear system of partial differential equations to solve, yet we can make use of acceleration techniques unsuited for unsteady computations because

[3] Computation made by M. Prosi.

they destroy time-accuracy. However, some important quantities (recirculation regions, oscillatory shear stress etc.) cannot be evaluated with high accuracy and only a general qualitative structure of the flow field can be inferred.

We mention that in some particular contexts, for instance in the hyperthermia treatment where some drugs are activated through an artificial localised increase in temperature (see [123, 219]), the variation of blood *temperature* may be relevant. Describing the evolution of temperature requires to introduce another partial differential equation which derives from the principle of energy conservation, and couple it with the Navier-Stokes equations. In large and medium sized vessel the coupling is weak, since here temperature variations have small influence in the flow field. Therefore, one may solve the energy equation (which is instead strongly influenced by the flow field because of the convection term) after having calculated the velocity field. The computational overhead is in this case minimal since we have to solve a single additional equation, moreover of linear type. Things are different in micro-circulation, where the combined effect of temperature on the blood apparent viscosity and on other mechanical properties of the vessel wall makes the situation more complex [178]. However, since in the physiological regime the temperature inside the human body is constant and the situations where temperature variations are relevant are rather special, we will not pursue this topic further in this book.

2.2 Mathematical models for biochemical transport processes

The transport of biochemicals by the arterial blood stream and its interaction with intra-wall transport is of great interest in the vascular physiology and biology. The local mass transfer between the blood and the arterial wall affects the transport of nutrients to the cells, the removal of metabolic wastes from the wall, and the accumulation of potentially atherogenic molecules [175]. The transendothelial mass transfer has been already explained in Section 1.1.3 of Chapter 1. One main aspect of the interest concerns the relation between haemodynamics and molecular transport and the development of pathological vessel alterations.

It has been observed that low density lipoprotein (LDL) accumulation in the intima at zones of low and oscillating wall shear stress is associated with the tendency to intimal thickening and the development of atherosclerotic diseases [64, 278].

The dynamics of dissolved gases (e.g., oxygen or carbon dioxide) and of macromolecules (e.g., lipoprotein or albumin) in arteries and in the arterial wall is strongly related to the flow dynamics of blood. Irregular blood flow patterns with flow stagnation, separation and recirculation, and resulting local low and oscillating wall shear stress, causes local disturbed mass transfer, e.g. [305, 381].

Several mathematical models have been developed for the study of biochemical transport processes in arteries. The simplest model considers solute transport only in the artery lumen and replaces the wall by means of an appropriate boundary condition at the inner surface of the arterial wall (blood-endothelium boundary). This model couples the Navier-Stokes equations with the advection-diffusion equation describing the dynamics of molecules transported in blood.

Improved models account for the arterial wall, where the mass transport in blood and in the wall are described applying physically appropriate laws to model the interaction between the blood flow and the biochemical transport. These models take into account the heterogeneous layers constituting the realistic arterial wall (from inside to outside) the endothelium, the intima, the internal elastic lamina (IEL) and the media. The physical behaviour of the different layers are approximated with the laws of mass transport in porous media (intima and media) and through plasma-permeable membranes (endothelium and IEL), see [251, 381]. In order to simplify the multilayer model the arterial wall can be treated as a single porous layer which is separated from the arterial lumen by a membrane.

2.2.1 Transport in the arterial lumen

The mathematical description of arterial mass transport requires to augment the Navier-Stokes equations (2.1) with the advection-diffusion-equation for the solute concentration c,

$$\frac{\partial c}{\partial t} + \boldsymbol{u} \cdot \boldsymbol{\nabla} c - \boldsymbol{\nabla} \cdot (D \boldsymbol{\nabla} c) = 0 \quad \text{in} \quad \Omega, \quad t > 0. \tag{2.3}$$

The velocity $\boldsymbol{u}$ couples the transport problem to the Navier-Stokes problem. A further coupling of the concentration field to the flow field occurs whenever the diffusivity D of the solute in plasma depends on the strain, see [411] and references therein.

The characterisation of the transport processes uses the Péclet number, defined as $Pe = \frac{UL}{2D}$, which relates the advective transport to the diffusion. Here, L is a typical length scale, for instance the length of the vessel under consideration.

Mass transport processes in medium-sized and large arteries are generally strongly advection dominated, which is reflected in rather large Péclet numbers. The resulting numerical problems are discussed in Chapter 7.

The solution of the time-dependent mass transport problem requires the prescription of an appropriate condition at the initial time $t = 0$, i.e. $c(\boldsymbol{x}, 0) = c_0(\boldsymbol{x})$ for $\boldsymbol{x} \in \Omega$, being c_0 a given function.

For flow domains with "artificial" inflow and outflow boundaries, in most cases a constant concentration profile is prescribed at the inflow cross-section Γ_{in} as Dirichlet boundary condition. At the outflow boundary zero diffusive flux can be assumed, i.e. a homogeneous Neumann condition, i.e. $\partial c/\partial n = 0$.

Appropriate boundary conditions at the inner surface of the arterial wall depends on the molecule size. The transfer of small molecules (dissolved gases) to and into the wall is controlled by diffusion in the boundary layer, as the endothelium is not an significant barrier to the motion of these molecules. Thus, the assumption of a Dirichlet boundary condition at the inner surface is in this case justified. However, in the transfer of macromolecules (LDL) from blood into the arterial wall the main resistance is the endothelial layer. The flux across the endothelium into the arterial wall is determined by the endothelial permeability and by the concentration differential. Therefore, a permeability boundary condition at the blood-endothelium surface Γ_w of the type

$$c\boldsymbol{u} \cdot \boldsymbol{n} - D\frac{\partial c}{\partial \boldsymbol{n}} = \mathcal{P}(c - c_i), \tag{2.4}$$

is appropriate to model the arterial macromolecule transport. $\mathcal{P}$ is the endothelial permeability, c_i is a prescribed concentration in the sub-endothelial intima, and $\boldsymbol{u} \cdot \boldsymbol{n}$ is the normal component of the filtration velocity of plasma at the lumen surface. It is either known or computed using the Darcy model presented in Chapter 7.

Expressing the fact that the endothelium is not a passive barrier to macromolecules, the permeability depends on the local shear stress at the endothelium, i.e $\mathcal{P} = \mathcal{P}(|\boldsymbol{t}^T \boldsymbol{\sigma} \boldsymbol{n}|)$, where the shear stress $\boldsymbol{t}^T \boldsymbol{\sigma} \boldsymbol{n}$ is the tangential component of the Cauchy stress tensor, defined in Chapter 3, equation (3.33).

This model is called *wall-free model* since we are not computing the transport inside the arterial wall. It is suitable to analyse the lumen concentration polarisation effect of large molecules directly at the wall, which happens when the equilibrium concentration at the fluid-endothelium boundary is higher than the concentration in the bulk of the blood stream.

A more realistic model of biochemical transport processes in arteries takes into account the heterogeneous wall, consisting of layers with strongly different thickness and physical properties, as shown in Fig. 1.4. This is called the *multilayer model* and it couples the solute concentration in the blood stream (lumen) and in the intima and media. For a complete derivation of such model, we remand to Chapter 7.

The multilayer model requires to determine a large number of parameters which characterise the physical properties of each layer. The transport parameters of the intima and the media (effective diffusivity, Darcy permeability and porosity) are obtained from the fibre matrix models of the arterial wall tissue. The parameters of the permeable membranes, the endothelium and the IEL (permeability, hydraulic conductivity and reflection coefficients), are calculated from the equations of pore theory. The literature concerning these topics is very extended. Among others, we refer to [11,106,233,234,270]. For the specific case of the multilayer model, we will present in Chapter 7 a brief overview, that is mainly inspired to [251].

2.3 Numerical solution of partial differential equations: a quick review

The mathematical models we have briefly illustrated in the previous sections cannot in general be solved analytically, a part simple cases. Thus we have to resort to numerical techniques to find approximated solutions. It is our intention to give in this section just an introductory glance on this topic. The interested reader can find details in the ample literature available, see for instance [343, 407, 498].

All models just presented are based on partial differential equations (PDEs) for an unknown u (which may be a scalar or a vector field) of the general form

$$\frac{\partial u}{\partial t} + L(u) = f, \quad \text{in } \Omega, \quad 0 < t < T, \tag{2.5}$$

where L indicates a (linear or non-linear) differential operator in the space variable $\boldsymbol{x}$. The former equation will be augmented by proper boundary and inital conditions. In some cases the time derivative is not present (steady problems). Even when the problem is originally set in a semi-infinite time domain, the numerical approximation deals with a bounded time interval, the time T indicating the final time of our simulation.

The most common techniques to solve numerically a PDE are based on a subdivision of the computational domain Ω into a grid, see Fig. 2.5. The solution u is replaced by an approximation u_h which depends on a finite number of parameters, typically (but not necessarily) the values of u_h at the nodes of the grid. The pedix h is here an indication of the grid spacing. Some details on the most common meshing strategies used for cardiovascular geometries are given in Chapter 4.

In the case of time-dependent problems, we will also need to advance the approximation in time, using a so called time-advancing (or time-stepping)

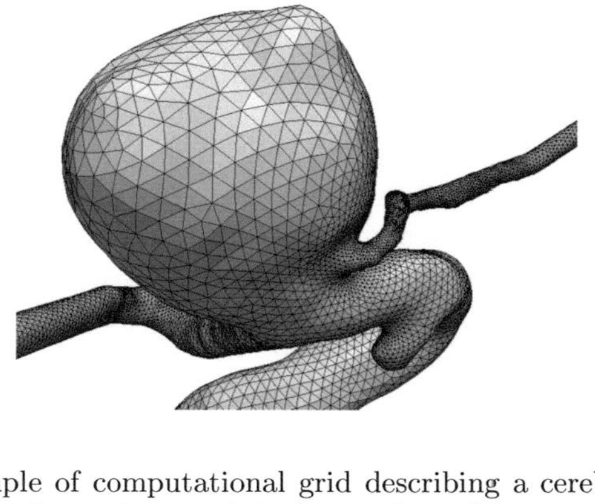

Fig. 2.5. An example of computational grid describing a cerebral artery with an aneurysm. Here only the surface mesh is shown, formed by triangles. The interior is covered by a tetrahedral grid (courtesy of T. Passerini, Aneurisk Project)

scheme. It is typically an iterative method that from the knowledge of the approximation u_h^n at a time t^n, for $n = 0, 1, \ldots, n$ builds the approximation u_h^{n+1} at time $t^{n+1} = t^n + \Delta t$, being $\Delta t > 0$ a chosen *time step*. Most frequently, one-step schemes are adopted, where the computation of u_h^{n+1} will involve just the knowledge of u_h^n.

Let us consider space discretisation first. The most common methods are finite difference, finite volume and finite elements.

2.3.1 Finite difference method (FDM)

When adopting finite differences, the approximated solution u_h is in fact a vector of values $\boldsymbol{u}_h = [u_1, \ldots, u_n]^T$ corresponding to the approximation at the nodes of the computational grid. The differential problem is *collocated* at the grid nodes by replacing the differential operator L with finite differences. For instance, the Laplace operator in two dimensions $\Delta u = \partial^2 u/\partial x^2 + \partial^2 y/\partial y^2$ at node $\boldsymbol{x}_i$ of the regular grid of Fig. 2.6 would be approximated as

$$\left(\frac{\partial^2}{\partial x^2} + \frac{\partial^2}{\partial y^2}\right) u(\boldsymbol{x}_i) \simeq \frac{u_e + u_w + u_s + u_n - 4u_i}{h^2},$$

being h the grid spacing in the x and y directions, here taken constant for simplicity.

Historically, finite differencing is probably the first technique adopted for spatial discretisation. Yet, its use is less common in modern solvers. The reason is manifold. The construction of the finite difference operator is rather complicated for grids that are not uniform and not structured (a structured grid is a grid made up by a regular pattern of nodes). Yet, these grids are mandatory to treat complex geometries, particularly in three dimensional problems. The handling of boundary conditions is also not always straightforward with finite differences, in particular boundary conditions of Neumann type which involve the normal derivative of u at the boundary.

2.3.2 Finite volume method (FVM)

The finite volume method makes use of an integral formulation of the equation. It can be employed whenever the operator L is written in the so called *divergence* or *conservation* form, that is

$$L(u) = \operatorname{div} \boldsymbol{F}(u), \tag{2.6}$$

where $\boldsymbol{F}$ is the so called *flux vector*, which depends on u and on spatial derivatives of u. Let us note that with a few manipulations, the Navier-Stokes equations (2.1) may be written in conservation form, where for the momentum equation

$$\boldsymbol{F}(\boldsymbol{u}, P) = \boldsymbol{u} \otimes \boldsymbol{u} + P\boldsymbol{I} - \mu \boldsymbol{D}(\boldsymbol{u}),$$

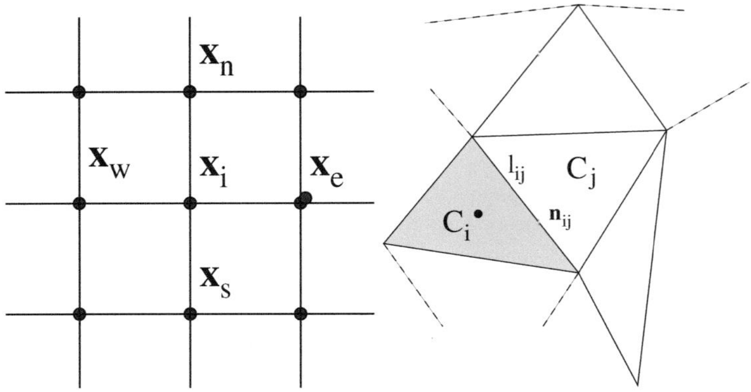

Fig. 2.6. On the left an example of a regular two dimensional grid used for approximation by finite differences. On the right, a generic control volume C_i used in a finite volume scheme. Although we show here a grid made of triangles, finite volumes methods con operate on control volume of general polygonal shape

while for the continuity equation $\boldsymbol{F}(\boldsymbol{u}) = \boldsymbol{u}$. Also equation (2.3) can be recast in conservation form, thanks to the continuity equation $\boldsymbol{u} \cdot \boldsymbol{\nabla} c = \operatorname{div}(c\boldsymbol{u})$.

In general, all differential problems that model a conservation law of physics can be cast in conservation form. We will address in more detail the conservation form of the Navier-Stokes equations in Chapter 3.

For what concerns finite volume methods, once the differential operator is written in conservation form, we integrate the equation on control volumes (usually of polygonal shape) built on the grid, like the one shown in Fig. 2.6. The unknowns are now the approximation of u at each control volume. By applying the divergence theorem we have

$$\int_{C_i} \operatorname{div} \boldsymbol{F}(u) d\boldsymbol{x} = \int_{\partial C_i} \boldsymbol{F}(u) \cdot \boldsymbol{n} d\gamma \simeq \sum_j \boldsymbol{F}_{l_{ij}}(u_h) \cdot \boldsymbol{n}_{ij}.$$

Here, $\boldsymbol{F}_{l_{ij}}$ is an approximation, called numerical flux, of the flux vector on the side l_{ij} of the control volume C_i. The latter has normal $\boldsymbol{n}_{ij}$. The numerical flux depends on the numerical solution u_h. In practise, it usually depends on the value of u_h at the control volume C_i and at the adjacent control volumes. In this way the previous expression actually involves a small number of unknowns. By applying it to all control volumes of the grid we can transform (2.6) into system of linear (or non-linear) equations.

Also in this case we can introduce a parameter h which accounts of the size of control volumes. Typically h is the maximum diameter of the control volumes of the grid. The smaller h the finer the approximation and the greater the computational cost (since we have a higher number of control volumes).

The finite volume method is probably nowadays the most used method for computational fluid dynamics (CFD). The reason is that it combines a high geometrical flexibility (it can operate on arbitrarily complex geometries, even using grids with control volumes of different shapes) with computational efficiency. Furthermore, the construction of the numerical fluxes can be done so that some physical properties (such as local conservation or monotonicity) are preserved also at numerical level. An account of finite volumes for CFD is given in [530].

2.3.3 Finite element method (FEM)

Finite elements are based on a different integral formulation. To describe it let first consider a simple steady problem where L is the Laplace operator with mixed boundary condition, more precisely

$$-\Delta u = f \quad \text{in } \Omega, \tag{2.7}$$

with

$$u = 0, \quad \text{on } \Gamma_D \quad \text{and } \boldsymbol{\nabla} u \cdot \boldsymbol{n} = \frac{\partial u}{\partial n} = g, \quad \text{on } \Gamma_N, \tag{2.8}$$

being Γ_N and Γ_D two parts of the boundary of Ω such that $\Gamma_N \cap \Gamma_D = \emptyset$ and $\Gamma_N \cup \Gamma_D = \partial\Omega$. We will also assume that $\Gamma_D \neq \emptyset$. The function h is a given datum (Neumann boundary condition), while on the Dirichlet boundary Γ_D we have assumed homogeneous conditions only for the sake of simplicity.

The weak formulation

We proceed formally by multiplying both members by a test function $v : \Omega \mapsto \mathbb{R}$, regular enough, integrating over Ω, and using integration by parts (by applying the Green formula) we get

$$\int_\Omega \boldsymbol{\nabla} u \cdot \boldsymbol{\nabla} v d\Omega - \int_{\partial\Omega} v \boldsymbol{\nabla} u \cdot \boldsymbol{n} d\gamma = \int_\Omega f v d\Omega.$$

If v is chosen so that it is zero on Γ_D, by applying the Neumann boundary condition finally we obtain

$$\int_\Omega \boldsymbol{\nabla} u \cdot \boldsymbol{\nabla} v d\Omega = \int_\Omega f v d\Omega + \int_{\Gamma_N} g v d\gamma. \tag{2.9}$$

This statement can be written in the general form $a(u, v) = F(v)$, by setting $a(u, v) = \int_\Omega \boldsymbol{\nabla} u \cdot \boldsymbol{\nabla} v$ and $F(v) = \int_\Omega f v d\Omega + \int_{\Gamma_N} g v d\gamma$.

To give sense to the formal steps made so far, we need to identify the correct functional space for the solution u and the test function v. We will postpone this aspect to Section 2.4. For the time being, we assume that u and v are regular enough so that all the previous steps are well defined and the integrals finite. We can then note that (a) if u is a solution of the original problem (2.7)-(2.8), then it satisfies (2.9); (b) the test function v and the solution u are subject to the same essential conditions on Γ_D, namely they are both zero.

It comes then natural to introduce the abstract problem

$$\textit{Find } u \in V \textit{ such that } \quad a(u,v) = F(v), \quad \forall v \in V, \tag{2.10}$$

being V a space of function regular enough and null on Γ_D, which we will make more precise later.

Formulation (2.10) is called *weak formulation* . We have obtained it for the Laplace problem (2.7)–(2.8), yet it is a rather general fact that a wide class of partial differential problems can be rewritten in the weak form (2.10), with obviously a different definition of $a(u,v)$ and $F(v)$, and possibly of the space V. The application $F(v)$ returns a real number for each $v \in V$ and is called a *functional*, while $a(u,v)$ returns a real number for each couple of functions u and v in V and is called a *form*. Under certain assumptions on the space V, the form a and the functional F it is possible to prove that the weak formulation is *well-posed*, that is it admits a unique solutions u which depends continuosly on the data of the problem (in our example g and f). This important result takes the name of Lax-Milgram lemma and its statement can be found, for instance, in [408]. Furthermore, it can be proved that regular solution of the weak formulation do indeed satisfy the original differential problem in what is called *strong form* (in contract to the weak form). However, the space of weak solutions is somehow larger than that of the problem in strong form.

Therefore, the weak formulation may be seen as a generalisation of the original problem. It gives a robust mathematical framework to differential problems, encompassing situations (e.g. rather irregular data or domains) which cannot be treated satisfactorily in the classical strong formulation. Even for more complex problems, like the Navier-Stokes equations or the fluid-structure interaction problem, a weak formulation may be found, as it will be illustrated in Chapter 8.

The Galerkin method

Moving from the weak formulation we can replace the space V, which is infinite dimensional, with a finite dimensional subspace V_h, that is we choose a $V_h \subset V$ with $\dim(V_h) = N_h$ and solve the problem:

$$\textit{Find } u_h \in V_h \textit{ such that } \quad a(u_h, v_h) = F(v_h), \quad \forall v_h \in V_h. \tag{2.11}$$

Being V_h finite dimensional the approximate solution u_h may be expanded with respect to a base of V_h as $u_h(\boldsymbol{x}) = \sum_{i=1}^{N_h} u_i \phi_i(\boldsymbol{x})$. In other words, V_h is spanned by the basis $\{\phi_i,\, i = 1, \dots, N_h\}$. The coefficients $u_i \in \mathbb{R}$ are called *degrees of freedom* and are indeed the unknowns of the discrete problem. Furthermore, we can choose $v_h = \phi_j$ for $j = 1, \dots N_h$ in (2.11) to produce linear system of equations $A\boldsymbol{u} = \boldsymbol{b}$, where

$$A_{ij} = a(\phi_j, \phi_i) = \int_\Omega \boldsymbol{\nabla}\phi_j \cdot \boldsymbol{\nabla}\phi_i \, d\Omega, \quad b_j = F(\phi_j) = \int_\Omega f\phi_j d\Omega + \int_{\Gamma_N} g\phi_j d\gamma.$$

Matrix A is traditionally called the *stiffness matrix.* The actual expression for stiffness matrix and source term may be more complex for problems more complicated than Laplace's, yet the way of deriving the discrete system remains fundamentally the same. In the case of a non-linear problem, the resulting system will be non-linear, typically this means that the matrix A will depend on u_h.

This technique of building the discrete problem by projection on a subspace and searching the solution in the same subspace takes the name of *Galerkin method.*

The finite element space

A last (but not the least) step is to choose the way of building V_h. To this aim, various different techniques are possible. In the classical spectral element method for periodic solutions a truncated Fourier series is used on the whole Ω. It is a valid method if the solution is very smooth and on very simple geometries (typically cubic or cylindrical domains). The other methods do require to subdivide the domain into a grid $\mathcal{T}_h$ of polygonal elements (or at least elements that can be mapped by simple transformations into a polygon), in a way similar to what is done in the finite volume method. Given the grid, the space V_h may be expressed by piecewise polynomial functions, for instance we could consider the space

$$X_h^r(\mathcal{T}_h) = \{v_h \in C^0(\overline{\Omega}), : \quad v_h|_K \in \mathbb{P}^r, \quad K \in \mathcal{T}_h\}$$

of piecewise polynomials of degree r on each grid element K. The space V_h is then taken as the subspace of $X_h^r(\mathcal{T}_h)$ that accounts for the constraints at the Dirichlet boundary. Methods of that sort are the *finite element method* (FEM) and the *spectral element method* (SEM). They differ on the choice of the basis for V_h and on the fact that the SEM adopts high order polynomials, while in the FEM rarely r exceeds 3 (and often is equal to 1, i.e linear finite elements). Another characteristic of the SEM method is the use of special quadrature rule to approximate the integrals which guarantee high convergence rate (for smooth solutions) while keeping the computational cost of building the linear system reasonably small. Thus, they are quite interesting when dealing with smooth solutions. However, are much less used than FEM in standard solvers, since often the solution is not as regular as needed to benefit from the method and their implementation on complex geometries may be rather complex. Indeed, SEM methods are usually (although not always) implemented on grids whose elements are hexahedra (quadrilaterals in 2D), while finite elements are also implemented on tetrahedral (triangular) grids, which are much more flexible. For more details on the spectral element method the reader may consult [60, 253].

The usual (though not exclusive) choice for the basis function ϕ_i in the FEM is such that the degrees of freedom u_i do correspond to the value of

u_h at some points of the grid called nodes. An important characteristic of the FEM is that the basis function ϕ_i has small support, i.e. is different from zero only on a limited connected portion of Ω. The main consequence is that the stiffness matrix A is *sparse*, since $A_{ij} = 0$ whenever the support of ϕ_i and ϕ_j has zero intersection, and this happens whenever nodes $\boldsymbol{x}_i$ and $\boldsymbol{x}_j$ are not shared by any element of the mesh. This fact is very relevant in applications since sparse matrices have a smaller memory requirement than their full counterpart. The computer implementation is also rather efficient, since the matrix and the right hand side can be built by looping over the mesh elements and performing local operations on each element.

The FEM is probably one of the most adopted numerical method for partial differential equations, especially in the field of structural mechanics, although, as already mentioned, in the field of CFD finite volume methods are probably more popular. Yet, finite elements are gaining grounds also in this field, particularly in the case of incompressible flow. The richness (and flexibility) of their mathematical formulation allows in fact to develop a large variety of numerical schemes, basically changing the discrete spaces where the solution is sought and the test functions chosen.

The parameter h in the finite element method is identified as the maximum diameter of the finite elements in the given mesh. The smaller h, the higher the number of elements necessary to cover Ω and the higher the number of degrees of freedom (and the dimension of the linear system).

In the case of non linear problems, like the Navier-Stokes equation, the application of the method leads to a non-linear system of equation, where the stiffness matrix is itself function of the discrete solution.

Convergence

In all methods shown so far we expect that the approximation u_h becomes more precise as h goes to zero. Indeed, a request we make is that a discretisation method be *convergent*, that is the error should go to zero as $h \to 0$. Furthermore, we say that the method converges with order p if it exists a constant $C = C(u) > 0$ so that, for h sufficiently small, the following inequality applies

$$||u - u_h|| \leq C\, h^p.$$

The error is measured in a suitable norm, here indicated by $||\cdot||$. The order of convergence typically depends on the particular method chosen, the regularity of the exact solution and the selected norm.

For instance, a standard FEM discretisation of the Laplace problem satisfies

$$||u - u_h||_{H^1(\Omega)} \leq C\|u\|_{H^s(\Omega)} h^p,$$

for a constant $C > 0$, where $p = \min(r, s-1)$, being r the degree of the finite element, and s a measure of the regularity of the solution u. More precisely, the error estimate is true whenever $u \in H^s(\Omega)$. The definition of the Sobolev spaces $H^k(\Omega)$ as well as that of the H^k norm $||\cdot||_{H^k(\Omega)}$ will be given in Section 2.4. Therefore, if we use linear finite elements, we have a method whose convergence is linear with respect to h when using the H^1 norm to measure the error.

We mention also the possibility of generating another class of schemes by replacing the original form $a(u_h, v_h)$ with an approximation $a_h(u_h, v_h)$. The simplest way by which this is done is by performing numerical quadratures to approximate the integrals which define the form. Methods of this sort are usually called *generalised Galerkin methods*. We give in Fig. 2.7 a synthesis of the main numerical techniques for PDEs which includes those mentioned here.

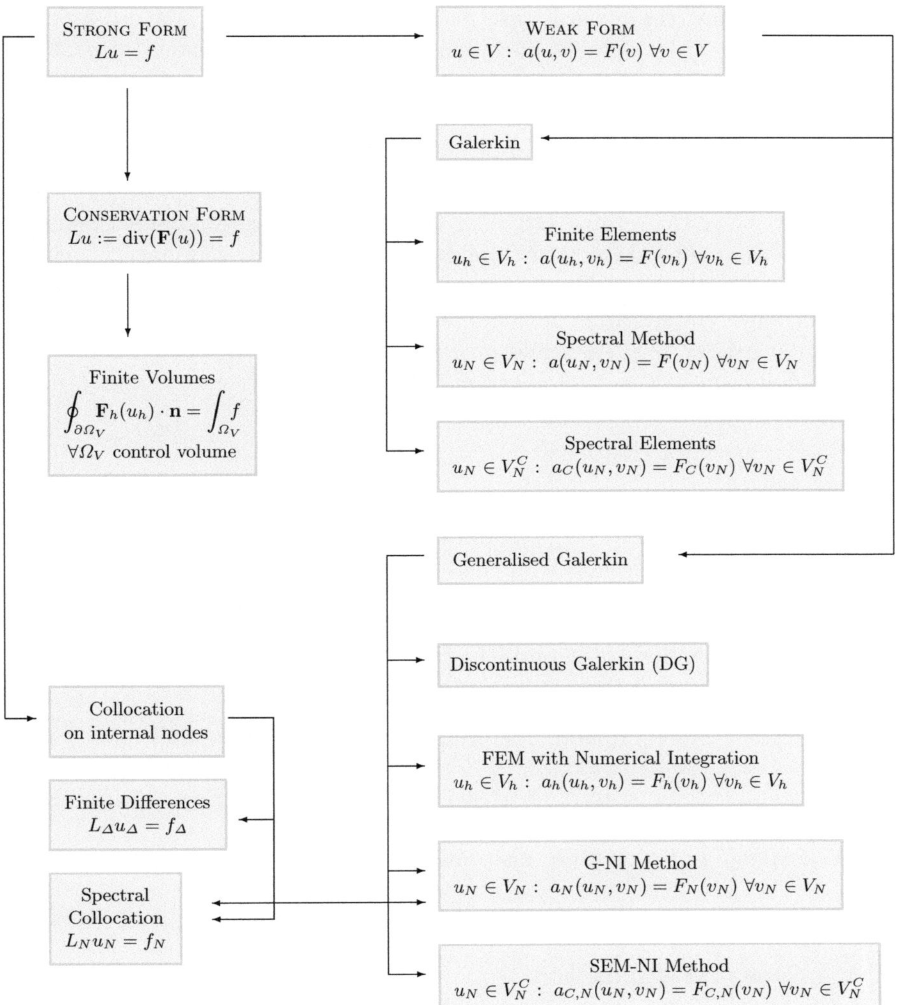

Fig. 2.7. A flow-chart of the main discretisation methods for PDEs

2.3.4 Time advancing schemes

In the previous paragraphs we have considered the discretisation with respect to the space variables. If we have a transient problem we need to consider the time as well. What is usually done in this case is to first discretise in space and then consider the time evolution. The reason why the two variables are treated differently is due to their different nature. The differential problems we will consider here are usually boundary value problems with respect to space, that is conditions are set on the whole boundary of the spatial domain Ω. On the contrary, they require a condition only at one end of the time axis, the initial condition. It is natural, then, to think of using a different numerical techniques to treat the time variable.

If we consider the general case of equation (2.5), after space discretisation with finite differences or finite volumes we obtain a system of ordinary differential equations on each node i, of the form

$$\frac{du_i}{dt}(t) + \boldsymbol{s}_i^T \boldsymbol{u}(t) = f_i(t), \quad 0 < t < T, \tag{2.12}$$

where $\boldsymbol{u}(t) = [u_1(t), \ldots, u_{N_h}(t)]^T$ are the degrees of freedom (here equal to the approximated solution at the nodes or at the control volumes), which are now function of the time. Furthermore, $f_i(t) = f(\boldsymbol{x}_i, t)$ and $\boldsymbol{s}_i$ is here a vector of coefficients. For instance, for the Laplace equation, finite differences on a the regular grid of Fig. 2.6 would give at any internal node i

$$\frac{du_i}{dt}(t) + \frac{4u_i(t) - u_e(t) - u_w(t) - u_s(t) - u_n(t)}{h^2} = f_i(t).$$

In matrix form

$$\frac{d\boldsymbol{u}}{dt}(t) + A\boldsymbol{u}(t) = \boldsymbol{f}(t),$$

where A is the matrix with the $\boldsymbol{s}_i$ as rows.

Schemes for this system of ordinary differential equations require to choose a time step Δt and solve a problem for $\boldsymbol{u}^n$, approximation of $\boldsymbol{u}(t^n)$, being $t^n = n\Delta t$. The most common are

- the *explicit Euler* method, also called *forward Euler* method

$$\boldsymbol{u}^{n+1} = \boldsymbol{u}^n + \Delta t \left[A\boldsymbol{u}^n + \boldsymbol{f}(t^n)\right]; \tag{2.13}$$

- the *implicit Euler* method, also called *backward Euler* method

$$(\boldsymbol{I} + \Delta t A)\boldsymbol{u}^{n+1} = \boldsymbol{u}^n + \Delta t \boldsymbol{f}(t^{n+1}); \tag{2.14}$$

- the *Crank-Nicolson* method,

$$(\boldsymbol{I} + \frac{1}{2}\Delta t A)\boldsymbol{u}^{n+1} = \boldsymbol{u}^n + \frac{\Delta t}{2}\left[A\boldsymbol{u}^n + \boldsymbol{f}(t^n) + \boldsymbol{f}(t^{n+1})\right]. \tag{2.15}$$

All methods compute in successive steps the sequence $\boldsymbol{u}^1, \boldsymbol{u}^2, \ldots$, being $\boldsymbol{u}^0$ known from the initial condition of the differential problem.

The main difference among (2.13) and (2.14) or (2.15) is that the former allows to compute the approximation at time step t^{n+1} without the need to solve a linear system. This is why is called explicit. Crank-Nicolson scheme is more accurate than the other two since it a second order method with respect to time. It means that assuming that the space operator is exact the error between the approximated solution and the exact one goes to zero as $(\Delta t)^2$ when $\Delta t \to 0$. The other two methods are just first order. Explicit methods are always subject to a stability condition, that is they provide a reasonable approximation only if $\Delta t \leq \widehat{\Delta t}$, where the *critical time step* $\widehat{\Delta t}$ depends on the particular method chosen and on the eigenvalues of the matrix A. The latter is normally a decreasing function of h. Thus, typically the finer the grid, the smaller the time step we have to adopt with an explicit scheme to satisfy the stability condition. The type of problems we have to face to solve haemodynamic applications usually exhibit a second order differential operator L and, in general, for this class of problems

$$\widehat{\Delta t} = Ch^{-2},$$

which penalises explicit schemes strongly. Therefore, despite their higher computational complexity, implicit and unconditionally stable schemes are often preferred for this class of problems. For instance, both implicit Euler and Crank-Nicolson schemes fall in this category.

Were the original differential problem non-linear, implicit schemes lend to non-linear problems, to be solved at each time step. A possibility is to resort to a Newton iteration or other fixed point strategies, see for instance [257,403].

When dealing with finite element computations, the ordinary differential equations stemming from space discretisation are in fact of the form

$$M\frac{du_i}{dt}(t) + S\boldsymbol{u}(t) = f_i(t),$$

where M is the so called *mass matrix*, of elements $M_{ij} = \int_\Omega \phi_i \phi_j \, d\Omega$. Consequently, we end up with a non trivial linear system even when adopting explicit schemes. Yet, often the mass matrix M can be replaced with a diagonal matrix, called *lumped mass matrix*, and we are able to write the differential system in the same form as in (2.12).

We mention that several other time advancing schemes are possible. In particular, for the class of problems we deal in this book, methods based on backward difference formulae (BDF) are quite interesting since they couple good stability and convergence properties with an acceptable computational cost. Interested readers can refer, for instance, to [403].

2.4 Some elements of functional analysis

We give here some elements of functional analysis to help the reader through some of the next chapters. Because of the scope of the book and the sake of space we will be very brief and rather informal. A more complete introduction in the context of partial differential equations is [424], while among the more advanced books on the subject we mention [552] and [438].

First of all with *functional space* we denote a *linear* space of functions $\Omega \subset \mathbb{R}^d \mapsto \mathbb{R}^n$, where n is typically 1 (scalar functions) or either 2 or 3 (vector functions), as well as d. We assume that the domain Ω is open and bounded. A common example of functional space is the space of continuous real functions on an interval $\Omega \subset \mathbb{R}$, usually denoted by $C^0(\Omega)$.

A norm is an application $V \mapsto \mathbb{R}$ such that

$$||v|| \geq 0, \quad \text{and} \quad ||v|| = 0 \quad \text{iff} \quad v = 0, \tag{2.16}$$

$$||v + w|| \leq ||v|| + ||w||, \qquad \forall v, w \in V, \tag{2.17}$$

$$||\alpha v|| = |\alpha| ||v||, \quad \forall v \in V, \quad \forall \alpha \in \mathbb{R}.$$

We recall that a normed and complete linear space V is also called a *Banach* space.

2.4.1 Functionals and bilinear forms

Given a functional space V an application

$$F : \quad V \mapsto \mathbb{R}$$

is called a *functional* on V. A functional is linear if $F(\alpha v + \beta w) = \alpha F(v) + \beta F(w)$, for all real numbers α and β and all v and w in V. A linear functional on a normed space V is *continuous* if and only if it is bounded, i.e. $\exists C > 0$ such that

$$|F(v)| \leq C ||v||_V, \quad \forall v \in V.$$

We have indicated by $||\cdot||_V$ the norm of V. The space of linear and continuous functionals on V is itself a normed space, called the dual space V'. The norm of a functional is in fact the smallest constant C in the previous inequality, or equivalently

$$||F||_{V'} = \sup_{\substack{v \in V \\ v \neq 0}} \frac{|F(v)|}{||v||_V}.$$

A linear and continuous functional applied to an element $v \in V$ is often indicated using the *crochet* symbol, that is $F(v)$ can be written alternatively as ${}_{V'}\langle F, v \rangle_V$ (or simply $\langle F, v \rangle$ whenever there is no ambiguity). This notation puts into evidence the duality between the two spaces.

An application

$$a : V \times V \mapsto \mathbb{R},$$

that maps two elements of V to a real number is called a form. It is a *bilinear* form if linear with respect to each argument (taken singularly), i.e

$$a(\lambda u + \mu w, v) = \lambda a(u, v) + \mu a(w, v), \quad \forall \lambda, \mu \in \mathbb{R}, \forall u, v, w \in V,$$

$$a(u, \lambda w + \mu v) = \lambda a(u, v) + \mu a(u, w), \quad \forall \lambda, \mu \in \mathbb{R}, \forall u, v, w \in V.$$

A bilinear form is continuous if there exists a constant $M > 0$ such that

$$|a(u, v)| \leq M \|u\|_V \|v\|_V, \quad \forall u, v \in V,$$

and is *coercive* if $\exists \alpha > 0$ such that

$$a(u, u) \geq \alpha \|u\|_V^2, \quad \forall u \in V.$$

A scalar product (u, v) of a space V is an application $V \times V \mapsto \mathbb{R}$ such that it is bilinear with respect to each argument, $||v|| = \sqrt{(u, u)}$ is a norm on V (called normed induced by the scalar product) and in addition the Cauchy-Schwarz inequality holds:

$$(u, v) \leq \|u\| \|v\|, \quad \forall u, v \in V.$$

In other words, the scalar product is a continuous bilinear form with respect to the induced norm, with continuity constant equal to 1. A complete functional space V equipped with a scalar product and the induced norm is called *a Hilbert space*. Hilbert spaces play a fundamental role in the analysis of partial differential equations.

2.4.2 Support of a function

The support of a function f is the closure of the subset of Ω where $f \neq 0$. A function is said to have compact support in Ω if its support is contained in a closed and bounded subset of Ω. In particular, if f has compact support in Ω is zero on the boundary of Ω.

2.4.3 Sobolev spaces

The space $L^2(\Omega)$ is the space of square integrable functions, that is

$$L^2(\Omega) = \{v : \Omega \mapsto \mathbb{R}, \quad \int_\Omega v^2 d\Omega < +\infty\}.$$

It is a Hilbert space with scalar product $(u, v)_{L^2(\Omega)} = \int_\Omega u, v \, d\Omega$ and norm $\|v\|_{L^2(\Omega)} = \left(\int_\Omega u, v \, d\Omega\right)^{1/2}$. Often, the L^2 scalar product is simply indicated as (u, v). To the sake of precision, we mention that the integral in the definition of $L^2(\Omega)$ (and of all the other functional spaces introduced in this section) is a Lebesgue integral. Lebesgue integration is a mathematical construction that extends the classical integral due to Riemann to a wider class of functions. From the practical point view there is little difference in using Lebesgue integrals, since bounded functions integrable in the classical sense are also Lebesgue integrable and the two integrals coincide.

The existence of the L^2 scalar product is based on the fact that if u and v are in $L^2(\Omega)$, then the integral $\int_\Omega uv\, d\Omega$ exists and is finite.

The space $H^s(\Omega)$ is defined as the space of function of $L^2(\Omega)$ such that all derivatives (partial derivatives if Ω is multidimensional) of order up to s belong to $L^2(\Omega)$ as well. For instance, in the case $\Omega \subset \mathbb{R}$,

$$H^1(\Omega) = \{v \in L^2(\Omega) : \quad \frac{dv}{dx} \in L^2(\Omega)\}.$$

The derivative in the definition has to be intended as generalised derivative (also called "distributional derivative"). In this context, $dv/dx \in L^2(\Omega)$ actually means that there exists a $g \in L^2(\Omega)$ such that for all functions $w \in C^\infty(\Omega)$ with compact support in Ω the following equality holds, i.e.

$$-\int_\Omega g w d\Omega = \int_\Omega v \frac{dw}{dx} d\Omega.$$

We will identify g with $\frac{dw}{dx}$. The notion of generalised derivative effectively extends the concept of derivative to non-differentiable functions in the classical sense. However, the two derivatives coincide for regular functions.

The Sobolev space $H^s(\Omega)$, with s a positive integer and $\Omega \subset \mathbb{R}^d$, is a Hilbert space when endowed with the scalar product

$$(u, v)_{H^s(\Omega)} = \sum_{|\boldsymbol{\alpha}| \le s} \int_\Omega \frac{\partial^{|\boldsymbol{\alpha}|} u}{\partial x^{\alpha_1} \dots \partial x^{\alpha_d}} \frac{\partial^{|\boldsymbol{\alpha}|} v}{\partial x^{\alpha_1} \dots \partial x^{\alpha_d}} d\Omega,$$

and the corresponding norm

$$\|u\|_{H^s(\Omega)} = \left[\sum_{|\boldsymbol{\alpha}| \le s} \int_\Omega \left(\frac{\partial^{|\boldsymbol{\alpha}|} u}{\partial x^{\alpha_1} \dots \partial x^{\alpha_d}} \right)^2 d\Omega \right]^{1/2}$$

Here, $\boldsymbol{\alpha} = [\alpha_1, \dots, \alpha_d]$ is a *multi-index* of non negative integers and $|\boldsymbol{\alpha}| = \alpha_1 + \dots + \alpha_n$, and we have also adopted the convention that $\frac{\partial^{|\boldsymbol{\alpha}|} u}{\partial x^{\alpha_1} \dots \partial x^{\alpha_d}} = u$ whenever $|\boldsymbol{\alpha}| = 0$. As a consequence of the definition, $\|u\|_{H^s(\Omega)} \le \|u\|_{L^2(\Omega)}$ and $H^s(\Omega) \subset L^2(\Omega)$, for all s. We can also conventionally set $H^0(\Omega) \equiv L^2(\Omega)$, so all previous definitions and properties extend trivially to the case $s = 0$ as well.

A most important space for the differential problems of our interest is $H^1(\Omega)$, where

$$(u,v)_{H^1(\Omega)} = \int_\Omega (uv + \nabla u \cdot \nabla v)\, d\Omega, \quad \|u\|_{H^1(\Omega)} = \sqrt{\int_\Omega (u^2 + ||\nabla u||^2)\, d\Omega}.$$

Here, $||\nabla u|| = \sqrt{\sum_{i=1}^3 (\partial u/\partial x_i)^2}$ indicates the Euclidean norm of the gradient. The H^s *seminorm*[4] is defined as

$$|u|_{H^s(\Omega)} = \sqrt{\sum_{|\alpha|=s} \int_\Omega \left(\frac{\partial^{|\alpha|} u}{\partial x^{\alpha_1} \dots \partial x^{\alpha_d}} \right)^2 d\Omega}.$$

We have that $H^{k+1}(\Omega) \subset H^k(\Omega)$ for $k = 0, 1, \dots$ with continuous injections, indeed if $u \in H^{k+1}(\Omega)$ then $\|u\|_{H^k(\Omega)} \le \|u\|_{H^{k+1}(\Omega)}$.

We mention that in the next chapters, the symbol $[H^k(\Omega)]^3$ will be used to indicate the space of vector functions whose components belong to $H^k(\Omega)$, i.e. $[H^k(\Omega)]^3 = H^k(\Omega) \times H^k(\Omega) \times H^k(\Omega)$.

2.4.4 Traces

Let us first notice that two square integrable functions u_1 and u_2 which differ only on a set of zero measure identify in fact the same member of $L^2(\Omega)$, as $\|u_1 - u_2\|_{L^2(\Omega)}$. Being the boundary of Ω of zero measure it is clear that we cannot in general give a meaning to the value on $\partial\Omega$ of a function of $L^2(\Omega)$. Yet, what about a function belonging to $H^s(\Omega)$ with $s \ge 1$?

A major result is that if Ω is sufficiently regular, for instance polygonal or having a C^1 boundary (more details in the cited bibliography) there exists a linear and continuous application

$$\gamma_0 : H^s(\Omega) \mapsto \mathrm{L}^2(\partial\Omega),$$

such that $\gamma_0 v = v|_{\partial\Omega}$, $\forall v \in H^s(\Omega) \cap C^0(\overline{\Omega})$. The application $\gamma_0 v$ is called *trace* of v on $\partial\Omega$.

The fact that γ_0 is linear and continuous implies that $\exists C > 0$ so that

$$\|\gamma_0 v\|_{L^2(\partial\Omega)} \le C \|v\|_{H^s(\Omega)}.$$

The result can be extended to the case of $\gamma_\Gamma : H^s(\Omega) \mapsto L^2(\Gamma)$ where $\Gamma \subset \partial\Omega$ is sufficiently regular and of non-null $d-1$ measure[5].

---

[4] A seminorm enjoys all properties of a norm a part that it can be zero when its argument is different from zero.

[5] $\partial\Omega$ is of zero d-measure, i.e. when considered as immersed in the space R^d, while in general has a non-zero $d-1$ measure. For instance the surface of a sphere has zero volume (3-measure) but a certain area (2-measure).

This result allows to give sense to the Dirichlet conditions whenever we seek a solution to a differential problem in $H^s(\Omega)$. We wish to point out that the operator γ_Γ is not onto $L^2(\Gamma)$. In particular, the functions of $L^2(\Gamma)$ which are traces of functions of $H^1(\Omega)$ is a subspace of $L^2(\Gamma)$ denoted as $H^{1/2}(\Gamma)$.

We can extend to functions in $H^s(\Omega)$ with $\Omega \subset \mathbb{R}^d$ and $d = 1, 2$ or 3 the well known Green integration and, consequently, the divergence theorem of classical vector calculus. In the following of the book for the sake of simplicity we will indicate $\gamma_0 u$ with $u_{|\partial\Omega}$, using the same notation adopted for a continuous function.

The space $H_0^1(\Omega)$

We can define the space $H_0^1(\Omega)$ as the space of functions with null trace on $\partial\Omega$

$$H_0^1(\Omega) = \{v \in H^1(\Omega) : \ \gamma_0 v = 0\}.$$

In fact, it is possible to define $H_0^1(\Omega)$ for arbitrary bounded domains Ω, using technicalities we prefer to avoid in this sketchy notes.

It is also possible to define $H_\Gamma^1(\Omega)$ as the space of function with null trace on $\Gamma \subset \partial\Omega$,

$$H_\Gamma^1(\Omega) = \{v \in H^1(\Omega) : \ \gamma_\Gamma v = 0\}.$$

An important result for what concerns the analysis of partial differential problems is the Poincaré inequality, which states that there exists a constant C_Ω such that

$$\|v\|_{L^2(\Omega)} \leq C_\Omega \|v\|_{H^1(\Omega)} \qquad \forall v \in H_0^1(\Omega).$$

2.4.5 Back to the weak formulation

We are now in the position of making expression (2.10) more precise. Indeed, by inspecting all the integrals that make up the bilinear form and the functional, we can note that the requirements we have to make so that all integrals exists and are finite is that $V = H_{\Gamma_D}^1$, provided that $f \in L^2(\Omega)$ and $h \in L^2(\Gamma_N)$. Actually, the conditions on the data indicated here are not the most general possible, yet are already quite broad to demonstrate the generality of the weak formulation.

We mention that with this choice problem (2.10) is well posed.

2.5 Conclusions

The objective of this chapter was twofold. On the one hand, we gave an overview of some basic mathematical models governing haemodynamics, with a greater emphasis on their physical significance and applicability rather than on a rigorous formal derivation. To the latter are dedicated some of next chapters.

One the other hand, we provided some basic notions on methods for their numerical solution. We have also introduced some of the notation that will be used throughout the book. The notions given here are only elementary and have only the aim of introducing the occasional reader to the subject. The bibliography provided could however serve as a complement.

3

The derivation of the equations for fluids and structure

Miguel A. Fernández, Luca Formaggia, Jean-Frédéric Gerbeau, and Alfio Quarteroni

In this chapter we derive the equations governing the mechanics of the fluid (the blood) and the structure (the vessel wall). The derivation will be made in a rigorous way, yet trying to provide the reader a physical understanding. Reason of space obliged us to focus on the most important models for haemodynamic computations and to omit several details and the proofs of the propositions. For instance, all issues related to energy conservation principles have been ignored and we have eventually considered only incompressible fluids.

The reader interested in a more in-depth analysis may refer to several books on continuum mechanics available in the literature. We give here some, non exhaustive, indications. Introductory general texts are [211,310] as well as [221], which is more focused on solid mechanics. More mathematical oriented texts are [92, 313], while a general introduction on non-linear mechanics is found in [512]. For what concerns shell theory, of which we are here giving just an outline, a rigorous mathematical introduction is found in [93,94], while a text more oriented on the numerical aspects is [75]. As for fluid mechanics, we mention [90].

The first part of the chapter is dedicated to the kinematics of continuum media. Kinematics is the part of mechanics that describe the motion. It forms the background enabling to derive the differential equations which "translate" into mathematical terms some fundamental principles of physics. Namely, mass and momentum balance. Up to this point there is no need to distinguish between solids and fluids (and gases, for what matters).

It is only when we characterise how the medium reacts internally to an exterior action that the behaviour of the two types of media diverge and we are able to finalise the derivation of the mathematical models.

In haemodynamic applications often fluid and structure interact, for instance when blood flows in a compliant vessel. This fact prompts the introduction of a particular point of view: the so-called Arbitrary Lagrangian Eulerian formulation, which is particularly convenient for the numerical computation of this type of problems. Reduced models for the structure are often used

Formaggia L, Quarteroni A, Veneziani A (Eds.): Cardiovascular Mathematics. Modeling and simulation of the circulatory system

in fluid/structure interaction computations to cut down on computational complexity. They will be illustrated together with the general formulation of the fluid-structure problem.

We will write the equations in the so called *tensorial form*, which is independent of the particular coordinate system used. Whenever is needed we will report the corresponding expression in terms of Cartesian components. When dealing with shell models we will need to introduce a curvilinear system of coordinates. We have tried to keep the notation as standard as possible, avoiding too technical details, yet the reader may find in appendix 12.4.4 an explanation of the main mathematical symbols used throughout the chapter.

3.1 The kinematics of continuum media

Let $\widehat{\Omega} \subset \mathbb{R}^3$ be a domain, that is a bounded, open and simply connected subset of $\mathbb{R}^3$, with smooth boundary, filled by a *continuum medium*. We shall refer to $\widehat{\Omega}$ as the *reference configuration* of the medium under consideration.

A *deformation* of $\widehat{\Omega}$ is a smooth one-to-one mapping

$$\widehat{\boldsymbol{\phi}} : \widehat{\Omega} \longrightarrow \Omega, \quad \widehat{\boldsymbol{x}} \longrightarrow \boldsymbol{x} = \widehat{\boldsymbol{\phi}}(\widehat{\boldsymbol{x}}),$$

associating each point $\widehat{\boldsymbol{x}}$ of $\widehat{\Omega}$ to new position $\boldsymbol{x} = \widehat{\boldsymbol{\phi}}(\widehat{\boldsymbol{x}})$ in the current configuration $\Omega \subset \mathbb{R}^3$. The vector quantity

$$\widehat{\boldsymbol{\eta}}(\widehat{\boldsymbol{x}}) = \widehat{\boldsymbol{\phi}}(\widehat{\boldsymbol{x}}) - \widehat{\boldsymbol{x}} \tag{3.1}$$

is called *displacement* of the *material point* $\widehat{\boldsymbol{x}}$. The local deformation is linked to the *deformation gradient*, defined as

$$\widehat{\boldsymbol{F}}(\widehat{\boldsymbol{x}}) = \boldsymbol{\nabla}_{\widehat{\boldsymbol{x}}} \widehat{\boldsymbol{\phi}}. \tag{3.2}$$

Here, the symbol $\boldsymbol{\nabla}_{\widehat{\boldsymbol{x}}}$ indicates the gradient with respect to the $\widehat{\boldsymbol{x}} = (\widehat{x}_1, \widehat{x}_2, \widehat{x}_3)$ coordinates. Sometimes we will omit the suffix when it is clear from the context which coordinate system we are adopting. The deformation gradient is a second order tensor field, therefore $\widehat{\boldsymbol{F}} : \widehat{\Omega} \rightarrow \mathbb{R}^{3\times 3}$ being $\mathbb{R}^{3\times 3}$ the space of three dimensional matrices. In Cartesian coordinates its value is given by the 3×3 matrix of components[1]

$$\widehat{F}_{ij} = \frac{\partial x_i}{\partial \widehat{x}_j}, \quad i, j = 1, 2, 3.$$

We also assume that its determinant

$$\widehat{J} = \det \widehat{\boldsymbol{F}}, \tag{3.3}$$

[1] In fact, to be a tensor the components have to satisfy certain rules with respect to coordinate transformation, see any elementary book on tensor analysis like [47].

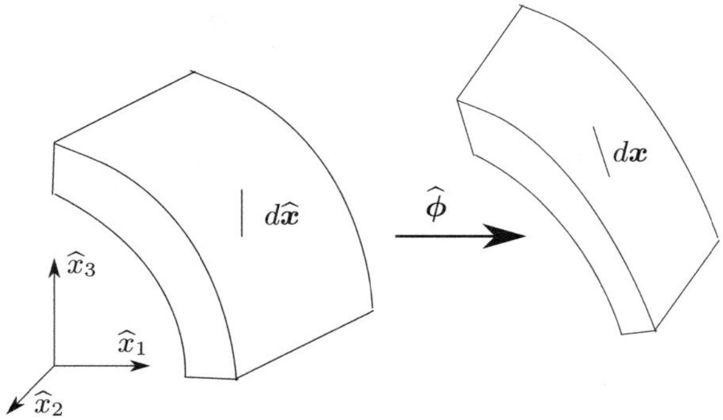

Fig. 3.1. Local deformation of a material neighbourhood. An infinitesimal vector $d\widehat{\boldsymbol{x}}$ is deformed into $d\boldsymbol{x}$

called the *Jacobian* of the deformation, is everywhere strictly positive. It means that the mapping is *orientation preserving*.

The link between $\widehat{\boldsymbol{F}}$ and the local deformation is made clear if we consider two arbitrary points $\widehat{\boldsymbol{a}}$ and $\widehat{\boldsymbol{b}} = \widehat{\boldsymbol{a}} + \widehat{\boldsymbol{\delta}}$ of $\widehat{\Omega}$, separated by the "small" vector $\widehat{\boldsymbol{\delta}}$ (refer to Fig. 3.1).

Let $\boldsymbol{a} = \widehat{\boldsymbol{\phi}}(\widehat{\boldsymbol{a}})$ and $\boldsymbol{b} = \widehat{\boldsymbol{\phi}}(\widehat{\boldsymbol{b}})$ be the corresponding points in Ω. The regularity of the map $\widehat{\boldsymbol{\phi}}$ allows us to write $\boldsymbol{b} = \boldsymbol{a}+\boldsymbol{\delta} = \widehat{\boldsymbol{a}}+\widehat{\boldsymbol{F}}(\widehat{\boldsymbol{a}})\widehat{\boldsymbol{\delta}}+o(\widehat{\boldsymbol{\delta}})$, where the symbol $o(\boldsymbol{h})$ stands for an infinitesimal of higher order than $\boldsymbol{h}$ for $||\boldsymbol{h}|| \to 0^+$, being $||\cdot||$ the Euclidean norm. The length of $\boldsymbol{\delta} = \boldsymbol{b} - \boldsymbol{a}$ is given by

$$||\boldsymbol{\delta}|| = \sqrt{\boldsymbol{\delta}^T\boldsymbol{\delta}} = \left[\widehat{\boldsymbol{\delta}}^T\widehat{\boldsymbol{F}}^T(\widehat{\boldsymbol{a}})\widehat{\boldsymbol{F}}(\widehat{\boldsymbol{a}})\widehat{\boldsymbol{\delta}}\right]^{1/2} + o(||\widehat{\boldsymbol{\delta}}||).$$

This relation is often expressed in the form

$$||d\boldsymbol{x}|| = \sqrt{d\widehat{\boldsymbol{x}}^T\widehat{\boldsymbol{F}}^T\widehat{\boldsymbol{F}}d\widehat{\boldsymbol{x}}}, \tag{3.4}$$

and it gives the change of the length of the "infinitesimal vector" $d\widehat{\boldsymbol{x}}$ due to the deformation. The tensor $\widehat{\boldsymbol{C}} = \widehat{\boldsymbol{F}}^T\widehat{\boldsymbol{F}}$ is called the *right Cauchy-Green* tensor.

In the following we will often indicate by $\widehat{V}$ a subdomain of $\widehat{\Omega}$ and by V its image $V = \widehat{\boldsymbol{\phi}}(\widehat{V}) = \{\boldsymbol{x} \in \Omega : \widehat{\boldsymbol{\phi}}^{-1}(\boldsymbol{x}) \in \widehat{V}\}$.

Then,

$$|V| = \int_V d\boldsymbol{x} = \int_{\widehat{V}} \widehat{J}(\widehat{\boldsymbol{x}})d\widehat{\boldsymbol{x}} \tag{3.5}$$

is the *measure* of V (i.e. its volume). The Jacobian thus measures the variation of volume due to the deformation.

To derive the equations of continuum mechanics we need to relate differential operators acting on the two configurations. For instance, by applying the usual rules for the gradient of composite functions we have

Proposition 3.1. *Let* $\widehat{f} : \widehat{\Omega} \to \mathbb{R}$ *be a regular function and* $f : \Omega \to \mathbb{R}$ *defined as* $f(\boldsymbol{x}) = \widehat{f}(\widehat{\boldsymbol{\phi}}^{-1}(\boldsymbol{x}))$*; then*

$$\boldsymbol{\nabla}_{\widehat{\boldsymbol{x}}}\widehat{f} = \widehat{\boldsymbol{F}}\boldsymbol{\nabla} f.$$

An important role in this context is played by the *Piola transformation*. Let us refer to Fig. 3.2, where we display a generic volume $\widehat{V} \subset \widehat{\Omega}$ and its image V, together with the corresponding normals to the boundary, indicated by $\widehat{\boldsymbol{n}}$ and $\boldsymbol{n}$, respectively. Let also assume that we have a sufficiently regular second order tensor field $\boldsymbol{\sigma} : \Omega \longrightarrow \mathbb{R}^{3\times3}$, defined on the deformed configuration.

The *Piola transformation* of $\boldsymbol{\sigma}$ associated to the given deformation $\widehat{\boldsymbol{\phi}}$ is the second order tensor field $\widehat{\boldsymbol{\Pi}} = \mathcal{P}_{\widehat{\boldsymbol{\phi}}}(\boldsymbol{\sigma}) : \widehat{\Omega} \to \mathbb{R}^{3\times3}$ given by

$$\widehat{\boldsymbol{\Pi}}(\widehat{\boldsymbol{x}}) = \widehat{J}(\widehat{\boldsymbol{x}})\boldsymbol{\sigma}\big(\widehat{\boldsymbol{\phi}}(\widehat{\boldsymbol{x}})\big)\widehat{\boldsymbol{F}}^{-T}(\widehat{\boldsymbol{x}}), \tag{3.6}$$

for all $\widehat{\boldsymbol{x}} \in \widehat{\Omega}$. Using a short hand notation we may write $\widehat{\boldsymbol{\Pi}} = \widehat{J}\widehat{\boldsymbol{\sigma}}\widehat{\boldsymbol{F}}^{-T}$.

The *inverse Piola transformation* of $\widehat{\boldsymbol{\Pi}}$ returns the tensor $\boldsymbol{\sigma}(\boldsymbol{x})$ according to

$$\boldsymbol{\sigma}(\boldsymbol{x}) = \widehat{J}^{-1}\big(\widehat{\boldsymbol{\phi}}^{-1}(\boldsymbol{x})\big)\widehat{\boldsymbol{\Pi}}\big(\widehat{\boldsymbol{\phi}}^{-1}(\boldsymbol{x})\big)\widehat{\boldsymbol{F}}^{T}\big(\widehat{\boldsymbol{\phi}}^{-1}(\boldsymbol{x})\big), \tag{3.7}$$

or, more simply, $\boldsymbol{\sigma} = J^{-1}\widehat{\boldsymbol{\Pi}}\boldsymbol{F}^T$.

The main property of the Piola transformation is given by the following important formula (see [92] for a proof).

Proposition 3.2. *Let* $\boldsymbol{\sigma}$ *be a regular tensor field in* Ω *and* $\widehat{\boldsymbol{\Pi}}$ *its Piola transformation, we have*

$$\mathbf{div}_{\widehat{\boldsymbol{x}}}\widehat{\boldsymbol{\Pi}} = J\,\mathbf{div}\boldsymbol{\sigma}, \tag{3.8}$$

where $\mathbf{div}_{\widehat{\boldsymbol{x}}}$ *is the divergence with respect to the* $\widehat{\boldsymbol{x}}$ *coordinates and the equality has to be understood on corresponding points in* $\widehat{\Omega}$ *and* Ω*, respectively.*

As a result, by the application of the divergence theorem, we have

$$\int_{\partial\widehat{V}} \widehat{\boldsymbol{\Pi}}\widehat{\boldsymbol{n}}\,\mathrm{d}\widehat{\gamma} = \int_{\partial V} \boldsymbol{\sigma}\boldsymbol{n}\,\mathrm{d}\gamma, \tag{3.9}$$

whenever $\widehat{\boldsymbol{\Pi}}$ and $\boldsymbol{\sigma}$ are related by (3.6). The use of this equality will be made clear in the next sections.

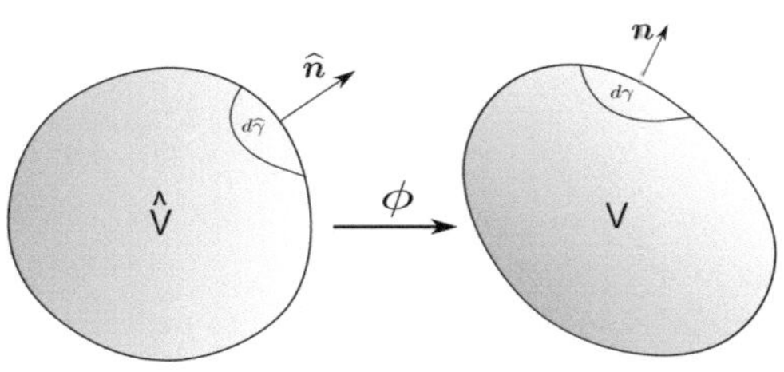

Fig. 3.2. The transformation of a material volume under deformation

It is also possible to derive the following relation for any scalar field f in Ω and $\widehat{f} = f \circ \widehat{\phi}$

$$\int_{\partial V} f \boldsymbol{n} \, \mathrm{d}\gamma = \int_{\partial \widehat{V}} \widehat{f} \widehat{J} \widehat{\boldsymbol{F}}^{-T} \widehat{\boldsymbol{n}} \, \mathrm{d}\widehat{\gamma}, \tag{3.10}$$

where

$$\mathrm{d}\gamma = \widehat{J} ||\widehat{\boldsymbol{F}}^{-T} \widehat{\boldsymbol{n}}|| \, \mathrm{d}\widehat{\gamma} \quad \text{and } \boldsymbol{n} = \frac{\widehat{\boldsymbol{F}}^{-T} \widehat{\boldsymbol{n}}}{||\widehat{\boldsymbol{F}}^{-T} \widehat{\boldsymbol{n}}||}. \tag{3.11}$$

The first relation in (3.11) is often called *Nanson's formula* and relates the measure of a surface element in the reference configuration to that of the corresponding element in the current configuration. The second expression relates the corresponding normals.

3.1.1 The motion

What we have shown so far is a static picture, to have motion we need to bring the time into play. A *motion* is a smooth map

$$\widehat{\varphi} : \widehat{\Omega} \times \mathbb{R}^+ \longrightarrow \mathbb{R}^3, \quad (\widehat{\boldsymbol{x}}, t) \longrightarrow \boldsymbol{x} = \widehat{\varphi}(\widehat{\boldsymbol{x}}, t),$$

such that, at any $t \geq 0$, $\widehat{\varphi}_t = \widehat{\varphi}(\cdot, t)$ is a deformation. In other words, a motion is one-parameter family of deformations, the parameter t being the time. Without loss of generality we have assumed here that the motion starts at $t = 0$ (initial time). The reference configuration $\widehat{\Omega}$ is in principle arbitrary, yet often it coincides with the initial configuration, i.e $\widehat{\Omega} = \Omega(0)$. When not otherwise stated, we will implicitly make this assumption.

The point $\boldsymbol{x} = \widehat{\varphi}(\widehat{\boldsymbol{x}}, t)$ is the position at time t of the *material point* (also called *material particle*) identified by $\widehat{\boldsymbol{x}}$, while $\Omega(t) = \widehat{\varphi}(\widehat{\Omega}, t)$ denotes the *current configuration* at time t.

In this context, the displacement is now also function of time, $\widehat{\boldsymbol{\eta}}(\widehat{\boldsymbol{x}}, t) = \widehat{\varphi}(\widehat{\boldsymbol{x}}, t) - \widehat{\boldsymbol{x}}$ being the displacement at time t.

All the kinematic quantities defined in the previous section can be extended to a motion. In particular, $\widehat{\boldsymbol{F}}$ and $\widehat{J}$ still indicate the deformation gradient and Jacobian, respectively, yet are now function also of time. For instance, $\widehat{\boldsymbol{F}}(\widehat{\boldsymbol{x}}, t) = \boldsymbol{\nabla}_{\widehat{\boldsymbol{x}}} \widehat{\varphi}(\widehat{\boldsymbol{x}}, t)$.

Given a subdomain $\widehat{V} \subset \widehat{\Omega}$, the set $V(t) = \{\boldsymbol{x} \in \Omega(t) : \boldsymbol{x} = \widehat{\varphi}(\widehat{\boldsymbol{x}}, t), \widehat{\boldsymbol{x}} \in \widehat{V}\}$ is formed by the same material particles as $\widehat{V}$ and is called a *material (sub)domain*, or also *material volume*. Thanks to (3.5), if $\widehat{J}$ is constant in time (i.e $\frac{\partial \widehat{J}}{\partial t} = 0$) the material subdomain does not change its measure during motion.

The *velocity* is indeed a major kinematic quantity and is the time derivative of the displacement:

$$\widehat{\boldsymbol{u}}(\widehat{\boldsymbol{x}}, t) = \frac{\partial}{\partial t} \widehat{\boldsymbol{\eta}}(\widehat{\boldsymbol{x}}, t) = \frac{\partial}{\partial t} \widehat{\varphi}(\widehat{\boldsymbol{x}}, t), \tag{3.12}$$

the last equality is obtained by using the definition (3.1), now referred to time t.

3.1.2 Lagrangian, Eulerian and ALE formulations

We can define all physical quantities alternatively on the reference or on the current configuration, the choice being a matter of convenience. For instance the field $\widehat{\rho} : \widehat{\Omega} \times \mathbb{R}^+ \to \mathbb{R}^+$ indicates the density, i.e. $\widehat{\rho}(\widehat{\boldsymbol{x}}, t)$ is the density at time t in the material point $\widehat{\boldsymbol{x}}$. Yet, the invertibility of the mapping allows us to refer the same quantity to the current configuration: for all $t > 0$

$$\rho(\boldsymbol{x}, t) = \widehat{\rho}(\widehat{\boldsymbol{\varphi}}_t^{-1}(\boldsymbol{x}), t), \quad \boldsymbol{x} \in \Omega(t),$$

is the density at the point $\boldsymbol{x} \in \Omega(t)$ occupied by the material particle $\widehat{\boldsymbol{x}}$ at time t.

The interplay between these two "points of view" is crucial in continuum mechanics. When we adopt $(\widehat{\boldsymbol{x}}, t)$ as independent variables we use a *Lagrangian formulation*, while when we refer to the $(\boldsymbol{x}, t)$ pair we employ the *Eulerian formulation*. In the Lagrangian formulation we focus on the material particle $\widehat{\boldsymbol{x}}$ and its evolution; in the Eulerian formulation we observe what happens at a given point $\boldsymbol{x}$ in the physical space. When a field is expressed in the Eulerian coordinates it is referred to as an *Eulerian field*, while a *Lagrangian field*, also called *material field*, is a field expressed in Lagrangian coordinates.

We will adopt the same symbol for a given physical quantity. Yet, the superscript $\widehat{\ }$ will denote a Lagrangian field. To summarise, for a quantity q we have

$$\widehat{q}(\widehat{\boldsymbol{x}}, t) = q(\boldsymbol{x}, t), \quad \text{with } \boldsymbol{x} = \widehat{\boldsymbol{\varphi}}(\widehat{\boldsymbol{x}}, t),\ \widehat{\boldsymbol{x}} \in \widehat{\Omega},\ t > 0. \tag{3.13}$$

We will also make use of the composition operator: $\widehat{q}(\cdot, t) = q(\cdot, t) \circ \widehat{\boldsymbol{\varphi}}_t$. Conversely,

$$q(\boldsymbol{x}, t) = \widehat{q}(\widehat{\boldsymbol{x}}, t), \quad \text{with } \widehat{\boldsymbol{x}} = \widehat{\boldsymbol{\varphi}}_t^{-1}(\boldsymbol{x}),\ \boldsymbol{x} \in \Omega(t),\ t > 0, \tag{3.14}$$

or, more simply, $q(\cdot, t) = \widehat{q}(\cdot, t) \circ \widehat{\boldsymbol{\varphi}}_t^{-1}$ (see Fig. 3.3 and Fig. 3.4).

Therefore, the velocity $\boldsymbol{u}$ in the Eulerian frame is simply obtained by mapping $\widehat{\boldsymbol{u}}$ in the current configuration, i.e.

$$\boldsymbol{u}(\boldsymbol{x}, t) = \widehat{\boldsymbol{u}}(\widehat{\boldsymbol{\varphi}}_t^{-1}(\boldsymbol{x}), t), \quad (\boldsymbol{x}, t) \in \Omega(t) \times \mathbb{R}^+. \tag{3.15}$$

Sometimes it is useful to describe the displacement as an Eulerian field, obtaining

$$\boldsymbol{\eta}(\boldsymbol{x}, t) = \boldsymbol{x} - \widehat{\boldsymbol{\varphi}}_t^{-1}(\boldsymbol{x}). \tag{3.16}$$

One formulation may be more convenient than the other, depending on the context. Let us make this aspect more precise. As already illustrated in Chapter 2 when we want to solve the differential equations governing the motion of a fluid or a solid we need to identify the *computational domain* where we want

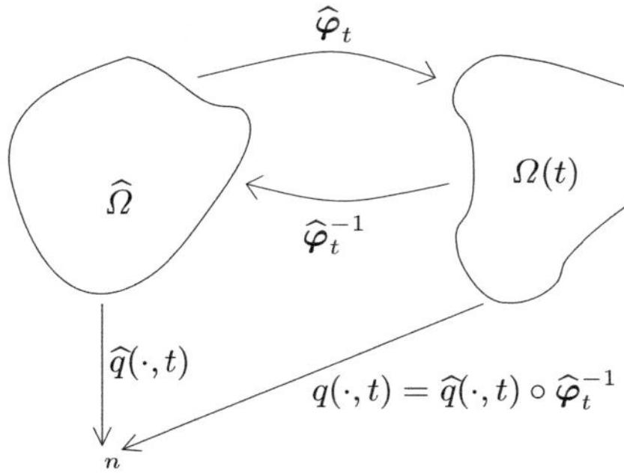

Fig. 3.3. Eulerian description of a Lagrangian field

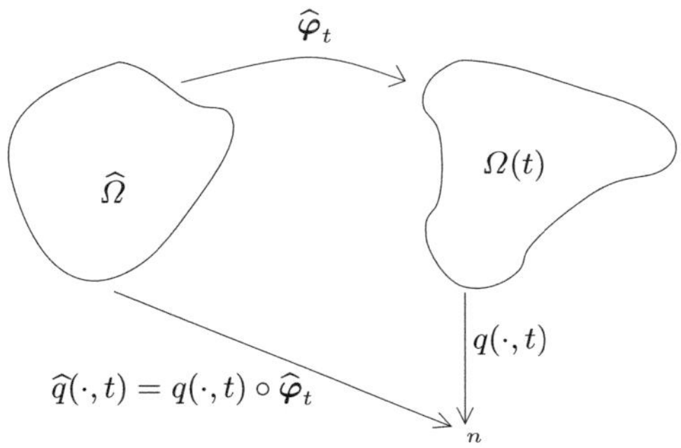

Fig. 3.4. Lagrangian description of an Eulerian field

to solve the equations, on the boundary of which we need to provide suitable boundary conditions. In a solid, where the displacements are often relatively small, the computational domain is often taken to be $\widehat{\Omega}$ and the Lagrangian formulation is thus preferred. This situation is sketched in Fig. 3.5.

In a fluid the situation is rather different. The displacements are extremely large and, moreover, usually irrelevant, since, as we will make clear in a later

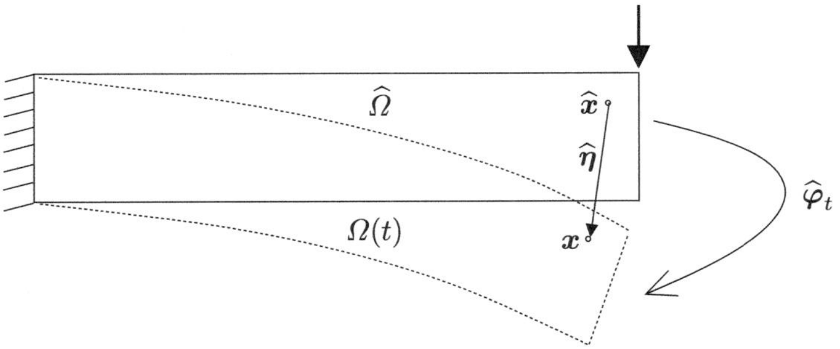

Fig. 3.5. Lagrangian description of the motion of a solid. The differential problem will be posed on $\widehat{\Omega}$, using a Lagrangian description

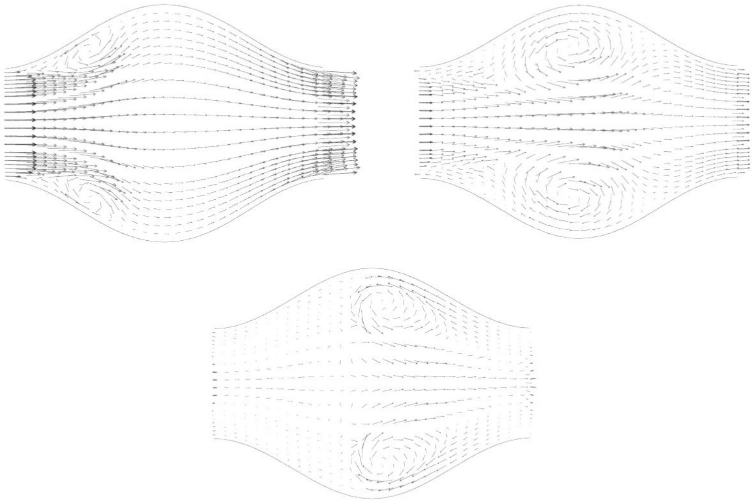

Fig. 3.6. Example of velocity field in the same region at three time instants

section, for a fluid we are normally interested in the velocity field, like the one in Fig. 3.6, or other related quantities, rather than the displacement itself. Therefore, the computational domain is normally chosen as a fixed, open bounded set $\Omega \subset \mathbb{R}^3$ located where we are interested to compute the solution. No special requirements is made on Ω apart that is should be "filled by the fluid", that is $\Omega \subset \Omega(t)$ for all times t we are observing the motion[2], see Fig. 3.7. The Eulerian framework is then here preferable. However, the Lagrangian frame is still useful as a tool to formally derive the equations from fundamental principles.
As already mentioned in Chapter 2, in many cases of practical interest in haemodynamics, such as blood flowing in a compliant artery, the computational domain for the fluid cannot be fixed in time, as it has to follow the displacements of the fluid-wall interface[3]. Yet, the Lagrangian frame is not of help here, since certainly we do not wish to follow the evolution of the blood particles as they circulate along the whole cardiovascular system! We usually wish to compute the flow field in a domain confined in the area of interest, yet following the movement of the wall interface, (see for instance Fig. 3.8).

The computational domain, which we will now indicate with $\omega(t)$, is neither fixed nor a material subdomain, since its evolution is not governed by the fluid motion, but has to comply by that of the boundary $\partial\omega(t)$, which

[2] For the sake of simplicity we have set as the time interval for our equations the whole positive real line, yet in practical computations the time interval of interest is obviously finite.

[3] Special computational techniques, like the immersed boundary method [385], may get around this fact, at the price of using more complex equations, see Chapter 9.

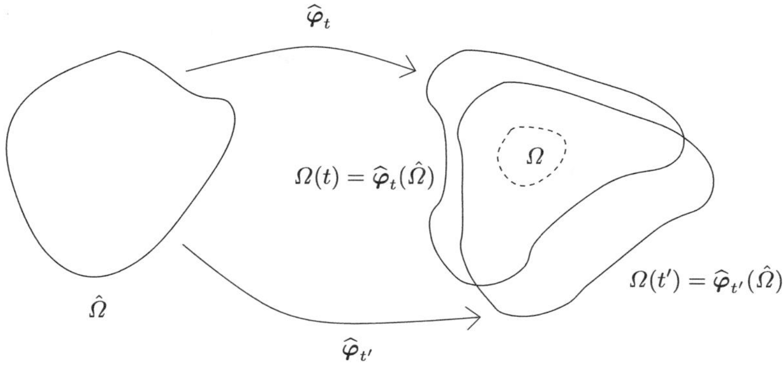

Fig. 3.7. The computational domain Ω in the Eulerian formulation. It is a fixed portion of space filled by the medium during its motion

is either given or the result of the coupling with a structural model. It is then necessary to introduce another, intermediate, frame of reference, called *Arbitrary Lagrangian Eulerian* (ALE).

We will show in Section 3.5 how it is possible to build from the evolution of $\partial\omega(t)$ an auxiliary motion

$$\widetilde{\mathcal{A}} : \widetilde{\omega} \times \mathbb{R}^+ \to \mathbb{R}^3 \quad (\widetilde{\boldsymbol{x}}, t) \to \boldsymbol{x} = \widetilde{\mathcal{A}}(\widetilde{\boldsymbol{x}}, t),$$

such that $\omega(t) = \widetilde{\mathcal{A}}(\widetilde{\omega}, t)$, for all $t > 0$, see Fig. 3.9. Here, $\widetilde{\omega} \subset \mathbb{R}^3$ is a reference (fixed) configuration, which in general (yet not necessarily) corresponds to the initial position at $t = 0$, i.e. $\omega(0)$. Fig. 3.9 gives a sketch of the situation.

In the ALE formulation we have then the interplay of (at least) two motions: the one of the medium under consideration and that of the computational domain. The former is governed by physical laws, the latter is rather arbitrary, provided that the given law for the domain boundary movement be respected.

Given an *ALE field*, that is a field defined in the ALE reference domain, $\widetilde{q} : \widetilde{\omega} \times \mathbb{R}^+ \longrightarrow \mathbb{R}$, its *Eulerian description* is given by

$$q(\boldsymbol{x}, t) = \widetilde{q}(\widetilde{\mathcal{A}}_t^{-1}(\boldsymbol{x}), t), \quad \forall \boldsymbol{x} \in \omega(t), \quad t > 0,$$

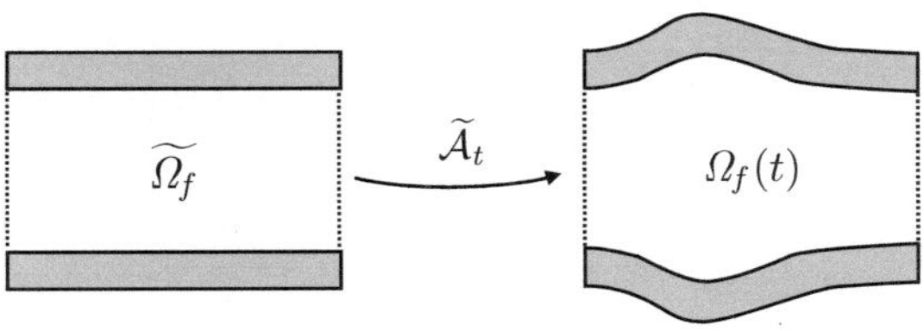

Fig. 3.8. The computational domain Ω_f for the fluid in a compliant artery. It deforms to follow the arterial wall movement, yet the axial position of its proximal and distal boundary is kept fixed. Its evolution is described by the ALE map

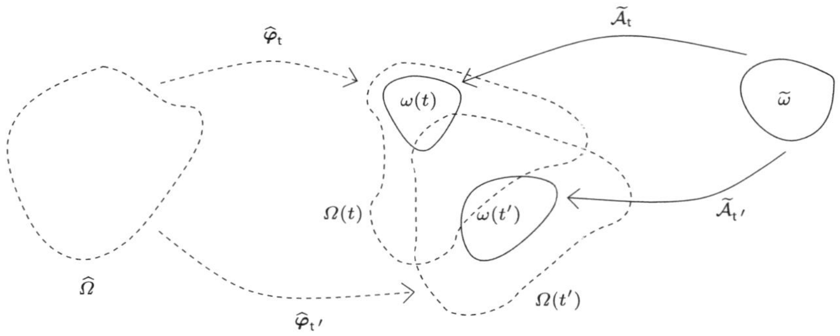

Fig. 3.9. The moving computational domain $\omega(t)$ and the ALE map. Here, for generality, we show an arbitrary reference computational domain $\widetilde{\omega}$. Most of the times, however, it is chosen to coincide with $\omega(0)$

also indicated as $q(\cdot,t) = \widetilde{q}(\cdot,t) \circ \widetilde{\mathcal{A}}_t^{-1}$. Conversely,

$$\widetilde{q}(\widetilde{\boldsymbol{x}},t) = q(\widetilde{\mathcal{A}}(\widetilde{\boldsymbol{x}},t),t), \quad \forall \widetilde{\boldsymbol{x}} \in \widetilde{\omega}, \quad t > 0, \tag{3.17}$$

or, equivalently $\widetilde{q}(\cdot,t) = q(\cdot,t) \circ \widetilde{\mathcal{A}}_t$. Here we have taken the case of a scalar field, yet the same rule applies to vector and tensor fields.

Analogously to what done before, we can define the *computational domain velocity*, also called *ALE velocity*, as

$$\widetilde{\boldsymbol{w}}(\widetilde{\boldsymbol{x}},t) = \frac{\partial \widetilde{\mathcal{A}}}{\partial t}(\widetilde{\boldsymbol{x}},t), \quad \forall \widetilde{\boldsymbol{x}} \in \widetilde{\omega}, \tag{3.18}$$

which can be mapped to the Eulerian frame by means of (3.17), in short hand notation $\boldsymbol{w}(.,t) = \widetilde{\boldsymbol{w}}(\cdot,t) \circ \widetilde{\mathcal{A}}_t^{-1}$.

Remark 3.1.1 *In general, $\boldsymbol{w}(\boldsymbol{x},t) \neq \boldsymbol{u}(\boldsymbol{x},t)$. However, we can note two particular cases:*

- $\boldsymbol{w} = \boldsymbol{0}$*: the computational domain is fixed as $\omega(t) = \omega(0)$ for all times; we recover the Eulerian formulation;*
- $\boldsymbol{w} = \boldsymbol{u}$*: the computational domain $\omega(t)$ is now a material domain; we recover the Lagrangian formulation.*

In analogy with what already done for the Lagrangian frame, we can define the Jacobian of the ALE movement $\widetilde{J}_{\widetilde{\mathcal{A}}} = \det \frac{\partial \widetilde{\mathcal{A}}}{\partial \widetilde{\boldsymbol{x}}}$ and with $J_{\widetilde{\mathcal{A}}}$ the corresponding quantity in the current configuration, obtained by composition with the inverse ALE map. Recasting the Euler expansion formula (3.26) to the ALE mapping we obtain

$$\left.\frac{\partial J_{\widetilde{\mathcal{A}}}}{\partial t}\right|_{\widetilde{\mathcal{A}}} = J_{\widetilde{\mathcal{A}}} \operatorname{div} \boldsymbol{w}. \tag{3.19}$$

For the sake of notation, we will follow the convention that if $F = F(\boldsymbol{x},t)$ then F_t indicates the function of the space variable only, defined as $F_t(\boldsymbol{x}) = F(\boldsymbol{x},t)$, at any fixed time t.

Eulerian, Lagrangian and ALE time-derivatives

We have already seen how to transform some space differential operators from different configurations, once we know the deformation. To complete the picture, we need now to understand how to relate time derivatives in the different formulations.

For a given scalar Eulerian field q (the discussion applies also to vector or tensor fields), we define the *Eulerian time-derivative* as simply

$$\frac{\partial q}{\partial t}(\boldsymbol{x}, t), \quad \boldsymbol{x} \in \Omega(t). \tag{3.20}$$

In other words, we look at the rate of change of q at a fixed point $\boldsymbol{x}$ in the physical space, where the current configuration lives. It is nothing else than the classical partial derivative.

Let now $\widehat{q}$ be the Lagrangian description of q. We define the *material time-derivative* $\frac{Dq}{Dt}$ of q as

$$\frac{Dq}{Dt}(\cdot, t) = \frac{\partial \widehat{q}}{\partial t}(\cdot, t) \circ \widehat{\boldsymbol{\varphi}}_t^{-1}. \tag{3.21}$$

We can give a different interpretation of the material derivative, with a more immediate physical meaning. Let us note that by recalling relation (3.13) we may write that

$$\begin{aligned}\frac{\partial}{\partial t}\widehat{q}(\widehat{\boldsymbol{x}}, t) &= \lim_{h\to 0} \frac{\widehat{q}(\widehat{\boldsymbol{x}}, t+h) - \widehat{q}(\widehat{\boldsymbol{x}}, t)}{h} \\ &= \lim_{h\to 0} \frac{q(\widehat{\boldsymbol{\varphi}}(\widehat{\boldsymbol{x}}, t+h), t+h) - q(\widehat{\boldsymbol{\varphi}}(\widehat{\boldsymbol{x}}, t), t)}{h} \\ &= \frac{\mathrm{d}}{\mathrm{d}t}(\widehat{\boldsymbol{\varphi}}(\widehat{\boldsymbol{x}}, t), t).\end{aligned}$$

Therefore, using (3.21),

$$\frac{D}{Dt}q(\boldsymbol{x}, t) = \frac{\mathrm{d}}{\mathrm{d}t}q(\widehat{\boldsymbol{\varphi}}(\widehat{\boldsymbol{x}}, t), t), \quad \text{with } \boldsymbol{x} = \widehat{\boldsymbol{\varphi}}(\widehat{\boldsymbol{x}}, t). \tag{3.22}$$

The material derivative of q at $(\boldsymbol{x}, t)$ is thus the rate of variation in time of q “experienced” by an observer which moves with the particle $\widehat{\boldsymbol{x}}$ located at time t in the point $\boldsymbol{x}$.

Standard application of the chain rule for the composition of functions in (3.22) yields the following result.

Proposition 3.3. *For any given Eulerian field q, the following identity holds*

$$\frac{Dq}{Dt} = \boldsymbol{u} \cdot \boldsymbol{\nabla} q + \frac{\partial q}{\partial t}. \tag{3.23}$$

It follows that the Lagrangian derivative is made of two contributions. A *transport term* $\boldsymbol{u} \cdot \boldsymbol{\nabla} q$ accounting for variations of q due to changes in the position of the particle and the standard Eulerian time derivative.

The same type of considerations may be extended to the ALE formulation. In particular the *ALE time-derivative* $\dfrac{\partial q}{\partial t}_{|\widetilde{\mathcal{A}}}$ of a field q may be defined in a way analogous to the material derivative. In particular, for each $\boldsymbol{x} \in \omega(t)$ and $t > 0$ we have

$$\frac{\partial q}{\partial t}_{|\widetilde{\mathcal{A}}} = \frac{\mathrm{d}}{\mathrm{d}t} q(\widetilde{\mathcal{A}}(\widetilde{\boldsymbol{x}}, t), t), \quad \text{with } \boldsymbol{x} = \widetilde{\mathcal{A}}(\widetilde{\boldsymbol{x}}, t). \tag{3.24}$$

In other words, we look at the rate of change of q in a point that moves with the computational domain. The importance of this relation emerges in the context of the numerical discretisation. When computing numerically a solution in a moving domain we are usually interested in the variation of quantities collocated at the nodes of a computational mesh, and the latter necessarily follows the evolution of the computational domain. In Fig. 3.10 we show one node at two different times, namely $\boldsymbol{x}_i(t)$ and $\boldsymbol{x}_i(t+\delta t)$, being i the node index. If q_i indicates the quantity of interest at the given node, its value at the two different times, $q_i(t)$ and $q_i(t + \delta t)$, have to be understood as

$$q_i(t) = q(\boldsymbol{x}_i(t), t), \quad q_i(t + \delta t) = q(\boldsymbol{x}_i(t + \delta t), t + \delta t).$$

As a result, their difference is related to the ALE time derivative, since

$$q_i(t + \delta t) - q_i(t) = q(\boldsymbol{x}_i(t + \delta t), t + \delta t) - q(\boldsymbol{x}_i(t), t) = \int_t^{t+\delta t} \frac{\partial q}{\partial t}_{|\widetilde{\mathcal{A}}}(\boldsymbol{x}_i, t)\, \mathrm{d}t.$$

The use of the Eulerian time-derivative would be in this case troublesome, because a fixed point $\boldsymbol{x}$ which at time t is inside a moving computational domain may well have fallen outside at time $t + \delta t$! This remark points out the advantage of using the ALE framework.

We can use the same arguments used to derive (3.23) to obtain the following proposition.

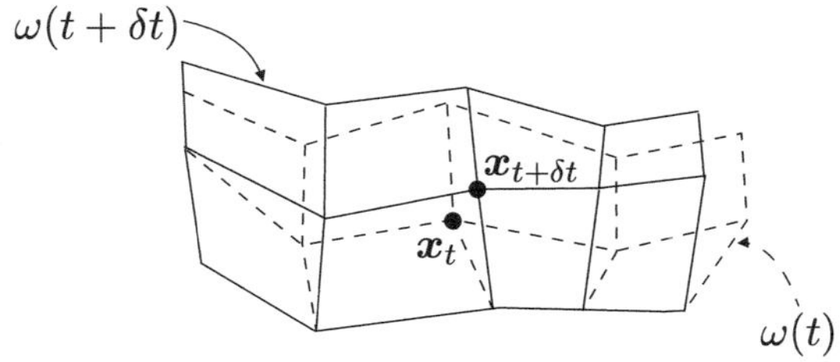

Fig. 3.10. Example of a moving mesh

Proposition 3.4. *The following identity holds*

$$\frac{\partial}{\partial t}_{|\widetilde{\mathcal{A}}} q = \boldsymbol{w} \cdot \boldsymbol{\nabla} q + \frac{\partial q}{\partial t}. \tag{3.25}$$

The transport term $\boldsymbol{w} \cdot \boldsymbol{\nabla} q$ accounts for the variations of q caused by the motion of the computational domain. It is clearly zero if the domain is fixed, while it coincides with the transport term in the material derivative (3.23) if $\boldsymbol{w} = \boldsymbol{u}$.

The Reynolds transport formula

An interesting property of the Jacobian is that its time derivative is linked to the divergence of the velocity field.

Proposition 3.5. *Let J denote the Jacobian (3.3) in the Eulerian frame. We have the relation*

$$\frac{D}{Dt} J = J \operatorname{div} \boldsymbol{u}, \tag{3.26}$$

sometimes called the *Euler expansion formula*. It allows to obtain the following fundamental result.

Proposition 3.6 (Reynolds transport formula). *Let $V(t)$ be a material domain, i.e. $V(t) = \{\boldsymbol{x} : \boldsymbol{x} = \widehat{\boldsymbol{\varphi}}(\widehat{\boldsymbol{x}}, t),\ \widehat{\boldsymbol{x}} \in \widehat{V}\}$, and f a continuously differentiable field. Then,*

$$\frac{\mathrm{d}}{\mathrm{d}t} \int_{V(t)} f \,\mathrm{d}\boldsymbol{x} = \int_{V(t)} \left(\frac{Df}{Dt} + f \operatorname{div} \boldsymbol{u} \right) \mathrm{d}\boldsymbol{x} = \int_{V(t)} \left(\frac{\partial f}{\partial t} + \operatorname{div}(f\boldsymbol{u}) \right) \mathrm{d}\boldsymbol{x}. \tag{3.27}$$

When working with the ALE formulation it might be useful to consider the Reynolds formula acting on the moving computational domain.

Proposition 3.7 (ALE transport formula). *Let $\widetilde{\omega}_0 \subset \widetilde{\omega}$ be a subdomain in the ALE reference configuration and $\omega_0(t) = \{\boldsymbol{x} : \boldsymbol{x} = \widetilde{\mathcal{A}}(\widetilde{\boldsymbol{x}}, t),\ \widetilde{\boldsymbol{x}} \in \widetilde{\omega}\}$ its image by the ALE map. Clearly $\omega_0(t)$ is always contained in the computational domain $\omega(t)$. We have that*

$$\frac{\mathrm{d}}{\mathrm{d}t} \int_{\omega_0(t)} f \,\mathrm{d}\boldsymbol{x} = \int_{\omega_0(t)} \left(\frac{\partial}{\partial t}_{|\widetilde{\mathcal{A}}} f + f \operatorname{div} \boldsymbol{w} \right) \mathrm{d}\boldsymbol{x} = \int_{\omega_0(t)} \left(\frac{\partial f}{\partial t} + \operatorname{div}(f\boldsymbol{w}) \right) \mathrm{d}\boldsymbol{x}\,, \tag{3.28}$$

for any continuously differentiable field f. Here $\boldsymbol{w}$ indicates the domain velocity defined in (3.18).

3.2 The equations of continuum mechanics

The basic equations of continuum mechanics provide some well known conservation principles in the form of differential problems.

3.2.1 Mass conservation

The *mass* of an arbitrary material domain $V(t)$ at time t is given by

$$\int_{V(t)} \rho \, \mathrm{d}\boldsymbol{x}, \tag{3.29}$$

being ρ the density (or volume mass) of the continuum medium. The units of measurement of density are $[\rho] = \mathrm{kg/m^3}$.

In classical mechanics the mass of a body does not change during the motion, a principle known as the *mass conservation*. Therefore,

$$\frac{\mathrm{d}}{\mathrm{d}t} \int_{V(t)} \rho \, \mathrm{d}\boldsymbol{x} = 0, \tag{3.30}$$

holds true for any $V(t)$ at any time. This is an integral statement, we want to express it "point-wise". To is aim, we use the Reynolds transport formula (3.6) to obtain

$$\frac{\mathrm{d}}{\mathrm{d}t} \int_{V(t)} \rho \, \mathrm{d}\boldsymbol{x} = \int_{V(t)} \left(\frac{\partial \rho}{\partial t} + \operatorname{div}(\rho \boldsymbol{u}) \right) \mathrm{d}\boldsymbol{x},$$

by which, due to the arbitrariness of $V(t)$, we get the following

Proposition 3.8 (Continuity equation). *If ρ indicates the density of a continuum medium, mass conservation implies that*

$$\frac{\partial \rho}{\partial t} + \operatorname{div}(\rho \boldsymbol{u}) = 0, \quad \mathit{in} \quad \Omega(t), \tag{3.31}$$

for all $t > 0$, that is

$$\frac{\partial \rho}{\partial t} + \sum_{i=1}^{3} \frac{\partial}{\partial x_i} (\rho u_i) = 0.$$

If the fluid has *constant density* then (3.31) implies the well known *incompressibility equation*

$$\operatorname{div} \boldsymbol{u} = 0 \quad \text{in} \quad \Omega(t), \quad t > 0. \tag{3.32}$$

On the other hand $\operatorname{div} \boldsymbol{u} = 0$ implies $\frac{DJ}{Dt} = 0$, thanks to the Euler expansion formula and the definition of material derivative. In turn, this is equivalent to $\dfrac{\mathrm{d}}{\mathrm{d}t}|V(t)| = 0$ for any material domain $V(t)$. That is, in a constant density fluid the volume of a material domain does not change during motion. In haemodynamics applications, blood is usually considered a constant density fluid. The continuity equation can be rewritten in the Lagrangian frame, we will give more details when we deal with the dynamics of a solid.

3.2.2 Conservation of momentum

The *conservation of (linear) momentum* is in fact the well known Newton's law. The rate of change of the momentum of a material domain $V(t)$, given by $\int_{V(t)} \rho \boldsymbol{u} \, \mathrm{d}\boldsymbol{x}$ equals the resultant of the external forces acting on it, that is

$$\frac{\mathrm{d}}{\mathrm{d}t} \int_{V(t)} \rho \boldsymbol{u} \, \mathrm{d}\boldsymbol{x} = \boldsymbol{F} = \boldsymbol{F}_v + \boldsymbol{F}_s.$$

Referring to Fig. 3.11, the force $\boldsymbol{F}$ is the composition of two terms: a *volume force* $\boldsymbol{F}_v$, and a *surface force* $\boldsymbol{F}_s$. The former acts on each particle of $V(t)$ (like the force of gravity) and is expressed as the integral of the density times a *specific force* (i.e. force per unit of weight) $\boldsymbol{f}$ which has the dimension of an acceleration, $[\boldsymbol{f}] = \mathrm{m/s^2}$.

The latter is instead responsible for the mutual interaction between the material contained in $V(t)$ and the exterior, through the boundary $\partial V(t)$. More precisely, $\boldsymbol{F}_s$ is equal to the surface integral of the so called *Cauchy stress* $\boldsymbol{t}$, which has the dimension of force per unit area, $[\boldsymbol{t}] = \mathrm{N/m^2}$, that is $\boldsymbol{F}_s = \int_{\partial V(t)} \boldsymbol{t} d\gamma$.

It was indeed Cauchy who also postulated that $\boldsymbol{t}$ can be computed by applying to the normal $\boldsymbol{n}$ of $\partial V(t)$ a symmetric second-order tensor[4] $\boldsymbol{\sigma} : \Omega(t) \to \mathbb{R}^{3\times 3}$, called the *Cauchy stress tensor*, i.e.

$$\boldsymbol{t} = \boldsymbol{\sigma n} \quad \text{on } \partial V(t), \quad \text{componentwise } t_i = \sum_{j=1}^{3} \sigma_{ij} n_j. \tag{3.33}$$

The *momentum conservation law* can then be expressed by the following equation,

$$\frac{\mathrm{d}}{\mathrm{d}t} \int_{V(t)} \rho \boldsymbol{u} \, \mathrm{d}\boldsymbol{x} = \int_{V(t)} \rho \boldsymbol{f} \, \mathrm{d}\boldsymbol{x} + \int_{\partial V(t)} \boldsymbol{\sigma n} \, \mathrm{d}\gamma = \int_{V(t)} \rho \boldsymbol{f} \, \mathrm{d}\boldsymbol{x} + \int_{V(t)} \mathbf{div} \boldsymbol{\sigma} d\boldsymbol{x}, \tag{3.34}$$

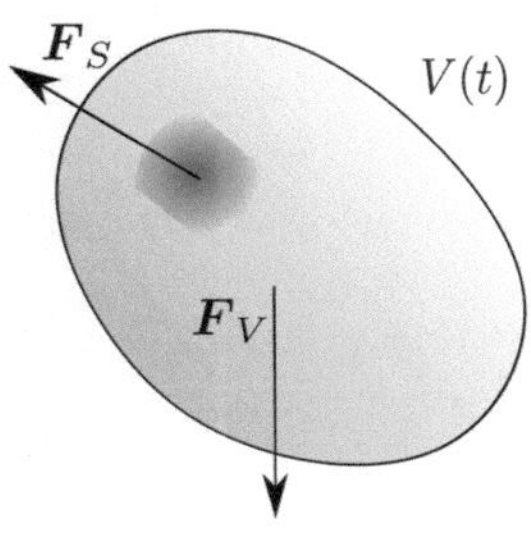

Fig. 3.11. Forces acting on a material volume $V(t)$

[4] The symmetry is in fact an implication of the conservation of angular momentum. We will not pursue this issue here, the interested reader may refer to the given bibliography. Note that the Cauchy postulate implies that the dependence of $\boldsymbol{t}$ on the geometry of $\partial V(t)$ is only through its normal. This holds true in most situations.

valid for all material domains $V(t)$. To obtain the last equality we have used the divergence theorem. Finally, by exploiting the Reynolds transport formula (3.6) we obtain

Proposition 3.9 (Momentum conservation). *Assume that* (3.30) *holds. Then* (3.34) *is equivalent to*

$$\rho\frac{\partial \boldsymbol{u}}{\partial t} + \rho(\boldsymbol{u}\cdot\boldsymbol{\nabla})\boldsymbol{u} - \mathbf{div}\boldsymbol{\sigma} = \rho\boldsymbol{f}, \quad in \quad \Omega(t), \quad t>0. \tag{3.35}$$

Componentwise, we have

$$\rho\frac{\partial u_i}{\partial t} + \rho\sum_{j=1}^{3} u_j\frac{\partial u_i}{\partial x_j} - \rho\sum_{j=1}^{3}\frac{\partial \sigma_{ij}}{\partial x_j} = f_i, \quad i=1,2,3.$$

The equations may be written in conservation form as

$$\frac{\partial(\rho\boldsymbol{u})}{\partial t} + \mathbf{div}\big(\rho\boldsymbol{u}\otimes\boldsymbol{u} - \boldsymbol{\sigma}\big) = \rho\boldsymbol{f}, \quad in \quad \Omega(t), \quad t>0, \tag{3.36}$$

which componentwise reads

$$\frac{\partial(\rho u_i)}{\partial t} + \sum_{j=1}^{3}\frac{\partial}{\partial x_j}\big(\rho u_i u_j - \sigma_{ij}\big) = \rho f_i, \quad i=1,2,3.$$

In contrast, (3.35) is generally said to be in *quasi-linear* form or sometimes in the *gradient form.*

Remark 3.2.1 *The transport term* $(\boldsymbol{u}\cdot\boldsymbol{\nabla})\boldsymbol{u}$ *(or* $\mathbf{div}\boldsymbol{u}\otimes\boldsymbol{u}$ *in the conservation form), is a* non-linear *term. This aspect makes the analysis, as well as the numerical solution more complex. Only in flow at very low Reynolds numbers* (≤ 10) *the non-linear term may be neglected.*

At each point of the boundary of a material domain $V(t)$ the Cauchy stress $\boldsymbol{t}$ can be decomposed into its components normal and tangential to the surface, given respectively by

$$t_n = \boldsymbol{t}\cdot\boldsymbol{n} = (\boldsymbol{\sigma}\boldsymbol{n})\cdot\boldsymbol{n}, \quad \text{and } \boldsymbol{t}_t = \boldsymbol{t} - t_n\boldsymbol{n}. \tag{3.37}$$

The latter is indeed a vector laying on the tangential plane and is called the *shear stress* vector. Componentwise, it may be computed as

$$[t_t]_i = \sum_{j=1}^{3}\sigma_{ij}n_j - \sum_{k,j=1}^{3}\sigma_{kj}n_j n_k n_i, \quad i=1,\dots 3.$$

It is an important parameter in haemodynamics since the endothelium cells are very sensitive to the shear stress at the vessel walls. Let us note that $(\boldsymbol{\sigma}\boldsymbol{n})\cdot\boldsymbol{n}$ is a scalar quantity which may also be written as $\boldsymbol{n}^T\boldsymbol{\sigma}\boldsymbol{n}$. In a Cartesian coordinate system it is readily computed as $\sum_{i,j=1}^{3} \sigma_{ij} n_i n_j$. The equations have been here written in Eulerian formulation.

In the case of a fixed computational domain Ω they can be used directly, just replacing $\Omega(t)$ with Ω (we recall that Ω is a subset of $\Omega(t)$ for all t). In the case of a moving domain it is preferable to use the ALE formulation. To this aim it is sufficient to employ identity (3.25). If instead one wants to use a full Lagrangian formulation it is necessary to transform also the space differential operators, in order to write the equations on $\widehat{\Omega}$ instead of $\Omega(t)$. The Piola formula (3.8) can then become handy. We postpone these issues to Section 3.3.2.

3.3 Fluids and solids

We need now to make precise how the Cauchy stress tensor is linked to the kinematics. It is indeed at this point where the behaviour of solids and fluids diverges.

As solids react to deformations, the Cauchy stress must depend on $\widehat{\boldsymbol{F}}$ (or on quantities which are directly related to $\widehat{\boldsymbol{F}}$). The reference configuration plays here an important role.

Fluids instead can adapt to a deformation, as a fluid can fill freely any arbitrary shape. Yet it takes time to fill it. And oil takes more time than water. It means that fluids react mechanically not to the deformation itself but to its rate. More precisely, the relevant quantity is here the *strain rate tensor* $\boldsymbol{D}$ defined in (2.2) of Chapter 2, and whose dimensions are $[\boldsymbol{D}] = \mathrm{s}^{-1}$. Componentwise, the strain rate reads

$$D_{ij} = \frac{1}{2}\left(\frac{\partial u_i}{\partial x_j} + \frac{\partial u_j}{\partial x_i}\right), \quad i, j = 1, \ldots 3.$$

In a fluid then $\boldsymbol{\sigma}$ is a function of $\boldsymbol{D}$, while it is independent of $\widehat{\boldsymbol{F}}$. A consequence is that the reference configuration is a concept useful for the derivation of the equations, yet it does not play any particular role for a fluid. Intermediate behaviours, like that of visco-elastic fluids, for instance, are possible; they will be addressed in detail in Chapter 6.

The relation between the Cauchy stress tensor $\boldsymbol{\sigma}$ and the kinematic quantities is called *constitutive relation*, or constitutive law, and is a characteristic of the type of material under consideration. To be physically correct, a constitutive relation must obey certain rules, like the principle of material frame indifference [512] which states that the relation should be invariant under a change of frame of reference. More details may be found also in the literature cited at the beginning of the chapter.

3.3.1 The Navier Stokes equations for a constant density fluid

We consider here the case of a constant density incompressible Newtonian fluid. As anticipated in Chapter 2, this is a limitation usually accepted for blood flow in large arteries, and we have discussed its consequences already in Section 3.2.1.

In a *Newtonian incompressible fluid*, the Cauchy stress tensor depends linearly on the strain rate. More precisely, we have

$$\boldsymbol{\sigma} = \boldsymbol{\sigma}(\boldsymbol{u}, P) = -P\boldsymbol{I} + 2\mu\boldsymbol{D}(\boldsymbol{u}) = -P\boldsymbol{I} + \mu(\boldsymbol{\nabla}\boldsymbol{u} + \boldsymbol{\nabla}\boldsymbol{u}^T), \tag{3.38}$$

where P is the *pressure*, $\boldsymbol{I}$ is the identity matrix, μ is the *dynamic viscosity* of the fluid and is a positive quantity.

The term $2\mu\boldsymbol{D}(\boldsymbol{u})$ is the *viscous stress* component of the stress tensor. We have that $[P] = \mathrm{N/m^2}$ and $[\mu] = \mathrm{kg/ms}$.

The viscosity may vary, for example it may depend on the fluid temperature. The assumption of Newtonian fluid, however, implies that μ is *independent of kinematic quantities.* Simple models for non-Newtonian fluids, often used for blood flow simulations, express the viscosity as function of the strain rate, that is $\mu = \mu(\boldsymbol{D}(\boldsymbol{u}))$. The treatment of such cases is considered in Chapter 6 and will not be covered here.

We now recall that, if P is a scalar and $\boldsymbol{\Sigma}$ a tensor field, then the following identity holds,

$$\mathbf{div}(P\boldsymbol{\Sigma}) = \boldsymbol{\nabla}P\boldsymbol{\Sigma} + P\mathbf{div}\boldsymbol{\Sigma},$$

and, therefore,

$$\mathbf{div}(P\boldsymbol{I}) = \boldsymbol{\nabla}P\boldsymbol{I} + P\mathbf{div}\boldsymbol{I} = \boldsymbol{\nabla}P.$$

The momentum equation(3.36) may then be written as

$$\rho\frac{\partial \boldsymbol{u}}{\partial t} + \rho\mathbf{div}(\rho\boldsymbol{u} \otimes \boldsymbol{u}) + \boldsymbol{\nabla}P - \mathbf{div}(\mu\boldsymbol{D}(\boldsymbol{u})) = \rho\boldsymbol{f}. \tag{3.39}$$

Since ρ is constant, it is sometimes convenient to introduce the kinematic viscosity $\nu = \mu/\rho$, with $[\nu] = \mathrm{m^2/s}$, and write

$$\frac{\partial \boldsymbol{u}}{\partial t} + \mathbf{div}(\boldsymbol{u} \otimes \boldsymbol{u}) + \boldsymbol{\nabla}P - \mathbf{div}[\nu(\boldsymbol{\nabla}\boldsymbol{u} + \boldsymbol{\nabla}\boldsymbol{u}^T)] = \boldsymbol{f}, \tag{3.40}$$

where $P = P/\rho$ is a scaled pressure (with $[P] = \mathrm{m^2/s^2}$).

Under the additional hypothesis that ν is constant, the momentum equation may be further elaborated by considering that $\mathbf{div}\boldsymbol{\nabla}\boldsymbol{u} = \boldsymbol{\Delta u}$ and $\mathbf{div}\boldsymbol{\nabla}\boldsymbol{u}^T = \boldsymbol{\nabla}(\mathrm{div}\boldsymbol{u}) = \boldsymbol{0}$, producing the alternative formulation

$$\frac{\partial \boldsymbol{u}}{\partial t} + \mathbf{div}(\boldsymbol{u} \otimes \boldsymbol{u}) + \boldsymbol{\nabla}P - \nu\boldsymbol{\Delta u} = \boldsymbol{f}. \tag{3.41}$$

However, for reasons that will appear clear in Chapter9, and have to do with the different natural boundary conditions associated with the two formulations, for fluid-structure interaction problems it is more convenient to use the momentum equation in the form (3.39), even when the viscosity is constant.

The Navier-Stokes equations in the Eulerian frame

The set of differential equations formed by the continuity equation and the momentum equation in the form derived in the previous section provides the *Navier-Stokes equations* for a constant density fluid.

They have been written in the Eulerian frame and if the computational domain Ω is time-independent they can be recast as the following system of equations for the unknowns velocity $\boldsymbol{u}$ and pressure P,

$$\begin{aligned}&\rho\frac{\partial \boldsymbol{u}}{\partial t} + \rho(\boldsymbol{u}\cdot\boldsymbol{\nabla})\boldsymbol{u} + \boldsymbol{\nabla}P - 2\,\mathbf{div}(\mu\boldsymbol{D}(\boldsymbol{u})) = \rho\boldsymbol{f},\\ &\operatorname{div}\boldsymbol{u} = 0,\end{aligned} \tag{3.42}$$

for any $t > 0$ and in Ω. Alternatively, one may use the conservative form (3.39).

Furthermore, we need to prescribe the initial status of the fluid velocity, for instance

$$\boldsymbol{u}(t = t_0, \boldsymbol{x}) = \boldsymbol{u}_0(\boldsymbol{x}) \qquad \boldsymbol{x} \in \Omega. \tag{3.43}$$

There is *no initial condition* for the pressure.

We have already introduced the issue of boundary conditions in Chapter 2. We here recall the more classical boundary conditions which are mathematically compatible with the Navier Stokes equations, namely

1. *Applied stresses* (or *Neumann* boundary condition)

   $$\boldsymbol{\sigma}\cdot\boldsymbol{n} = -P\boldsymbol{n} + 2\mu\boldsymbol{D}(\boldsymbol{u})\cdot\boldsymbol{n} = \boldsymbol{h} \quad \text{on } \Gamma_N \subset \partial\Omega, \tag{3.44}$$

   where Γ_N is a measurable subset (possibly empty) of the whole boundary $\partial\Omega$ and $\boldsymbol{h} = \boldsymbol{h}(\boldsymbol{x}, t)$ a given vector defined on Γ_N and (possibly) function of time. This is a typical condition at distal boundaries, where often $\boldsymbol{h} = P_{ext}\boldsymbol{n}$, being $= P_{ext}$ a prescribed "external" pressure.
2. *Prescribed velocity* (or *Dirichlet* boundary condition).

   $$\boldsymbol{u} = \boldsymbol{g} \qquad \text{on } \Gamma_D,$$

   where $\boldsymbol{g} : \Gamma_D \times \mathbb{R}^+ \to \mathbb{R}^3$ is a given function. Since $\operatorname{div}\boldsymbol{u} = 0$ in Ω, it must be noted that if $\Gamma_D = \partial\Omega$ then $\boldsymbol{g}$ must satisfy

   $$\int_{\partial\Omega} \boldsymbol{g}\cdot\boldsymbol{n} = 0, \tag{3.45}$$

   at any time. This condition is applied at the vessel wall interface and usually also at the proximal boundaries.

Clearly for a proper boundary condition specification we must have $\Gamma_N \cup \Gamma_D = \partial\Omega$. Other boundary conditions are possible, they will be discussed whenever appropriate.

The conditions to apply are normally inspired by physical considerations. For instance, for a viscous fluid ($\mu > 0$) like the one we are considering here, it is appropriate to impose the Dirichlet condition $\boldsymbol{u} = \frac{\partial}{\partial t}\boldsymbol{\eta}$ at a solid boundary, being η the displacement of the boundary. In the case of a fixed wall the condition is homogeneous and is also called *no-slip* condition. When dealing with an artificial boundary the choice of appropriate conditions in the context of haemodynamic problems is more delicate and should in any case guarantee the well-posedness of the resulting differential problem. In particular, the imposition of a Neumann condition in a distal section may cause instabilities in the presence of flow reversal, since this condition is most appropriate in outflow sections.

As mentioned, at distal sections (like Γ^{out} in Fig. 2.1) one often imposes a constant (possibly homogeneous) Neumann condition. Yet, this would indeed simulate a discharge into a reservoir at constant pressure. A rather unphysical situation for the case of a human vessel as it neglects the presence of the remaining part of the circulatory system completely. In Chapter 11 we will address this problem in more depth presenting some possible solutions.

After having computed the solution using the numerical scheme of choice, we may wish to estimate the wall shear stresses using the second relation in (3.37). In a Newtonian fluid the Cauchy stress at each point of the surface of interest Γ may be computed from the flow field solution as

$$\boldsymbol{t} = -P\boldsymbol{n} + \mu\frac{\partial \boldsymbol{u}}{\partial n} + \mu\boldsymbol{\nabla}\boldsymbol{u}^T\boldsymbol{n}. \tag{3.46}$$

Here, $\frac{\partial \boldsymbol{u}}{\partial n} = \boldsymbol{\nabla}\boldsymbol{u}\,\boldsymbol{n}$ is the normal derivative of $\boldsymbol{u}$. If the surface is flat then $\boldsymbol{n}$ is constant on Γ and thus $\boldsymbol{\nabla}\boldsymbol{u}^T\boldsymbol{n} = \boldsymbol{\nabla}u_n$, being $u_n = \boldsymbol{u}\cdot\boldsymbol{n}$ the component of the velocity normal to the surface. If in addition Γ is a fixed wall surface, then $\boldsymbol{u} = \boldsymbol{0}$ on Γ and thus $\boldsymbol{\nabla}\boldsymbol{u}^T\boldsymbol{n} = \boldsymbol{0}$. We will see in Chapter 9 how it is possible to recover this quantity when adopting finite elements for the numerical solution. The shear stress acting on the wall is readily obtained from $\boldsymbol{t}$ by using relation (3.37). Note that the shear stress does not depend on the pressure term, since it cancels out.

The Navier-Stokes equations in the ALE frame

When dealing with a moving computational domain $\omega(t)$ it is preferable to use the Navier-Stokes equations in the ALE framework introduced in Section 3.1.2. By using (3.25) on the momentum equation we derive that

$$\begin{aligned} &\rho\frac{\partial \boldsymbol{u}}{\partial t}_{|\widetilde{\mathcal{A}}} + \rho[(\boldsymbol{u}-\boldsymbol{w})\cdot\boldsymbol{\nabla}]\boldsymbol{u} + \boldsymbol{\nabla}P - 2\mathbf{div}(\mu\boldsymbol{D}(\boldsymbol{u})) = \rho\boldsymbol{f}, \\ &\operatorname{div}\boldsymbol{u} = 0, \end{aligned} \tag{3.47}$$

in $\omega(t)$. We may note that the introduction of the ALE time-derivative induces a correction in the transport term by subtracting to the "transport velocity" $\boldsymbol{u}$ the domain velocity $\boldsymbol{w}$ given by (3.18).

A conservation form may be devised as well. Recalling (3.19) we have

$$J_{\widetilde{\mathcal{A}}} \frac{\partial \boldsymbol{u}}{\partial t}_{|\widetilde{\mathcal{A}}} = \frac{\partial}{\partial t}_{|\widetilde{\mathcal{A}}} (J_{\widetilde{\mathcal{A}}} \boldsymbol{u}) - J_{\widetilde{\mathcal{A}}} \boldsymbol{u} \operatorname{div} \boldsymbol{w},$$

by which, with simple manipulations, we get the following conservation form for the Navier-Stokes equations in the ALE frame,

$$\begin{aligned} & J_{\widetilde{\mathcal{A}}}^{-1} \rho \frac{\partial}{\partial t}_{|\widetilde{\mathcal{A}}} (J_{\widetilde{\mathcal{A}}} \boldsymbol{u}) + \mathbf{div}\big(\rho \boldsymbol{u} \otimes (\boldsymbol{u} - \boldsymbol{w})\big) + \boldsymbol{\nabla} P - 2\mathbf{div}(\mu \boldsymbol{D}(\boldsymbol{u})) = \rho \boldsymbol{f}, \\ & \operatorname{div} \boldsymbol{u} = 0. \end{aligned} \tag{3.48}$$

3.3.2 The equations for a solid

We describe now the motion of the structure in terms of its displacement field $\widehat{\boldsymbol{\eta}}$ with respect to a given material reference configuration $\widehat{\Omega}$. Mapping back the continuity equation in integral form (3.30) to the reference domain we obtain

$$0 = \frac{\mathrm{d}}{\mathrm{d}t} \int_{\widehat{V}} \widehat{J} \widehat{\rho} d\widehat{\boldsymbol{x}} = \int_{\widehat{V}} \frac{\partial (\widehat{J} \widehat{\rho})}{\partial t} d\widehat{\boldsymbol{x}}.$$

From the arbitrariness of $\widehat{V}$ we derive the continuity equation in the Lagrangian frame, namely

$$\frac{\partial}{\partial t} \widehat{\rho}_0 = 0, \quad \text{in } \widehat{\Omega}, \quad t > 0, \tag{3.49}$$

where we have set

$$\widehat{\rho}_0 = \widehat{J} \widehat{\rho}. \tag{3.50}$$

Note that for a constant density material (3.49) together with the definition of reference domain, implies that $\widehat{J} = 1$ for all $t \geq 0$.

The momentum equation in integral form (3.34) can also be rewritten in the Lagrangian frame by mapping all integrals back on the reference domain and using (3.12) to obtain

$$\frac{\mathrm{d}}{\mathrm{d}t} \int_{\widehat{V}} \widehat{J} \widehat{\rho} \frac{\partial \widehat{\boldsymbol{\eta}}}{\partial t} \, \mathrm{d}\widehat{\boldsymbol{x}} - \int_{\widehat{V}} \widehat{J} \widehat{\mathbf{div} \boldsymbol{\sigma}} \, \mathrm{d}\widehat{\boldsymbol{x}} = \int_{\widehat{V}} \widehat{J} \widehat{\rho} \widehat{\boldsymbol{f}} \, \mathrm{d}\widehat{\boldsymbol{x}}.$$

Yet, (3.50) and (3.49) give

$$\frac{\mathrm{d}}{\mathrm{d}t} \int_{\widehat{V}} \widehat{J} \widehat{\rho} \frac{\partial \widehat{\boldsymbol{\eta}}}{\partial t} \, \mathrm{d}\widehat{\boldsymbol{x}} = \int_{\widehat{V}} \widehat{\rho}_0 \frac{\partial^2 \widehat{\boldsymbol{\eta}}}{\partial t^2} \, \mathrm{d}\widehat{\boldsymbol{x}}.$$

Thus, by considering the arbitrariness of $\widehat{V}$ we obtain the following differential equation

$$\widehat{\rho}_0 \frac{\partial^2 \widehat{\boldsymbol{\eta}}}{\partial t^2} - \widehat{J} \widehat{\mathbf{div} \boldsymbol{\sigma}} = \widehat{\rho}_0 \widehat{\boldsymbol{f}}, \quad \text{in } \widehat{\Omega}, \, t > 0.$$

This form is still not satisfactory as $\widehat{\mathbf{div}\boldsymbol{\sigma}}$ is in a "mixed form" because the divergence is still taken with respect to $\boldsymbol{x}$. We now use the Piola transform and Proposition 3.2 to get

$$\widehat{\rho}_0 \frac{\partial^2 \widehat{\boldsymbol{\eta}}}{\partial t^2} - \mathbf{div}_{\widehat{\boldsymbol{x}}} \widehat{\boldsymbol{\Pi}} = \widehat{\rho}_0 \widehat{\boldsymbol{f}}, \quad \text{in } \widehat{\Omega}, \quad t > 0. \tag{3.51}$$

The tensor $\widehat{\boldsymbol{\Pi}} = \mathcal{P}_{\widehat{\varphi}}(\boldsymbol{\sigma}) = \widehat{J}\widehat{\boldsymbol{\sigma}}\widehat{\boldsymbol{F}}^{-T}$ is called the *first Piola-Kirchhoff tensor* and (3.51) is the *momentum equation* written in the Lagrangian frame. It is also known as the equation of *elastodynamics.*

Unlike the Cauchy stress tensor $\boldsymbol{\sigma}$, the first Piola-Kirchhoff tensor $\widehat{\boldsymbol{\Pi}}$ is non-symmetric. Since constitutive laws are often better expressed in terms of symmetric stress tensors, it is natural to introduce the *second Piola-Kirchhoff tensor* $\widehat{\boldsymbol{\Sigma}}$

$$\widehat{\boldsymbol{\Sigma}} = \widehat{\boldsymbol{F}}^{-1}\widehat{\boldsymbol{\Pi}} = \widehat{J}\widehat{\boldsymbol{F}}^{-1}\widehat{\boldsymbol{\sigma}}\widehat{\boldsymbol{F}}^{-T} \tag{3.52}$$

which is symmetric.

For an *elastic material* the stress is a function of the deformation (and possibly of thermodynamic variables such the temperature) but is independent on the deformation history (and thus on time). The material characteristics may still vary in space. In an *homogeneous* material the mechanical properties do not vary with $\boldsymbol{x}$. As a consequence the strain energy function depends only on the deformation. A material is mechanically *isotropic* if its response to deformation is the same in all directions.

The constitutive equation is usually written in terms of the *Green-Lagrange strain tensor*, defined as

$$\widehat{\boldsymbol{E}} = \frac{1}{2}\left(\widehat{\boldsymbol{F}}^T\widehat{\boldsymbol{F}} - \boldsymbol{I}\right), \tag{3.53}$$

where $\boldsymbol{I}$ is the identity tensor. Componentwise,

$$\widehat{E}_{ij} = \frac{1}{2}\left(\sum_{l=1}^{3} \widehat{F}_{li}\widehat{F}_{lj} - \delta_{ij}\right),$$

being δ_{ij} the Kronecker's symbol. Applying (3.2) and (3.1) we have also

$$\widehat{\boldsymbol{E}} = \frac{1}{2}\left(\boldsymbol{\nabla}_{\widehat{\boldsymbol{x}}}\widehat{\boldsymbol{\eta}} + \boldsymbol{\nabla}_{\widehat{\boldsymbol{x}}}^T\widehat{\boldsymbol{\eta}}\right) + \frac{1}{2}\boldsymbol{\nabla}_{\widehat{\boldsymbol{x}}}^T\widehat{\boldsymbol{\eta}}\boldsymbol{\nabla}_{\widehat{\boldsymbol{x}}}\widehat{\boldsymbol{\eta}}, \tag{3.54}$$

which componentwise reads $\widehat{E}_{ij} = \frac{1}{2}\left(\frac{\partial \widehat{\eta}_i}{\partial \widehat{x}_j} + \frac{\partial \widehat{\eta}_j}{\partial \widehat{x}_i}\right) + \sum_{l=1}^3 \frac{\partial \widehat{\eta}_l}{\partial \widehat{x}_i}\frac{\partial \widehat{\eta}_l}{\partial \widehat{x}_j}$.

The tensor $\widehat{\boldsymbol{E}}$ is not affected by a superimposed rigid body motion, and in particular by rigid rotations. Indeed, from a geometric point of view $\widehat{\boldsymbol{E}}$ is directly related to the difference of the squared length of a elemental vector $d\widehat{\boldsymbol{x}}$ and its image: by recalling (3.4) we have that

$$\frac{1}{2}(||d\boldsymbol{x}||^2 - ||d\widehat{\boldsymbol{x}}||^2) = d\widehat{\boldsymbol{x}}^T\widehat{\boldsymbol{E}}d\widehat{\boldsymbol{x}}.$$

Many constitutive laws can be devised for a solid. For a *hyperelastic material* we first define a *density of elastic energy* $W : \mathbb{R}^{3\times 3} \longrightarrow \mathbb{R}^+$, and then set

$$\widehat{\boldsymbol{\Sigma}}(\widehat{\boldsymbol{E}}) = \frac{\partial W}{\partial \widehat{\boldsymbol{E}}}(\widehat{\boldsymbol{E}}). \tag{3.55}$$

Componentwise, $\widehat{\Sigma}_{ij} = \frac{\partial W}{\partial \widehat{E}_{ij}}, \quad i,j = 1,2,3.$

A simple example of energy density for a *homogeneous isotropic material* whose reference configuration is the natural state[5] is the Saint-Venant Kirchhoff model, where

$$W(\widehat{\boldsymbol{E}}) = \frac{L_1}{2}(\mathrm{tr}\,\widehat{\boldsymbol{E}})^2 + L_2\,\mathrm{tr}\,\widehat{\boldsymbol{E}}^2, \tag{3.56}$$

which componentwise reads (by exploiting the symmetry of $\widehat{\boldsymbol{E}}$)

$$W = \frac{L_1}{2}\left(\sum_{i=1}^{3} \widehat{E}_{ii}\right)^2 + L_2 \sum_{i=1}^{3}\sum_{j=1}^{3} \widehat{E}_{ij}^2.$$

Here, L_1 and L_2 denote the first and second *Lamé coefficients*[6]. Correspondingly, we have

$$\widehat{\boldsymbol{\Sigma}}(\widehat{\boldsymbol{E}}) = L_1(\mathrm{tr}\,\widehat{\boldsymbol{E}})\boldsymbol{I} + 2L_2\widehat{\boldsymbol{E}}. \tag{3.57}$$

This relation is often written componentwise in terms of a fourth order symmetric tensor, called the elasticity tensor, $\boldsymbol{H} = (H_{ijkl})$, defined by

$$H_{ijkl} = L_1\delta_{ij}\delta_{kl} + L_2\left(\delta_{ik}\delta_{jl} + \delta_{il}\delta_{jk}\right), \tag{3.58}$$

so that

$$\widehat{\Sigma}_{ij} = \sum_{1\le i,j\le 3} H_{ijkl}E_{kl}, \tag{3.59}$$

which is commonly known as (generalised) *Hook's law*. In tensorial form it reads $\widehat{\boldsymbol{\Sigma}} = \mathbf{H} : \widehat{\boldsymbol{E}}$.

Note the in fact the only components of $\boldsymbol{H}$ which are different from zero are $H_{1111} = H_{2222} = H_{3333} = L_1 + 2L_2$ and $H_{stst} = H_{stts} = L_2$, for $s \neq t$.

More complex constitutive relations for hyperelastic materials may be found in [221], and in particular models specially tailored for biological tissues and blood vessels are reported in [178] and [222].

Often an elastic material is characterised by its *Young modulus* E and *Poisson coefficient* ξ. Indeed, these quantities are inferred from experiments more directly than the Lamé coefficients. We have the following relations

$$E = L_2\frac{3L_1 + 2L_2}{L_1 + L_2}, \qquad \xi = \frac{1}{2}\frac{L_1}{L_1 + L_2}, \tag{3.60}$$

---

[5] The natural state is a configuration where the Cauchy stress tensor is zero everywhere.

[6] In the literature L_1 and L_2 are usually denoted by λ and μ, respectively. We have used different symbols to avoid repetitions.

and

$$L_1 = \frac{E\xi}{(1-2\xi)(1+\xi)}, \qquad L_2 = \frac{E}{2(1+\xi)}. \tag{3.61}$$

Specific models for the arterial wall

A simple Saint-Venant Kirchhoff elasticity model can be adopted only when one is not really interested in the details of the stress inside the arterial wall but only on its effect of the Haemodynamics. The development of reduced models detailed in Section 3.4 does indeed make use of this type of modelling.

However, in reality the internal structure of the wall of an arterial vessel is rather complex, an account has been given in Chapter 1. The presence of different layers and of collagen fibres which activate when the strain has reached a critical level makes a homogeneous isotropic models clearly inadequate for a detailed analysis of stresses inside the arterial wall.

Furthermore, it is often assumed that biological tissues, and thus the wall of a blood vessel, are incompressible. The case of an incompressible material is rather special. Indeed the Saint-Venant Kirchhoff model in its original formulation fails, since $\xi = 1/2$ in an incompressible material. The constitutive relation has to take into account the incompressibility constraints, a general account is given in [243, 558]. We here only mention that it is convenient to factor the deformation gradient $\widehat{\boldsymbol{F}}$ into his spherical and distortional part,

$$\widehat{\boldsymbol{F}} = \left(\widehat{J}^{1/3}\boldsymbol{I}\right)\widehat{\boldsymbol{F}}^*,$$

and use this decomposition to define a modified strain measure $\widehat{\boldsymbol{E}}^*$ as

$$\widehat{\boldsymbol{E}}^* = \frac{1}{2}(\widehat{\boldsymbol{F}}^{*T}\widehat{\boldsymbol{F}}^* - \boldsymbol{I}) = \frac{1}{2}(\widehat{J}^{-2/3}\widehat{\boldsymbol{F}}^T\widehat{\boldsymbol{F}} - \boldsymbol{I}).$$

When the motion is incompressible $\widehat{J} = 1$ during the whole motion and indeed in this case $\widehat{\boldsymbol{F}} = \widehat{\boldsymbol{F}}^T$ and $\widehat{\boldsymbol{E}} = \widehat{\boldsymbol{E}}^*$. In general,

$$\widehat{\boldsymbol{E}}^* = \widehat{J}^{-2/3}\widehat{\boldsymbol{E}} + \frac{1}{2}(\widehat{J}^{-2/3} - 1)\boldsymbol{I},$$

and thus

$$\frac{\partial \widehat{\boldsymbol{E}}^*}{\partial \widehat{\boldsymbol{E}}} = \widehat{J}^{-2/3}\left[\mathcal{I} - \frac{1}{3}\widehat{\boldsymbol{F}}^T\widehat{\boldsymbol{F}} \otimes \left(\widehat{\boldsymbol{F}}^T\widehat{\boldsymbol{F}}\right)^{-1}\right].$$

where $\mathcal{I}$ is the fourth order identity tensor with components $I_{ijkl} = (\delta_{ik}\delta_{jl} + \delta_{il}\delta_{jk})/2$.

The elastic energy density may then be expressed as the sum of two terms,

$$W(\widehat{\boldsymbol{E}}) = U(\widehat{J}) + W^*(\widehat{\boldsymbol{E}}^*),$$

where the dependence of $\widehat{\boldsymbol{E}}^*$ and $\widehat{J}$ on $\widehat{\boldsymbol{E}}$ is understood. The first term represent the volumetric elastic energy, which is constant in an incompressible material, the second term is associated to the volume preserving deformations. Correspondingly, the second Piola Kirchhoff stress tensor becomes

$$\widehat{\boldsymbol{\Sigma}} = \frac{\partial U}{\partial \widehat{\boldsymbol{E}}} + \frac{\partial W^*}{\partial \widehat{\boldsymbol{E}}} = P\widehat{J}(\widehat{\boldsymbol{F}}^T\widehat{\boldsymbol{F}})^{-1} + \widehat{\boldsymbol{\Sigma}}^*, \tag{3.62}$$

and the Cauchy stress tensor

$$\boldsymbol{\sigma} = P\boldsymbol{I} + \boldsymbol{\sigma}^*,$$

P being the *pressure*, while $\boldsymbol{\sigma}^*$ and $\widehat{\boldsymbol{\Sigma}}^*$ are related by the inverse Piola transformation.

Pressure in an incompressible material plays the role of the Lagrange multiplier that enforces the incompressibility constraint $\widehat{J} = 1$. It is a role identical to that played by the fluid pressure in an incompressible flow. As for the distortional energy density W^*, several expressions specifically targeted to biological tissues are found in [23] and a critical review is available in [223].

The actual model to be adopted in practise may depend on the type of investigation to be carried out. For instance, in physiological situations the collagen fibres are not activated and the arterial wall behaves largely like an isotropic hyperelastic material. A possible constitutive law in this case can be derived from the model presented in [114], that is

$$W^* = \frac{a}{b}\left[e^{\frac{b}{2}(I_1-3)} - 1\right]. \tag{3.63}$$

Here, a and b are two parameters to be fitted by experiments and I_1 indicates the first invariant of the right Cauchy-Green tensor, which in terms of $\widehat{\boldsymbol{E}}^*$ is defined as $I_1 = 2\,\mathrm{tr}(\widehat{\boldsymbol{E}}^*) + 3$.

However, if we are interested to study situations where the strains go beyond the physiological range, like during balloon angioplasty, the hypothesis of isotropic behaviour is not realistic. The collagen fibres in this case enter into action, after a critical strain level. Since they are aligned principally along two directions, they introduce a markedly anisotropy. In [223] a model was proposed to account for this fact. The fibre directions are indicated by $\boldsymbol{a}_1$ and $\boldsymbol{a}_2$, respectively, and are in general a function of $\widehat{\boldsymbol{x}}$. Correspondingly we may define the tensors $\boldsymbol{A}_1 = \boldsymbol{a}_1 \otimes \boldsymbol{a}_1$ and $\boldsymbol{A}_2 = \boldsymbol{a}_2 \otimes \boldsymbol{a}_2$. The energy density is expressed as function of the modified right Cauchy green tensor $\boldsymbol{C}^*$, which is related to $\widehat{\boldsymbol{E}}^*$ by $\boldsymbol{C}^* = 2\widehat{\boldsymbol{E}}^* + \boldsymbol{I}$. More precisely, the important variables are the first invariant $I_1 = \mathrm{tr}\,\boldsymbol{C}^*$, which we have already introduced, and $I_{a_1} = \boldsymbol{C}^* : \boldsymbol{A}_1$ and $I_{a_2} = \boldsymbol{C}^* : \boldsymbol{A}_2$. The distortional energy density is then expressed as $W^* = W^*_{iso} + W^*_{aniso}$, where

$$W^*_{iso} = W^*_{iso}(I_1) = \frac{c}{2}(I_1 - 3),$$

corresponds to a so-called neo-Hookean elestic model, and $c > 0$ is a suitable parameter. While

$$W^*_{aniso} = W^*_{aniso}(I_{a_1}, I_{a_2}) = \frac{k_1}{2k_2}\left[e^{k_2(I_{a_1}-1)^2} + e^{k_2(I_{a_2}-1)^2}\right].$$

Here, $k_1 > 0$ is a stress-like material parameter and $k_2 > 0$ a dimensionless parameter, both to be fitted by experiments. The dependance of W^*_{aniso} More details may be found in the cited reference.

We anticipate that another important characteristics of arterial walls is that they are normally in a pre-stressed state. We postpone the discussion on this issue to Section 3.3.2.

Finally, viscoelastic behaviour may be relevant in muscular arteries (i.e. arterioles) [180, 224]. Moreover, when undergoing major strains plasticity effects should be taken into account as well [183]. These types of modelling go beyond the scope of this book and will not be investigated any further.

Boundary conditions

Also in this case we have a second order system of partial differential equations and we need to provide proper boundary conditions on $\partial\widehat{\Omega}$. The two main conditions are again:

- *Dirichlet conditions.* The displacements are imposed on part of the boundary
$$\widehat{\boldsymbol{\eta}} = \widehat{\boldsymbol{g}}, \qquad \text{on } \widehat{\Gamma}_D,$$
being $\widehat{\boldsymbol{g}}$ a given function;
- *Neumann conditions.* Surface stresses are applied on a portion of the boundary. Notice that often the given data are on the current configuration, so they have to be recast to $\partial\widehat{\Omega}$. For instance, we might want to enforce
$$\boldsymbol{\sigma n} = \boldsymbol{h}, \qquad \text{on} \quad \Gamma_N(t) \subset \partial\Omega(t).$$
Using relations (3.9) and (3.11) we have
$$\widehat{\boldsymbol{\Pi}}_{\boldsymbol{\sigma}}\widehat{\boldsymbol{n}} = \widehat{J}||\widehat{\boldsymbol{F}}^{-T}\widehat{\boldsymbol{n}}||\widehat{\boldsymbol{h}} \quad \text{on } \widehat{\Gamma}_N, \tag{3.64}$$
which is the relation which is needed in practise to enforce the Neumann condition in the Lagrange frame.

Other conditions may be of interest for cardiovascular applications, for instance non-reflecting boundary conditions. They are meant to minimise the spurious reflections appearing when improper boundary conditions are imposed on a computational domain which is in fact representing a small portion of a larger body. For instance, an artery separated from the rest of the circulatory system. This issue is rather complex and its treatment goes beyond the scope of this chapter. Some considerations on special boundary conditions for cardiovascular problems may be found in Chapter 11 in the context of multiscale modelling.

The linear elasticity from a pre-stressed configuration

The equations written so far are rather general. Yet, even if we employ a linear relation between $\widehat{\boldsymbol{\Sigma}}$ and $\widehat{\boldsymbol{E}}$, like for instance (3.57), they give rise to a non-linear problem in the displacement $\widehat{\boldsymbol{\eta}}$, because of the presence of the deformation gradient in the relation between $\widehat{\boldsymbol{\Sigma}}$ and $\widehat{\boldsymbol{\Pi}}$, as well as the quadratic term in (3.54).

However, when both strains and displacements are small we may derive a simpler, linear form of the equation. In haemodynamics, the hypothesis of small displacements can be accepted in small arteries. Yet, it is sometimes used also in larger vessels when deriving reduced models of structure dynamics, since it is assumed that this approximation is of the same importance as the others introduced by the model reduction process.

Yet, things are complicated by the fact that usually displacements may be assumed to be small with respect to a configuration which is not a natural one. Indeed, it has been observed that a vessel when extracted from its natural site tends to shrink, and it opens up when cut longitudinally [177, 178]. This is an indication that the Cauchy stresses in an *in vivo* artery are not zero even when the artery is "at rest". The presence of a circumferential pre-stress may help in better equilibrating the stress state inside the arterial wall when the vessel is subject to the intramural pressure. Therefore, to be correct the linearisation procedure has to be carried out with respect to a pre-stressed reference state.

Since hyperelastic constitutive equations are written assuming instead a natural (i.e. zero stress) reference state, the problem is not straightforward. We proceed then by assuming the existence of a natural configuration $\widehat{\Omega}_0$ from which the actual reference configuration $\widehat{\Omega}$ is displaced by $\widehat{\boldsymbol{\eta}}_0 = \widehat{\boldsymbol{\eta}}_0(\widehat{\boldsymbol{x}}_0)$, being $\widehat{\boldsymbol{x}}_0 \in \widehat{\Omega}_0$. The current configuration $\Omega(t)$ is then obtained as usual from $\widehat{\Omega}$ by applying the displacement $\widehat{\boldsymbol{\eta}}$, which is assumed small and to have small gradients $\partial\widehat{\boldsymbol{\eta}}/\partial\widehat{\boldsymbol{x}}$. The total displacement from the natural configuration is $\widehat{\boldsymbol{\eta}}_t = \widehat{\boldsymbol{\eta}}_0 + \widehat{\boldsymbol{\eta}}$, and in general it is not small (see Fig. 3.12). For the sake of notation, here and in the following we will use the hat ($\widehat{\ }$) sign to indicate quantities referred either to the natural or the pre-stressed configuration, the ambiguity being resolved by the context.

The motion of $\Omega(t)$ is the superposition of a time-independent deformation from $\widehat{\Omega}_0$ to $\widehat{\Omega}$ and the motion from $\widehat{\Omega}$ to $\Omega(t)$. That is, a point $\boldsymbol{x}$ in the current configuration is associated to a point $\widehat{\boldsymbol{x}}$ in the natural configuration by $\boldsymbol{x} = \widehat{\boldsymbol{x}} + \widehat{\boldsymbol{\eta}}_0 + \widehat{\boldsymbol{\eta}} = \widehat{\boldsymbol{x}} + \widehat{\boldsymbol{\eta}}_t$. Finally, the Cauchy stress $\boldsymbol{\sigma}^0$ in the reference domain is self-equilibrating, i.e.

$$\mathbf{div}_{\widehat{\boldsymbol{x}}}\boldsymbol{\sigma}^0 = \mathbf{0}, \quad \text{in } \widehat{\Omega}. \tag{3.65}$$

To get the linearised equations we will write the elastodynamics equations with respect to $\widehat{\Omega}_0$ and then apply a linearisation procedure around the reference configuration $\widehat{\Omega}$. We define the deformation gradient with respect to the natural state as $\widehat{\boldsymbol{F}}_0(\boldsymbol{\eta}) = \boldsymbol{I} + \boldsymbol{\nabla}_{\widehat{\boldsymbol{x}}_0}\boldsymbol{\eta}$, being $\boldsymbol{\nabla}_{\widehat{\boldsymbol{x}}_0}\boldsymbol{\eta} = \dfrac{\partial \boldsymbol{\eta}}{\partial \widehat{\boldsymbol{x}}_0}$, and $\widehat{\boldsymbol{F}}^0 = \widehat{\boldsymbol{F}}_0(\widehat{\boldsymbol{\eta}}_0)$ its value at the reference configuration. Accordingly, we have

$$\widehat{\boldsymbol{E}}_0(\boldsymbol{\eta}) = \frac{1}{2}(\widehat{\boldsymbol{F}}_0^T(\boldsymbol{\eta})\widehat{\boldsymbol{F}}_0(\boldsymbol{\eta}) - \boldsymbol{I}) = \frac{1}{2}(\boldsymbol{\nabla}_{\widehat{\boldsymbol{x}}_0}\boldsymbol{\eta} + \boldsymbol{\nabla}^T_{\widehat{\boldsymbol{x}}_0}\boldsymbol{\eta}) + \frac{1}{2}\boldsymbol{\nabla}^T_{\widehat{\boldsymbol{x}}_0}\boldsymbol{\eta}\boldsymbol{\nabla}_{\widehat{\boldsymbol{x}}_0}\boldsymbol{\eta}$$

and $\widehat{\boldsymbol{E}}^0 = \widehat{\boldsymbol{E}}_0(\widehat{\boldsymbol{\eta}}_0)$. We will consider a hyperelastic constitutive law given by

$$\widehat{\boldsymbol{\Sigma}}_0(\boldsymbol{\eta}_t) = \frac{\partial W}{\partial \widehat{\boldsymbol{E}}_0}(\widehat{\boldsymbol{E}}_0(\boldsymbol{\eta}_t)), \tag{3.66}$$

being W a suitable energy function. The equations of elastodynamics written with respect to the natural configuration then read

$$\widehat{\rho}^0\frac{\partial^2\widehat{\boldsymbol{\eta}}_t}{\partial t^2} - \mathbf{div}_{\widehat{\boldsymbol{x}}_0}\widehat{\boldsymbol{F}}_0(\widehat{\boldsymbol{\eta}}_t)\widehat{\boldsymbol{\Sigma}}_0(\widehat{\boldsymbol{\eta}}_t) = \widehat{\rho}^0\widehat{\boldsymbol{f}}, \quad \text{in } \widehat{\Omega}_0, \quad t > 0, \tag{3.67}$$

where $\widehat{\rho}^0$ is the density referred to the natural state configuration.

To linearize the differential operators in (3.67) around the reference configuration $\widehat{\Omega}$ we introduce the symbol $D_{\widehat{\boldsymbol{\eta}}_0}f(\boldsymbol{\eta})$ to indicate the Gateaux derivative in $\widehat{\boldsymbol{\eta}}_0$ and applied to $\boldsymbol{\eta}$, being $\boldsymbol{\eta}$ a displacement field on Ω_0 [92], i.e.

$$D_{\widehat{\boldsymbol{\eta}}_0}f(\widehat{\boldsymbol{\eta}}) = \lim_{\epsilon\to 0}\frac{f(\widehat{\boldsymbol{\eta}}_0 + \epsilon\widehat{\boldsymbol{\eta}}) - f(\widehat{\boldsymbol{\eta}}_0)}{\epsilon}.$$

We assume that the displacement are sufficiently regular to guarantee its existence and continuity everywhere.

The most troublesome term in (3.67) is the one containing the divergence operator, since we need to rewrite it with respect to the $\widehat{\boldsymbol{x}}$ coordinates. To this aim, we use the Piola transform (3.6) and property 3.2 to write

$$\mathbf{div}_{\widehat{\boldsymbol{x}}_0}\widehat{\boldsymbol{F}}_0\widehat{\boldsymbol{\Sigma}}_0 = \widehat{J}_0\mathbf{div}_{\widehat{\boldsymbol{x}}}\left[\widehat{J}_0^{-1}\left(\widehat{\boldsymbol{F}}_0\widehat{\boldsymbol{\Sigma}}_0\right)\widehat{\boldsymbol{F}}^{0T}\right],$$

where $\widehat{\boldsymbol{F}}^0$ and $\widehat{J}_0 = |\widehat{\boldsymbol{F}}^0|$ are independent from $\widehat{\boldsymbol{\eta}}$. Therefore,

$$D_{\widehat{\boldsymbol{\eta}}_0}\left(\mathbf{div}_{\widehat{\boldsymbol{x}}_0}\widehat{\boldsymbol{F}}_0\widehat{\boldsymbol{\Sigma}}_0\right)(\widehat{\boldsymbol{\eta}}) = \widehat{J}_0\mathbf{div}_{\widehat{\boldsymbol{x}}}\left[\widehat{J}_0^{-1}D_{\widehat{\boldsymbol{\eta}}_0}(\widehat{\boldsymbol{F}}_0\widehat{\boldsymbol{\Sigma}}_0)(\widehat{\boldsymbol{\eta}})\widehat{\boldsymbol{F}}^{0T}\right].$$

By standard derivation rule and setting $\widehat{\boldsymbol{\Sigma}}^0 = \widehat{\boldsymbol{\Sigma}}_0(\widehat{\boldsymbol{\eta}}_0)$ we can write

$$D_{\widehat{\boldsymbol{\eta}}_0}(\widehat{\boldsymbol{F}}_0\widehat{\boldsymbol{\Sigma}}_0)(\widehat{\boldsymbol{\eta}}) = D_{\widehat{\boldsymbol{\eta}}_0}\widehat{\boldsymbol{F}}_0(\widehat{\boldsymbol{\eta}})\widehat{\boldsymbol{\Sigma}}^0 + \widehat{\boldsymbol{F}}^0 D_{\widehat{\boldsymbol{\eta}}_0}\widehat{\boldsymbol{\Sigma}}_0(\widehat{\boldsymbol{\eta}}). \tag{3.68}$$

Since

$$D_{\widehat{\boldsymbol{\eta}}_0}\widehat{\boldsymbol{F}}_0(\widehat{\boldsymbol{\eta}}) = \boldsymbol{\nabla}_{\widehat{\boldsymbol{x}}_0}\widehat{\boldsymbol{\eta}} = \boldsymbol{\nabla}_{\widehat{\boldsymbol{x}}}\widehat{\boldsymbol{\eta}}\widehat{\boldsymbol{F}}^0,$$

thanks to the inverse Piola transform and the relation between the Cauchy and the second Piola-Kirchhoff stress tensor, we have

$$\widehat{J}_0^{-1}D_{\widehat{\boldsymbol{\eta}}_0}\widehat{\boldsymbol{F}}_0(\widehat{\boldsymbol{\eta}})\widehat{\boldsymbol{\Sigma}}^0\widehat{\boldsymbol{F}}^{0T} = (\boldsymbol{\nabla}_{\widehat{\boldsymbol{x}}}\widehat{\boldsymbol{\eta}})(\widehat{J}_0^{-1}\widehat{\boldsymbol{F}}^0\widehat{\boldsymbol{\Sigma}}^0\widehat{\boldsymbol{F}}^{0T}) = \boldsymbol{\nabla}_{\widehat{\boldsymbol{x}}}\widehat{\boldsymbol{\eta}}\boldsymbol{\sigma}^0.$$

Indeed, $\boldsymbol{\sigma}^0 = \widehat{J}_0^{-1}\widehat{\boldsymbol{F}}_0\widehat{\boldsymbol{\Sigma}}^0\widehat{\boldsymbol{F}}^{0T}$.

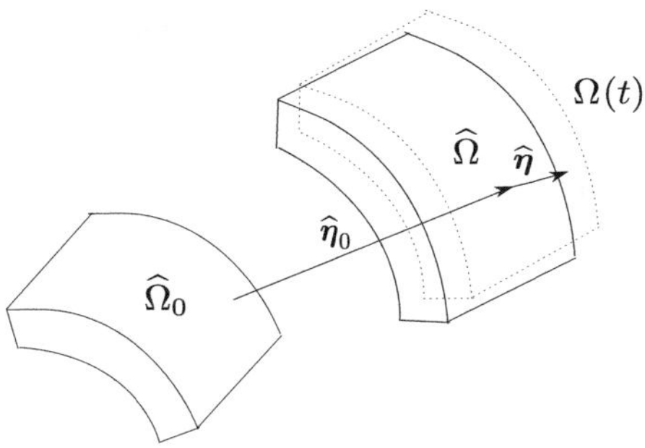

Fig. 3.12. The reference and natural state configurations together with the current configureation in dashed lines

The second term in (3.68) is elaborated further as

$$D_{\widehat{\eta}_0}\widehat{\boldsymbol{\Sigma}}_0(\widehat{\boldsymbol{\eta}}) = \frac{\partial^2 W}{\partial \widehat{\boldsymbol{E}}^2}(\widehat{\boldsymbol{E}}^0) D_{\widehat{\eta}_0}\widehat{\boldsymbol{E}}_0(\widehat{\boldsymbol{\eta}}) = \widehat{\boldsymbol{H}} : \left(\widehat{\boldsymbol{F}}^{0T}\varepsilon(\widehat{\boldsymbol{\eta}})\widehat{\boldsymbol{F}}^0\right),$$

where

$$\widehat{\boldsymbol{H}} = \frac{\partial^2 W}{\partial \widehat{\boldsymbol{E}}^2}(\widehat{\boldsymbol{E}}_0(\widehat{\boldsymbol{\eta}}_0)), \quad \text{componentwise } \widehat{H}_{ijkl} = \frac{\partial^2 W}{\partial \widehat{E}_{ij}\widehat{E}_{kl}}(\widehat{\boldsymbol{E}}^0), \tag{3.69}$$

while

$$\varepsilon(\widehat{\boldsymbol{\eta}}) = \frac{1}{2}\left(\boldsymbol{\nabla}_{\widehat{\boldsymbol{x}}}\widehat{\boldsymbol{\eta}} + \boldsymbol{\nabla}_{\widehat{\boldsymbol{x}}}^T\widehat{\boldsymbol{\eta}}\right) \tag{3.70}$$

is the well known *linearised* strain tensor.

Note that if we adopt the Saint-Venant Kirchhoff model (3.56) the components of the elasticity tensor defined in (3.69) are exactly those given in (3.58).

We now exploit the tensor identity $\widehat{\mathbf{H}} : (\widehat{\boldsymbol{F}}^{0T}\varepsilon\widehat{\boldsymbol{F}}^0) = \widehat{\mathbf{H}} : (\widehat{\boldsymbol{F}}^{0T}\widehat{\boldsymbol{F}}^{0T}) : \varepsilon$, which can be easily verified when written componentwise since

$$\widehat{H}_{ijkl}(\widehat{F}^0_{sk}\varepsilon_{st}\widehat{F}^0_{tl}) = (\widehat{H}_{ijkl}\widehat{F}^0_{sk}\widehat{F}^0_{tl})\varepsilon_{st}$$

to finally write,

$$\widehat{J}_0^{-1}\widehat{\boldsymbol{F}}^0 D_{\widehat{\eta}_0}\widehat{\boldsymbol{\Sigma}}_0(\widehat{\boldsymbol{\eta}})\widehat{\boldsymbol{F}}^{0T} = \widehat{J}_0^{-1}\widehat{\boldsymbol{F}}^0\left[\widehat{\mathbf{H}} : \left(\widehat{\boldsymbol{F}}^{0T}\widehat{\boldsymbol{F}}^{0T}\right) : \varepsilon(\widehat{\boldsymbol{\eta}})\right]\widehat{\boldsymbol{F}}^{0T} = \widehat{\mathbf{H}}^{\mathrm{P}} : \varepsilon(\widehat{\boldsymbol{\eta}})$$

where

$$\widehat{\mathbf{H}}^{\mathrm{P}} = \widehat{J}_0^{-1}\left(\widehat{\boldsymbol{F}}^0\widehat{\boldsymbol{F}}^0\right) : \widehat{\mathbf{H}} : \left(\widehat{\boldsymbol{F}}^{0T}\widehat{\boldsymbol{F}}^{0T}\right) \tag{3.71}$$

is the linear elasticity fourth order tensor in the reference pre-stressed configuration $\widehat{\Omega}$. Componentwise, $\widehat{H}^{\mathrm{P}}_{ijkl} = \widehat{J}_0^{-1}\widehat{F}^0_{is}\widehat{F}^0_{jt}\widehat{H}_{stpq}\widehat{F}^0_{kp}\widehat{F}^0_{lq}$, where all repeated indexes are implicitly summed from 1 to 3.

We now recognise that $\widehat{\rho}^0/\widehat{J}^0$ is nothing else than $\widehat{\rho}_0$, the density in the reference configuration $\widehat{\Omega}$. Using the expressions found so far and exploiting (3.65), we are now able to write the linearised equations in the pre-stressed state as

$$\widehat{\rho}_0 \frac{\partial^2 \widehat{\boldsymbol{\eta}}}{\partial t^2} - \mathbf{div}_{\widehat{\boldsymbol{x}}} \left[\nabla_{\widehat{\boldsymbol{x}}} \widehat{\boldsymbol{\eta}} \boldsymbol{\sigma}^0 + \widehat{\mathbf{H}}^{\mathrm{P}} : \boldsymbol{\varepsilon}(\widehat{\boldsymbol{\eta}}) \right] = \widehat{\rho}_0 \widehat{\boldsymbol{f}}, \quad \text{in } \widehat{\Omega}, \quad t > 0. \tag{3.72}$$

We can make the following remarks:

- Whenever $\widehat{\Omega}$ is a natural state $\boldsymbol{\sigma}^0 = \mathbf{0}$ and $\widehat{\mathbf{H}}^{\mathrm{P}}$ reduces to the standard linear elasticity tensor $\mathbf{H}$. System (3.72) becomes then the usual system of equations of linear elastodynamics,

$$\widehat{\rho}_0 \frac{\partial^2 \widehat{\boldsymbol{\eta}}}{\partial t^2} - \mathbf{div}_{\widehat{\boldsymbol{x}}} \big(\mathbf{H} : \boldsymbol{\varepsilon}(\widehat{\boldsymbol{\eta}}) \big) = \widehat{\rho}_0 \widehat{\boldsymbol{f}}, \tag{3.73}$$

  where if we adopt (3.58) we have

$$\mathbf{H} : \boldsymbol{\varepsilon}(\widehat{\boldsymbol{\eta}}) = L_1 (\operatorname{tr} \boldsymbol{\varepsilon}(\widehat{\boldsymbol{\eta}})) \boldsymbol{I} + 2 L_2 \boldsymbol{\varepsilon}(\widehat{\boldsymbol{\eta}}). \tag{3.74}$$

- Even if the material is homogeneous and isotropic with respect to the natural configuration, the same material in the pre-stressed configuration $\widehat{\Omega}$ is in general neither isotropic nor homogeneous. Indeed, these two properties depend not only on the material internal structure but also on the chosen reference state [92]. Homogeneity is retained whenever $\widehat{\boldsymbol{F}}^0$ (and thus $\boldsymbol{\sigma}^0$) is constant, while maintaining isotropy requires that $\widehat{\boldsymbol{F}}^0 = a\mathbf{I}$, for a non negative scalar field a, and (consequently) that $\boldsymbol{\sigma}^0$ be proportional to the identity tensor $\mathbf{I}$.
- An interesting case is when the deformation gradient $\widehat{\boldsymbol{F}}^0$ is *diagonal* and the material complies with the Saint-Venant Kirchhoff model (3.58) (w.r.t. the natural state). Then also $\boldsymbol{\sigma}^0$ is diagonal and it may be verified that $\widehat{\mathbf{H}}^{\mathrm{P}}$ conforms to that of an orthotropic material with axis of symmetry coinciding with the chosen coordinate axis.
  Now, it is well known that the mechanical behaviour of the arterial wall can be approximated as orthotropic [178]. The analysis carried out here suggests that this behaviour can be caused not only by the particular structure of the material composing a blood vessel, but also by its pre-stressed state.
- Thanks to the symmetry of $\boldsymbol{\sigma}^0$ we have $\nabla_{\widehat{\boldsymbol{x}}} \widehat{\boldsymbol{\eta}} \boldsymbol{\sigma}^0 = \boldsymbol{\sigma}^0 \boldsymbol{\varepsilon}(\widehat{\boldsymbol{\eta}}) - \boldsymbol{\sigma}^0 \boldsymbol{\omega}(\widehat{\boldsymbol{\eta}})$, where $\boldsymbol{\omega}(\widehat{\boldsymbol{\eta}}) = \frac{1}{2}(\nabla_{\widehat{\boldsymbol{x}}} \widehat{\boldsymbol{\eta}} - \nabla^T_{\widehat{\boldsymbol{x}}} \widehat{\boldsymbol{\eta}})$ is the *rotation tensor*. It means that in a pre-stressed state the material may react also to pure rotations.

The results reported in this section are consistent with the findings in [23], where the authors considered an incompressible material and followed a different linearisation procedure by writing the elasticity tensor on the current configuration.

It is worth to point out that the expressions derived in this section are not relevant if one carries out a full non-linear analysis. However, even in this case it is necessary to account of pre-stress. What is done in common practise is to derive the pre-stress state from measurements of the opening angle and of the shrinking (when such invasive experiments are not feasible one may refer to reference data contained in the cited literature). How to introduce the pre-stress in the actual computation may depend on the numerical technique adopted.

Weak formulation of the equations of elastodynamics

We have introduced in Chapter 2 the weak formulation of a differential problem. We will here sketch that associated to (3.73). For the sake of simplicity we consider a homogeneous Dirichlet condition, i.e we set $\widehat{\boldsymbol{g}} = \mathbf{0}$ on $\widehat{\Gamma}_D$. Indeed the non-homogeneous case may be reduced to an homogeneous problem by a lifting technique [407] and more complex situations will be treated in Chapter 9. If we consider the space of vector functions

$$\widehat{\boldsymbol{V}} = [H_0^1(\widehat{\Omega})]^3 = \{\widehat{\boldsymbol{v}} \in [H^1(\widehat{\Omega})]^3 : \quad \widehat{\boldsymbol{v}} = \mathbf{0} \quad \text{on } \widehat{\Gamma}_D\},$$

following a route similar to that indicated in Chapter 2 we obtain the following formulation:

For any $t > 0$ find $\widehat{\boldsymbol{\eta}} = \widehat{\boldsymbol{\eta}}(t) \in \widehat{\boldsymbol{V}}$ such that

$$\int_{\widehat{\Omega}} \widehat{\rho}_0 \frac{\partial^2 \widehat{\boldsymbol{\eta}}}{\partial t^2} \cdot \widehat{\boldsymbol{v}} + a(\widehat{\boldsymbol{\eta}}, \widehat{\boldsymbol{v}}) = F(\widehat{\boldsymbol{v}}), \quad \forall \widehat{\boldsymbol{v}} \in \widehat{\boldsymbol{V}}, \tag{3.75}$$

where

$$a(\widehat{\boldsymbol{\eta}}, \widehat{\boldsymbol{v}}) = \int_{\widehat{\Omega}} \widehat{\boldsymbol{\Pi}} : \widehat{\boldsymbol{v}} d\Omega, \quad F(\widehat{\boldsymbol{v}}) = \int_{\widehat{\Omega}} \widehat{\boldsymbol{f}} \cdot \widehat{\boldsymbol{v}} d\Omega + \int_{\widehat{\Gamma}_N} \widehat{\boldsymbol{h}} \cdot \widehat{\boldsymbol{v}}\, d\widehat{\gamma}.$$

Here, given two tensors $\boldsymbol{A}$ ad $\boldsymbol{B}$, the symbol $\boldsymbol{A} : \boldsymbol{B}$ indicates the scalar $\sum_{i,j=1}^{3} A_{ij} B_{ij}$.

Relation (3.75) is indeed a scalar equation. We can however recover three equations for each component of $\widehat{\boldsymbol{\eta}}$ by selecting $\widehat{\boldsymbol{v}} = (\widehat{v}, 0, 0)^T$, $\widehat{\boldsymbol{v}} = (0, \widehat{v}, 0)^T$ and $\widehat{\boldsymbol{v}} = (0, 0, \widehat{v})^T$, respectively, with $\widehat{v} \in H_0^1(\widehat{\Omega})$.

3.4 Reduced structural models

As mentioned in Chapter 2, sometimes we can use reduced models for the structure. This choice may reduce computational costs when we are interested in the effects of the structure mechanics on the fluid, rather than on an accurate evaluation of the stresses inside the vessel tissue.

A possibility often used for haemodynamic computations is to adopt shell models, even if the thickness of the wall of blood vessels would not justify them in full, since they assume that the structure is very thin. The basic notions of linear shell theory can be found in [75] and the treatment of the non-linear case may be found in [286].

For the sake of completeness, we give a brief account of the derivation of the equations of linear shells in a rather general setting, yet at the same time we will specialise them for the case of a cylindrical surface, an important paradigm for blood vessels and discuss the effects of pre-stress, following the derivation found in [352], in the context of fluid-structure interaction problems.

3.4.1 The geometrical description of a shell

In this section we will use the following summation convection: quantities with repeated indexes appearing at the same side of an equation are automatically summed up. Furthermore, Greek indexes will run in the set $\{1, 2\}$ whereas Latin indexes in $\{1, 2, 3\}$.

A shell is a solid medium whose reference configuration, $\widehat{\Omega}$, can be defined by a mid-surface, $\mathcal{S}$, and a thickness $h_s > 0$. More precisely, we shall assume that the mid-surface is the image of a two-dimensional domain $\omega \subset \mathbb{R}^2$ by an injective mapping (or chart) $\boldsymbol{\psi} : \omega \subset \mathbb{R}^2 \longrightarrow \mathbb{R}^3$, i.e.,

$$\mathcal{S} = \boldsymbol{\psi}(\omega),$$

see Fig. 3.13. We also assume that the chart $\boldsymbol{\psi}$ is such that the tangent vectors

$$\boldsymbol{a}_\alpha(\xi_1, \xi_2) = \frac{\partial \boldsymbol{\psi}}{\partial \xi_\alpha}(\xi_1, \xi_2), \quad (\xi_1, \xi_2) \in \omega,$$

are linearly independent. Thus we may define the unit normal vector to the mid-surface

$$\boldsymbol{a}_3 = \frac{\boldsymbol{a}_1 \times \boldsymbol{a}_2}{\|\boldsymbol{a}_1 \times \boldsymbol{a}_2\|}.$$

Finally, we parametrise the reference domain $\widehat{\Omega}$ by the mapping $\boldsymbol{\Psi}$ given by

$$\boldsymbol{\Psi}(\xi_1, \xi_2, \xi_3) = \boldsymbol{\psi}(\xi_1, \xi_2) + \xi_3 \boldsymbol{a}_3(\xi_1, \xi_2), \tag{3.76}$$

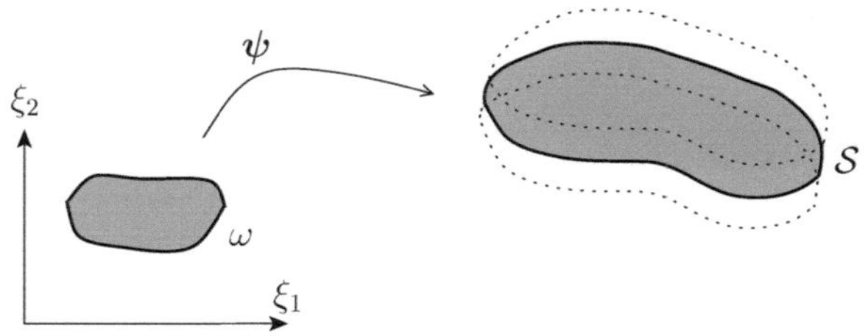

Fig. 3.13. Parametrisation of the shell mid-surface

for all $(\xi_1, \xi_2, \xi_3) \in \Theta$, where

$$\Theta = \left\{ (\xi_1, \xi_2, \xi_3) \in \mathbb{R}^3 \ : \ (\xi_1, \xi_2) \in \omega, \, \xi_3 \in \left(-\frac{h_s}{2}, \frac{h_s}{2} \right) \right\}.$$

As a result, we have $\widehat{\Omega} = \boldsymbol{\Psi}(\Theta)$, see Fig. 3.14. Note that h_s could vary along the mid-surface, however, for the sake of clarity we assume that h_s is constant.

The parametrisation of the domain given by the map $\boldsymbol{\Psi}$ induces a three-dimensional curvilinear coordinate system. We can introduce the so-called covariant basis $\{\boldsymbol{g}_1, \boldsymbol{g}_2, \boldsymbol{g}_3\}$ defined by

$$\boldsymbol{g}_i(\xi_1, \xi_2, \xi_3) = \frac{\partial \boldsymbol{\Psi}}{\partial \xi_i}(\xi_1, \xi_2, \xi_3), \quad \forall (\xi_1, \xi_2, \xi_3) \in \Theta.$$

and the associated local contravariant basis $\{\boldsymbol{g}^1, \boldsymbol{g}^2, \boldsymbol{g}^3\}$ defined by the relation

$$\boldsymbol{g}_i \cdot \boldsymbol{g}^j = \delta_i^j,$$

being δ_i^j the Kronecker's symbol. Tensors of arbitrary order can be expressed in terms of either basis. For instance, $\mathbf{f} = f_i \boldsymbol{g}^i = f^i \boldsymbol{g}_i$, f_i and f^i being called the *covariant* and *contravariant* components of the vector $\mathbf{f}$, respectively. The *metric tensor* $g_{ij} = \boldsymbol{g}_i \cdot \boldsymbol{g}_j$ and its inverse $g^{ij} = \boldsymbol{g}^i \cdot \boldsymbol{g}^j$ allow to perform the change of basis, whenever needed. For instance, we have $v_i = g^{ij} v^j$. If the coordinate system is orthonormal, then $g_{ij} = g^{ij} = \delta_{ij}$, i.e. the transformation reduces to the identity and there is no distinction between covariant and contravariant components.

We now introduce some symmetric surface tensors which are fundamental in shell analysis. The first, second and third fundamental forms of the mid-surface are tensors defined on the surface here indicated by $\boldsymbol{a}$, $\boldsymbol{b}$ and $\boldsymbol{c}$, whose covariant components are given by

$$a_{\alpha\beta} = \boldsymbol{a}_\alpha \cdot \boldsymbol{a}_\beta, \quad b_{\alpha\beta} = \boldsymbol{a}_3 \cdot \frac{\partial \boldsymbol{a}_\alpha}{\partial \xi_\beta} \quad \text{and } c_{\alpha\beta} = b_{\alpha\gamma} a^{\gamma\lambda} b_{\lambda\beta}, \tag{3.77}$$

respectively. The first fundamental form is also called *surface metric tensor*.

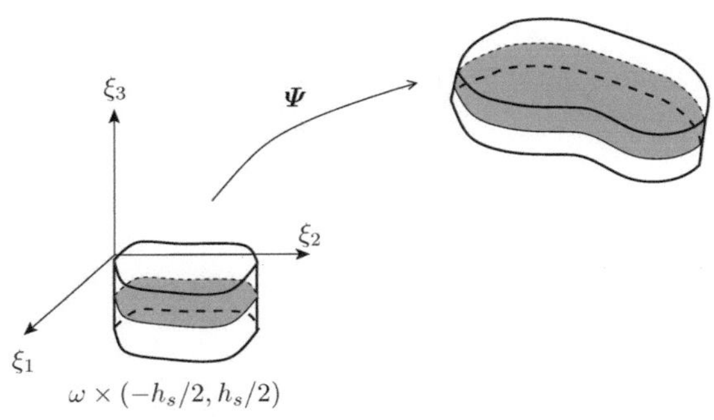

Fig. 3.14. Geometric description of a shell, which might represent a portion of the wall of a blood vessel

A function indexed by Greek letter is assumed to lay on the mid-surface $\xi_3 = 0$. Let us also note that at $\xi_3 = 0$ we have that $\boldsymbol{g}_\alpha = \boldsymbol{a}_\alpha$ and $g_{\alpha\beta} = a_{\alpha\beta}$.

There is the need to give a meaning to the derivation of a surface tensor field. Given a vector field $\boldsymbol{f} = \boldsymbol{f}(\xi_1, \xi_2)$ on the mid-surface we denote by $f_{\alpha|\beta}$ the *surface covariant derivative* of its covariant component f_α defined as

$$f_{\alpha|\beta} = \frac{\partial f_\alpha}{\partial \xi_\beta} - \Gamma^\lambda_{\alpha\beta} f_\lambda. \tag{3.78}$$

Here, $\Gamma^\lambda_{\alpha\beta}$ stands for the Christoffel's symbol defined as

$$\Gamma^\lambda_{\alpha\beta} = \frac{\partial \boldsymbol{a}_\alpha}{\partial \xi_\beta} \cdot \boldsymbol{a}^\lambda. \tag{3.79}$$

Relation (3.78) is readily extended to a tensor field of any order.

For the sake of illustration, let us consider a cylindrical shell of constant radius R_0 and length L aligned along the canonical base vector $\boldsymbol{e}_3$. It can be parametrised by the chart

$$\boldsymbol{\Psi}(\xi_1, \xi_2, \xi_3) = \begin{bmatrix} (R_0 + \xi_3)\cos\xi_1 \\ (R_0 + \xi_3)\sin\xi_1 \\ \xi_2 \end{bmatrix}, \tag{3.80}$$

where

$$(\xi_1, \xi_2) \in \omega = [0, 2\pi] \times [0, L], \quad \text{and} \qquad \xi_3 \in [-h_s/2, h_s/2].$$

One may immediately associate the selected independent variables with the standard cylindrical coordinates (r, θ, z): $\theta = \xi_1$, $r = R_0 + \xi_3$ and $z = \xi_2$.

The covariant base vector are thus given by

$$\boldsymbol{g}_1 = \begin{bmatrix} -(R_0 + \xi_3)\sin\xi_1 \\ (R_0 + \xi_3)\cos\xi_1 \\ 0 \end{bmatrix}, \quad \boldsymbol{g}_2 = \begin{bmatrix} 0 \\ 0 \\ 1 \end{bmatrix}, \quad \boldsymbol{g}_3 = \begin{bmatrix} \cos\xi_1 \\ \sin\xi_1 \\ 0 \end{bmatrix},$$

and the surface vectors by

$$\boldsymbol{a}_1 = \begin{bmatrix} -R_0\sin\xi_1 \\ R_0\cos\xi_1 \\ 0 \end{bmatrix}, \quad \boldsymbol{a}_2 = \begin{bmatrix} 0 \\ 0 \\ 1 \end{bmatrix}, \quad \boldsymbol{a}_3 = \begin{bmatrix} \cos\xi_1 \\ \sin\xi_1 \\ 0 \end{bmatrix}.$$

It then follows that

$$\frac{\partial \boldsymbol{a}_1}{\partial \xi_1} = \begin{bmatrix} -R_0\cos\xi_1 \\ -R_0\sin\xi_1 \\ 0 \end{bmatrix}, \quad \frac{\partial \boldsymbol{a}_1}{\partial \xi_2} = \frac{\partial \boldsymbol{a}_2}{\partial \xi_1} = \frac{\partial \boldsymbol{a}_2}{\partial \xi_2} = \boldsymbol{0}.$$

On the other hand, as covariant surface vectors we have

$$\boldsymbol{a}^1 = \begin{bmatrix} -\frac{1}{R_0}\sin\xi_1 \\ \frac{1}{R_0}\cos\xi_1 \\ 0 \end{bmatrix}, \quad \boldsymbol{a}^2 = \boldsymbol{a}_2, \quad \boldsymbol{a}^3 = \boldsymbol{a}_3.$$

Therefore,

$$\begin{aligned}
&a_{11} = R_0^2,\ a_{12} = a_{21} = 0,\ a_{22} = 1, && a^{11} = R_0^{-2},\ a^{12} = a^{21} = 0,\ a^{22} = 1,\\
&b_{11} = -R_0,\ b_{12} = b_{21} = b_{22} = 0, && c_{11} = 1,\ c_{12} = c_{21} = c_{22} = 0.
\end{aligned} \tag{3.81}$$

In particular, all the Christoffel's symbols are zero

$$\Gamma^\lambda_{\alpha\beta} = \frac{\partial \boldsymbol{a}_\alpha}{\partial \xi_\beta} \cdot \boldsymbol{a}^\lambda = 0,$$

so that the covariant and standard derivation coincide in this particular case.

3.4.2 Shell kinematics

In general, shell models are based on some kinematic assumptions relating the displacement of points located in a material line orthogonal to the mid-surface, i.e. when ξ_1, ξ_2 are kept fixed, while $\xi_3 \in (-h_s/2, h_s/2)$. For instance, under the *Reissner-Mindlin kinematics assumption* [335, 425], it is assumed that such material line remains unstretched during the motion. As a consequence the displacement $\widehat{\boldsymbol{\eta}}$ of a point belonging to the shell may be expressed by the following equation:

$$\widehat{\boldsymbol{\eta}}(\xi_1, \xi_3, \xi_3) = \boldsymbol{d}(\xi_1, \xi_2) + \xi_3 \theta_\lambda(\xi_1, \xi_2) \boldsymbol{a}^\lambda(\xi_1, \xi_2), \tag{3.82}$$

where $\boldsymbol{d}(\xi_1, \xi_2)$ is the displacement of the mid-surface and θ_λ the rotation of a line normal to the mid-surface.

Using this assumption, the covariant components of the linearised strain tensor $\boldsymbol{\varepsilon}(\widehat{\boldsymbol{\eta}})$, whose general definition in terms of the shell metric is

$$\varepsilon_{ij}(\widehat{\boldsymbol{\eta}}) = \varepsilon(\widehat{\boldsymbol{\eta}}) : \boldsymbol{g}_i \otimes \boldsymbol{g}_j = \frac{1}{2}\left(\frac{\partial \widehat{\boldsymbol{\eta}}}{\partial \xi_j} \cdot \boldsymbol{g}_i + \frac{\partial \widehat{\boldsymbol{\eta}}}{\partial \xi_i} \cdot \boldsymbol{g}_j \right),$$

becomes

$$\begin{aligned}
\varepsilon_{\alpha\beta}(\widehat{\boldsymbol{\eta}}) &= \gamma_{\alpha\beta}(\boldsymbol{d}) + \xi_3 \chi_{\alpha\beta}(\boldsymbol{d}, \boldsymbol{\theta}) - \xi_3^2 \kappa_{\alpha\beta}(\boldsymbol{\theta}),\\
\varepsilon_{\alpha 3}(\widehat{\boldsymbol{\eta}}) &= \zeta_\alpha(\boldsymbol{d}, \boldsymbol{\theta}), \quad \text{and} \quad \varepsilon_{33}(\widehat{\boldsymbol{\eta}}) = 0,
\end{aligned}$$

with $\boldsymbol{\gamma}$, $\boldsymbol{\chi}$ and $\boldsymbol{\kappa}$ being the so-called *membrane*, *bending* and *shear* parts of the strain tensor, whose covariant components are

$$\begin{aligned}
\gamma_{\alpha\beta}(\boldsymbol{d}) &= \frac{1}{2}\left(d_{\alpha|\beta} + d_{\beta|\alpha}\right) - b_{\alpha\beta} d_3,\\
\chi_{\alpha\beta}(\boldsymbol{d}, \boldsymbol{\theta}) &= \frac{1}{2}\left(\theta_{\alpha|\beta} + \theta_{\beta|\alpha} - b^\lambda_\beta d_{\lambda|\alpha} - b^\lambda_\alpha d_{\lambda|\beta}\right) + c_{\alpha\beta} d_3,\\
\kappa_{\alpha\beta}(\boldsymbol{\theta}) &= \frac{1}{2}\left(b^\lambda_\beta \theta_{\lambda|\alpha} + b^\lambda_\alpha \theta_{\lambda|\beta}\right),
\end{aligned}$$

respectively, while

$$\zeta_\alpha(\boldsymbol{d},\boldsymbol{\theta}) = \frac{1}{2}\left(\theta_\alpha + \frac{\partial d_3}{\partial \xi_\alpha} + b_\alpha^\lambda d_\lambda\right). \tag{3.83}$$

The tensor $\boldsymbol{\gamma}$ is also called *change of metric* tensor, since it is related to the change in the surface metric tensor caused by the deformation. Often an additional kinematic condition is adopted which takes the name of *Kirchhoff-Love* kinematics condition. It states that during the motion any material line orthogonal to the (reference) mid-surface remains straight, unstretched and orthogonal to the mid-surface. The Kirchhoff-Love assumption introduces the following relation between the translation and rotation displacements, see [75],

$$\theta_\lambda = -\frac{\partial d_3}{\partial \xi_\lambda} - b_\lambda^\mu d_\mu, \tag{3.84}$$

by which

$$\zeta_\alpha = 0, \quad \text{and} \quad \varepsilon_{\alpha 3} = 0.$$

Thanks to the Kirchhoff-Love conditions we have eliminated the rotations θ_α.

In addition, it is often assumed that the term of order ξ_3^2 may be neglected. This is the term responsible to shear strain, which can indeed be considered small for the target application. The resulting shell model is called *membrane-bending model*.

3.4.3 Shell dynamics

In curvilinear coordinates, Hook's law is still written in the form (3.59) where now to account for the fact that we are not using curvilinear coordinates we have

$$H^{ijkl} = L_1 g^{ij} g^{kl} + L_2\left(g^{ik} g^{jl} + g^{il} g^{jk}\right). \tag{3.85}$$

In shell models we make the further assumption of *plane stresses*. That is, because of the small thickness we assume zero stresses along the normal direction, namely $T^{33} = 0$. We thus obtain the modified constitutive equation

$$T^{\alpha\beta} = C^{\alpha\beta\lambda\mu}\varepsilon_{\lambda\mu}, \quad \sigma^{\alpha 3} = \frac{1}{2} D^{\alpha\lambda}\varepsilon_{\lambda 3},$$

with

$$C^{\alpha\beta\lambda\mu} = \frac{E}{(1+\xi)}\left(g^{\alpha\lambda} g^{\beta\mu} + \frac{\xi}{1-\xi} g^{\alpha\beta} g^{\lambda\mu}\right) \quad \text{and} \quad D^{\alpha\lambda} = \frac{2E}{1+\xi} g^{\alpha\lambda}.$$

We indicate by $\hat{\rho}_{s,0}$ the density of the material composing the shell, measured in kg/m^3. We assume that external stresses $\boldsymbol{s}_1$ and $\boldsymbol{s}_2$ act on the boundaries of $\widehat{\Omega}$ given by the image of $\omega \times \{-h_s/2\}$ and $\omega \times \{h_s/2\}$, respectively. Clearly we have $\boldsymbol{s}_1 = \boldsymbol{s}_1(\xi_1, \xi_2)$ and $\boldsymbol{s}_2 = \boldsymbol{s}_2(\xi_1, \xi_2)$, and with the symbol $\boldsymbol{f}$ we indicate the resultant $\boldsymbol{f}(\xi_1,\xi_2) = \boldsymbol{s}_2(\xi_1,\xi_2) - \boldsymbol{s}_1(\xi_1,\xi_2)$, f being a force per unit area $[\boldsymbol{f}] = \mathrm{N/m^2}$ (in our applications $\boldsymbol{f}$ is directly related to the transmural pressure across the blood vessel),

The equations governing the dynamics of a shell is better written directly using the weak formulation. We here give just the sketch of the procedure. We assume a membrane-bending model and, for the sake of simplicity we take homogeneous Dirichlet conditions on the lateral boundaries, image of $\partial\omega \times (-h_s/2, h_s/2)$. On the remaining boundaries we have the action of the stresses $\boldsymbol{s}_1$ and $\boldsymbol{s}_2$, which induce a Neumann-type boundary condition. Starting from (3.75)[7], since here $\widehat{\Omega} = \boldsymbol{\Psi}(\Theta)$ we can rewrite the integrals over Θ. Then, as $\Theta = \omega \times (-h_s/2, h_s/2)$ we can reduce all the integrals on ω by integrating along the ξ_3 direction. The final result is the variational formulation of the membrane-bending model, which reads: *For all $t > 0$, find $\boldsymbol{d}$ such that*

$$\int_\omega h_s \hat{\rho}_{s,0} \frac{\partial^2 \boldsymbol{d}}{\partial t^2} \cdot \boldsymbol{q} d\omega + \int_\omega \widetilde{C}^{\alpha\beta\lambda\mu} \left[h_s \gamma_{\alpha\beta}(\boldsymbol{d}) \gamma_{\lambda\mu}(\boldsymbol{q}) + \frac{h_s^3}{12} \rho_{\alpha\beta}(\boldsymbol{d}) \rho_{\lambda\mu}(\boldsymbol{q}) \right] d\omega = \int_\omega \boldsymbol{f} \cdot \boldsymbol{q} d\omega, \qquad (3.86)$$

for all test function $\boldsymbol{q}$ regular enough and with zero trace on the Dirichlet portion of the boundary. Here,

$$\widetilde{C}^{\alpha\beta\lambda\mu} = \frac{E}{2(1+\xi)} \left(a^{\alpha\lambda} a^{\beta\mu} + a^{\alpha\mu} a^{\beta\lambda} + \frac{2\xi}{1-\xi} a^{\alpha\beta} a^{\lambda\mu} \right)$$

and

$$\rho_{\alpha\beta}(\boldsymbol{d}) = d_{3|\alpha\beta} + b^\mu_{\alpha|\beta} d_\mu + b^\mu_\alpha d_{\mu|\beta} + b^\mu_\beta d_{\mu|\alpha} - c_{\alpha\beta} d_3.$$

An advantage of the shell model is that now we are effectively operating on a two dimensional domain. The discretisation by finite elements of (3.86) then leads, in principle at least, to cheaper solution schemes than with a 3D formulation on $\widehat{\Omega}$. Examples of suitable finite element spaces for shell models can be found in the cited literature.

We consider again the example of the cylinder illustrated in the previous section and we make the additional hypotheses of axi-symmetric displacements, that is that $d_1 = 0$ as well as all derivatives w.r.t. ξ_1. Furthermore, for the sake of clarity, we will indicate with the suffixes θ and z the first and second component of the displacement vector: $\boldsymbol{d} = (d_\theta, d_r)$. Under these hypothesis we have

$$\gamma_{11}(\boldsymbol{d}) = R_0 d_r, \quad \gamma_{22}(\boldsymbol{d}) = \frac{\partial d_z}{\partial z}, \quad \gamma_{12}(\boldsymbol{d}) = \gamma_{21}(\boldsymbol{d}) = 0,$$

$$\rho_{11}(\boldsymbol{d}) = -d_r, \quad \rho_{22}(\boldsymbol{d}) = \frac{\partial^2 d_r}{\partial z^2}, \quad \rho_{12}(\boldsymbol{d}) = \rho_{21}(\boldsymbol{d}) = 0.$$

[7] In (3.75) $\boldsymbol{f}$ was a volume force, which is here taken equal to zero. The symbol $\boldsymbol{f}$ is here used instead to indicate the surface stress resultant acting on the shell.

Therefore, we have

$$
\begin{aligned}
\widetilde{C}^{\alpha\beta\lambda\mu}\gamma_{\alpha\beta}(\boldsymbol{d})\gamma_{\lambda\mu}(\boldsymbol{q}) =& \frac{E}{2(1+\xi)}\left(\frac{1}{R_0^2}d_r q_r + \frac{\partial d_z}{\partial z}\frac{\partial q_z}{\partial z}\right) \\
&+ \frac{E\xi}{1-\xi^2}\left(\frac{d_r}{R_0^2} + \frac{\partial d_z}{\partial z}\right)\left(\frac{q_r}{R_0^2} + \frac{\partial q_z}{\partial z}\right),
\end{aligned}
$$

while

$$
\begin{aligned}
\widetilde{C}^{\alpha\beta\lambda\mu}\rho_{\alpha\beta}(\boldsymbol{d})\rho_{\lambda\mu}(\boldsymbol{q}) =& \frac{E}{2(1+\xi)}\left(\frac{1}{R_0^4}d_r q_r + \frac{\partial^2 d_r}{\partial z^2}\frac{\partial^2 q_r}{\partial z^2}\right) \\
&+ \frac{E\xi}{1-\xi^2}\left(-\frac{d_r}{R_0^2} + \frac{\partial^2 d_r}{\partial z^2}\right)\left(-\frac{q_r}{R_0^2} + \frac{\partial^2 q_r}{\partial z^2}\right).
\end{aligned}
$$

Replacing these expressions into (3.86) and counter-integrating by parts (for simplicity let us assume homogeneous Dirichlet boundary conditions) we may recognise that the corresponding strong differential form is nothing else than the well known system of equation for a cylindrical Koiter-type shell, that is

$$
\begin{aligned}
h_s\widehat{\rho}_{s,0}\frac{\partial^2 d_z}{\partial t^2} - \frac{h_s E}{1-\xi^2}\left(\frac{\partial^2 d_z}{\partial z^2} + \xi\frac{1}{R}\frac{\partial d_r}{\partial z}\right) &= f_z, \\
h_s\rho_0\frac{\partial^2 d_r}{\partial t^2} + \frac{h_s E}{R(1-\xi^2)}\left(\xi\frac{\partial d_z}{\partial z} + \frac{d_r}{R}\right) + \frac{h_s^3 E}{12(1-\xi^2)}& \\
\left(\frac{\partial^4 d_r}{\partial z^4} - \frac{2\xi}{R^2}\frac{\partial^2 d_r}{\partial z^2} + \frac{d_r}{R^4}\right) &= f_r. \qquad (3.87)
\end{aligned}
$$

3.4.4 One-dimensional reduced structural models

One dimensional models are a very simple way to describe the dynamics of a single vessel. We assume that the artery is of cylindrical shape and the only space dimension considered is the axial one. There are different ways to derive them. For instance, directly from physical principles, as done in [401] or [406], or from shell models like in [522]. By further simplification assumptions that lead to simple algebraic relationship between the vessel section area and the average pressure, they are often used to develop 1D models for blood flow in compliant arteries like those illustrated in Chapter 10.

Here we will sketch the derivation starting from a shell model and accounting for pre-stress.

To this aim, we will follow [352], alternative derivations may be found, for instance, in [401], [406], or in [523], where some viscoelastic effects are accounted for.

We will consider the situation of Fig. 3.15 where the reference configuration is a cylindrical surface. In the case of a standard cylinder, the map

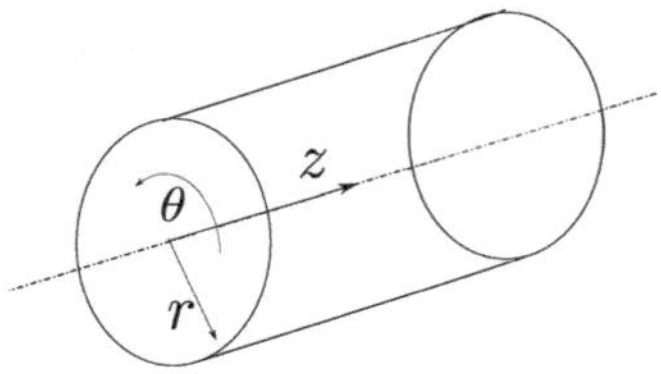

Fig. 3.15. Cylindrical map. $\xi_1 = \theta$, $\xi_2 = r$ and $\xi_3 = z$

will coincide with that indicated in (3.80). We may then identify ξ_1, ξ_2 and ξ_3 with the circumferential, the axial and the radial physical coordinates, and for this reason we will alternatively use the indexes θ, z, and r, respectively. Furthermore the surface is the image of $\theta \in (0, 2\pi)$, $z \in (0, L)$ and $r \in (R_0 - h_s/2, R_0 + h_s/2)$.
The main assumptions are:

- The ratio h_s/R_0 of the vessel wall is small so that we can neglect bending terms (which indeed scale with higher order than membrane terms with respect to this ratio). In other words we will set to zero the last term in the left hand side of (3.86) and consider only membrane effects.
- The wall displaces in the normal direction, i.e. $\boldsymbol{d} = (0, 0, \eta)$. Correspondingly we have
$$\gamma_{\alpha\beta}(\boldsymbol{d}) = -b_{\alpha\beta}\eta. \tag{3.88}$$
The assumption that longitudinal and circumferential displacements are negligible compared to the radial ones is usually accepted in the biomedical literature.
- The vessel is subject to a time varying transmural pressure $\Delta P = P - P_{ext}$ across the surface. Consequently we take
$$\boldsymbol{f} = \Delta P \boldsymbol{n}, \tag{3.89}$$
being $\boldsymbol{n}$ the outward oriented normal. For the sake of simplicity, we assume homogeneous Dirichlet boundary condition (i.e. a clamped vessel). Yet accounting for conditions of other type is rather straightforward.
- The reference configuration is pre-stressed, yet the deformation gradient $\widehat{\boldsymbol{F}}^0$ is assumed to be diagonal (in the shell local reference system) and constant. More precisely we set
$$\widehat{\boldsymbol{F}}^0 = \mathrm{diag}(F^0_{\theta\theta}, F^0_{zz}, 1),$$
being $F^0_{\theta\theta}$ and F^0_{zz} constants. In correspondence we assume a diagonal (and constant) pre-stress tensor $\boldsymbol{\sigma}^0 = \mathrm{diag}(\sigma^0_{\theta\theta}, \sigma^0_{zz}, 0)$. The value of the parameters may be inferred from measurements of the opening angle and shrinking of an extracted vessel, or by considerations on how the pre-stressed configuration has been generated [23, 115, 391, 523].

We first have to find out the modifications induced by the pre-stress state to the standard shell model. We have seen that pre-stressing induces two modifications to the standard linearised elasticity equations: a change in the stress-strain tensor $\boldsymbol{H}$ and the appearance of an extra term in the stress, of the form $\nabla_{\widehat{\boldsymbol{x}}}\widehat{\boldsymbol{\eta}}\boldsymbol{\sigma}^0$. Being $\widehat{\boldsymbol{F}}^0$ diagonal the former modification is readily accounted for by replacing g^{ij} with $F^0_{ii}F^0_{jj}g^{ij}$ (no implied sum) in (3.85). We are able to carry out the standard derivation that led to (3.86) also in this case, however now the tensor $\widetilde{\boldsymbol{C}}$ becomes

$$\widetilde{C}^{\alpha\beta\lambda\mu} = \frac{E}{2(1+\xi)}F^0_{\alpha\alpha}F^0_{\beta\beta}F^0_{\lambda\lambda}F^0_{\mu\mu}\left(a^{\alpha\lambda}a^{\beta\mu}+a^{\alpha\mu}a^{\beta\lambda}+\frac{2\xi}{1-\xi}a^{\alpha\beta}a^{\lambda\mu}\right).$$

Thanks to (3.88) we may derive that in (3.86)

$$h_s\widetilde{C}^{\alpha\beta\lambda\mu}\gamma_{\alpha\beta}(\boldsymbol{d})\gamma_{\lambda\mu}(\boldsymbol{q}) = a_0\eta q_r, \tag{3.90}$$

where

$$a_0 = \frac{h_sE}{1-\xi^2}\left[(1-\xi)\widetilde{a}^{\alpha\lambda}\widetilde{a}^{\beta\delta}b_{\alpha\beta}b_{\lambda\delta}+\xi\widetilde{a}^{\alpha\beta}\widetilde{a}^{\lambda\delta}b_{\alpha\beta}b_{\lambda\delta}\right],$$

while

$$\widetilde{a}^{\alpha\beta} = F^0_{\alpha\alpha}F^0_{\beta\beta}a^{\alpha\beta} \quad \text{(no sum implied)}.$$

Finally, we account also for the term $\nabla_{\widehat{\boldsymbol{x}}}\widehat{\boldsymbol{\eta}}\,\boldsymbol{\sigma}^0$ and we make the additional assumption of axial symmetry, i.e. we set to zero all derivatives w.r.t. ξ_1. Under this hypothesis the radial component of $\mathbf{div}(\nabla\eta\widehat{\boldsymbol{\sigma}}^0)$ reduces to $T^0_{zz}\frac{\partial^2\eta}{\partial z^2}$.

We have then

$$h_s\hat{\rho}_{s,0}\frac{\partial^2\eta}{\partial t^2}+a\eta-b\frac{\partial^2\eta}{\partial z^2} = P-P_{ext}, \quad z\in(0,L), \quad t>0, \tag{3.91}$$

with $\eta=0$ at $z=0$ and $z=L$ (or other suitable boundary conditions) while $\eta=\eta_0$ and $\partial\eta/\partial t=\eta_1$ at $t=0$, η_0 and η_1 being suitable initial data.

Here,

$$a = a_0+\sigma^0_{\theta\theta}b_{\gamma1}b_{\gamma1}+\sigma^0_{zz}b_{\gamma2}b_{\gamma2}. \tag{3.92}$$

is the elastic coefficient modified to account for the pre-stress and $b=\sigma^0_{zz}$.

A notable case if that of the regular cylinder, where we may apply (3.81). We may for instance assume that the circumferential pre-stress has been caused by an external pressure P^+ originally applied to the unstressed cylinder (this value is sometimes assumed to be equal to the mean arterial pressure). By using the simple Poisson's law for the stress in a pressurised cylinder we have then $\sigma^0_{\theta\theta}=P^+R_0/h_s$. As for the term $F^0_{\theta\theta}$, it might be estimated from the measurements of the opening angle $\widehat{\Theta}$ of artery specimens opened up longitudinally so that they can recover a zero-stress configuration, i.e. $F^0_{\theta\theta}=1+\frac{\pi}{\widehat{\Theta}}$.

Gathering all this information the expression for a simplifies into

$$a = (F^0_{\theta\theta})^4\frac{h_sE}{R_0(1-\xi^2)}+\frac{P^+}{R_0}.$$

In several works however, the effect of the pre-stress in the coefficient a is neglected. Either because the value of the a is estimated from measurements taken *in vivo*, thus already accounting for the pre-stress, or because it is felt that pre-stress introduces a correction of the same order of the incertitude on the value of E and R_0. In the latter case the simpler formula $a = \frac{h_s E}{R_0(1-\xi^2)}$ is used instead, and this is the expression we will adopt in the sequel of the book whenever model (3.91) is adopted.

Model (3.91) is called *string model*, since it is akin to the one governing the motion of a string under tension. Some authors link the presence of the second order space derivative in this model not to the pre-stress but to the Timoshenko shear factor, an empirical term introduced to better account for shear deformation and rotatory inertia effects in the theory of thin structures [510]. In fact, probably both effects are present at the same time.

A more complete reduced one-dimensional model for the vessel structure takes the general form (see [406], [525])

$$h_s\hat{\rho}_{s,0}\frac{\partial^2\eta}{\partial t^2} + a\eta - b\frac{\partial^2\eta}{\partial z^2} + c_1\frac{\partial\eta}{\partial t} - c_2\frac{\partial^3\eta}{\partial t\partial z^2} = P - P_{ext}, \quad z \in (0,L), \quad t > 0. \tag{3.93}$$

Here, c_1 and c_2 are two non-negative parameters accounting for the viscoelastic property of the vessel wall, see also [523], [33]. We will call (3.93) a *generalised string model* and it is often used as a simplified (yet rather complete) model for the study of fluid structure interaction problems in a single artery (see Chapters 8 and 9).

A whole class of models can be derived by setting to zero some of the parameters. In particular, the simplest model is obtained by neglecting all derivative terms (including the inertial term), obtaining the simple algebraic expression

$$a\eta = P - P_{ext} \tag{3.94}$$

used for the derivation of the basic one-dimensional model for blood flow in arteries, as illustrated in Chapter 10.

3.5 Modelling fluid-structure interaction problems

In this section we describe the general non-linear fluid-structure system in large displacements arising in blood flows in large arteries. We consider as computational domain a model of a portion of an artery, see Fig. 3.16. It consists of a deformable structure $\Omega_s(t)$ (vessel wall) surrounding a moving domain $\Omega_f(t)$ filled by a fluid under motion (blood). The fluid structure interface, *i.e.* the common boundary between $\Omega_s(t)$ and $\Omega_f(t)$, is denoted by $\Gamma(t) = \partial\Omega_f(t) \cap \partial\Omega_s(t)$. In the sequel, variables with a sub-script s or f shall refer to quantities within the fluid or the solid domains, respectively.

We will ignore body forces, i.e. we take $\boldsymbol{f} = \boldsymbol{0}$ both for the fluid and the structure. For haemodynamic applications this corresponds in practise to ignore the effects of gravity.

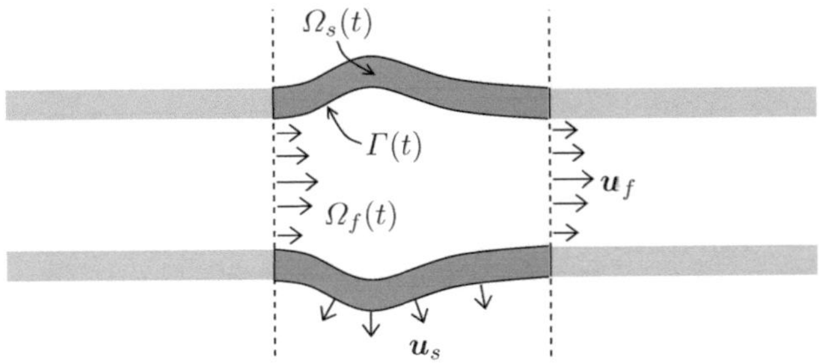

Fig. 3.16. Geometric configuration (2D section)

We assume the motion of the control volume $\Omega_f(t)$ to be parametrised by an ALE map $\widetilde{\mathcal{A}} : \widetilde{\Omega_f} \times \mathbb{R}^+ \longrightarrow \mathbb{R}^3$ (see Section 3.1.2), *i.e.* $\Omega_f(t) = \widetilde{\mathcal{A}}(\widetilde{\Omega_f}, t)$. The reference domain $\widetilde{\Omega_f}$ being the position of the control volume at the initial time. We assume that the inlet $\Gamma_{f,D}$ and outlet $\Gamma_{f,N}$ boundaries are at a fixed axial position along the artery model of Fig. 3.17.

As showed in Section 3.1.2, when dealing with moving domains it is natural to work with ALE time-derivatives. More precisely, we will use formulation (3.48).

The differential equations have to be completed with proper boundary conditions on $\partial\Omega_f(t)\backslash\Gamma(t)$. For instance, we can enforce

$$\begin{aligned} \boldsymbol{u}_f &= \boldsymbol{u}_D, \quad \text{on} \quad \Gamma_{f,D}, \\ \boldsymbol{\sigma}_f(\boldsymbol{u}_f, P)\boldsymbol{n}_f &= \boldsymbol{g}_N, \quad \text{on} \quad \Gamma_{f,N}, \end{aligned} \tag{3.95}$$

with $\boldsymbol{u}_D$ a given velocity and $\boldsymbol{g}_{f,N}$ a given density of surface load.

To summarise, we have

$$\begin{aligned} \rho_f \frac{\partial \boldsymbol{u}_f}{\partial t}_{|\widetilde{\mathcal{A}}} + \rho_f(\boldsymbol{u}_f - \boldsymbol{w}) \cdot \boldsymbol{\nabla}\boldsymbol{u}_f - \mathbf{div}\boldsymbol{\sigma}_f(\boldsymbol{u}_f, P) &= \mathbf{0}, \quad \text{in} \quad \Omega_f(t), \\ \operatorname{div} \boldsymbol{u}_f &= 0, \quad \text{in} \quad \Omega_f(t). \\ \boldsymbol{u}_f &= \boldsymbol{u}_{f,D}, \quad \text{on} \quad \Gamma_{f,D}, \\ \boldsymbol{\sigma}_f(\boldsymbol{u}_f, P)\boldsymbol{n}_f &= \boldsymbol{g}_{f,N}, \quad \text{on} \quad \Gamma_{f,N}. \end{aligned} \tag{3.96}$$

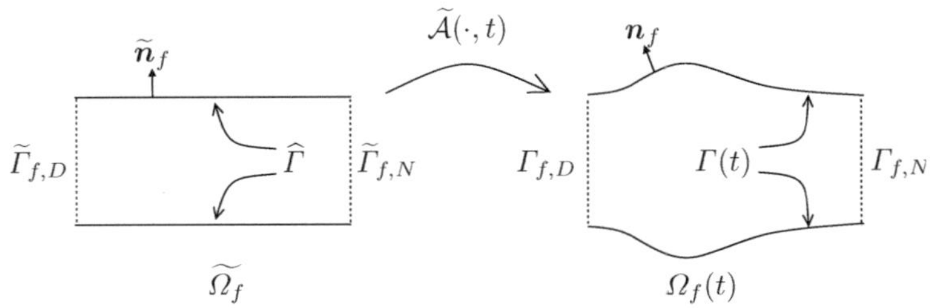

Fig. 3.17. Description of the motion of the computational domain for the fluid via the ALE map $\widetilde{\mathcal{A}}$

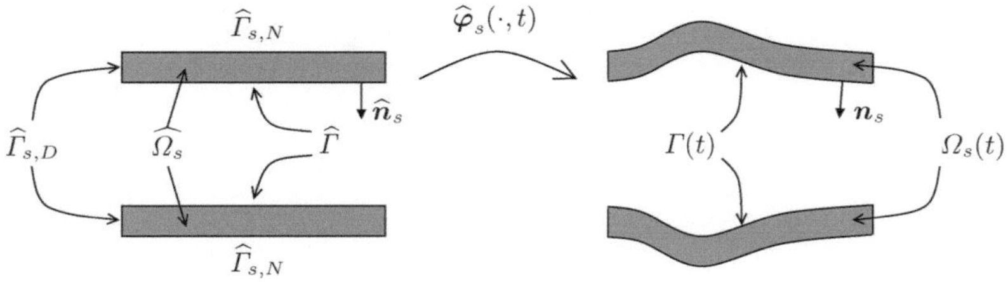

Fig. 3.18. Description of the motion of the solid (2D section)

Remark 3.5.1 *So far, we have assumed the ALE map $\widetilde{\mathcal{A}}$, and in particular the ALE velocity field $\boldsymbol{w}$, to be known. As wee shall see in the next section that we can define the ALE map as an extension of the boundary position with a technique that can be extended readily to the numerical computation.*

As anticipated in Section 3.3.2, we consider a Lagrangian description of the motion of the structure, where $\widehat{\Omega_s}$ is a given material reference configuration (see Fig. 3.18). We describe the motion of the structure in terms of its displacement field $\widehat{\boldsymbol{\eta}}_s : \widehat{\Omega_s} \times \mathbb{R}^+ \longrightarrow \mathbb{R}^3$. For the sake of simplicity, we here assume the structure to be clamped on the boundaries $\widehat{\Gamma}_{s,D}$.

The differential problem for the structure part then reads

$$\begin{aligned} \hat{\rho}_{s,0} \frac{\partial^2 \widehat{\boldsymbol{\eta}}_s}{\partial t^2} - \mathbf{div}_{\widehat{\boldsymbol{x}}} \big(\widehat{\boldsymbol{F}}_s \widehat{\boldsymbol{\Sigma}} \big) &= \mathbf{0}, \quad \text{in} \quad \widehat{\Omega_s}, \\ \widehat{\boldsymbol{\eta}}_s &= \mathbf{0}, \quad \text{on} \quad \widehat{\Gamma}_{s,D}, \\ \widehat{\boldsymbol{F}}_s \widehat{\boldsymbol{\Sigma}} \widehat{\boldsymbol{n}}_s = \widehat{J}_s \| \widehat{\boldsymbol{F}}^{-T} \widehat{\boldsymbol{n}}_s \| \widehat{\boldsymbol{g}}_{s,N}, &\quad \text{on} \quad \widehat{\Gamma}_{s,N}, \end{aligned} \tag{3.97}$$

with $\widehat{\boldsymbol{\Sigma}}$ related to $\widehat{\boldsymbol{\eta}}_s$ through a constitutive law of the form (3.55).

The fluid and solid problems (3.96) and (3.97) must be coupled ensuring a global energy balance. This is achieved by imposing three interface coupling conditions: geometry, velocity and stress.

Geometry coupling: construction of the ALE map

We first enforce that the moving control volume follows the interface motion, *i.e.*

$$\widetilde{\mathcal{A}} = \widehat{\boldsymbol{\varphi}}_s, \quad \text{on} \quad \widehat{\Gamma}, \tag{3.98}$$

this is a geometry coupling condition. Since we describe the motion of the solid in terms of its displacement $\widehat{\boldsymbol{\eta}}_s$, it is also useful to describe the ALE map in terms of the displacement of the control volume, $\widetilde{\boldsymbol{\eta}}_f : \widetilde{\Omega_f} \times \mathbb{R}^+ \longrightarrow \mathbb{R}^3$, defined by

$$\widetilde{\boldsymbol{\eta}}_f(\widetilde{\boldsymbol{x}}, t) = \widetilde{\mathcal{A}}(\widetilde{\boldsymbol{x}}, t) - \widetilde{\boldsymbol{x}},$$

for all $\widetilde{\boldsymbol{x}} \in \widetilde{\Omega_f}$. Thus, (3.98) reduces to

$$\widetilde{\boldsymbol{\eta}}_f = \widehat{\boldsymbol{\eta}}_s, \quad \text{on} \quad \widehat{\Gamma}. \tag{3.99}$$

By differentiating this equality with respect to t, it follows that

$$\widetilde{\boldsymbol{w}} = \widehat{\boldsymbol{u}_s}, \quad \text{on} \quad \widehat{\Gamma}. \tag{3.100}$$

On the other hand, since the inlet and outlet boundaries remain fixed along the motion, we also have

$$\widetilde{\boldsymbol{\eta}}_f = \mathbf{0}, \quad \text{on} \quad \widetilde{\Gamma}_{f,D} \cup \widetilde{\Gamma}_{f,N}. \tag{3.101}$$

Notice that (3.99) and (3.101) provide the value of $\widetilde{\boldsymbol{\eta}}_f$ on the boundary of $\widetilde{\Omega_f}$. However, inside $\widetilde{\Omega_f}$, f $\widetilde{\boldsymbol{\eta}}_f$ (and hence $\widetilde{\mathcal{A}}$) is arbitrary: it can be any reasonable extension of $\widehat{\boldsymbol{\eta}}_{s|\widehat{\Gamma}}$ over $\widetilde{\Omega_f}$ (subjected to (3.101)). In the sequel we will denote this operation by

$$\widetilde{\boldsymbol{\eta}}_f = \mathrm{Ext}(\widehat{\boldsymbol{\eta}}_{s|\widehat{\Gamma}}). \tag{3.102}$$

For instance, the operator Ext can be given in terms of an harmonic extension, by solving:

$$\begin{aligned} -\Delta\widetilde{\boldsymbol{\eta}}_f &= \mathbf{0}, && \text{in} \quad \widetilde{\Omega_f}, \\ \widetilde{\boldsymbol{\eta}}_f &= \mathbf{0}, && \text{on} \quad \widetilde{\Gamma}_{f,D} \cup \widetilde{\Gamma}_{f,N}, \\ \widetilde{\boldsymbol{\eta}}_f &= \widehat{\boldsymbol{\eta}}_s, && \text{on} \quad \widehat{\Gamma}. \end{aligned} \tag{3.103}$$

Continuity of velocity and stress

Since the fluid is assumed to be viscous, it perfectly sticks to the interface (or solid) boundary. This means that the whole velocity field must be continuous at the interface. Thus, we set

$$\boldsymbol{u}_f = \boldsymbol{w}, \quad \text{on} \quad \Gamma(t). \tag{3.104}$$

Finally, in order to ensure the balance of stresses on the interface, we enforce the continuity of stress at the interface. Thus, using the properties of the Piola transform (Proposition 3.2) we get the coupling condition

$$\widehat{\boldsymbol{F}}_s \widehat{\boldsymbol{\Sigma}} \widehat{\boldsymbol{n}}_s + J_{\widetilde{\mathcal{A}}} \widetilde{\boldsymbol{\sigma}}_f(\boldsymbol{u}_f, P) \widetilde{\boldsymbol{F}}_{\widetilde{\mathcal{A}}}^{-T} \widetilde{\boldsymbol{n}}_f = 0, \quad \text{on} \quad \widehat{\Gamma}. \tag{3.105}$$

The coupled fluid-structure problem

Using the coupling conditions (3.102), (3.104) and (3.105) the coupled fluid-structure interaction problem reads: find $\widetilde{\boldsymbol{\eta}}_f : \widetilde{\Omega_f} \times \mathbb{R}^+ \longrightarrow \mathbb{R}^3$, $\widetilde{\boldsymbol{u}_f} : \widetilde{\Omega_f} \times \mathbb{R}^+ \longrightarrow \mathbb{R}^3$, $\widetilde{p} : \widetilde{\Omega_f} \times \mathbb{R}^+ \longrightarrow \mathbb{R}$ and $\widehat{\boldsymbol{\eta}}_s : \widehat{\Omega_s} \times \mathbb{R}^+ \longrightarrow \mathbb{R}^3$, such that

- Fluid sub-problem:

$$\left\{ \begin{aligned} \rho_f \frac{\partial \boldsymbol{u}_f}{\partial t}_{|\widetilde{\mathcal{A}}} + \rho_f(\boldsymbol{u}_f - \boldsymbol{w}) \cdot \boldsymbol{\nabla} \boldsymbol{u}_f - \mathbf{div} \boldsymbol{\sigma}_f(\boldsymbol{u}_f, P) &= \mathbf{0}, \quad \text{in} \quad \Omega_f(t), \\ \operatorname{div} \boldsymbol{u}_f &= 0, \quad \text{in} \quad \Omega_f(t), \\ \boldsymbol{\sigma}_f(\boldsymbol{u}_f, P)\boldsymbol{n}_f &= \boldsymbol{g}_{f,N}, \quad \text{on} \quad \Gamma_{f,N}. \end{aligned} \right. \tag{3.106}$$

- Solid sub-problem:

$$\begin{cases} \hat{\rho}_{s,0}\dfrac{\partial^2\widehat{\boldsymbol{\eta}}_s}{\partial t^2} - \mathbf{div}_{\hat{\boldsymbol{x}}}(\widehat{\boldsymbol{F}}_s\widehat{\boldsymbol{\Sigma}}) = \mathbf{0}, & \text{in } \widehat{\Omega_s}, \\ \widehat{\boldsymbol{\eta}}_s = \mathbf{0}, & \text{on } \Gamma_{s,D}, \\ \widehat{\boldsymbol{F}}_s\widehat{\boldsymbol{\Sigma}}\widehat{\boldsymbol{n}}_s = \mathbf{0}, & \text{on } \widehat{\Gamma}_{s,N}. \end{cases} \tag{3.107}$$

- Coupling conditions:

$$\begin{cases} \widetilde{\boldsymbol{\eta}}_f = \mathrm{Ext}(\widehat{\boldsymbol{\eta}}_{s|\widehat{\Gamma}}), \quad \Omega_f(t) = \widetilde{\mathcal{A}}(\widetilde{\Omega_f}, t), \quad \widetilde{\boldsymbol{w}} = \dfrac{\partial\widetilde{\boldsymbol{\eta}}_f}{\partial t}, & \text{in } \widetilde{\Omega_f}, \\ \boldsymbol{u}_f = \boldsymbol{w}, & \text{on } \Gamma(t), \\ \widehat{\boldsymbol{F}}_s\widehat{\boldsymbol{\Sigma}}\widehat{\boldsymbol{n}}_s + \widetilde{J}_{\widetilde{\mathcal{A}}}\tilde{\boldsymbol{\sigma}}_f(\boldsymbol{u}_f, P)\widetilde{\boldsymbol{F}}_{\widetilde{\mathcal{A}}}^{-T}\widetilde{\boldsymbol{n}}_f = 0, & \text{on } \widehat{\Gamma}. \end{cases} \tag{3.108}$$

This is a complex non-linear system of equations whose numerical treatment is addressed in Chapter 9. Some elements for its mathematical analysis, under some simplifying hypotheses, are reported in Chapter 8.

3.6 Conclusions

We have derived the equations that governs the dynamics of fluid and structure, in the hypothesis of a continuum media. If this is a reasonable assumption for the structure and for blood flow in the main vessels, the continuum hypothesis may become questionable for the flow in small capillaries, where the dimension of the vessel becomes comparable to that of blood cells.

This issue is treated partly in Chapter 6 and we will not investigate it further in this book. We will see in other chapters, in particular Chapter 10, how models of the global circulation may account for the haemodynamics in the capillary bed by using suitable lumped parameter models. Indeed, the details of the flow in the capillaries is needed only in specific microcirculation studies.

Even if we have assumed a Newtonian behaviour for the fluid, we have derived the flow equations in generality, and they may be easily adapted to the more complex rheological models presented in Chapter 6.

As for the models for the vessel wall, the actual structure of a blood vessel is rather complex, as explained in Chapter 1. We have preferred giving here the most basic models, giving reference to the interested reader of the specialised literature where more sophisticated modelling may be found. In fact, if one is interested mainly on the effect of the structure movements on the haemodynamics there is no need of using complex models for the latter. They are instead mandatory if one is interested in having the details of the stress fields inside the vessel wall.

We wish to warn the reader that usually the more complex a model is the higher number of parameters it requires. Experiments to determine those parameters are often complex, in particular if one wishes to fit them to a specific person. In this case only indirect measurements are at disposal, *ex vivo* experiments being obviously out of question.

4

From image data to computational domains

Luca Antiga, Joaquim Peiró, and David A. Steinman

The advent of high-resolution imaging systems and powerful computational resources has made it possible to obtain information about the *in vivo* anatomy of blood vessels in a non invasive way. By employing this information as the domain definition for computational fluid dynamics, it is now possible to model hemodynamics in realistic geometric configurations on a subject-specific basis. Since geometry has a strong influence on hemodynamics, as will shown extensively in Chapter 5, the procedure used to model the geometry of a blood vessel from medical images plays a primary role in determining the reliability of haemodynamic predictions and, ultimately, their clinical significance.

In this chapter we will describe the process of defining domains for hemodynamics modelling from clinically acquired images. The solution of the equations of flow, transport and structure (see Chapter 2 and 3). in realistic geometries requires the use of numerical approximation methods, such as finite elements and finite volumes [371, 407]. Such methods are based on the discretisation of the physical domain in elements of simple shape and finite size (e.g. tetrahedra or hexahedra), which constitute the so-called computational mesh. The process from images to computational meshes representing realistic vascular geometries involves several separate steps (which are summarised in the flow chart of Fig. 4.1): i) Sets of images are first acquired using one of the clinically available imaging techniques. Imaging datasets typically come in the form of sets of 2D images each having a well defined position and orientation in space. Such sets can either be formed by contiguous images that can be stacked along a spatial direction, thus defining a volume, or be constituted by disjoint images. In addition, series of images of the same anatomical structure can be taken at several instants in time, effectively increasing the dimensionality of the data-set. ii) According to image quality and acquisition technique characteristics, images eventually undergo an enhancement step, during which vascular structures are made clearer at the expense of noise and non-vascular content. iii) Image segmentation, which is the process by which the regions of the belonging to vascular structures are identified, is then performed. Depend-

Formaggia L, Quarteroni A, Veneziani A. (Eds.): Cardiovascular Mathematics. Modeling and simulation of the circulatory system

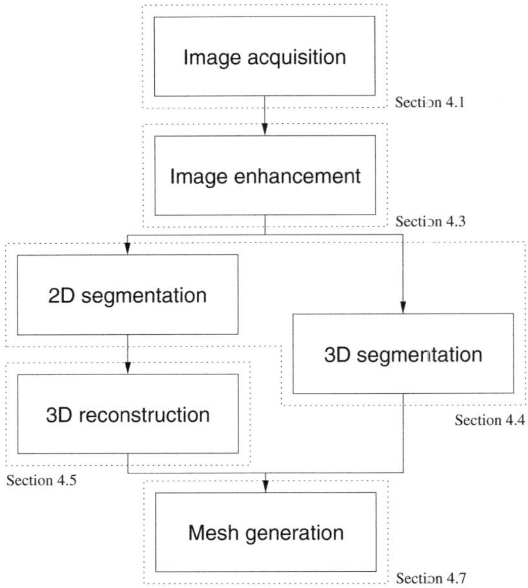

Fig. 4.1. Flow chart depicting the typical workflow from medical images to computational meshes. References to sections in the present chapter covering the enclosed topics are also reported

ing on the nature of the source images and on the geometric complexity of the 3D vascular structure of interest, segmentation can take place on single 2D planes or directly in 3D. In the first case, a 3D reconstruction phase is needed in order to generate the final 3D shape of the vessel from the information defined on the separate 2D planes. Finally, in case of time-resolved acquisitions, the segmentation have to adapt to the changes in shape occurring over time. iv) Finally, the definition of the vessel surface is employed for the generation of the computational mesh onto which the hemodynamics modelling problem can be solved numerically. For this purpose, well-shaped 2D elements are generated over the surface, and the model interior is then filled with 3D elements of appropriate density for the haemodynamic modelling problem.

While in the past several works have dealt with the description of the process from images to computational models as a whole, the tendency of current methodological publications on the subject is to focus on particular aspects of the process. Indeed, the way the single steps of the process are performed is potentially interchangeable (e.g. image segmentation is typically independent of mesh generation), and not all the possible combinations of techniques have actually been documented within a description of the whole process. We will therefore try to draw a sketch of the most relevant techniques today available for generating subject-specific models of blood vessels from medical images, including, for each step, the techniques that have been or could be potentially employed for the purpose.

4.1 Vascular imaging

Before reviewing the techniques involved in turning medical image data into geometries, it is important to appreciate the underlying physics, capabilities and limitations of the three main vascular imaging modalities available: X-ray, i.e. digital subtraction angiography and computerised tomography [206,284,389], magnetic resonance [203,327,369], and ultrasound [45,144,228] imaging. In the interest of space these are only briefly discussed below; for further information the reader is referred to the recent reviews cited. In general, however, it should be appreciated throughout that superior image quality and resolution invariably come at the expense of invasiveness and acquisition time.

4.1.1 X-ray imaging

Akin to casting a shadow, x-ray imaging records the projection of x-ray beams through the body and onto a radiographic film, fluoroscopic screen, or digital detector. Differential absorption of x-rays by the various body structures produces contrast in the resulting 2D images, though it is usually only possible to discriminate among bone, soft tissue and air. Highlighting the vascular lumen anatomy at the expense of the wall and surrounding tissue – angiography – typically requires the introduction of a radio-opaque dye into the blood stream.

Traditionally, x-ray angiography highlights the lumen by injecting an iodine-based contrast agent via a catheter placed directly into the artery of interest, which serves to effectively replace the blood within the artery for a few seconds. This results in superior contrast, and so permits the real-time acquisition of the projections. Such "fluoroscopic" imaging is particularly suited to mobile vessels like the coronary arteries (see Fig. 4.2 A), and so can be useful for prescribing time-varying motions for blood flow simulations (see Chapter 9). For relatively static vessels like the cerebral or peripheral arteries, digital subtraction angiography (DSA), which acquires an image prior to the contrast agent injection and then subtracts it digitally, can be used to better discriminate the opacified lumen from surrounding bone and soft tissue. Either way, real time or at least high temporal resolution (cine) angiography allows for the visualisation of contrast agent as it flows into the vascular tree. Although in principle this makes it possible to quantify blood flow rates and residence times [463], in practise it is most often used clinically to identify late or absent filling of distal and collateral vessels.

Owing to its superior contrast and spatial resolution ($\sim 0.2\,\mathrm{mm}$), projection x-ray angiography remains the gold standard for most vascular imaging applications. Still, its projective nature means that often-tortuous 3D lumen geometries can only be properly reconstructed from multiple projections, typically coupled with simplifying assumptions about the shape of the lumen cross-section (see Section 4.5). Such assumptions are unsuitable for truly 3D vascular structures like cerebral aneurysms (Fig. 4.2 B), so to get around this, rotational angiography techniques (RA) have been developed in which the gantry supporting the x-ray source and detector is rotated rapidly around the patient, allowing for the acquisition of many projections within the few seconds that contrast agent is being injected. From these multiple projections it is then possible to reconstruct high quality, high resolution (~ 0.4 mm isotropic, meaning the same resolution in all three directions) 3D images of the artery.

As with all catheterisation procedures, intra-arterial angiography carries with it a small but non-negligible risk of emboli (blood clots, air bubbles, etc.) travelling downstream and getting lodged in smaller arteries, a risk often higher than that associated with ionising radiation itself [36]. A less invasive alternative is to inject the contrast agent intravenously – any emboli must first pass through the lungs, where, for air bubbles especially, they can be filtered out. The downside is that the contrast agent mixes with the rest of the blood volume before it reaches the arteries via the heart. This serves to dilute its effect, and so higher contrast agent or x-ray doses may be required. Intravenous injection also restricts the temporal window available for imaging: too early and the contrast agent has not yet reached the artery of interest; too late and adjacent veins become enhanced, which ultimately makes it difficult to discriminate the arteries from veins.

While projection angiography still relies on intra-arterial injection, computed tomography (CT) angiography takes advantage of intravenous injections. Building upon the principles of computed axial tomography (i.e., CAT scans), a ring incorporating one or more x-ray sources and opposing detectors is rotated rapidly around the patient, producing and then reconstructing into an image the projections from multiple fan beams. By moving the patient axially through the donut-shaped scanner during this process, volumetric (3D) images can be reconstructed (Fig. 4.2 C). Owing to the short temporal window available for purely arterial enhancement, such "helical" CTA has typically been forced to sacrifice axial for in-plane resolution by using relatively long spiral pitches, resulting in anisotropic spatial resolutions despite the nominal 3D nature of the image data (see Section 4.3). The recent availability of scanners with multiple rings of sources and detectors now makes it possible to achieve sub-millimetre isotropic resolutions. With appropriate gating (i.e., synchronisation) of the acquisition to the heartbeat, temporally-resolved 3D imaging – often referred to as 4D CT – becomes feasible. This makes possible the reconstruction of time-resolved 3D lumen boundaries, or the validation of motions predicted by fluid-structure interaction models (see Chapter 9).

4.1.2 Magnetic Resonance Imaging (MRI)

MRI exploits the phenomenon of nuclear magnetic resonance, whereby atomic nuclei possessing spin can be made to resonate at their so-called Larmor frequency, proportional to the strength of an applied magnetic field. In MRI, protons, which resonate at radiofrequencies (RF) for clinical-strength scanners, are first aligned by placing the patient within a powerful superconducting magnet. (For this reason, MRI is contraindicated for patients with metallic or electronic implants; getting within metres of an MRI scanner can also stop your watch and erase your bank cards.) Brief application of RF energy sets the protons resonating, after which the RF signals decay at rates characteristic to the tissue in which the protons are bound. By simultaneously applying magnetic field gradients, it becomes possible to effectively encode position into the frequency of the signal. As such, MR images are actually acquired in frequency space (often referred to as k-space), and images are obtained by inverse Fourier transforms. Since the strength and evolution of the MR signal are related to the tissue properties, contrast can be generated by judicious selection and timing of the RF pulses and magnetic field gradients, collectively referred to as a pulse sequence. Thus the chief advantage of MRI is that it can achieve soft tissue contrast far superior to other imaging modalities. On the other hand, since the MRI signal is relatively weak, usually sensitive RF coils (i.e., antennae) must be placed close to the body surface, often to the unease of patients already anxious after being placed within a long cylindrical magnet (c.f., the shorter, donut-shaped configuration used for CT). Because signal strength is proportional to the voxel volume – a voxel is the 3D version of a 2D image pixel – high in-plane resolutions are usually only achievable by acquiring 2D images over relatively thick slices, which has implications on the way in which the 3D vascular geometries can be reconstructed, as will be explained throughout the chapter (see Sections 4.3 and 4.5). Even then, relatively long scan times are often required to traverse k-space: a single image can take up to several minutes depending on the type of contrast required. Patient motion then becomes a major challenge, especially since acquisition in frequency space can produce non-intuitive artifacts in the transformed image.

For vascular imaging, MRI has an important advantage over x-ray-based techniques: contrast can be generated without the need for exogenous agents. In time-of-flight (TOF) MRA angiography, static tissue is suppressed by saturating it with RF energy within a desired slice or volume, and then unsaturated blood flows in, appearing bright against the suppressed static tissue (Fig. 4.2 D). The timing of TOF angiograms must therefore be done carefully, unsaturated blood must be allowed enough time to flow in, but not so much that it becomes suppressed itself. This can be a problem for volumetric (3D) acquisitions, and so, even though less time-efficient, TOF angiograms are often acquired as a series of contiguous or overlapping thick (2D) axial slices. Still, artefactual signal voids can appear even in 2D images when complex, recirculating blood flow is present, confounding the segmentation of the lumen boundaries. Care must also be exercised in choosing the image resolution: too coarse and the blood signal is weakened by so-called phase dispersion caused by the presence of large velocity gradients; too fine and there are not enough protons to return adequate signal, thus necessitating longer scan times and/or thicker slices. These limitations can be largely overcome by contrast-enhanced (CE)-MRA, which resorts to the intravenous injection of a paramagnetic contrast agent to shorten the relaxation time of blood relative to background tissue. This results in a stronger blood signal within a shorter acquisition time, and minimises the saturation of slow flow. Like CTA, the intravenous injections must be timed carefully to avoid venous contamination. Unlike CTA, however, CE-MRA cannot yet be accomplished within a few seconds, and so pulse sequences must be designed carefully so as to minimise the effects of variable contrast agent concentration during the traversal of k-space.

In what amounts to the inverse of TOF-MRA, black blood (BB)-MRI seeks to suppress all signal, including that of blood, from *outside* the imaging slice or volume. As shown in Fig. 4.2 E, this makes it possible to see not only the (black) vessel lumen but also the (bright) vessel wall and surrounding tissue. As a result, BB-MRI – by definition imaging, not strictly angiography – is particularly attractive for characterising the vascular wall pathologies that can usually only be inferred from the presence of tortuosity or stenosis in traditional angiograms. In the context of vascular modelling, BB-MRI can be used to reconstruct both the lumen *and* wall simultaneously [480], which is particularly advantageous for providing outer wall (or simply wall thickness) boundary conditions for structural or fluid-structure interaction analyses (see Chapter 9). Like TOF-MRA, BB-MRI is based on the assumption that blood leaves the imaging region before it has time to recover its signal, so flow artifacts can also occur, albeit appearing as the inverse of those in TOF-MRA.

An alternative less susceptible to saturation/recovery effects is phase contrast (PC)-MRA, which relies on the fact that the velocity of moving spins can be encoded into the phase of the complex MR signal. Not only does this produce bright blood angiograms from the magnitude of the signal; as Fig. 4.2 F shows, the blood velocities themselves can be encoded into images of the signal phase, in principle one image for each direction of flow. By gating the acquisition to the cardiac rhythm, it becomes possible to produce time-resolved (cine) images of the blood velocities. In principle, this allows for the acquisition of a complete "4D" velocity field [43] ; in practise, such scans can be very time-consuming and so are not always tolerated by patients. PC-MRA tends not to be used for angiographic purposes alone, since for a given resolution and coverage, more scan time is required relative to TOF-MRA and especially CE-MRA.

4.1.3 Ultrasound (US) imaging

Relative to x-ray and MR imaging, US is the least expensive and least invasive. Similar to sonar and other echolocation techniques, US works by transmitting beams of low power, high frequency sound waves (on the order of a few MHz) into the body via a hand-held probe coupled to the skin through a conductive gel. Normally, this same probe receives the echoes caused by the strong reflections at tissue boundaries, and the weaker reflections within the tissues themselves. The distance between the probe and the reflections can then be calculated from the known speed of sound through tissue (1540 m/s) and the measured delay between transmission and each echo.

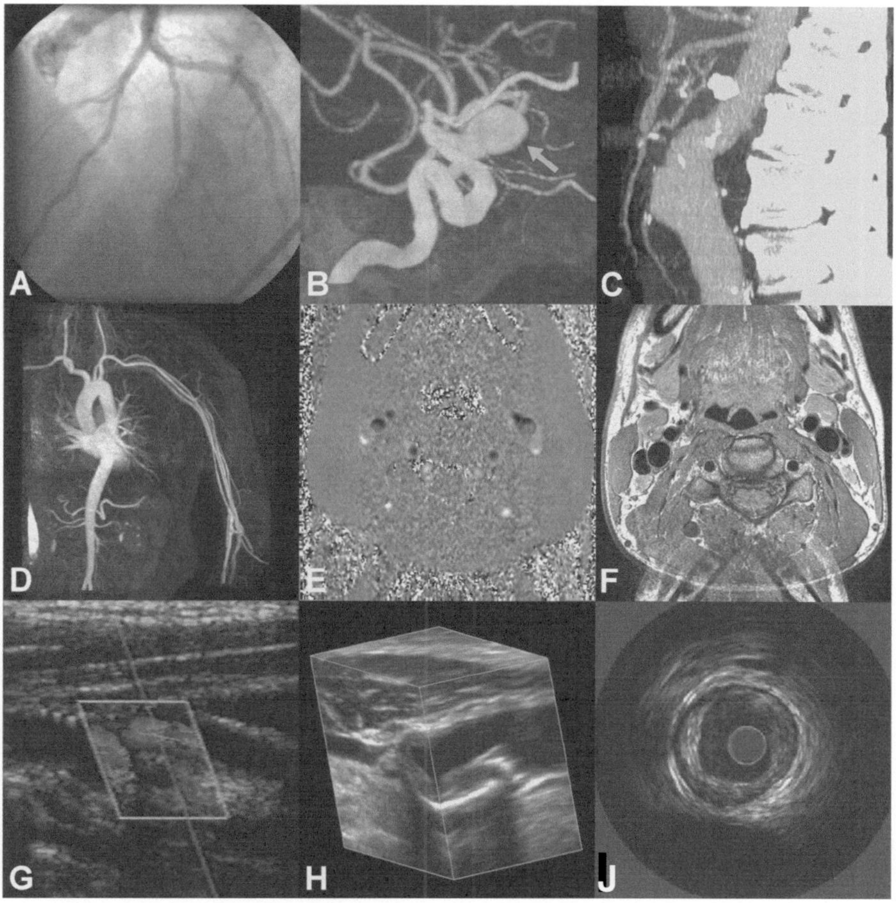

Fig. 4.2. Representative vascular images from the various modalities discussed. A. 2D x-ray angiogram of a coronary artery tree. B. Maximum intensity projection (MIP) through a 3D x-ray angiogram of a cerebral aneurysm (arrow). C. MIP through a 3D CTA of an abdominal aortic aneurysm. D. MIP through a 3D CE-MRA of the major arteries from neck to abdomen. E. 2D PC and F. BB-MRI images of the carotid arteries at the level of the bifurcation. G. Duplex US image of a carotid artery bifurcation. H. 3DUS image of a carotid artery bifurcation. J. IVUS image of a coronary artery in cross-section. Panels A&J courtesy of Dr. Jolanda Wentzel, Erasmus University. Panel D courtesy of Dr. Nils Planken, Department of Radiology, Amsterdam Medical Center. Panel G courtesy of Dr. David Spence, Robarts Research Institute. Panel H courtesy of Dr. Aaron Fenster, Robarts Research Institute

For typical depths of penetration, echo delays are less than a millisecond, and so US offers a remarkable facility for real-time imaging. For example, the amplitude of each echo can be assigned a grayscale value and displayed on screen at its respective depth from the probe. With the beam fixed this produces a M-mode image, so named because it sensitively depicts tissue motions at high ($\sim$ 1000 Hz) temporal resolution. More commonly, the US beam is swept, either mechanically or electronically, through a plane or sector to produce real-time ($\sim$ 100 Hz) 2D B-mode images, so named because their brightness reflects the distribution of tissue throughout the slice. By virtue of the Doppler effect, blood flow in the direction of the US beam produces shifts in the frequencies of the returned echoes, which can be converted into velocities and mapped onto a near-real-time ($\sim$ 15 Hz) colour Doppler image, as shown in the duplex US (i.e., combined B-mode and colour Doppler) image shown in Fig. 4.2 G.

An obvious limitation of conventional US imaging is the 2D nature of the acquisition, which, as noted earlier, makes visualisation of tortuous arteries difficult. (Remember that these are actual slices through the vessel, not projections.) This can be overcome via three-dimensional US (3DUS), which reconstructs an image volume from conventional 2D slices acquired during freehand or mechanical translation of the US probe (Fig. 4.2 H). Although 3DUS B-mode volumes can be acquired in less than a minute, longer scan times are required for 3D colour Doppler US images. Moreover, this approach is sensitive to vessel motion between individual 2D slices: 3DUS images can exhibit so-called "sawtooth" artifacts if the artery is pulsating as the probe is translated. These limitations, however, may soon be overcome through the development of 2D array transducers, which will permit real-time acquisition of 3D (and possibly 4D) US images.

As evidenced in Figs. 4.2 G and 4.2 H, ultrasound image quality and resolution are typically coarse relative to the other imaging modalities. Moreover, constructive and destructive interference of the scattered sound waves results in a form of multiplicative noise referred to as "speckle". As with MRI, image quality in US is also inextricably tied to the proximity of the vessel to the transducer at the surface: with increasing depth, less acoustic power is available for reflection. Similarly, tissue behind a calcification can be entirely masked because all of the acoustic power is reflected, leading to well-known shadowing artifacts. This also precludes the use of US for imaging cerebral vessels within the skull, except those visible through the thin temporal bone. Similarly, because the US also does not transmit well through air (hence the need for coupling gel between the transducer and the skin surface), imaging of abdominal vessels can be challenging. Image quality and artifacts cannot simply be overcome by increasing the power deposited, for this would risk heating the tissue. Instead, for deep or shadowed vessels like the coronaries, one resorts to intravascular ultrasound (IVUS), which places the transducer within the artery via a catheter (Fig. 4.2 J). Although this results in an invasiveness equal to that of x-ray angiography, it does provide information that angiography does not, namely, the surrounding tissue. As with BB-MRI, this is useful for providing the necessary boundaries for fluid-structure interaction analyses (see Chapter 9); however, because imaging planes follow the orientation of the (usually tortuous) vessel [261], adjacent slices are not parallel, potentially complicating the reconstruction of the 3D geometry (see Section 4.5).

4.2 Geometric modelling of blood vessels

Regardless the specific imaging modality, medical images contain information in the form of multidimensional arrays of numeric values, which are correlated with one or more physical properties of the imaged anatomical structures. Modelling the geometry of a vessel from medical images consists in extracting the location of the vessel wall from the values contained in the image volume. Since the image formation process in general alters the underlying anatomical information, and since the resolution with which the latter is acquired is bound to be finite, medical images are *coarse* representations of the underlying anatomy. Modelling the surface of an anatomical object from an image can therefore be regarded as an inverse problem.

More formally, a medical image can be seen as the scalar function $I : \Omega \rightarrow \mathbb{R}$ which associates an intensity value to every point in the acquisition volume $\Omega \subset \mathbb{R}^3$. In this framework, an image is not a collection of isolated samples, but rather a continuous function known at the nodes of a regular grid, whose values are interpolated over space with suitable shape functions (e.g. linear, cubic). On the basis of I, we are ultimately interested in finding a representation of the surface corresponding to the lumen wall boundary, or, in case the imaging technique allows it, as in the case of black blood MRI, to the inner and outer boundaries of the vessel wall. In both cases, we will generically indicate the obtained surface representations with $\mathbf{S}$, which will then serve as the definition of the boundary of the computational domain for the haemodynamic or fluid-structure interaction problem at hand, as introduced in Chapter 3.

Before we can face the problem of determining the location of $\mathbf{S}$ from I, it is necessary to describe how a generic 3D surface can be mathematically represented.

4.2.1 Explicit surface representations

A surface $\mathbf{S}$ corresponding to the vascular wall can be represented explicitly as a bivariate parametric function with values in $\mathbb{R}^3$ (as shown in Fig. 4.3, left). A common choice in computer graphics is expressing $\mathbf{S}$ as a set of adjacent polygons (e.g. triangles) whose vertexes have a known position. The surface in this case is given by

$$\mathbf{S} = \bigcup_i \mathbf{S}_i \tag{4.1}$$

with

$$\mathbf{S}_i(u, v) = \sum_{j=1}^{N_i} \phi_{i,j}(u, v)\, \mathbf{p}_{i,j} \tag{4.2}$$

where i indicates the i-th element, N_i is the number of nodes in the i-th element, $\phi_{i,j}$ is the shape function on element i, relative to node j, and $\mathbf{p}_{i,j}$

is the position of the j-th node in the i-th polygon. In general, the shape functions employed are linear Lagrangian basis functions satisfying

$$\phi_{i,j}(u_l, v_l) = 1 \qquad \text{for } l = j \tag{4.3}$$

$$\phi_{i,j}(u_l, v_l) = 0 \qquad \text{for } l \neq j \tag{4.4}$$

$$\sum_j \phi_{i,j}(u, v) = 1 \qquad \forall\ (u, v) \in \mathbf{U}_i \tag{4.5}$$

where U_i is the parametric space of the i-th element. In the case of triangular elements, suitable shape functions are barycentric coordinates. Due to the linear nature of the interpolation, a large number of small polygonal elements are required in order to represent a realistic anatomical structure. The representation does not offer any built-in control over the regularity of the surface apart from its continuity. However, given the simplicity of the formulation, it is very flexible with respect to the possible topologies that can be represented.

An alternative way of explicitly representing a surface is to use adjacent high-degree polynomial patches, such as NURBS (non-uniform rational B-splines) (as shown in Fig. 4.3, right) [403]. In this case, the surface takes the form of a union of patches each defined by a tensor product rule

$$\mathbf{S}_i(u, v) = \frac{\sum_{j=1}^{N} \sum_{k=1}^{M} \phi_{i,j}^{p}(u) \phi_{i,k}^{q}(v) w_{i,j,k} \mathbf{p}_{i,j,k}}{\sum_{j=1}^{N} \sum_{k=1}^{M} \phi_{i,j}^{p}(u) \phi_{i,k}^{q}(v) w_{i,j,k}} \tag{4.6}$$

where i indicates the i-th patch, $\mathbf{p}_{i,j,k}$ is one of the $M \times N$ control points, $w_{i,j,k}$ is the weight associated to the j,k-th point and $\phi_{i,j}^{p}$ a B-spline basis function of degree p, defined recursively as

$$\phi_{i,j}^{0}(u) = \begin{cases} 1 & u_j \leq u < u_{j+1} \\ 0 & \text{otherwise} \end{cases} \tag{4.7}$$

$$\phi_{i,j}^{p}(u) = \frac{u - u_j}{u_{j+p} - u_j}\, \phi_{i,j}^{p-1}(u) + \frac{u_{j+p+1} - u}{u_{j+p+1} - u_{j+1}}\, \phi_{i,j+1}^{p-1}(u) \tag{4.8}$$

where the values $u_1 \ldots u_{N+p+1}$ are called *knots* and satisfy $u_j \in [0, 1]$ and $u_{j-1} \leq u_j$. A realistic surface is obtained by employing several adjacent patches and expressing continuity conditions at their boundaries. Such conditions can reflect different degrees of continuity, namely positional continuity (C0), tangential continuity (C1) or curvature continuity (C2), which respectively require continuity of zeroth, first and second derivatives of adjacent parametric patches.

The degree p of the B-spline basis function controls the smoothness of the resulting surface and must be cautiously chosen in order to properly reproduce the desired surface features while avoiding high-degree artifacts, which appear as spurious oscillations typically located in the vicinity of patch boundaries. Compared to polygonal representations, an anatomically realistic surface can be represented by a lower number of NURBS patches and its smoothness, and

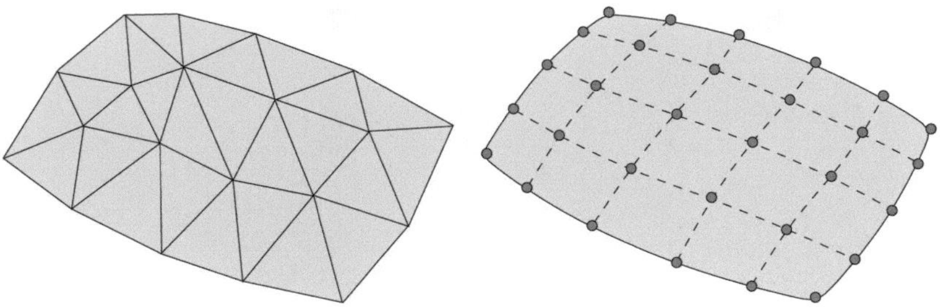

Fig. 4.3. Left, polygonal surface; right, NURBS surface (dashed lines represent isolines of the parameters u, v, while dots represent knots)

consequently the size of the smaller surface features, can be controlled more directly. However, the use of larger patches leads to reduced flexibility in the representable surface topology.

The advantages of the NURBS representation is the interpretation of the vertexes $p_{i,j}$ as a control polygon that permits an intuitive modification of the surface through changes in their position. Additionally, changes in the position of one of the vertexes affects the surface only locally, a desirable feature for CAD systems.

A representation that offers both topological flexibility and direct control over surface smoothness is constituted by *subdivision surfaces.* Since their description is not critical for the contents of this chapter, we refer the reader to specific publications on this matter [561].

4.2.2 Implicit surface representations

In addition to the explicit representation described so far, a surface can also be thought of as embedded in a function $F : \mathbb{R}^3 \to \mathbb{R}$, and represented by describing its embedding. For example, the surface $\mathbf{S}_s$ of a sphere of centre $\mathbf{c}$ and radius r is the locus of points $\mathbf{x} \in \mathbb{R}^3$ where the function $F_s(\mathbf{x}) = (\mathbf{x} - \mathbf{c})^2 - r^2$ is zero. In this case, the surface of the sphere is embedded in the 3D function F_s, that is, $\mathbf{S}_s$ is an isosurface (or the zero level-set) of F_s. The implicit representation of a surface $\mathbf{S}$ therefore becomes

$$\mathbf{S} = \left\{\mathbf{x} \in \mathbb{R}^3 : F(\mathbf{x}) = k\right\} \tag{4.9}$$

where k is a value of choice.

For a realistic vascular surface, the function F is likely not known in closed form. Instead, it can either be given at the nodes of a regular grid or it can be defined as a superposition of analytical basis functions. The simplest example of the first case occurs when the surface of a vessel is assumed to coincide with a particular value of intensity on a clinical image. In this situation, the embedding function F is the image itself I, of which the vascular surface is an isosurface (as shown in Fig. 4.4). Embedding functions known at the nodes of

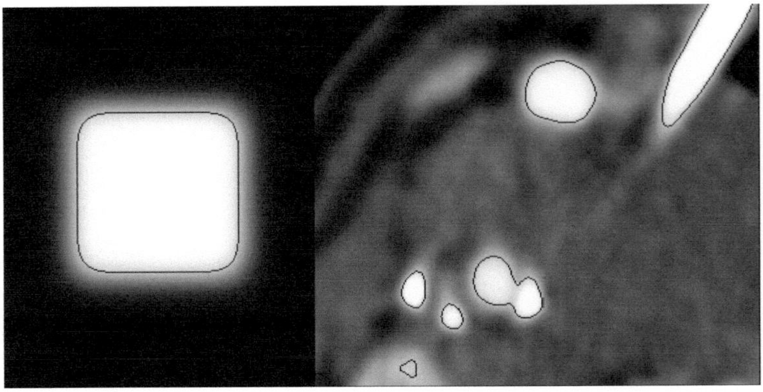

Fig. 4.4. Traces of embedding functions on single imaging planes, along with an explicit representation of one isolevel: left, analytic embedding function; right, medical image as an embedding function

a grid can also be obtained as the result of modelling procedures guided by image features, as shown later in the chapter. For example, in the case of *level sets* (see 4.4.4), the embedding function is generated as the finite differences solution of a PDE [453].

The embedding function is defined as the superposition of analytic functions in the case of *radial basis functions* (RBF), for which the value of a single radial basis function depends solely on the distance from a given location (hence their name). The embedding function in this case is given by

$$F(\mathbf{x}) = P(\mathbf{x}) + \sum_{i=1}^{N} w_i \, \phi(\|\mathbf{x} - \mathbf{x}_i\|) \tag{4.10}$$

where P is a low-degree polynomial function, w_i is a set of weights corresponding to the locations $\mathbf{x}_i$ and ϕ is the basis function. For modelling 3D shapes, radial basis functions take one of the following forms [375]

$$\phi(r) = \begin{cases} r & \text{linear} \\ r^3 & \text{cubic} \\ \exp(-Cr^2) & \text{Gaussian} \\ (r^2 + C^2)^{\frac{1}{2}} & \text{multiquadratic} \\ (r^2 + C^2)^{-\frac{1}{2}} & \text{inverse multiquadratic} \end{cases} \tag{4.11}$$

where $C > 0$ in all expressions. The choice among the various possibilities is performed on the basis of smoothness of the result and on the convergence properties of the numerical method employed to determine the coefficients w_i in Eq. 4.10, as shown in Section 4.5.3. Common choices for representing 3D surfaces have been the linear and the cubic RBFs, the former exhibiting better convergence properties, the latter resulting in a greater surface smoothness [67].

4.2.3 From implicit to explicit surface representations

Most numerical techniques for modelling hemodynamics require explicit geometric representations of the physical domain on which problems are solved. Therefore, we will here describe the operation that allows to obtain explicit representations from implicit ones. Contouring, or isosurface extraction, is the procedure by which an explicit representation of a surface $\mathbf{S}$ is generated from the 3D scalar function F that embeds it.

Marching cubes [299] is a widely used algorithm for generating polygonal explicit surface representations from embedding functions sampled on a regular grid. As already noted, medical images are embedding functions for their isosurfaces, so, provided the isolevel associated to the vascular wall is known (which is usually not true for real world images) Marching Cubes can be used to directly obtain the surface of a vessel (the limitations of this approach will be explained in Section 4.4.2).

The algorithm works on the basic idea that a polygonal surface whose vertexes lie on grid edges can intersect a cubical neighbourhood of the grid and partition its vertexes in a finite number of configurations, 64 reduced to 15 by symmetry, called topological cases.

Thanks to this property, the polygonal surface can be constructed, one cubical neighbourhood at a time, by selecting the topological case corresponding to the local partition of above and below vertexes. Compatibility of the surface from cube to cube is obtained owing to the fact that each couple of neighbouring cubes presents the same vertex partition on the shared face. After the selection of the proper topological case, the exact position of polygon vertexes is obtained by linearly interpolating the values of F along the intersected edges. Once each cubical neighbourhood has been visited, the polygonal explicit surface representation is generated (an example is shown in Fig. 4.5).

A potential problem with this algorithm is that, in a limited number of topological cases, two distinct polygon configurations can give rise to the same cube vertex partition. Since this could break surface continuity if incompatible choices were made for two neighbouring cubes, additional criteria have been proposed to select the case which guarantees topological consistency. This is an acceptable solution in most cases, when the surface to be reconstructed is regular. As an alternative, other methods have been proposed to solve the topological consistency problem, such as Marching Tetrahedra, in which space is subdivided in tetrahedra rather than in cubes, resulting in 16 possible polygonisations reduced to 3 by symmetry [299].

The previous algorithm can be applied whenever the function F is available at the vertexes of a regular grid. If the implicit representation is given analytically under the form of a radial basis function, a possibility for constructing an explicit surface is to sample the radial basis function over a regular grid and extract the isosurface of zero level using marching cubes. Alternatively, it is possible to exploit the analytic nature of F [42]. Instead of relying on

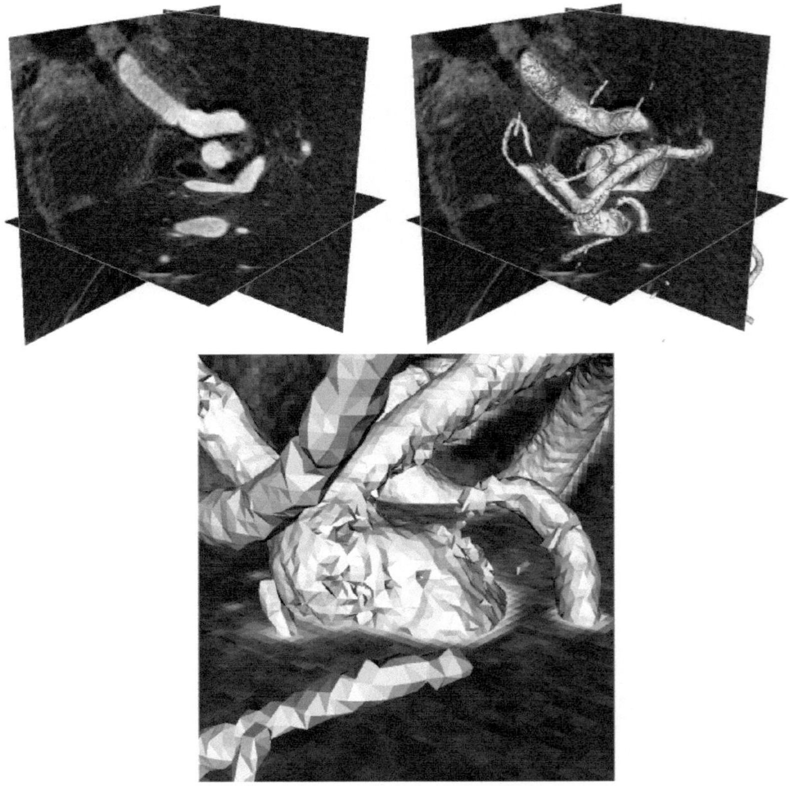

Fig. 4.5. Example of 3D contouring performed with the Marching Cubes algorithm on a CRA image of a cerebral aneurysm. Left, the 3D image; middle, the result of contouring at the level of the transition between the contrast-enhanced vascular lumen and the surrounding tissue; right, a detail showing the appearance of the resulting polygonal surface

a grid of predefined samples which are then linearly interpolated from grid point to grid point, the method takes advantage of the fact that values of F are available at all locations without interpolation, and accurately locates surface points by means of a root finding method in the vicinity of the desired contour value. Aside from this, the polygonisations method utilises similar concepts to those used in marching cubes and marching tetrahedra.

4.3 Image enhancement

In dealing with the problem of building representations of the geometry of blood vessels, we have assumed that the location of their surface was known. We will now start to face the problem of how to actually derive such information from medical images.

Medical images can be affected by noise and artifacts that may interfere with the segmentation process, or the image data may be provided in a form not suitable for the segmentation method of choice, as in the case of anisotropic resolutions, for which the spacing of the imaging grid along different axes is different. In order to alleviate these problems, an imaging enhancement step can be performed prior to segmentation. The introduction of such a step can substantially alter the information contained in an image and potentially play a role in the outcome of haemodynamic modelling. Since such influence is associated in general with a set of user-dependent parameters, care must be taken at defining the minimum amount of image enhancement operations needed for segmentation to be successful.

4.3.1 Resampling

A first pre-segmentation operation we describe is image resampling. Its goal is to change the resolution of the image in one or more imaging axis directions. For modality-dependent reasons, images can be acquired with resolutions that do not match the requirements imposed by the segmentation method of choice. This leads to the need of changing (in most cases, increasing) the spacing of the imaging grid in one or more directions, granted that this operation will in no case increase the information content of the image.

Image resampling therefore consists in projecting image intensity values onto a different grid than the original one. The most common way of performing resampling is to obtain the image values at the new grid points by interpolation from the original imaging grid. The choice of the interpolation operator affects the accuracy of the resampling. If subsampling is needed, interpolation can be preceded by low-pass filtering (see next section) of the original image in order to avoid the generation of artifacts.

Among the available interpolation methods, the most common are nearest neighbour and linear interpolation, which correspond to constant and first order shape functions over the imaging grid. More sophisticated interpolation

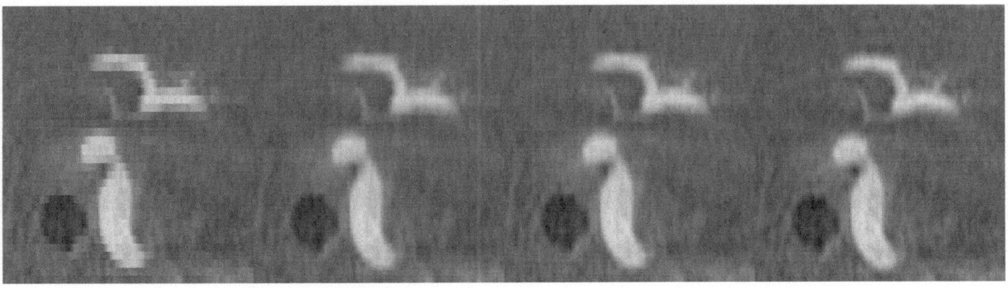

Fig. 4.6. From left to right, CRA image with anisotropic resolution (the number of points along the horizontal direction is four times greater than along the vertical direction), resampled with nearest neighbour, linear, cubic and sinc interpolation

methods include B-spline [514] and windowed sinc interpolation. In the former, a representation of the image based on bell-shaped high-order (typically cubic) polynomials centred at the imaging grid points is first obtained by least squares approximation. The image is then resampled onto the new grid by linear combination of the polynomial basis functions. In the latter, off-grid values are obtained by convolution of the image with a cardinal sine kernel. Convolution of the image I with a kernel K is defined as

$$I * K(\mathbf{x}) = \int_{-\infty}^{\infty} \int_{-\infty}^{\infty} I(\mathbf{x}) \, K(\mathbf{x} - \bar{\mathbf{x}}) \, d\bar{\mathbf{x}}, \tag{4.12}$$

where in this case the kernel is defined as

$$K(\mathbf{x}) = \mathrm{sinc}(\mathbf{x}) = \frac{\sin \mathbf{x}}{\mathbf{x}}. \tag{4.13}$$

For the convolution kernel to have finite support, the cardinal sine function is restricted to a suitable window, hence the name. Since the Fourier transform of the sinc function is the box function, and since the convolution of two functions corresponds to a product in frequency space, this interpolation method corresponds to extending the periphery of the Fourier transform of the original image by a zero-padded region. Although theoretically optimal in terms of Shannon's sampling theory[1], the latter interpolation method can give rise to ringing artifacts around sharp edges. A sample evaluation of the described image interpolation method is shown in Fig. 4.6.

A more sophisticated interpolation method is *adaptive control grid interpolation* [166], which borrows concepts from motion estimation and frame prediction algorithms and aims at reconstructing missing inter-slice information for datasets suffering from highly anisotropic resolutions.

4.3.2 Noise reduction

Noise is generally identified as a random high-frequency signal added or multiplied to the image content. Noise is inherent in any acquisition process and it is ascribable to thermal noise in the signal processing electronics or to physical undesired signal sources. Reduction of noise can be obtained either by means of a smoothing filter, which removes the high-frequency components of the image, or by modelling noise characteristics and filtering them out. In the first case, no prior knowledge about the noise generation process is required, but, on the other hand, meaningful high-frequency image content can be filtered together with noise. In the second case, noise reduction is more specific, even if this depends on the accuracy of noise modelling. The first approach is

---

[1] The Shannon sampling theorem is a well-known result in information theory. Conversion of a continuous function into a numeric sequence is called *sampling*. Shannon theorem (or Nyquist-Shannon theorem) states that a continuous function featuring the highest frequency ν_M is completely determined by a sampling with frequency $2\nu_M$.

the most widely used in vascular modelling from CT and MR images, probably because noise for these modalities has simpler characteristics and signal-to-noise ratio (SNR) is usually fairly high. Moreover, the typical scale of the anatomical structures of interest in CT or MR is often much larger than that of noise. In contrast, more specific approaches are used for B-mode ultrasound image enhancement, which are affected by speckle noise, already introduced in Sect 4.1, whose scale is potentially similar to that of the observed structures.

One of the simplest and most used forms of noise reduction in images is Gaussian filtering. It consists in performing a convolution of the image $I(\mathbf{x})$ with a Gaussian kernel

$$G_\sigma(\mathbf{x}) = \frac{1}{\sqrt{(2\pi\sigma^2)^3}} e^{-\frac{\mathbf{x}^2}{2\sigma^2}} \tag{4.14}$$

where σ is the width of the Gaussian kernel and controls the amount of smoothing, i.e. the maximum spatial frequency represented in the filtered image. An equivalent approach is the simulation of a diffusion process for image intensity values governed by a PDE of the form

$$\frac{\partial I(\mathbf{x},t)}{\partial t} = c\, \Delta I(\mathbf{x},t) \tag{4.15}$$

where c is the diffusivity coefficient which regulates the strength of diffusion. We here underline that this formulation is made possible by the fact that the image is considered as a continuum of intensity values rather than a collection of isolated samples. The PDE is then solved numerically, for instance by using finite differences (see Chapter 2), over the imaging grid up to a time $\bar{t}$. Solving the diffusion equation with c and $\bar{t}$ is analogous to performing a convolution with a Gaussian kernel having $\sigma^2 = 2\,c\,\bar{t}$.

The drawback of the previous approaches is the potential loss of information that results from filtering an image in which signal and noise have similar spatial scales. In particular, objects in images are ideally separated from the background by sharp borders, which have a high frequency content. Smoothing can therefore result in edge blurring and displacement, which can affect both the estimation of surface geometry and alter the topology of the resulting object. In order to limit the effect of smoothing on relevant edges, anisotropic diffusion filtering has been introduced. The idea behind this approach is that smoothing should be stronger in regions dominated by noise, while it should preserve regions in which image features, such as object boundaries, are predominant. Obviously, this would require the definition of object boundaries, which in turn is our ultimate goal. Instead, image features are estimated from the gradient magnitude of the intensity values or by more sophisticated edge-detection techniques. In the standard formulation [384], the anisotropic diffusion equation is given by the following PDE

$$\frac{\partial I}{\partial t} = \nabla \cdot c(|\nabla I|)\, \nabla I \tag{4.16}$$

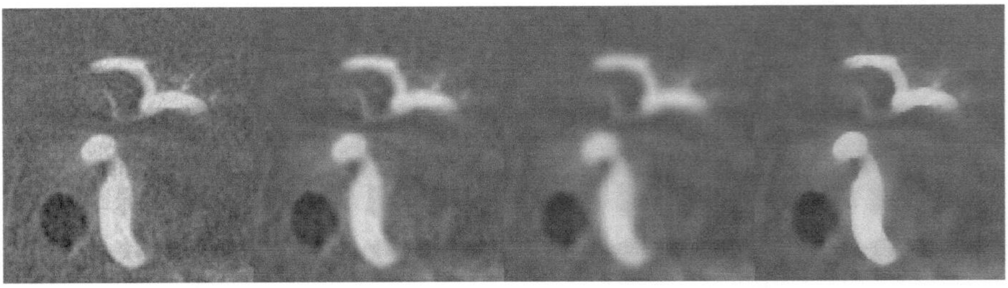

Fig. 4.7. From left to right, CRA image affected by noise, convolved with a Gaussian kernel with $\sigma = 2.5$ pixels, with a Gaussian kernel with $\sigma = 5$ pixels and filtered with anisotropic diffusion with the equivalent of $\sigma = 5$ pixels

where the diffusivity can be expressed as a decreasing function of the image gradient magnitude, such as

$$c(\mathbf{x}, t) = e^{-\left(\frac{|\nabla I|}{k}\right)^2} \tag{4.17}$$

or

$$c(\mathbf{x}, t) = \frac{k^2}{(k^2 + |\nabla I|^2)} \tag{4.18}$$

where k is used to control the relative influence of image features over the diffusion process [384]. This way, the diffusion process preserves those regions at which intensity values vary more rapidly, such as at object edges. The filter must be tuned for specific applications in terms of k and $\bar{t}$. Since the interpretation of the parameters is less straightforward than in the linear case, empirical evaluation of the effects of the filter is necessary.

An interesting variation of the classical anisotropic diffusion equation above is constituted by the *modified curvature diffusion equation* (MCDE) [541]

$$\frac{\partial I}{\partial t} = \nabla \cdot \left(c \, \frac{\nabla I}{|\nabla I|} \right) |\nabla I| \tag{4.19}$$

where diffusivity can take the same form as in the previous case. This equation, which is regarded as the evolution of a *level set* (see Section 4.4.4) analogous to anisotropic diffusion, can be interpreted as a feature-dependent flow of intensity isosurfaces controlled by their curvature, represented by the term $\nabla \cdot \frac{\nabla I}{|\nabla I|}$. This results in a flattening effect on high-curvature image isosurfaces, such as the ones produced by small-scale noise. This filter does not exhibit a feature edge enhancement effect as in the previous case. A sample evaluation of the described noise reduction methods is shown in Fig. 4.7.

4.3.3 Vessel enhancement

While the techniques presented so far can be applied to images independently from their specific content, *a priori* assumptions on the expected appearance of the structures of interest allow to formulate methods targeted at highlighting those structures only, such as *multiscale vessel enhancement* [167]. The aim of this method is to enhance vessel-shaped structures with respect to the rest of the anatomical structures based on the analysis of the eigenvalues of the Hessian matrix $\mathcal{H}$, of the image intensity.

Let's first recall the definition of Hessian matrix of an image at one point,

$$\mathcal{H}_\sigma = \begin{bmatrix} I_{xx} & I_{xy} & I_{xz} \\ I_{yx} & I_{yy} & I_{yz} \\ I_{zx} & I_{zy} & I_{zz} \end{bmatrix} \tag{4.20}$$

where

$$I_{\alpha\beta}(\mathbf{x}) = \sigma^2 \frac{\partial^2 G_\sigma(\mathbf{x})}{\partial\alpha\,\partial\beta} * I(\mathbf{x}) \tag{4.21}$$

that is, the convolution of the image with the second derivative of the Gaussian kernel with width σ. This corresponds to a convolution of $I(\mathbf{x})$ with $G_\sigma(\mathbf{x})$ and taking the second derivatives of the resulting image, which selects from the image the spatial scales above σ.

The basic idea behind the filtering technique is that a tubular structure should be characterised by low intensity variations along the axis of the vessel and by a certain degree of cross-sectional symmetry. In terms of Hessian matrix eigenvalues, denoted as λ_1, λ_2, λ_3 and sorted so that $|\lambda_1| \le |\lambda_2| \le |\lambda_3|$, the idea translates into the fact that, at points inside tubular structures, λ_1 should be low, and λ_2 and λ_3 should be high and of equal sign (negative for bright intensity vessels and positive for dark intensity vessels).

Based on these considerations, vessel enhancement for bright intensity vessels of scale σ can be obtained as the output of the following function

$$\mathcal{V}_\sigma(\mathbf{x}) = \begin{cases} 0 & \text{if } \lambda_2 > 0 \text{ or } \lambda_1 > 0, \\ \left(1 - e^{-\frac{\mathcal{R}_A^2}{2\alpha^2}}\right) e^{-\frac{\mathcal{R}_B^2}{2\alpha^2}} \left(1 - e^{-\frac{\mathcal{S}^2}{2c^2}}\right) & \text{otherwise} \end{cases} \tag{4.22}$$

where $\mathcal{R}_A = \frac{|\lambda_2|}{|\lambda_3|}$, $\mathcal{R}_B = \frac{|\lambda_1|}{\sqrt{|\lambda_2\lambda_3|}}$ and $\mathcal{S} = |\mathcal{H}_\sigma| = \sqrt{\sum_j \lambda_j^2}$. Parameters α, β and c are scaling factors. Since Equation (4.22) depends on the scale σ at which second derivatives are computed, the filter is applied at multiple scales and the optimal scale is selected as the one which yields the maximum filter response, that is $V(\mathbf{x}) = \max_\sigma \mathcal{V}_\sigma(\mathbf{x})$.

Besides being used for highlighting vessels in image datasets, the filter has been successfully employed for automated centreline detection [167], stenosis grading [168, 520], and level sets initialisation for segmentation [119]. Indeed, although effective for vessel detection, the filter does not ensure that the shape of the lumen is not altered, therefore it is more suited in initial phases of vessel identification than in precise location of the vessel wall.

Lastly, it must be noted that this image enhancement approach relies on assumptions that may not be verified for all imaging modalities and vascular segments. For example, the presence of non tubular vascular geometries, like aneurysms, complex bifurcations or calcifications, which in CT images appear brighter than the contrast medium, may give rise to low filter output inside vessels. Moreover, in black blood MRI imaging, the lumen appears dark, the wall is in general bright and the surrounding tissue may again appear dark, which does not lead to cylindrical structures but rather to thick walled hollow ones, which does not comply with the method assumptions.

4.4 Image segmentation for vascular modelling

The task of deriving the shape of an object from a digital image is commonly referred to as image segmentation. In its most classical acception, image segmentation implies that the pixels constituting an image are partitioned into classes corresponding to the objects represented in the image and to the background. In our context, however, the identification of the boundary of a vessel needs to be carried out at sub-pixel precision, for the resulting model to be suitable as the physical domain of a CFD simulation. In this sense, the automatic identification of vessels in an angiographic image is not as important as the accurate determination of the location of the lumen boundary. In fact, while a user can robustly identify the *presence* of a vessel on an image, a *precise* definition of its boundary is a challenging task for an operator in the absence of objective criteria, the implications of which are discussed in the next paragraph. Since the reconstruction of the vessel shape has a great influence in the modelled hemodynamics, as it will be clear in Chapter 5, we will focus on those segmentation techniques geared at accurately and precisely estimating the shape of the lumen rather than those designed for automatically identifying the presence of vessels in an image.

4.4.1 Manual segmentation

Manual placement of points or delineation of contours on single image planes is the first form of segmentation we take into account. This approach is based upon the decisions of an operator who identifies the boundaries of the structures of interest based on visual perception of image content. Obviously, this method is affected by a potentially low reproducibility of the results, especially when the image is of difficult interpretation. On the other hand, for images heavily affected by artifacts of low signal-to-noise ratios this might be the only option, as automated methods may not perform as well as human perception in filling missing information, or, if they did, they may require a large number of user-defined parameters that practically make segmentation completely operator dependent, only in a less intuitive way.

While the use of corrupted images for hemodynamics modelling is questionable regardless of whether manual or automated segmentation is performed, in most cases user-driven point placement or contour delineation is useful as an initial approximation for automated segmentation methods shown in the following sections. For several of such methods, in fact, the closer the initial segmentation is to the target shape, the more straightforward is the segmentation process, although a good segmentation method should be reasonably robust to initialisation.

In general, although operator dependency has to be minimised, completely automated segmentation of real-world medical images is arguably not a strict requirement for haemodynamic modelling, at least not as the requirement of locating the position of the vessel wall as accurately and reproducibly as possible. Rather, this is achieved by adopting a segmentation method based on mathematical methods, while allowing the user to steer the segmentation process, therefore integrating human perception with objective image-based criteria.

4.4.2 Thresholding and classification

The term thresholding refers to the identification of one or more image intensity values that separate the anatomical structures of interest from the background. The determination of thresholds can be performed manually or algorithmically, and it can take place once for the whole 3D image or on a slice-by-slice basis. The latter approach is necessary when the signal is not uniform among the slices, such as in TOF-MRA, in which the signal depends on the amount of flowing blood, or in CTA, in which the density of the contrast agent can vary during the acquisition, resulting in a change in intraluminal signal along the z-axis. Once one or more thresholds have been selected, thresholding can either proceed by generating a classified image containing discrete labels based on the relative positions of the original image intensities with respect to the threshold set, or, in case only one threshold has been defined, by performing contouring on the image at the threshold isolevel and generating an explicit representation of the corresponding surface.

Since clinical imaging techniques do not associate a precise intensity value to a particular tissue class, manual thresholding can present several shortcomings if geometry has a great impact on the subsequent analysis, as in the case of vascular modelling. The choice of a threshold intensity level strongly affects the size and the topology of the resulting surface, since the vascular lumen is characterised by strong spatial variations of image intensity compared to uniform tissue regions, and therefore the sensitivity of the resulting surface to the chosen threshold is high.

It is therefore of crucial importance to identify objective criteria capable to define thresholds corresponding to the vascular lumen boundaries. One of them, and the most used in the clinical setting, is the *full width at half maximum* (FWHM) criterion, which identifies the lumen boundary at an intensity level, I_{FWHM}, halfway between the peak intensity within the lumen and the intensity of the background (see Fig. 4.8). This criterion is mostly used for measuring vessel diameters by plotting image intensity along a line that crosses a vessel and measuring the distance between points at I_{FWHM} on both sides of

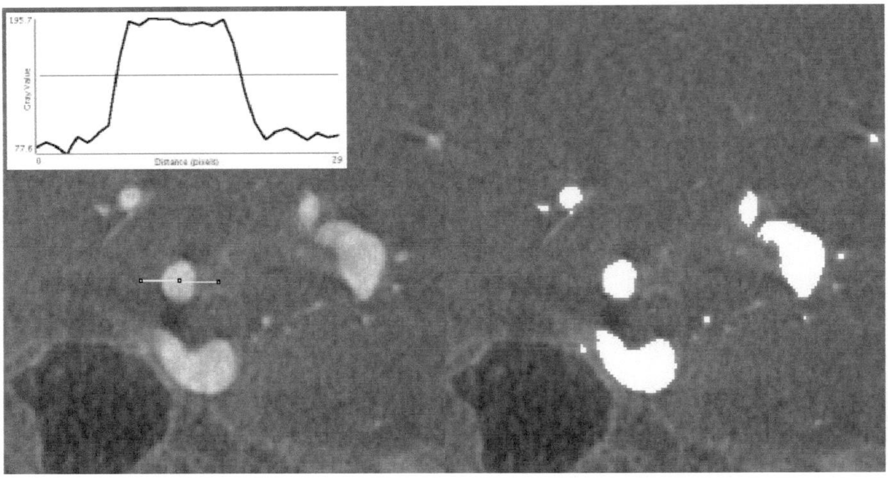

Fig. 4.8. Full width at half maximum (FWHM) criterion applied to a CRA image. Image intensities along the traced line are plotted at the upper left corner. On the right, the image is thresholded at the FWHM value

the lumen. This method has been proven to yield accurate estimates of diameters even for small vessels, for example, in TOF-MRA, while in PC-MRA the *full width at 10 %* criterion has been shown to be more accurate [225]. However, the FWHM criterion is sensitive to the definition of the peak lumen intensity, which could change with the location and the vessel size, and of the background, which in clinical images might consist of anatomical structures of heterogeneous intensities.

In contrast to the FWHM criterion, which is a local criterion, statistical thresholding methods seek to determine optimal thresholds from the distribution of intensity values over the whole image. A popular choice among statistical thresholding methods is Otsu's algorithm [362]. The method seeks to partition the image intensity histogram into classes in such a way that the between-class variance is maximised, where the between-class variance is defined as

$$\sigma_b^2 = \sum_{i=1}^{N_c} \omega_i (\mu_i - \mu)^2 \qquad (4.23)$$

where N_c is the number of classes, ω_i is the probability of a pixel of belonging to the i-th class, μ_i is the mean intensity of the i-th class and μ the overall image intensity. This method has been employed in [375] to segment vessels from TOF-MRA images.

Several other statistical criteria can be used for determining thresholds that respond to different optimality criteria, such as K-means and expectation maximisation for the estimation of mixture models, to cite a few [386].

Available statistical methods for pixel classification differ widely from pure thresholding methods, and assign each pixel to a particular anatomical tissue class based on other criteria, such as adjacency relationships, Markov random fields, or prior information about shape [386]. The vast amount of literature on this topic cannot be covered here. It only has to be stressed that most classification criteria work at the pixel level, so that the sub-pixel positioning of the vessel boundary must be sought in a post-classification stage, following smoothness criteria or optimising the position of the surface on the basis of image features, as with deformable models, described later on. In this sense, classification methods can also be employed as automatic initialisation for deformable models.

4.4.3 Region growing and front propagation

While classification methods typically produce a segmentation of the whole image, the interest in vascular modelling is typically to segment vascular structures. Region growing methods generate selective segmentations starting from a pre-segmented region (or single pixel) and iteratively add neighbouring pixels to the region if they satisfy specified homogeneity criteria. The procedure stops when no more pixels can be added to the region. The initialisation is usually performed interactively, and the resulting segmentation clearly depends on the homogeneity criterion adopted. Such criterion is commonly related to the intensity of the pixel under scrutiny with respect to the pixels belonging to the segmented region. The simplest criterion consists of accepting the pixel if its intensity lies between a pair of user-defined thresholds. A more conservative criterion states that a pixel is included if its intensity and that of its neighbours fall between user-defined thresholds. In both these cases, the criterion does not vary throughout the growth. In a more sophisticated approach, the pixel is accepted if its probability of belonging to the region is above a certain threshold. For instance, under the assumption that the intensities of the pixels belonging to the segmented structure are normally distributed around a central value, a pixel is accepted in the region if its intensity lies in the interval $[\mu - f\sigma, \mu + f\sigma]$, where μ and σ are the mean and standard deviation of the pixel intensity in the segmented region and f a user-defined factor expressing the permissiveness of the criterion [241]. Since they consist in adding individual pixels to the segmented region, region growing methods are not capable of delivering sub-pixel precision. However, the final shape can eventually be smoothed (which does not ensure sub-pixel precision, but at least produces a realistic surface) and they can also be fruitfully employed as initialisation tools for deformable models.

A conceptually related approach to region growing is represented by front propagation methods. This approach is based on tracking the propagation of a wavefront from a seed point over the image. The speed of the wave is regulated by image features, and is typically set to be lower in regions where the image intensity varies more rapidly and higher where the image is uniform. The purpose is to make the front move rapidly towards the vessels while slowing down as it approaches vessel boundaries. The most popular front propagation algorithm is represented by the fast marching method, which provides an efficient solution to the eikonal equation

$$\|\nabla T(\mathbf{x})\| = F(\mathbf{x}) \qquad \text{with } F(\mathbf{x}) > 0 \tag{4.24}$$

where $T(\mathbf{x})$ represents the first arrival time of the wave at a point of the domain and $F(\mathbf{x})$ is the reciprocal of the local wavefront speed. In other words, we are looking for the spatial distribution of the arrival times of a wave of given local speed. Once the initial front and $F(\mathbf{x})$ are defined, the eikonal equation is solved on the image grid using upwind finite differences. A more efficient solution of the eikonal equation can be achieved by only tracking the solution in a narrow band of pixels defined around the front. Once computed, the isocontours of $T(\mathbf{x})$ represent a collection of surfaces describing the shape of the waveform during the propagation. It is the user's responsibility to select the value of $T(\mathbf{x})$ that captures the desired surface. Since it produces a continuous function, this front propagation method is able to deliver sub-pixel precision. In practise, though, the fact that the front only slows down without actually stopping on the vessels boundary makes the use of this method alone not particularly robust for segmentation, since the shape of the segmented vessel will depend on the choice of the contouring value of $T(\mathbf{x})$. In other words, the method lacks an objective criterion for defining the location of the boundary of vessels based on image intensity. Nevertheless, this method is very effective for the initialisation of deformable models, which will be the subject of the next section.

4.4.4 Deformable models

Deformable models are curves or surfaces defined in the image space which change their shape on the basis of image features, external constraints and internal deformation laws [319]. This way, the position of a curve or a surface can be optimised to identify the position of lumen boundary with sub-pixel precision.

Deformable models are not conceptually different from other segmentation methods: they serve to identify the position of the boundary of the shape of interest from the information contained in an image. Their peculiarity lies in the fact that the segmentation problem is treated as an energy minimisation problem, where the energy depends on the position and shape of the curve or surface and on image features. The fact that the minimisation process proceeds through deformation of the model towards its final shape presents two main advantages: the evolution can be followed and eventually steered in an intuitive way, and the initialisation can be performed by providing a good geometric approximation to the final shape. Being an optimisation process, segmentation with deformable models makes it possible to establish a trade-off between local adherence to image features and global criteria (e.g. regularity of the resulting shape), thus allowing a control over the single contributions to the final result.

From a formal point of view, the energy functional can be expressed as the sum of an internal and an external energy

$$\mathcal{E} = \mathcal{E}_{int} + \mathcal{E}_{ext}. \tag{4.25}$$

The internal energy term governs how the model changes its shape, for example it can confer a membrane or thin plate-like behaviour to the model, or control its regularity in terms of smoothness. External energy terms include image-based terms and positional constraints. The former drive the deformation based on the features the underlying image, for example inflating the model with different speeds according to image intensity, or attracting the model towards edges, while the latter serve to steer the evolution of the model with user-defined rules, e.g. to avoid specific regions of the image in the presence of artifacts or to help the convergence of the model to the features of interest.

Deformable models can be employed both in 2D, i.e. deformable contours on planar images, or in 3D, i.e. deformable surfaces in a 3D image, depending on the nature of the data (disjoint images or thick slice imaging typically require 2D deformable models) and the geometry of the structures to reconstruct (vascular networks of complex geometry are more challenging to segment in sequences of 2D sections). Furthermore, the choice is also dictated by the need of user interaction for steering the evolution of the deformable model, e.g. in order to avoid the erroneous segmentation of flow-related artifacts arising in black blood MRI. Since interaction with a contour on a 2D slice is simpler than that with a surface within a 3D volume, 2D segmentation is often preferred in this case.

There are two major classes of deformable models, which correspond to the way the curve or surface is represented, namely *explicit* and *implicit* deformable models. Recalling the distinction made in Section 4.2, a surface $\mathbf{S}$ can be given by explicitly describing the position of its points or by describing an embedding function the surface is an isosurface of. In this perspective, the evolution of a deformable model can either be represented by explicitly tracking the position of its points, of by tracking changes in the embedding function. In the next two sections, the two approaches, along with their strengths and limitations, will be described independently from the specific form that $\mathcal{E}_{int}$ and $\mathcal{E}_{ext}$ can take. Subsequently, a description of image-based and internal forces applicable for both deformable model approaches will be provided.

Explicit deformable models

For explicit deformable models the position of surface points is explicitly represented and tracked during the evolution. In this case, the minimisation of Equation (4.25) acts on $\mathbf{S}(\mathbf{u})$, that is, on the way points in the parametric space are mapped onto the image space.

Two popular versions of explicit deformable models in 2D are *discrete dynamic contours* (DDC) and deformable splines, both commonly referred to as *snakes*. DDC are polylines, i.e. nodes connected by straight segments, whose deformation is expressed in terms of the change in the nodal coordinates. Deformable splines are instead piecewise polynomials with continuity constraints, each polynomial piece described by a set of control points. DDC are in general more flexible in terms of topology and easier to handle from a computational point of view, being described by nodal coordinates expressed in physical space. On the other hand, splines require fewer control points and implicitly incorporate internal constraints on their smoothness during the evolution. The choice between the two is in general application-dependent.

The general expression of the internal energy of a 2D snake is

$$\mathcal{E}_{int} = \int (w_1|\frac{\partial \mathbf{S}}{\partial u}|^2 + w_2|\frac{\partial^2 \mathbf{S}}{\partial u^2}|^2)du, \tag{4.26}$$

where u is the arclength, the first and second terms in the integral represent the snake's tension and stiffness, respectively. The relative contributions of the two terms are controlled by the weights w_1, w_2, chosen by the user on the basis of image characteristics. The external energy is in general expressed through the definition of a image-dependent potential

$$\mathcal{E}_{ext} = \int w_3 P(\mathbf{S})du. \tag{4.27}$$

More details on the choice of P will be given in Section 4.4.4. An example of snake evolution is shown in Fig. 4.9.

The minimisation of $\mathcal{E}$ in Equation (4.25) can be worked out either directly in its energetic form, e.g using a gradient descent minimisation approach on $\mathcal{E}$, or in its local form, by directly expressing the problem in terms of the evolution of the position of physical points of $\mathbf{S}$ with respect to u, leading to the evolution equation

$$\frac{\partial \mathbf{S}}{\partial t} = w_1\frac{\partial^2 \mathbf{S}}{\partial u^2} - w_2.\frac{\partial^4 \mathbf{S}}{\partial u^4} - w_3\nabla P(\mathbf{S}). \tag{4.28}$$

For DDC, a simple way to discretise equation 4.28 is by means of finite differences in the form of a *spring-mass* analogy, by which nodes are assigned a mass m, and the linear segments linking adjacent nodes are associated a stiffness. The nodal evolution equation for DDC is then expressed as [266]

$$m\,\mathbf{a} = w_{ext}\,\mathbf{f}_{ext} + w_{int}\,\mathbf{f}_{int} + w_d\,\mathbf{x}' \tag{4.29}$$

where $\mathbf{a}$ is the acceleration of nodes, $\mathbf{f}_{ext}$ and $\mathbf{f}_{int}$ are the external and internal forces applied to them, and the last term represents damping, introduced in order to avoid the set up of oscillations during the DCC evolution. The weights w_{ext}, w_{int} and w_d are again user-defined parameters.

The 3D counterparts of 2D snakes, commonly regarded as *balloons*, comprise deformable meshes and deformable spline surfaces. The considerations for the 3D case as well as the mathematical treatment of the energy terms

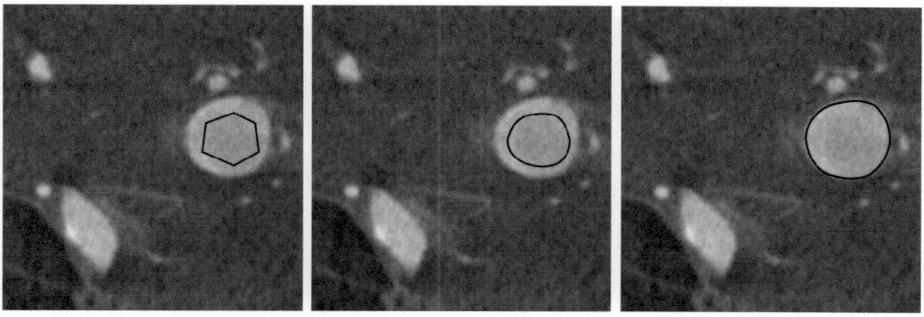

Fig. 4.9. Evolution of a 2D snake. Left, initialisation by interactive definition of the vertexes of a polygonal line; middle, refinement (or spline interpolation) under a smoothness constraint; right, deformation under the action of external image-based forces

and the minimisation problem are not substantially different from the 2D case. The parameter space is now represented by a bidimensional vector (u, v), and the internal energy terms represent local surface stretching and bending. As in the 2D case, the evolution of deformable meshes has been implemented resorting to the spring-mass analogy, although more sophisticated approaches based on the same idea assign a stiffness to the triangular mesh elements considered as solid surface elements rather than to their edges only [97, 318]. A typical evolution equation for an explicit 3D deformable model is

$$\frac{\partial \mathbf{S}}{\partial t} = w_1 G(\mathbf{S})\,\mathbf{N} + w_2 \Delta \mathbf{S} - w_3 \nabla P(\mathbf{S}) \tag{4.30}$$

in which the first term models inflation, by which the surface deforms along its normals with speed $G(\mathbf{S})$, the second term represents rigidity and the third term the action of an external force expressed as the gradient of a potential P, in general function of image features.

Specialised deformable models have been proposed for segmentation of vascular structures [167, 551]. In particular, Frangi et al [167] proposed the use of tensor-product B-splines in which one dimension is periodic and whose control points are constrained to move radially with respect to the estimated centreline, so that the deformable model maintains a cylindrical shape throughout the evolution. Similarly, but improving the behaviour of the model to bending, Yim et al [551] presented a *tubular deformable model*, consisting in a deformable mesh whose surface points are described in terms of radial distance and angle around the vessel axis, and are constrained to deform along radial lines. The main strength of these approaches is also their limitation, in that non-tubular vascular structures, such as complex bifurcations or aneurysms, are not easily reconstructed.

The main difficulty when dealing with explicit deformable models is the fact that they rely on specific parametric representations of $\mathbf{S}(\mathbf{u})$. In principle, the parametric space is fixed during the evolution; only the mapping from

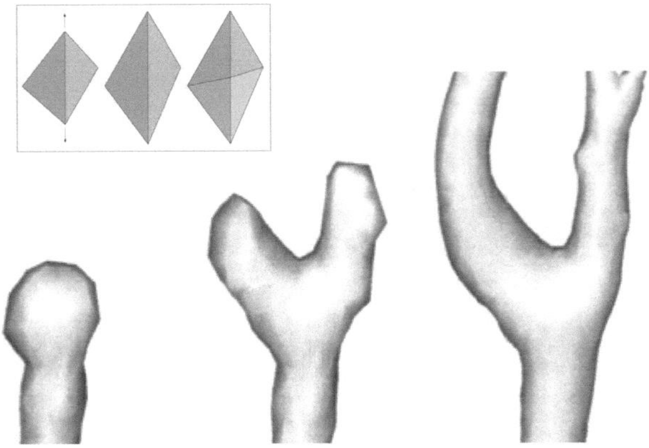

Fig. 4.10. Evolution of a polygonal balloon inflating under image-dependent forces. The surface is re-parametrised during the evolution to account for large deformations: if a triangle has one edges exceeding a threshold length, the two triangles sharing the edge are replaced by four smaller triangles (shown in the box)

the parametric space to the physical space is updated. In other words, a triangle in a polygonal balloon is allowed to have its nodal coordinates, but not its connectivity relationships with neighbouring triangles, updated during evolution. When the deformable model evolves, large deformations can occur, and the mapping from parametric to physical space can degenerate, or not be sufficiently refined to properly represent the underlying geometry. This issue is overcome with the introduction of re-parametrisation criteria, such as those employed by Ladak et al [265], which allow the mesh to be dynamically refined as the model undergoes large deformations. In particular, if the length of a triangle edge exceeds a user-defined threshold, the edge is split in two by the insertion of an additional node, and the two triangles sharing the edge are replaced by four triangles sharing the inserted node, as shown in Fig. 4.10 (see also Section 4.11.4).

The need for re-parametrisation is not only linked to large deformations. The initial topology of the deformable model may not correspond to that of the target shape. As an example, when an initially spherical model enters into two separate branches that merge back together, the model topology must change from that of a sphere to that of a torus, requiring an intersection detection phase followed by a global re-parameterisation. The problem of merging triangulated surface meshes has been addressed by Cebral et al [71] as a post-processing step. Topology-adaptive deformable models have also been proposed [320], for which the position of the deformable model is tracked on a background regular grid made up of simplexes (triangles in 2D and tetrahedra in 3D). Collision detection is performed by keeping track of the intersections of the surface on the grid; topology changes are then obtained by re-triangulating the surface from the grid once self-intersections have been removed.

Implicit deformable models

As discussed previously, a surface $\mathbf{S}$ can be represented implicitly as the iso-surface of a function F defined over $\mathbb{R}^3$ with values in $\mathbb{R}$. Therefore, the description of an implicitly represented deformable surface is given by tracking changes in the embedding function. The resulting implicit deformable model is commonly referred to as level set [453].

The link between the deformation of $\mathbf{S}$ and the evolution of F is given by the fact that, by definition, $\mathbf{S}$ remains a level set of F over time. Therefore,

$$\frac{\partial F(\mathbf{S})}{\partial t} = -\nabla F(\mathbf{S}) \cdot \frac{\partial \mathbf{S}}{\partial t} = -\left|\nabla F(\mathbf{S})\right| \frac{\partial \mathbf{S}}{\partial t} \cdot \mathbf{N} \tag{4.31}$$

where $\mathbf{N} = \frac{\nabla F}{|\nabla F|}$.

By substituting Equation (4.30) into Equation (4.31) and re-expressing all the terms in terms of F, the evolution of explicit 3D deformable models is turned in implicit form

$$\frac{\partial F(\mathbf{x})}{\partial t} = w_1 G(\mathbf{x})|\nabla F| - 2w_2 H(\mathbf{x})|\nabla F| - w_3 \nabla P(\mathbf{x}) \cdot \nabla F \tag{4.32}$$

in which $G(\mathbf{x})$ is inflation speed, $H(\mathbf{x}) = \nabla \cdot \frac{\nabla F}{|\nabla F|}$ is level set curvature and $P(\mathbf{x})$ a scalar potential whose gradient is the external force. The weights w_1, w_2 and w_3 are user-defined parameters controlling the influence of the respective terms. The evolution equation for implicit deformable models is solved over the whole image domain by means of upwind finite differences, a numerical approximation scheme which takes into account the direction of propagation of level sets when computing derivatives, avoiding smearing out of the solution. Once an implicit deformable model has completed its evolution, contouring can be performed on $F(\mathbf{x})$ at its zero level to obtain an explicit representation of the vessel surface. An example of level set evolution is shown in Fig. 4.11.

Implicit deformable models offer some advantages relative to their explicit counterparts. The most evident among these is topology independence, as there is no restriction on the evolution of the model in terms of representable topology or topology changes: a branch can merge with a neighbour at no computational cost or increased algorithmic complication during evolution. Another key advantage is that large deformations can be achieved without the need of re-parameterisation, since deformation is simply expressed as a change in the value of $F(\mathbf{x})$. Moreover, the evolution equation does not depend on the dimensionality of the problem, so an implicit deformable model can easily be described in N dimensions (e.g. space and time), allowing to write evolution equations for segmenting 3D time-resolved datasets. One last advantage is that the notion of surface interior and exterior is known throughout the evolution, making it easier to eventually incorporate region-based terms in the evolution equations.

Computational cost is one of the disadvantages of this approach, since in the general level sets framework a whole 3D volume must be evolved to

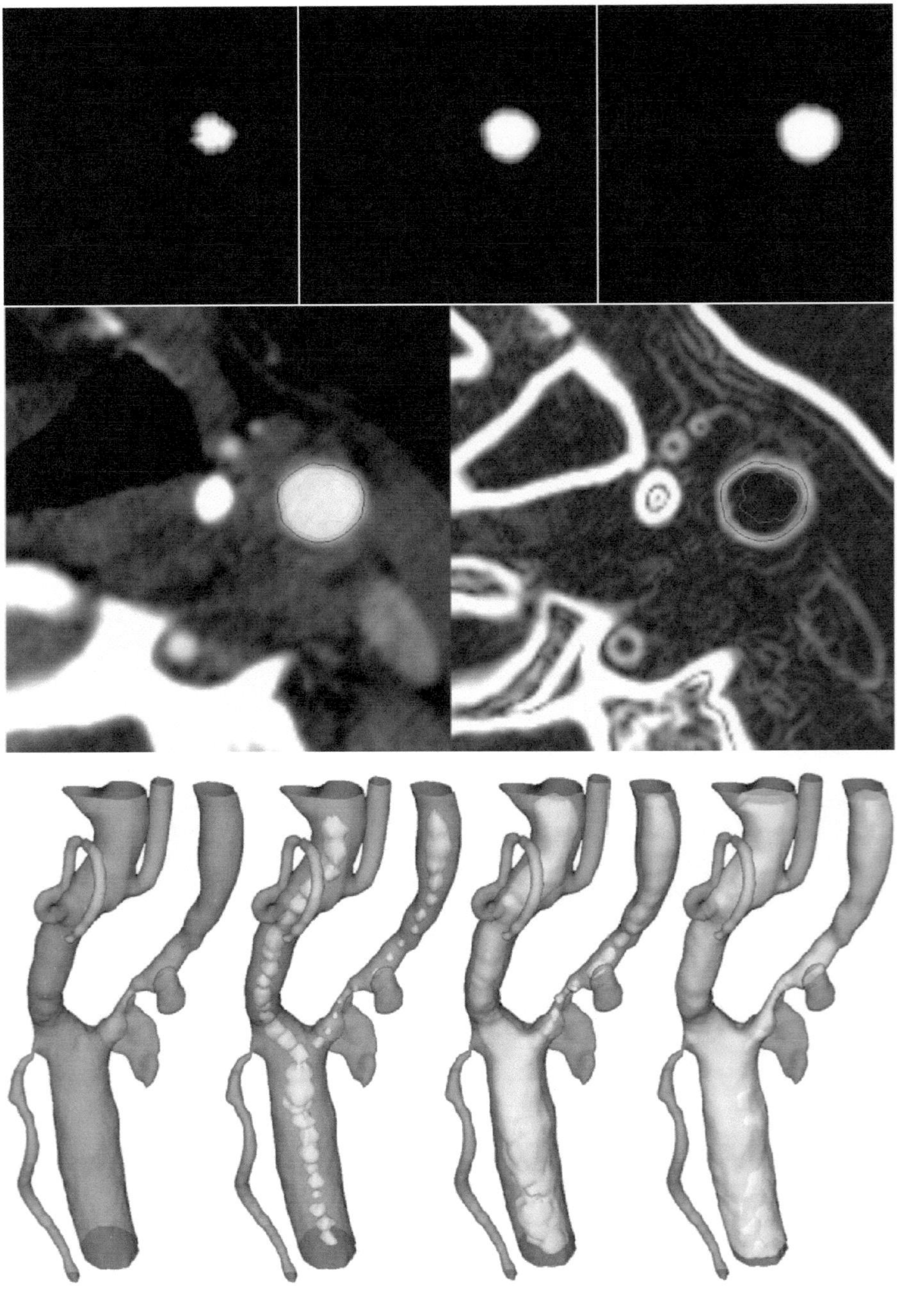

Fig. 4.11. Evolution of level sets under inflation dependent on image gradient magnitude. The top row shows the evolution of the embedding function $F(\mathbf{x})$; the mid row the corresponding zero level sets over the image (top left) and the image gradient magnitude (top right); the bottom row shows the 3D results of level set evolution, initialised from a set of disjoint seeds

track a 2D surface. In order to gain in efficiency, sparse field and narrow band methods have been proposed [540], in which only a few layers of grid points are evolved around the level set of interest, making computational cost depend on the 2D surface size rather on the size of the whole 3D embedding. One more disadvantage, which is a flip side of topology independence, is the fact that control over topology (e.g. in order to avoid self intersections or merging of neighbouring vessels) is not handled naturally by the framework.

Driving forces for deformable models

Here we now describe the image-based external force terms driving the evolution of both explicit and implicit deformable models by inflation and attraction. As a general modelling strategy, inflation terms serve to make the deformable model approach the vessel boundary from its initial shape, while attraction terms are used to make the model converge on the vessel boundary. Inflation speed terms must be crafted so that the expansion is faster in homogeneous regions (i.e. inside the lumen) and slower on vessel boundaries, while attraction terms have to be expressed as vectors pointing to image features with sub-voxel precision. In this framework, it must be noted that the role of inflation terms can be partially or completely replaced with proper initialisation strategies, such as thresholding, region growing or front propagation.

The formulation of external forces depends on the definition of image feature, which in our case must coincide with the boundary of the vessels. The most widely employed image feature definition for the segmentation of angiographic images is image gradient magnitude, $|\nabla I(\mathbf{x})|$, which quantifies the variations in local image intensity and thus highlights tissue interfaces, such as vessel boundaries. Being based on first derivatives of image intensity, gradient magnitude is likely to be sensitive to noise. Moreover, the *capture radius* of gradient magnitude can be small, that is, the model surface must be close to the vessel boundary for a gradient magnitude-based force to have an effect. For these reasons, smoothed versions of gradient magnitude are eventually employed, generated by convolving $I(\mathbf{x})$ with the gradient of a Gaussian kernel with width σ. This reduces noise and increases the capture radius to σ. Alternatively, in order to reduce the effect of noise, edge preserving smoothing can be employed [309]. In any case, the use of effective initialisation strategies can mitigate the need for an increase in capture radius and decrease the influence of noise in the deformable model evolution.

For the formulation of inflation speed terms, it is necessary to associate lower speeds to higher gradient magnitude values, as shown in Fig. 4.12. Possible choices are therefore

$$G(\mathbf{x}) = \frac{1}{1 + |\nabla I(\mathbf{x})|} \tag{4.33}$$

or

$$G(\mathbf{x}) = e^{-|\nabla I(\mathbf{x})|}. \tag{4.34}$$

As alternative formulations of the speed term, we cite the use of the function $V(\mathbf{x})$ previously presented in Section 4.3.3. With this approach, the deformable model is allowed to inflate at a higher speed in regions of high $V(\mathbf{x})$, while its inflation is slowed down as V decreases. Model speed is therefore adequately expressed by $G(\mathbf{x}) = V(\mathbf{x})$, as in [119]. In [519], the authors employ an intensity-based speed term by first fitting two normal distributions, $\mathcal{N}_v$ and $\mathcal{N}_b$, to the histograms of CE-MRA images, modelling vessel and background voxel statistics separately. Inflation speed is then expressed by

$$G(\mathbf{x}) = \frac{p_v(\mathbf{x}) - p_b(\mathbf{x})}{p_v(\mathbf{x}) + p_b(\mathbf{x})} \tag{4.35}$$

where p_v and p_b are the probabilities of a voxel of belonging to background and voxel classes, respectively, computed on the basis of $\mathcal{N}_v$ and $\mathcal{N}_b$. In another work, van Bemmel et al [520] translated the FWHM approach used in clinical settings (see Section 4.4.2) into a level set term which replaces the usual gradient based inflation speed term. The justification is to increase robustness to noise and outliers, although constraints on image acquisition modality (CE-MRA) and on the absence of flow artifacts have to be introduced. The proposed speed term is

$$G_{\text{FWHM}}(\mathbf{x}) = -1 + \frac{2}{\sigma\sqrt{2\pi}} \int_0^{I(\mathbf{x})} e^{-\frac{1}{2}(\xi - \frac{1}{2}\frac{I_{\max}(\mathbf{x})}{\sigma})} \, d\xi \tag{4.36}$$

that is the error function scaled between -1 and 1. $I_{\max}(\mathbf{x})$ is the maximum intensity value in a circular region measured in a plane perpendicular to the vessel centreline.

In contrast to inflation speed terms, attraction terms are usually formulated as gradients of a potential. Model evolution is aimed at minimising energy, therefore at seeking potential minima. Such potential can be expressed as a decreasing function of image features. The classical formulation is made in terms of image gradient magnitude as $P(\mathbf{x}) = |\nabla I(\mathbf{x})|$. Regions corresponding to at greater spatial variations in intensity levels are therefore valleys of the potential. The resulting image-based force field

$$\nabla P(\mathbf{x}) = \nabla |\nabla I(\mathbf{x})| \tag{4.37}$$

has its vectors pointing towards the valleys of $-|\nabla I(\mathbf{x})|$ (as shown in Fig. 4.12). This formulation therefore translates the criterion according to which the transition between two tissues coincides with the steepest variation in intensity values. Although this is not necessarily verified for all acquisition modalities and resolutions, this constitutes a well-accepted and rather accurate criterion. Again, the distance at which the force field acts depends on the width of the ridges, which can be increased by smoothing, at the price of a lower accuracy in the identification of boundaries. A multiresolution approach can also be employed in which the width σ of smoothing kernels is initially high, and is then decreased to regain accuracy.

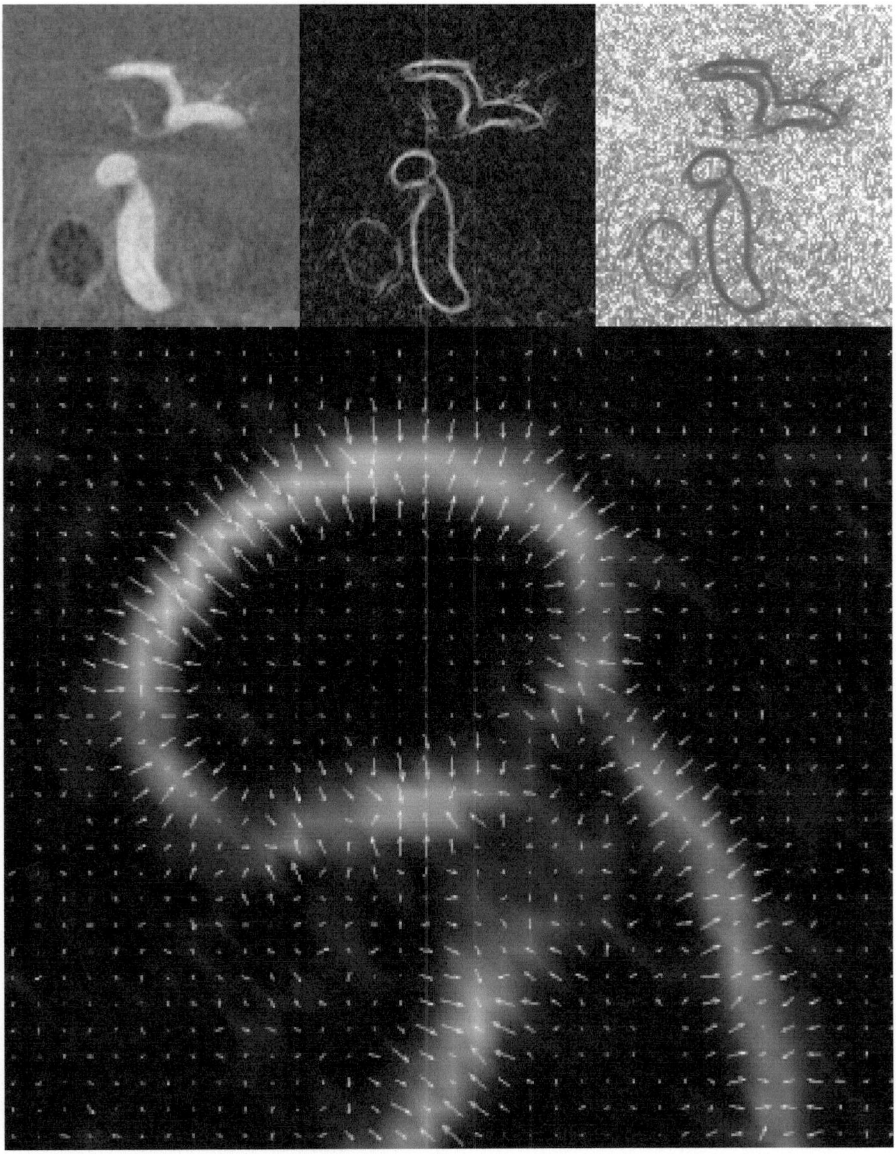

Fig. 4.12. Top left, original image; top mid, gradient magnitude image; top right, inflation speed image, obtained as $(1 + |\nabla I(\mathbf{x})|)^{-1}$; bottom, attraction field vectors $(\nabla(|\nabla I(\mathbf{x})|))$ superimposed to the gradient magnitude image, pointing to the ridges of gradient magnitude

4.5 Surface reconstruction

As extensively showed in the previous sections, the identification of the geometry of vascular structures on images can be either performed directly in 3D, or performed on a sequence of 2D images and subsequently reconstructed in 3D. In this latter case, the position of the vascular surface is known at disjoint locations, such as at a series of lines or a set of points in space, e.g. arising from tracing contours or from placing points on 2D images. In these cases, continuous representations of 3D surfaces must be generated from sparse data, a problem commonly referred to as surface reconstruction.

4.5.1 Lofting

Lofting is the procedure by which an explicit representation of a continuous surface is obtained from a set of disconnected lines. Such lines can for example be obtained as contours of the vascular lumen identified on different 2D imaging planes. These can in turn be parallel to each other, such as in conventional MR or CT, or non-parallel, as in intravascular ultrasound or freehand 3D ultrasound.

A simple lofting procedure consists in connecting each couple of successive contours by straight lines defining triangle edges. Corresponding triangle vertexes can be located along the contours based on their mutual distance, although this criterion can lead to distortion of the resulting surface in presence of abrupt changes in the shape of successive contours. One more difficulty is the generation of the lofted surface in presence of bifurcations, when one contour in one plane splits into two in the following plane.

A similar lofting technique consists in fitting a bivariate polynomial surface patch to the contour set. The surface patch is defined as a tensor-product bivariate polynomial $\mathbf{S}(u, v)$ where the parametric space is rectilinear in the longitudinal direction, $u \in [0, 1]$, and periodic in the circumferential direction, $v \in [0, 2\pi]$. The patch is fitted along the whole vessel with a least squares technique. Similar to the lofting procedure described above, geometric criteria are introduced in order to avoid that the circumferential parameterisation twists around the vessel [536]. The smoothness of the polynomial function allow the contours to be spaced by a greater amount than in the linear lofting case described above. This technique can notably deal with contours lying on non parallel planes, such as those obtained from IVUS images (see Section 4.1).

As already noted, the lofting approaches introduced so far are not suited to handle bifurcations. In other words, the topology of the surface has the requirement of being cylindrical, that is, it must be parameterisable by a rectangular parametric space in which one coordinate is periodic. Several approaches have been introduced to deal with the problem of bifurcating contours.

A technique used in [536] consists in fitting each bifurcation branch separately and prolonging it into the parent vessel. The interpenetrating surfaces are then clipped and stitched at the intersection lines. This method has the disadvantage of yielding non-smooth surfaces at seam lines. For this reason, this method is not recommended for modelling Y-shaped bifurcations, while it can be used to model T-shaped branches in which the parent vessel is much larger than the side branch. Even in this case, the non-realistic discontinuities in the orientation of normals at seam lines lead to models in which locations of particular physio-pathological interest, such as branches, are non-realistically reproduced.

Generic lofting algorithms capable of handling complex topologies are available in several CAD packages, and permit the user to generate free-form surfaces by controlling the shape of a set of contours. As such, they can be employed to generate surfaces from contours delineated on medical images. However, the generic nature of these solutions requires a certain degree of interaction and user skill to generate the desired surfaces, such as the placement of landmarks and editing of surface topology, at the expense of operator-independence and reproducibility.

A lofting technique that has gained popularity for 3D reconstruction of anatomical shapes from sets of parallel contours is the one proposed by Geiger [185] and implemented in the public domain software Nuages. Contours are first filled with triangles by means of a Delaunay tessellation approach (see next paragraph and Section 4.11) [165]. Subsequently, triangles on every contour are connected to the adjacent contour to form a set tetrahedra whose boundary, after a clean-up step, forms the final surface. Since one layer of tetrahedra is generated between each couple of contours, the smoothness of the final surface depends on the spacing between contours. This aspect can be improved with the use of subdivision methods in a post-processing step.

One more possibility for obtaining a continuous surface from a series of parallel contours is represented by *shape based interpolation* [422]. This method generates an implicit surface representation either from a series of closed contours or from a series of binary images generated using a segmentation technique. The implicit representation is given as a set of 2D images containing the value of the minimum distance of each pixel to the contours, referred to as the distance function. Since the contours are assumed to be closed, each distance value is given a positive or negative sign depending on whether the pixel is located inside or outside the contour, resulting in the so-called signed distance function. The computed signed distance function is then interpolated in 3D space by means of trilinear or higher-order interpolants. The final surface is the zero level-set of the resulting interpolated signed distance field.

4.5.2 Polygonisations of point sets

In a typical surface reconstruction, the position of the surface can be known at isolated points whose topological relationships are not available. As an example, this occurs when the geometry of a physical replica of a vascular segment is acquired by laser scanning techniques, but it can also occur in image-based modelling in those cases in which it does not make sense to define 2D contours due to complexity of the underlying shape (e.g. in case of a vascular network whose segments are diversely oriented with respect to the imaging plane). In this case, a continuous representation of the surface has to be reconstructed from the cloud of unorganised points.

A solution to this problem has been proposed in [226], and consists of constructing the signed distance function D to the surface approximated by the data points and then extracting the reconstructed surface by contouring D. In order to compute D, a set of tangent planes is first constructed at each data point by least squares fitting of the positions of the neighbouring points. The normals to the tangent planes are then consistently reoriented with a graph optimisation approach. The signed distance function is then obtained as

$$D(\mathbf{x}) = (\mathbf{x} - \mathbf{o}_i) \cdot \mathbf{n}_i \tag{4.38}$$

where $\mathbf{o}_i$ and $\mathbf{n}_i$ are the origin and normal of the i-th plane which is closest to the evaluation point $\mathbf{x}$.

An alternative solution for surface reconstruction from scattered points is offered by tessellation methods, which consist in filling space with simple 3D elemental volumes, typically tetrahedra, whose vertexes are the data points. The tessellation is performed in such a way that the boundary of the set of tetrahedra approximates the surface the data points have been obtained from.

At the basis of most tessellation methods is Delaunay tessellation. A tetrahedralisation of a set of points is a Delaunay tessellation when no point falls inside the circumsphere of any tetrahedron in the set. Delaunay tessellation and its dual geometric construction, the Voronoi diagram, share a variety of interesting geometric properties and they find wide application in reconstruction and shape description, see for example [165] where several methods for constructing the Delaunay tessellation of a set of points in 3D, are also described. By construction, the Delaunay tessellation of a set of points results in a convex set of tetrahedra, called a *convex hull*, irrespective of the original shape of the object whose surface points have been sampled. Therefore, its boundary does not in general correspond to the boundary of the object. What makes Delaunay tessellations attractive for surface reconstruction is the fact that, if the sampling density is sufficiently high, the original surface is approximated by subset of the faces of Delaunay tetrahedra. This means that it is possible to obtain the reconstructed surface by properly peeling external tetrahedra off the convex hull. The challenge here is the correct identification of external tetrahedra, since such information must be inferred without the help of topological information. In case the orientation of normals to the original surface is known for every point, a tetrahedron T can be classified as external when

$$(\mathbf{p}_j - \mathbf{c}) \cdot \mathbf{n}_j \geq 0 \qquad \forall \mathbf{p}_j \in T \tag{4.39}$$

where $\mathbf{p}_j$ is the j-th vertex of T, $\mathbf{c}$ its circumsphere and $\mathbf{n}_j$ the known normal to the j-th vertex. After elimination of external tetrahedra, the boundary of the resulting set of tetrahedra constitutes the reconstructed surface. Conversely, in case surface normals are not known the reconstruction method has select external tetrahedra by inferring the object shape from the 3D geometric distribution of data points. A vast literature deals with this problem (see for example [8, 9, 125, 131]).

Last, we mention the method of Boissonnat and Cazals [44], which follows the same idea of Hoppe's method described at the beginning of this section [226], but utilises the Delaunay tessellation of data points to infer neighbourhood relationships and robustly construct the signed distance function.

4.5.3 Interpolation by radial basis functions

It has already been described in 4.2.2 how a 3D surface can be implicitly represented as a superposition of analytical radial basis functions. Each RBF is centred at a predetermined location in space, which is in general associated with the known location of the surface to reconstruct, and has an expression chosen among the possibilities listed in Equation 4.11. Once the location and the expression of RBFs are determined, the implicit surface is fully determined by the coefficients w_i in Equation 4.10, as well as by the low-order polynomial function $P(\mathbf{x})$ (As suggested in [375], the latter can be omitted if the number of data points is large ($N > 10$); for this reason, in the following we will assume $P(\mathbf{x}) = 0$).

At this point, the problem is that of determining coefficients w_i from a set of N data points $\mathbf{p}_i$ of known location such that the resulting embedding function F is zero at the data points and smoothly interpolates between them. This implies the imposition of a set of conditions of the type

$$F(\mathbf{p}_i) = d_i \qquad i = 1, \ldots, N \tag{4.40}$$

which leads to a linear system of equations of the form

$$A \cdot \mathbf{w} = \mathbf{d} \tag{4.41}$$

where $A_{ij} = \phi(|\mathbf{p}_i - \mathbf{p}_j|)$ is a symmetric $N \times N$ matrix, $\mathbf{w}$ is the vector of N weights w_i and $\mathbf{d}$ is the right hand side vector containing the values that F has to take at the data points. The matrix A is non singular if $N \geq 2$ and $\mathbf{p}_i \neq \mathbf{p}_j$ for $i \neq j$. In theory, since the data points should lie on the surface, $\mathbf{d}$ should be identically zero. In practise, this would lead to a linear system that, if non singular, would only admit the trivial solution $\mathbf{w} = 0$. Therefore, one or more data points must be specified in such a way that $d_i \neq 0$. These points are referred to as *offset points*, and can be generated by moving data points away from the surface of a fixed amount. As an example, if data points are generated from closed planar contours, offset points can be generated by shrinking the contours along their normals of a fixed amount, as shown in [375].

Depending on the choice of RBF and the distribution of data points, the system needed for the computation of $\mathbf{w}$ can be badly conditioned or not positive definite. For this reason, robust iterative methods such as GMRES are employed. In order to improve convergence properties, ad-hoc preconditioners or regularisation techniques have been proposed [375].

In general, the choice of linear or cubic RBFs (see Equation 4.11), leads to smooth implicit functions and good convergence rates.

4.6 Overview of vascular modelling strategies

In the previous sections we briefly overviewed some of the main techniques available for accomplishing the several steps involved in modelling vascular segments from medical images. We will now give an overview on how these techniques have been combined to provide full-fledged image-based modelling strategies.

As anticipated previously, the choice of a modelling strategy depends on image modality (2D vs. 3D, bright blood vs. black blood), image quality (presence of noise or artifacts), vascular segment geometry and topology (simple vs. complex), purpose of analysis (pure geometry, hemodynamics or fluid-structure interaction), and it must take into account the issues of accuracy, reproducibility, robustness, automation. Automation has in general been considered a key feature in proposing tools for clinical contexts, such as for stenosis grading, while accuracy has been assigned a higher priority over automation for applications such as geometric or haemodynamic modelling, at the price of user interaction. In some situations the intervention of a trained operator is hardly replaceable, like in the case black blood MR imaging, when the presence of complex haemodynamic patterns gives rise to plaque-mimicking flow artifacts which are difficult to automatically discern from the vessel wall.

As already mentioned, the dimensionality of the imaging modality contributes to the choice of the dimensionality of the technique. For example, if the acquired images are made up of strongly anisotropic voxels, for which in-plane resolution is much greater than along the imaging plane normal, 2D segmentation followed by a 3D reconstruction offers more flexibility in handling typological and geometric changes occurring from one slice to the next. On the other hand, 3D segmentation provides a more straightforward possibility on datasets with a more isotropic resolution, allowing modelling of vascular segments with complex geometry. In general, initialisation and specification of user-defined constraints require more sophisticate approaches if directly performed in 3D.

Two representative studies in which vascular models were generated by 2D segmentation followed by 3D reconstruction are Milner et al [333] and Long et al [297]. In the former, carotid bifurcation models were generated from black blood MR images. 2D outlines were first generated by means of a region growing algorithm, which provided a sequence of oriented points around the lumen. Point position was eventually interactively adjusted based on the degree of fit to the wall and smoothness of a B-spline surface fitted to the points. Contours were finally lofted with B-spline surface patches, one for each vessel branch (common, internal and external carotid artery). Each surface patch was bounded by a contour; in particular, all surface patches were attached to the same contour at the bifurcation level, so to ensure surface continuity. Long et al instead resorted to 2D snakes for the segmentation of TOF-MRA images or abdominal aorta bifurcations. A two-stage smoothing procedure was applied to the generated lumen contours in order to correct misalignment of subsequent contours due to subject movement, and to improve global surface appearance. Four surface B-splines were generated from lumen contours, two of them following the outer wall of the bifurcation, from the parent vessels to the two daughters respectively, and two on the inner side of the daughter branches, meeting at the bifurcation apex.

A 2D segmentation technique geared towards the delineation of both lumen and wall boundaries in black blood MR images was presented by Ladak et al [266], based on a DDC model. Steinman et al [482] employed this method to generate 2D contours of carotid bifurcations. The contours were then filled to create a binary volume, inside which a 3D balloon was inflated, in order to generate a 3D mesh of triangular elements, whose smoothness was imposed through internal forces. In the same work, owing to the acquisition technique employed, the outer boundary of the vascular wall was also segmented using the same deformable model, and a 3D model of the vascular wall was derived. Besides allowing to test hypotheses on the correlations between hemodynamics and wall thickening, as introduced in Chapter 1, this technique might in principle be used for generating fluid-structure interaction models (see Chapter 3 and 9) based on patient-specific lumen and wall geometry.

Wang et al [536] addressed the problem of performing 2D outline generation for geometrically complex vessels by extracting approximated vessel centrelines from 3D image datasets, generating images oriented normally to vessel centrelines and performing level set-based 2D segmentation on the resulting images. The outlines were then lofted to produce analytical explicit representations of single branch surfaces, which were then merged together to obtain a complete model of a branching vascular structure.

Giordana et al [194] employed a 2D segmentation method based on edge detection and thresholding followed by cubic spline fitting to segment TOF-MRA images of distal bypass grafts. 3D reconstruction was then performed by means of implicit RBF. The same group [375] recently proposed automated segmentation of TOF-MRA by means of Otsu's thresholding followed by RBF reconstruction.

Kaazempur-Mofrad et al [248] employed nonlinear image enhancement and snake-based 2D segmentation followed by 3D surface lofting to reconstruct diseased carotid bifurcations from black blood MR images.

As for 3D explicit deformable models, Ladak et al [265] proposed the use of balloons initialised as a simple 3D shape (e.g. a sphere) and then evolved with a two-stage procedure, during which the model is first inflated under the effect of a gradient-dependent term until it approaches the vessel wall and then optimised under the effect of a gradient-based advection field. This technique was successfully employed for the segmentation of a cerebral aneurysms from RA [478] which constituted the first patient-specific model of hemodynamics in cerebral aneurysms. As an alternative to this approach, Yim et al [550] proposed to initialise explicit deformable models with isointensity surfaces built using a 3D contouring algorithm directly on the images. This provides easier generation of topologically complex initialisations, although the exclusion of unwanted structures requires further processing.

Last, 3D implicit deformable models have been employed in [119] [12,518] with different initialisation strategies. In [119], a front propagation approach based on the solution of the eikonal equation was employed in order to initialise level sets near the vessel wall. In [518] initialisation is provided by the estimation of centrelines performed on the basis of vesselness (see Section 4.3.3), and image-dependent inflation terms are then employed in conjunction with stopping criteria. In [12], centrelines were estimated from a surface extracted by contouring and again employed for initialisation of level sets. A first inflation stage was then performed, followed by attraction of level sets to vessel boundaries. Segmentation was carried out separately for branches of different scales, in order to avoid scaling problems in the evolution parameters. Final level sets relative to different branches were then merged together to obtain the complete model.

In short, the problem of defining the geometry of a computational domain representing a vascular segment from medical images has several possible solutions. The choice has to be made based on image characteristics and on the expected geometry and topology of the vascular segment under consideration. Since the outcome of this step is the definition of the computational domain upon which the modelling problem will be carried out, a careful choice of the technique and of the involved parameters is of primary importance for ensuring the significance of the final predictions.

4.7 Mesh Generation

The last step in the generation of computational domains from image data for the numerical approximation of PDEs introduced in Chapter 2 and 3, is the discretisation of the physical domain in small elements of simple shape and finite size (the computational mesh), as illustrated in Fig. 4.1.

To this end, this section contains a brief description of available mesh generation techniques that we consider to be particularly useful for cardiovascular geometries. The reader should be aware that there is no such thing as a "general" mesh generation technique; the most efficient or appropriate technique for mesh generation depends on the geometrical and physical complexity of the problem being solved as well as on the method of discretisation chosen. In what follows, the term mesh will be used to refer to the spatial discretisation required for the numerical approximation of PDEs. The term grid is often used in the literature with the same meaning, but here the word grid is reserved to denote a lattice of voxels/pixels of an image, as in the previous sections.

The literature in mesh generation is extensive. The reader could consult the general review articles [365,474,501], the textbooks [172,260,499,500], the special journal issues [59,366], and the "Meshing Research Corner" website maintained by S. Owen to expand on the necessarily brief coverage of the topic provided here.

4.8 B-Rep model of the computational domain

A general framework for the definition of a computational domain is the so called boundary representation, or B-Rep, where the domain is viewed as a polyhedron bounded by curved faces defined on surfaces. The faces in turn are polygons bounded by edges defined on curves that, in what is commonly referred to as a manifold representation, are common to two surfaces (see Fig. 4.13). Non-manifold representations are discussed elsewhere, e.g. [312].

The surfaces in the B-Rep definition of the computational domain can be defined as NURBS surfaces, implicit or level set surfaces, or triangulations, as discussed previously in Section 4.2. The edges are represented by the intersections between these surfaces.

A common practise is to generate the mesh in a bottom-up fashion, namely, starting from a division of the edges into segments, followed by a discretisation of the faces, and finally the generation of a volume mesh in the interior of the domain.

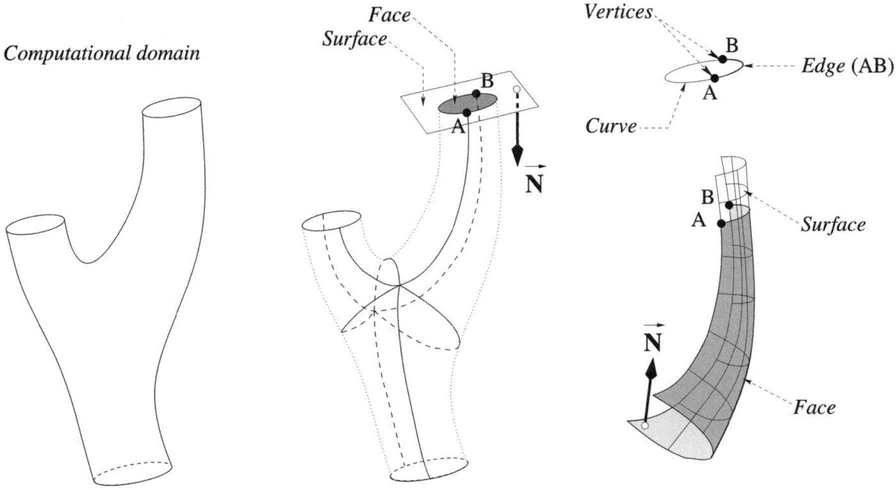

Fig. 4.13. Boundary representation (B-Rep) model of the computational domain

4.9 Structured versus unstructured meshes

Structured meshes are usually associated with numerical approximations by finite differences. The nodes of such meshes follow a regular repeatable pattern where each interior node is always connected to the same number of neighbouring nodes, as shown in Fig. 4.14(a). The presence of such a pattern means that the data structures required to represent the mesh are trivial, and the neighbour nodes can be easily identified by a suitable numbering of the nodes consistent with this pattern.

On the other hand, unstructured meshes do not show such a pattern and the number of neighbours to a node changes from node to node in the mesh. An example of such meshes is shown in Fig. 4.14(b). The data structures required to represent unstructured meshes are more involved as we need to store additional information to identify the neighbours of each node in the mesh. Finite elements and finite volumes are the techniques commonly used for numerical simulations in this type of meshes.

The mesh structure affects the efficiency of numerical algorithms for the solution of PDEs. The neighbouring values required for the construction of numerical approximations at a node of a structured mesh can be easily identified by direct addressing in the array storing the variables. A similar construction on an unstructured mesh requires the use of a connectivity array to identify the nodes neighbouring a given node. Its implementation requires indirect addressing of the array of variables. The implications for efficiency are significant: loops implemented using indirect addressing are at least twice as expensive as similar loops where direct addressing is used. Therefore, whenever the complexity of the geometry permits the generation of an structured mesh in a reasonable time, we could use numerical algorithms that take advantadge of this structure to produce solvers that are faster and more efficient than those implemented on unstructured meshes.

In what follows and without significant loss of generality, we will restrict our discussion mainly to structured meshes that are topologically square lattices of points and to unstructured meshes of triangles and tetrahedra. Other lattice topologies and element types are possible but we refer to the literature cited in Section 4.7 for a discussion.

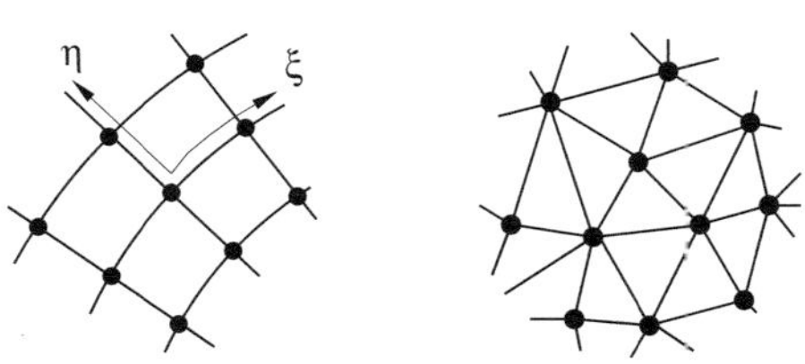

(a) (b)

Fig. 4.14. Structured and unstructured mesh discretisation of a computational domain

4.10 Structured mesh generation

Finite difference approximations are easily implemented on a Cartesian system of reference by defining an orthogonal network of lines parallel to the axes. The mesh nodes then correspond to the intersection of the coordinate lines. The application of boundary conditions is easy if the nodes are located on the boundary. However, this is often not the case in the presence of curved boundaries. It is still possible to impose boundary conditions at the intersection points of the network of lines with the boundary. This means that the finite difference approximations use unevenly distributed points which typically increases the truncation error of the approximation at boundary when compared with that of the interior points where the intervals are evenly spaced. Neumann boundary conditions, such as those described in Chapter 2, are difficult to implement since they involve the normal to the boundary and require additional points to construct the approximation.

To reduce the errors when applying boundary conditions one could use higher order approximations at the boundary, but this increases the computational cost and complicates the implementation as requires additional bookkeeping to construct the boundary approximations. An alternative method is to increase the resolution at the boundary using *recursive subdivision* methods, called *quadtree* in 2D and *octree* in 3D for reasons that will become clear in the next section.

4.10.1 Quadtree and octree Cartesian meshes

The main idea behind these methods is to selectively refine the mesh, i.e. reduce the mesh size, near the boundary to reduce approximation errors. The procedure starts by defining a coarse Cartesian mesh (e.g. 3×3 points) which contains the domain Ω. Cells that contain the boundary are identified and, if the discretisation error is larger than a certain prescribed value, the cell is divided into four. This subdivision is recursively applied to the newly created cells until the discretisation error is such that no further subdivision is required, as illustrated in Fig. 4.15.

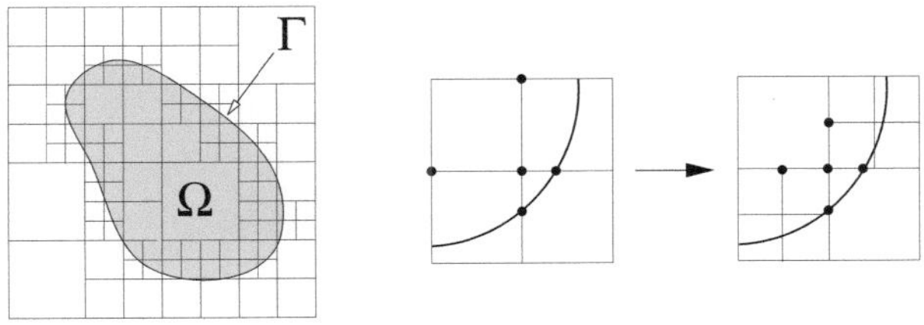

Fig. 4.15. Quadtree structured mesh: (a) general view; (b) improving the truncation error via subdivision near boundaries

An efficient way of implementing the method is the use of a tree structure in which the initial four cells are at the root and each cell is associated either the four cells that result from a splitting by half in both directions, or none if the cell is not broken up any more. These type of structures are well known and documented in the computer science literature [446], where they are extensively employed, e.g., for compiler parsing and image processing.

The use of a quadtree structure increases the amount of memory required as the tree needs to be stored. The discretisation of the PDE requires a complex housekeeping which involves a tree searching to form the finite difference approximations. The ideas described in 2D for the quadtree structure are readily applied in 3D (octree), where each cell is now subdivided into eight.

The added complexity required for the treatment of curved boundaries and the difficulty in applying boundary conditions in the normal direction has limited his application for viscous flows on complex geometries.

The favoured approach for structured meshes in the presence of curved boundaries is the use of *boundary conforming* meshes. These are meshes in which their boundary nodes are on the boundary of the computational domain thus eliminating the need for interpolation at intermediate points and reducing the associated discretisation errors.

4.10.2 Mesh generation by mapping

A method for generating structured boundary conforming meshes is the use of a suitable mapping. The idea of using a mapping $(x, y) \rightarrow (\xi, \eta)$, yet to be defined, is therefore to transform the domain Ω with boundary Γ into a rectangular region Ω^* with boundary Γ^* as shown in Fig. 4.16.

The original PDE is also transformed into a new PDE, which is solved in a square region where the application of boundary conditions is greatly simplified and the discretisation can be easily and accurately performed using standard finite difference approximations. An alternative option is to use the inverse mapping to transform a network of orthogonal lines in Ω^* into a net of coordinate lines (a mesh) in Ω which is boundary conforming. This mesh in Ω is boundary conforming and can be employed to discretise the PDE and boundary conditions using finite volume or finite element methods.

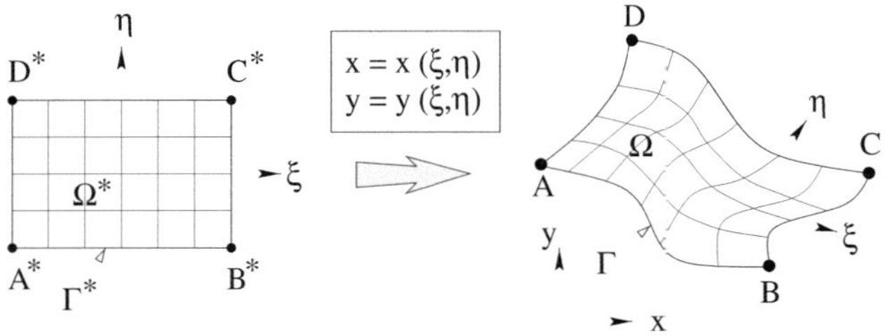

Fig. 4.16. Mapping of a region into a square region

The problem of this approach is that of finding a suitable mapping. The main types of structured mesh generation methods are either algebraic methods or based on the solution of elliptic, parabolic or hyperbolic PDEs.

Algebraic methods define the mapping via an explicit mathematical expression. For instance, the method of transfinite interpolation [134,470] obtains the mapping via the interpolation of polynomials through a set of points along the coordinate directions. Their main advantage of these methods is their simplicity and efficiency. However they often do not afford the user sufficient control to cluster points in regions where a finer mesh is required or to avoid mesh overlapping occuring for certain geometries.

Mesh generation by means of elliptic PDEs is discussed in the next section.

4.10.3 Elliptic mesh generation

The mapping that will transform a Cartesian mesh in the parameter space (η^1, η^2, η^3) into a mesh in the physical space $\mathbf{r} = (x, y, z)$ is defined as the solution of the system of elliptic PDEs of the form

$$\sum_{i=1}^{N}\sum_{j=1}^{N} g^{ij}\frac{\partial^2\mathbf{r}}{\partial\eta^i\partial\eta^j} + \sum_{k=1}^{N} P^k\frac{\partial\mathbf{r}}{\partial\eta^k} = \mathbf{0} \tag{4.42}$$

where N is the number of dimensions and

$$g_{ij} = \frac{\partial\mathbf{r}}{\partial\eta^i}\cdot\frac{\partial\mathbf{r}}{\partial\eta^j}; \quad \sum_{j=1}^{n} g^{ij}g_{jk} = \begin{cases} 1 & i = k \\ 0 & i \neq k \end{cases}. \tag{4.43}$$

The terms $P^k(\eta^1, \eta^2, \eta^3)$ are mesh control functions that are suitably defined to increase or decrease the mesh resolution about nodes or lines in the mesh.

The equations 4.42 are solved numerically. The unknowns are the coordinates of the interior mesh nodes. The boundary conditions are the coordinates of the mesh nodes in the boundary obtained in the previous step of the discretisation of the B-Rep of the computational domain. The PDE is discretise using centred finite differences and the resulting system of equations solved using iterative techniques.

The method has been applied to the generation of some very complex 3D geometries. However, finding a suitable mapping or sequence of mappings to transform the topologically square computational domain into a square it is often very difficult and requires a high degree of ingenuity. A strategy that, to a large extent, remedies this problem is the use multiblock meshes.

4.10.4 Multiblock techniques

In the multiblock method the computational domain is divided into a number of subdomains or blocks that are topologically square. These subdomains are

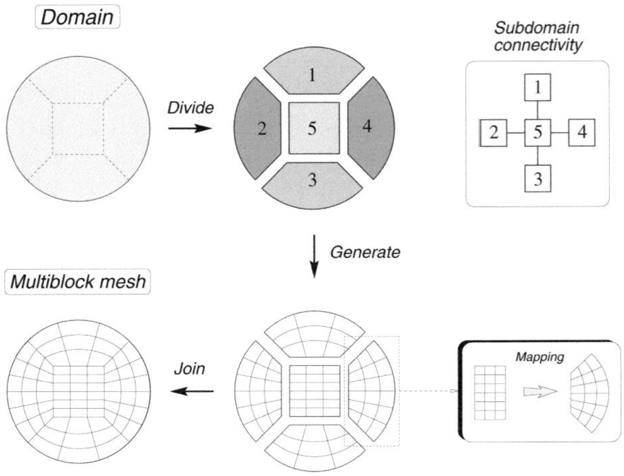

Fig. 4.17. Multiblock mesh generation

individually discretise using a mapping into a square or cube. Continuity across the interfaces between the blocks is ensured by requiring that the points (and perhaps tangent vectors) at the interfaces are shared by adjacent blocks. The different steps involved in the discretisation procedure by the multiblock approach are illustrated in Fig. 4.17.

This method has been very successful in producing structured meshes for complex 3D geometries. However, there are two main drawbacks. The first is an increase in computer memory for storage of the connectivity between the blocks and the additional information from neighbouring blocks that is required (usually in the form of halo cells) to form the approximations at the block interface boundaries. The second, and also the main bottleneck of the method at present, is the lack of a general method for the automatic subdivision of the computational domain into topologically square regions. This process often requires some form of user intervention that makes the task very difficult and time-consuming.

A way to ease the process of automatically generating meshes for complex geometries is the use of *composite overlapping* or, alternatively, *unstructured* meshes.

Composite overlapping meshes, also known as overset or chimera meshes, consist of separate boundary conforming meshes for each of the different components of the boundary, but without defining a precise interface with common points. Figure 4.18 shows a simple 2D example.

These methods facilitate considerably the generation of meshes for very complex geometries, but require the use of special interpolation procedures to transfer information between meshes. This could result in a loss of accuracy at the interfaces. For instance, properties such as conservation are difficult to preserve, particularly in 3D. Further information about these methods can be found in [81].

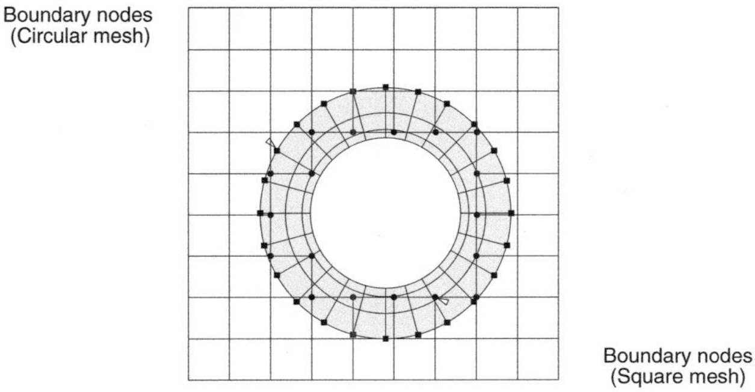

Fig. 4.18. Composite overlapping meshes

As discussed in Section 4.9, unstructured meshes do not have a predefined node and element arrangement, this lack of structure eases greatly the mesh generation and permits a better automatisation of the process. Their use has lead to a considerable reduction of the time required to generate a mesh for a complex geometry as compared to multiblock.

4.11 Unstructured mesh generation

In this section we discuss three of the most commonly used methods for generating unstructured meshes: Delaunay, advancing front and octree.

4.11.1 Delaunay mesh generation

This method is based in the construction of the Voronoi diagram for a given set of nodes. This is a spatial partition of the domain into regions, each of which is associated to a node in the set and contains the points that are closer to that node than to any other node in the set. A Delaunay triangulation, already introduced in Section 4.5, is uniquely defined by joining, with a straight line, nodes in regions sharing an edge. An example of a Voronoi partition and its dual Delaunay triangulation is shown in Fig. 4.19(a).

An important property of the Delaunay mesh is that circumcircles (circumspheres) of a triangle (tetrahedron) do not contain other nodes in the mesh. This is depicted in Fig. 4.19(b) and it will be referred to as the in-circle test in what follows. The algorithm proposed by Watson [537] uses this property to generate a mesh as follows. Assume that we have an existing Delaunay mesh where we want to introduce a new node. Those triangles in the mesh that do not satisfy the in-circle test, i.e. their circle contains the new point, are eliminated from the mesh. A new Delaunay mesh is then generated by connecting the new node to the nodes in the boundary of the (convex) hole created in the mesh in the previous step. This process is repeated for all the nodes in the set. An illustration of the algorithm is shown in Fig. 4.20.

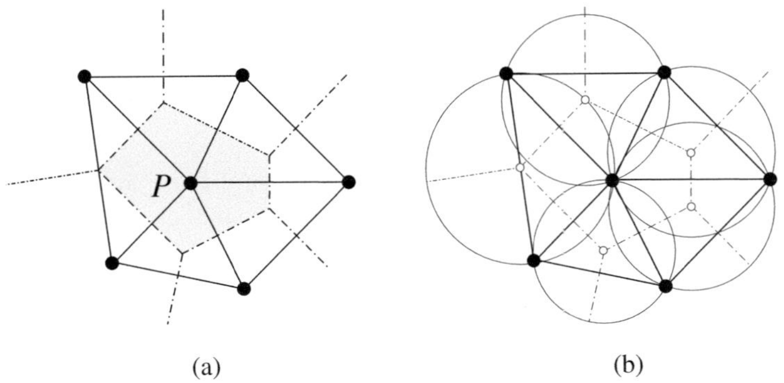

Fig. 4.19. Delaunay triangulation: (a) Voronoi diagram of a set of points. The shaded region indicates the Voronoi region associated with the point P. The dashed lines represent the boundary edges of the Voronoi regions. The Delaunay triangulation is obtained by joining those point that share a boundary edge. The Voronoi edges are the median lines of the sides of the triangulation. (b) The in-circle criterion: the circumcircles of the triangles in a Delaunay mesh do not contain any other nodes

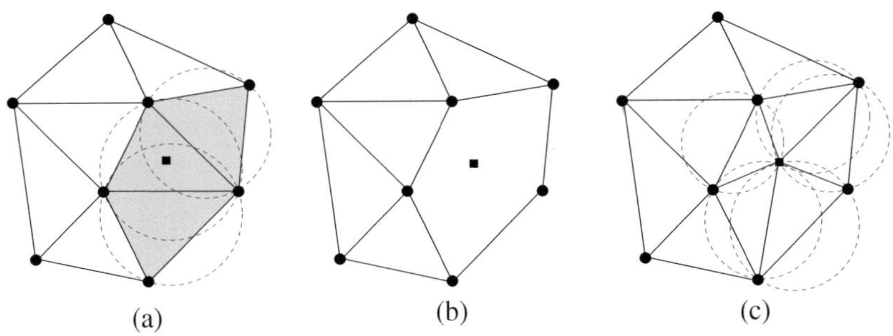

Fig. 4.20. An illustration of the Watson's algorithm for Delaunay mesh generation: (a) a new node is introduced into an existing Delaunay mesh, the triangles that do not satisfy the in-circle test are shaded; (b) the triangles that do not verify the in-circle test are deleted and (c) the new node is connected to the nodes in the boundary of the hole created to produce a new Delaunay mesh

A reliable implementation of this technique requires the use of robust algorithms that provide unambiguous answers for the in-circle test. These is required to handle degenerate cases, such as for instance four or more nodes in the same circumcircle, that will lead to topological incompatibilities (self-intersection) if the in-circle test is affected by round-off error. Robust algorithms for the in-circle test and other geometrical tests are discussed in [18, 461]. If the set of points is given, the main cost of the algorithm is the search for the circles that contain a point to be inserted in the mesh. A much more efficient version of the method is obtained is the search is reduced to a local search as proposed by [538]. The main idea is to automatically generate a point within a triangle if this is consistent with a specified mesh size distribution. As a result, the verification of the in-circle condition requires only a *local* search that is easily implemented by storing a list of neighbour triangles to a triangle.

Another very important property of the Delaunay triangulation is that its boundary is the convex hull of the set of nodes. If the boundary of the computational domain is not convex, an additional post-processing of the mesh is required for recovering a suitable discretisation of the boundary. Boundary recovery is the main difficulty associated with this generation technique, particularly if we require the mesh that conforms to the boundary discretisation to be Delaunay. This could be achieved, to some extent, by boundary point insertion but this might lead to a mesh which is too fine at the boundary. If obtaining a Delaunay mesh is not a requirement, mesh modification techniques could be employed to recover the surface discretisation [186].

4.11.2 Advancing front mesh generation

The advancing front method is based on the use of a generation front formed by facets that will be used to construct elements using a facet of the front as the element base. For a tetrahedral mesh, the facets are triangles and the elements are tetrahedra. The mesh elements are generated in sequence and, at a given stage of the generation process, the generation front is the discretise boundary of the region in the computational domain that remains to be meshed. The facets are consistently orientated so their normal could be used to determine the relative position of that region with respect to the front.

The generation front is a dynamic data structure which changes continuously during the generation process. The initial front is the set of facets generated in the previous stage of the discretisation of the B-Rep of the computational domain. During the generation process a facet is selected from the front and an element is generated. This may involve creating a new node or simply connecting to an existing node in the front. The validity of the element is verified by checking that this element does not intersect the generation front. After a valid element has been generated, the front is updated by deleting the facets of the newly generated element that are present in the current front and inserting the facets that are not. This updating process is illustrated in Fig. 4.21 for a two-dimensional domain.

The advancing front method preserves the boundary discretisation and also permits a straightforward implementation of mesh control. However, it is an heuristic method. A successful implementation requires procedures that are robust, i.e. insensitive to computer round-off error, to verify the validity of the element, a suitable strategy for the selection of facets and points to generate new elements, and the use of suitable range searching and sorting algorithms and data structures for efficiency [34].

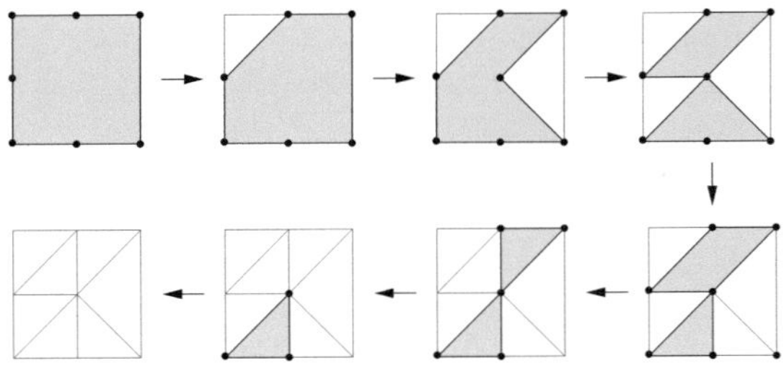

Fig. 4.21. Advancing front mesh generation. The shaded region represents the region that remains to be meshed. Its boundary is the generation front. The arrows indicate the generation sequence

The main advantadge of the method is that it preserves the boundary triangulation and thus there is no need for boundary recovery. The quality of the meshes it generates is very similar to that obtained by the Delaunay method when the same mesh distribution is prescribed. The cost is also comparable if a range search is required to insert points in the Delaunay mesh. However, the Delaunay method with automatic point insertion is more efficient.

This method can also be employed for the generation of unstructured meshes of quadrilaterals in reference [40, 559] and of hexahedra as described in references [41].

4.11.3 Octree and quadtree unstructured mesh generation

The starting point is the definition of a box, or cell, that contains the computational domain. This cell is recursively subdivided into smaller cells, usually four in 2D or eight in 3D. The subdivision is applied until the smallest cells permit to represent the boundary accurately. To ensure good mesh quality, the size of neighbouring cells is required not to differ by more than a factor of two. If the boundary discretisation is an input, then the vertices of the tree are moved to recover it. Otherwise, the intersections of the cells with the geometry are calculated and the discretisation of the boundary obtained in a manner similar to the marching cubes technique described in Section 4.2.3. In the final step, we triangulate the portions of the cells that are interior to the domain and exclude those that are exterior. An illustration of quadtree mesh generation is depicted in Fig. 4.22.

The octree technique is fast, conceptually simple and works reasonably well even with an inaccurate B-Rep of the boundaries. On the other hand, it introduces artificially preferred directions and produces poor elements near the boundary. This is due to the limited control on refinement near boundaries which must occur by factors of two. The quality of the mesh can be improved by the use of mesh enhancement techniques which are described in the next section.

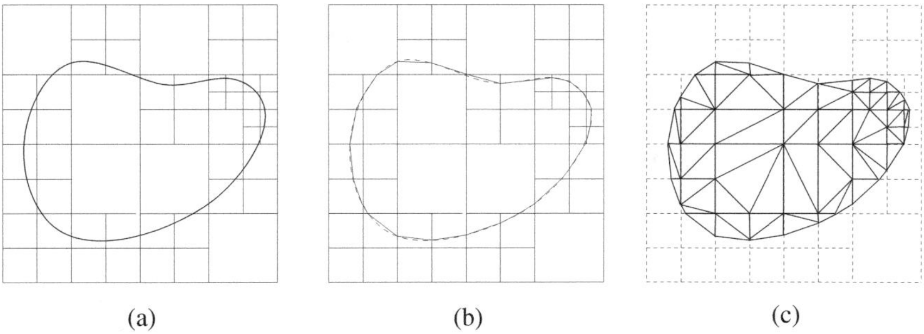

Fig. 4.22. Quadtree mesh generation: (a) spatial partition of the cells; (b) boundary discretisation; (c) triangulation of the interior portions of the cells

4.11.4 Mesh control, enhancement and adaption

The geometrical properties of the mesh play an important role in the efficiency and accuracy of numerical simulations performed on it. The cost of a flow simulation on a given mesh is proportional to the number of elements or nodes in the mesh. The quality of the flow solution at a given location is affected by the local discretisation errors that depend both on the mesh size and the smoothness of the solution. Finally, mesh distortion, e.g. the presence of very small angles, could have a detrimental impact on the convergence of algorithms for the solution of the discretise PDEs. It is therefore very important to incorporate mesh *control* strategies in mesh generation to achieve an optimal mesh, i.e. the one that produces the best accuracy for a given number of nodes.

Mesh control is usually implemented by requesting that the mesh to be generated conforms to a given spatial distribution of element size and shape. This distribution could be given as a user-defined function. Alternatively we could use techniques for mesh *adaption* where the mesh control function is automatically inferred from the geometry of the domain, a flow simulation on the current mesh, or both.

Mesh control is easily incorporated into any of the unstructured mesh generation techniques previously described. In the octree mesh generation this is achieved by splitting a cell only if the children cells have a length larger than the mesh size specified by the mesh control function at the cell centre. In the advancing front method, the characteristics of the element to be generated could be obtained by the evaluation of the mesh control function at the centroid of the front facet used as its base. In the Delaunay triangulation, a new point is inserted in the mesh only if its insertion leads to elements of a size larger than that specified by the mesh control function.

Due to algorithmic and geometrical constraints it is not always possible to achieve, using the previously described techniques, a mesh without distorted elements. The quality of an element of the mesh is almost always evaluated by comparison with its equilateral equivalent. Several quality indexes or metrics have been proposed in the literature and most of them are discussed in [462]. If a mesh control function is specified, the quality index must be computed in a suitable normalised space as described in [172,374].

The quality of the mesh can be improved through the use of mesh *enhancement* techniques such as mesh smoothing, side splitting, side collapsing and side swapping. These techniques are of a local nature and modify only a few nodes and elements in the mesh. The enhancement of the mesh is often achieved by locally applying them in sequence whilst sweeping through the mesh.

Mesh smoothing moves a node of the mesh to a new position that is a weighted average of the positions of the nodes that belong to the elements in the mesh surrounding the node. *Side splitting* inserts a new node in a side of the mesh and divide all the elements sharing the side in two to produce elements that contain the new node. *Side collapsing* takes a side of the mesh and eliminates it from the mesh by collapsing its two nodes into a new node. As a result, all the elements sharing the side also disappear from the mesh. *Side swapping* a side is eliminated from the mesh, leaving a cavity bounded by a polyhedron formed by the faces of the elements surrounding the side. A new mesh topology for this cavity is obtained by first constructing a triangulation using the nodes in the polyhedron that did not belong to the deleted side and then connecting these triangles to the nodes of the eliminated side. There might be many ways of constructing this triangulation and the obvious choice is to select the one leading to the best mesh quality. All these procedures could lead to the generation of invalid elements for certain meshes. In practise this is avoided by applying these operations only if the modified mesh is valid.

4.11.5 High-order mesh generation

High-order elements, despite their increased computational cost with respect to linear elements, can efficiently achieve high accuracy for a given computational work. When used in the frame of a spectral element method to solve the differential problem at hand, they exhibit exponential convergence for smooth solutions as the order of the polynomial is increased, and are particularly efficient for the long time integration of unsteady flows, see for instance [60,253].

The generation of a mesh of boundary conforming high-order elements can be achieved through the modification of a previously generated mesh by creating the additional points required for the high order interpolation and projecting them on the edges and surfaces of the boundary of the computational domain.

The construction of such elements starts with a discretisation of the edges of the tetrahedral mesh into N points as required by a Lagrangian polynomial interpolation of degree $N-1$. There are three possible cases to consider. If the end points of the mesh edge belong to an edge of the of the domain, the interpolation points are generated on the edge. If the mesh edge is on the boundary surface, the interpolation points are generated in a suitable projec-

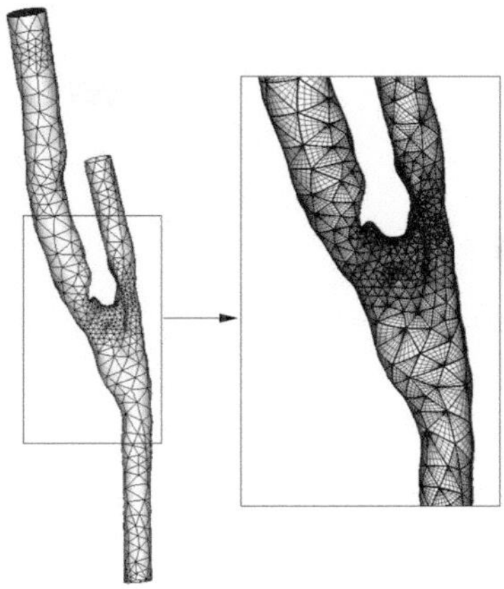

Fig. 4.23. Unstructured mesh of high-order elements: the figure on the left shows the coarse mesh representing the projection of the edges of the linear mesh on the boundary. The enlarged figure includes the interior points used in defining the high-order approximation within the elements

tion of the mesh edge onto the surface. In all other cases, the edge is taken to be straight and the interpolation points are equally spaced along its length.

The next step requires the subdivision of the faces of the tetrahedral elements. This involves two possible situations. If the mesh face is on the boundary surface, a transfinite interpolation from the interpolation points on the edges of the face followed by a projection on the surface is used to calculate their 3D coordinates. For all the other faces, a transfinite interpolation between the 3D coordinates of the interpolation points on the edges is employed to compute the position of the interior points. The final splitting of the tetrahedral elements involves a transfinite interpolation between the coordinates of the points previously generated on the faces of the element. An example of a high-order mesh is shown in Fig. 4.23. More details about these techniques can be found in [124, 459].

4.12 Conclusions

The purpose of this chapter was to give an overview on the existing techniques for generating patient-specific computational domains representing vascular segments starting from image data. Rather than providing a comprehensive list all the available approaches, we tried to organise this wide matter into a unified framework, focussing on the fundamental concepts and terminology. Our aim was to provide the reader with the means for choosing the best techniques for the specific problem at hand. What has been described in this chapter enables the application of the mathematical techniques presented in the reminder of the book to patient-specific cases.

5

Geometry and flow

Denis Doorly and Spencer Sherwin

Arterial disease, in the form of atheromatous plaques, is found to occur preferentially in regions where arteries bend and in the vicinity of branches, as discussed in Chapter 1. The changes in vessel shape due to pathology clearly affect blood flow, but there is a mutual interaction between haemodynamics and vascular biology. For example the traction (i.e. the force per unit area) exerted by the flowing blood on the vascular conduit walls directly affects how the endothelial cells function. Admittedly we do not yet fully understand the mechanisms through which haemodynamics and vascular biology interact. Nevertheless since any internal flow is strongly affected by the geometry of its conduit, we are motivated to explore how this is manifested in arteries.

In this chapter therefore we seek to uncover characteristic features of the relation between flow and vessel geometry. For the major part, we focus on simplified geometries rather than patient-specific vascular anatomies, and briefly touch on how the nature of the response depends on the pulsatile character of the flow. The flow regimes modelled are appropriate only for the larger arteries $d > 1\,\mathrm{mm}$, and it is assumed that the vessel walls can be taken as rigid and the viscosity as constant (i.e. Newtonian flow). Clearly errors are introduced by the latter simplifications, though as found by Moore et al. [340], Perktold and Rappitsch [419], Steinman and Ethier [481], assumptions of a rigid wall and Newtonian flow replicate the dominant features of large artery flows. In smaller vessel a non-Newtonian rheology would instead be more appropriate, as explained in Chapter 6.

The primary attributes we investigate are thus the geometric form of the vascular flow conduit and the inflow and outflow boundary conditions. The examples we present demonstrate characteristic flow patterns that occur where conduits bend, branch or narrow; in selecting examples we wish to illustrate how the flow response varies according to the temporal and spatial length scales of the problem. We distinguish between *global* and *local* characteristic features of the conduit geometry: global features are identifiable attributes extending over many diameters, whereas local features represent abrupt changes. A gradual bend or series of bends may be identified as a

Formaggia L, Quarteroni A, Veneziani A (Eds.): Cardiovascular Mathematics. Modeling and simulation of the circulatory system

global feature since the radius of curvature of an arterial bend is usually several times the diameter of an artery, whereas a stenosis often displays rapid changes in lumen diameter. Likewise in considering temporal boundary conditions, the flow may be modelled as effectively steady, quasi-steady or fully unsteady, depending on the quantity under investigation and the part of the cardiovascular system considered (c.f. Table 1.7 in Chapter 1).

The system of equations describing the model flow may be solved for particular values of viscosity μ, density ρ, and of the parameters specifying the geometry and inflow. However there exist group transformations that leave the system invariant, so that all solutions for arbitrary parameter values can be generated from a restricted subset, [74]. We begin by identifying certain dimensionless parameter combinations, termed similarity parameters, and discuss their physical significance at the outset.

We will then review some basic relations from the differential geometry of three-dimensional curves. These relations facilitate both precise descriptions of the bending and twisting of arteries, and the analysis of flow in curved vessels and along curved pathlines.

The concept of vorticity, and techniques to identify vortical regions or structures in a flow are next introduced. Together these tools prove especially useful in identifying the mechanisms responsible for the complex flow phenomena observed.

Having outlined the essential physical and analytic concepts, we begin the study by reviewing some key results in the viscous and inviscid analysis of steady flow in a bend. For the physiologically relevant range of parameters, direct numerical solution of the equations is however needed to provide accurate results. We thus apply computational methods to determine first of all the flow in an isolated bend, and subsequently the flow in sequences of relatively weak (45°) and strong (90°) bends respectively. We then move on to investigate flows at a graft anastomosis, including cases where the outflow bifurcates. The effects of varying temporal scales on the flow structures in unsteady flows are considered, both for a double bend and at a stenosis.

Finally we consider a few anatomically realistic geometries, and discuss the relative significance of global and local attributes in determining the flow characteristics in representative cases.

5.1 Similarity parameters: Re_D, De, Wo, U_{red} and their physical meaning

It is obvious that to model the *in vivo* flow environment computationally, a necessary starting point is to recover a geometrically similar definition, as discussed in Chapter 4. However in addition to geometric similarity, we need to assure dynamic similarity, that is the dynamics of the model system must match the real dynamics. It is not necessary that all the governing parameter values in the model match those in the real case, but only that the relevant dimensionless similarity parameters of the flow agree.

In curved pipes important parameters are the Reynolds and Dean numbers, whilst for unsteady flows the Womersley number and/or Reduced Velocity are also relevant. We now discuss the physical interpretation of these parameters, to complement their mathematical role in establishing invariant group transformations.

5.1.1 Reynolds number

As previously defined in Chapter 1, the Reynolds number, Re_D in an internal flow of mean sectional velocity U within a pipe or vessel of characteristic diameter D is given by

$$Re_D = \frac{\rho U D}{\mu}$$

where μ is the dynamic viscosity of the Newtonian fluid. We have here used the suffix D to indicate that the reference length used in the definition of the Reynolds number is the vessel diameter. Indeed, it is sometimes possible to use other length scales. The diameter is the most important length scale for fluid-dynamic phenomena in a vessel. The Reynolds number parameter naturally arises in the non-dimensionalisation of the Navier-Stokes equations. However it may physically be thought of as the ratio of inertial forces to viscous forces, as is more evident if we re-arrange the above definition into the form

$$Re_D = \frac{\rho U D}{\mu} = \frac{\rho U^2}{\mu U/D} \approx \frac{\text{Mom. flux}}{\text{wall shear stress}} = \frac{\text{inertial forces}}{\text{viscous forces}}.$$

In the first step we observe that Reynolds number can be interpreted as a ratio of the momentum flux ρU^2 over the pipe (i.e. momentum ρU crossing the diameter at speed U, see also Fig. 5.1(a)) to $\mu U/D$ which is an estimate of wall shear stress. Since inertial flux is related to the concept of an inertial force, we can argue that Reynolds number is a measure of inertial forces to viscous forces. When we have a larger Reynolds number inertial forces are therefore dominant over viscous forces and vice versa. This naturally leads us to the role of Reynolds number as the key parameter which identifies the transition of the flow to turbulence.

5.1.2 Dean number

A useful parameter for curved, planar pipes is the Dean number, De, which we define here as

$$De = 4\sqrt{\frac{D}{R_C}} Re_D$$

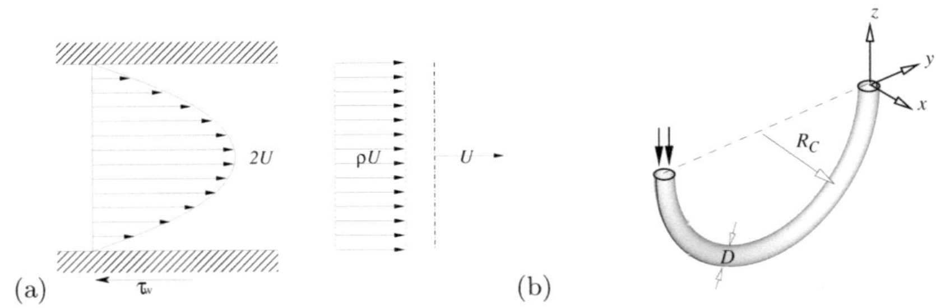

Fig. 5.1. (a) Interpretation of the Reynolds number as the ration of momentum flux ρU^2 to wall shear stress τ_W. (b) Definition of length parameters in the Dean number

where R_C is the radius of curvature (see Fig 5.1(b)), D is the pipe diameter and Re_D is the Reynolds number based on mean velocity and diameter. As noted by Berger et al. [35], the definition of the Dean number is not always consistent and so care must be taken when comparing values of the Dean number. As for the Reynolds number, we can provide a physical interpretation of the Dean number in terms of the balance between the forces due to inertia and centripetal acceleration and the viscous forces by re-arranging the terms as follows:

$$De = 4\sqrt{\frac{D}{R_C}}Re_D = 4\frac{\sqrt{\rho \bar{R}_C \frac{U^2}{\bar{R}_C^2} \times \rho U^2}}{\mu U/D} \approx \frac{\sqrt{\text{centripetal forces} \times \text{inertial forces}}}{\text{viscous forces}}.$$

In the above we have defined $\bar{R}_C = R_C/D$ and consequently the term $\rho \bar{R}_C \frac{U^2}{\bar{R}_C^2}$ is an approximation of the force to produce the centripetal acceleration since $U/\bar{R}_C$ is a measure of the angular velocity. As for the Reynolds number, ρU^2 represents an inertial contribution from the fluid whilst $\mu U/D$ represents the viscous forces.

Thus far we assume the curve to be planar; if we allow the pipe to possess torsion, additional similarity parameters may be introduced. For example, the Germano number Gn

$$Gn = (D/2)\tau Re_D$$

is introduced, where τ is the torsion (defined below) though Liu and Masliyah [295] also introduce the parameter:

$$\gamma = \frac{Gn}{De^{3/2}}$$

which is found to be important in determining the nature of the flow response to torsion.

5.1.3 Womersley number and Reduced Velocity/Strouhal number

When considering unsteady flows a commonly used flow parameter is the (Sexl)-Womersley number, Wo, defined as

$$Wo = \frac{D}{2}\sqrt{\frac{2\pi}{\nu T}}$$

where we recall that $\nu = \mu/\rho$ and T is normally taken as the fundamental period of the oscillatory flow. The problem of interest to Womersley [546] (and T. Sexl prior to this work [454]) was oscillatory flow in a straight pipe. Physically we can interpret the Womersley number as the ratio of pipe diameter to the laminar boundary layer growth over the pulse period T, i.e.

$$Wo = \frac{D}{2}\sqrt{\frac{2\pi}{\nu T}} \propto \frac{D}{\sqrt{\nu T}} = \frac{\text{Diameter}}{\text{Bndry. length growth in time T}}.$$

We arrive at this interpretation by considering the example shown in Fig. 5.2 (a,b).

If we consider a flow in a pipe at initial time τ with a boundary layer of thickness $\delta(\tau)$ then over a time T we expect the action of viscosity to cause the boundary layer to increase in size to $\delta(\tau + T)$. A dimensional argument commonly used in laminar boundary growth over flat plates is that the boundary layer growth is proportional to $\sqrt{\nu T}$ and hence our interpretation of this parameter.

The choice of appropriate dimensionless numbers is typically motivated by identifying parameters which collapse non-dimensionalised data into identifiable regimes. The relevance of the Womersley number is linked to the exact solution of a Newtonian fluid in a straight circular pipe subject to a periodic pressure difference. If $\delta P = A\cos(2\pi t/T)$ is the expression of the pressure difference applied at the two vessel ends, Womersley [546] (note also the cited work by T. Sexl) found that the the fully developed solution, when all components of the flow do not vary with streamwise distance, is periodic with only the axial velocity component u_z different from zero. For a given Womersley

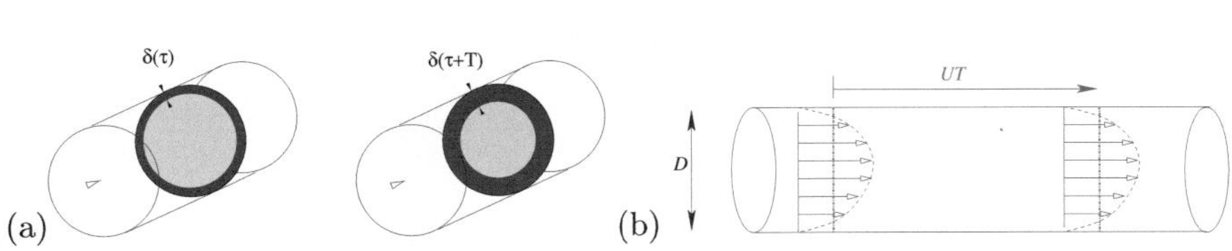

Fig. 5.2. (a) Physical interpretation of the Womersley number as the ratio of the diameter of the vessel, D, to the temporal growth of the laminar boundary layer δ betweenthe instants τ and $\tau + T$ due to the action of viscosity. (b) Physical interpretation of the reduced velocity which can be understood as the distance travelled by the mean flow, U, in one pulsatile period, T, divided by the diameter, D

number, the u_z velocity component depends only on the ratio of the radial coordinate over the vessel diameter, r/D, and on t/T and is given by

$$u_z = u_z(r,t) = \mathrm{Re}\left[\frac{AT}{2i\pi\rho}\left(1 - \frac{\mathrm{J}_0(i^{3/2}2Wo\frac{r}{D})}{\mathrm{J}_0(i^{3/2}Wo)}\right)e^{i2\pi\frac{t}{T}}\right]. \tag{5.1}$$

Here Re is the real part of a complex number, i indicates the imaginary unit and J_0 the Bessel function of order zero.

One of the potential limitations of the Womersley number is that it is related to physical scales within a given cross section of the pipe and not to any axial length scales. Therefore in problems involving variation of the flow in the streamwise direction and hence axial length scales, such as flow within double bends or stenoses, the role of the longitudinal geometry is not represented. Consequently meaningful ways to present the data may not easily be identified. An alternative non-dimensionalisation of the time scale, commonly used in other fields such as bluff body flows, is the Strouhal number (or frequency), St,

$$St = \frac{D}{UT}$$

the inverse of which is sometimes referred to as the reduced velocity

$$U_{red} = \frac{UT}{D} = \frac{\text{Distance travelled by mean flows}}{\text{Diameter}}.$$

As illustrated in Fig. 5.2, the reduced velocity has a physically straightforward interpretation as the ratio of the distance travelled by the mean flow along the pipe to the diameter. This number can also be interpreted as a non-dimensionalised pulsatile period. Clearly it explicitly introduces an axial length scale into the similarity parameter set and as we shall demonstrate in Section 5.4.4 this can prove useful in interpreting different flow regimes.

The reduced velocity and Womersley number are not independent and can be related through the Reynolds number by the relationship

$$U_{red} = \frac{\pi}{2}\frac{Re_D}{Wo^2}. \tag{5.2}$$

Finally we note that in their investigation of the formation strength of a vortex ejected from an orifice such as the aortic root, Gharib and co-workers [191, 432], have defined a formation number which is closely related to the reduced velocity.

5.2 The geometry of curves and pipes

5.2.1 The Frenet frame

Arteries follow a curved, and sometimes highly tortuous path, along their length with frequent branching or bifurcation. In the healthy state, the arterial lumen (the flow conduit) is reasonably circular. Each segment of artery

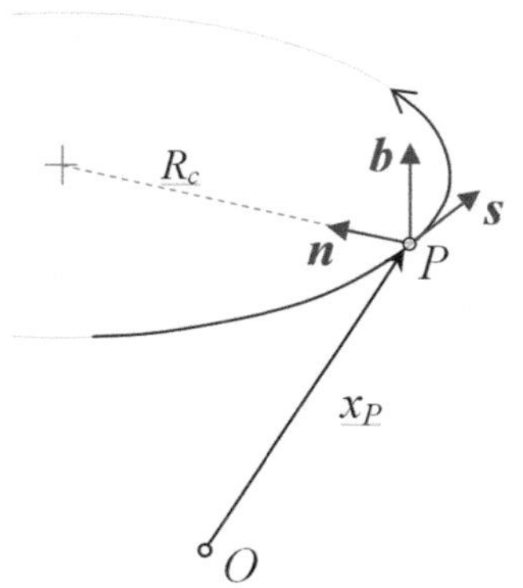

Fig. 5.3. Frenet frame: tangent $\mathbf{s}$, normal $\mathbf{n}$ and binormal $\mathbf{b}$ at point P

can thus be modelled as a curved pipe, and of constant cross-section if we neglect taper for the present. Such a geometry can be defined in terms of a centerline curve and a radius. Even where the arterial cross-section varies in area, or is non-circular, the locus of the centroid of the arterial lumen is a useful geometric attribute in characterisation and modelling. The differential geometry of curves provides a compact means to describe such geometry and an essential framework for theoretical analysis of the flow.

Let us consider a point P traversing a curved pathline in three dimensional space, as shown in Fig. 5.3.

The instantaneous position of P can be given either in terms of arc length s along the curve, $P(s(t))$, or by its position vector $\mathbf{x}_P$ with respect to axes centred at O. The unit tangent to the curve at P, which we write as $\mathbf{s}$ is given by:

$$\mathbf{s} = \frac{d\mathbf{x}_P}{ds} = \dot{\mathbf{x}_P}/v,$$

where v denote the speed at which P traverses the curve, i.e. $v = ds/dt = \dot{s} = \|\mathbf{x}_P\|$. At any point P, we can construct the Frenet frame of unit orthogonal vectors comprising $\mathbf{s}$, together with the principal normal $\mathbf{n}$, and the binormal $\mathbf{b}$. These are related according to the Frenet-Serret formulae:

$$\frac{d\mathbf{s}}{ds} = \kappa\mathbf{n} = \frac{1}{R_c}\mathbf{n}; \quad \mathbf{s}\times\mathbf{n} = \mathbf{b}; \quad \frac{d\mathbf{n}}{ds} = -\kappa\mathbf{s} + \tau\mathbf{b}.$$

The curvature κ is the reciprocal of the radius of curvature $\kappa = 1/R_c$; in physical terms, the curve passing through three nearby points is closely approximated by a circle with radius of curvature R_c. If $\tau = 0$, the curve is planar, so τ represents the rate at which the curve twists out of the plane spanned by $(\mathbf{s}, \mathbf{n})$, termed the *osculating* plane. The tangent is orthogonal to the *normal* plane spanned by $(\mathbf{n}, \mathbf{b})$, and the plane spanned by $(\mathbf{s}, \mathbf{b})$ is known as the *rectifying* plane.

A familiar example of a non-planar curve is the regular helix, $C(t) = (a\cos t/c, a\sin t/c, bt/c)$. The helix has curvature $\kappa = a/(a^2 + b^2)$ and torsion

$\tau = b/(a^2 + b^2)$, and can be thought of as a line wrapped around a cylinder of radius a, with a spacing between turns or pitch $c = (a^2 + b^2)$. We will call a the "wrapping radius" of the helix.

To analyse flow in a curved pipe, we naturally look to the Frenet frame to define a co-ordinate system. In a toroidal pipe, a co-ordinate system can be defined in terms of arc length s along the pipe cross-sectional centreline, and position (r, θ) in the normal plane, i.e. orthogonal to the centreline tangent. In the normal plane, x and y axes are usually taken respectively anti-parallel and parallel to $(\mathbf{n}, \mathbf{b})$ of the Frenet frame associated with the centreline. It is thus straightforward to arrive at an orthogonal co-ordinate system for a toroidal geometry.

For a helical tube however, a co-ordinate system set up in this way will not be orthogonal due to the constant twisting of the cross-section. Germano [190] introduced a rotation of the co-ordinate axes normal to the centreline to cancel the non-orthogonal terms. As stated compactly by Huttl and Wagner, [240], the position of a point in the Germano co-ordinate system is

$$\mathbf{x} = \mathbf{s}(s) - r\sin(\theta - \tau s)\mathbf{n}(s) + r\cos(\theta - \tau s)\mathbf{b}(s).$$

An alternative to the use of such a system is to recast the problem in helically symmetric form as shown by Zabielski and Mestel [554]. This is computationally highly efficient, as the problem is effectively reduced to two dimensions.

In the context of helical tube geometries we can define the helix amplitude as the ratio of wrapping radius (defined above) to pipe radius; helical pipes where the value of this ratio is of order one or less can be described as being of small amplitude. Recently small amplitude loosely coiled helical pipes been investigated for potential application to vascular prostheses, [61]. A loosely coiled small amplitude helical tube is similar to a helicoidal tube formed by translating the tube cross-section along the axis of the wrapping cylinder. However the latter geometry can easily be represented by a co-ordinate mapping, facilitating numerical solution of the flow.

5.2.2 Vorticity transport, generation and dynamics

Vorticity, defined as the curl of the velocity,

$$\boldsymbol{\omega} = \nabla \times \mathbf{u}$$

has several advantages as a primary variable in physical descriptions of fluid flow.

Firstly, the dynamics of vorticity can be related to the motion of neighbouring elements as we describe below.

Secondly, in incompressible flow, the traction exerted by the flow on an element of the wall surface with normal $\mathbf{n}$ is given by

$$\mathbf{t} = -p\mathbf{n} + \mu\boldsymbol{\omega} \times \mathbf{n}.$$

The viscous component of the stress in the fluid evaluated at the wall is known as the wall shear stress. The wall shear stress is responsible for the tangential component of the traction exerted by the flow on the wall surface, also known as the skin friction vector. From the above relation it is clear that not only is the wall vorticity directly proportional to the skin friction vector, but that curves tangential to the surface vorticity are orthogonal to the curves tangent to the skin friction field.

Thirdly the eruption of the near wall fluid layer which occurs in flow separation can be elegantly described and visualised using vorticity.

Writing $q^2 = \mathbf{u} \cdot \mathbf{u}$, and using the vector identity

$$\frac{1}{2}\nabla(\mathbf{u} \cdot \mathbf{u}) = \mathbf{u} \times (\nabla \times \mathbf{u}) + (\mathbf{u} \cdot \nabla)\mathbf{u},$$

the momentum equation for an incompressible Newtonian fluid (Ref. Chapter 2) can be written in the alternative form:

$$\frac{\partial \mathbf{u}}{\partial t} - \mathbf{u} \times \boldsymbol{\omega} = -\nabla(\frac{q^2}{2} + p) + \frac{1}{Re}\nabla^2 \mathbf{u}.$$

If the vorticity is non-zero, the flow is termed rotational. We can see from the above form of the momentum equation that in steady, inviscid, rotational flow, the gradient of total pressure is orthogonal to the velocity and vorticity fields. The tangent lines to the velocity and vorticity fields, which are respectively the streamlines and vortex lines of the flow, thus lie in a surface of constant total pressure known as a Bernoulli surface.

The essential properties of vorticity are summarised by the three Helmholtz laws. Taking the curl of the momentum equation, and using the constraints $\nabla \cdot \mathbf{u} = 0 = \nabla \cdot \boldsymbol{\omega}$ we obtain an equation for the transport of vorticity,

$$\frac{\partial \boldsymbol{\omega}}{\partial t} + \mathbf{u} \cdot \nabla \boldsymbol{\omega} = \frac{d\boldsymbol{\omega}}{dt} = \boldsymbol{\omega} \cdot \nabla \mathbf{u} + \frac{1}{Re}\nabla^2 \boldsymbol{\omega}. \tag{5.3}$$

If $\boldsymbol{\omega} = 0$ everywhere initially, the equation above shows it will remain so, provided we neglect transport by viscous diffusion.

Next consider the velocity $\mathbf{u}(\mathbf{x}_P)$ in the neighbourhood of a point P. The velocity field at any point a short distance $\boldsymbol{\delta}\mathbf{x}$ away can be approximated as:

$$\mathbf{u}(\mathbf{x}_P + \boldsymbol{\delta}\mathbf{x}) = \mathbf{u}(\mathbf{x}_P) + \boldsymbol{\delta}\mathbf{x} \cdot \nabla \mathbf{u}\,|_P + O(\delta x^2) \simeq \mathbf{u}(\mathbf{x}_P) + \boldsymbol{\delta}\mathbf{x} \cdot (\mathbf{D} + \boldsymbol{\Omega})$$

where

$$\mathbf{D} = \frac{1}{2}[\nabla \mathbf{u} + (\nabla \mathbf{u})^T] \quad \text{and} \quad \boldsymbol{\Omega} = \frac{1}{2}[\nabla \mathbf{u} - (\nabla \mathbf{u})^T]$$

are the symmetric and anti-symmetric components of the velocity gradient tensor; it can be shown that $\boldsymbol{\Omega}$ and $\boldsymbol{\omega}$ are related according to $\boldsymbol{\Omega} = -\frac{1}{2}\mathbf{I} \times \boldsymbol{\omega}$.

Imagine an elemental line of marked particles in the flow, or material line element denoted($\boldsymbol{\delta}\mathbf{x}_P$) at P, which is aligned with the local vorticity vector at some instant, i.e., $\boldsymbol{\delta}\mathbf{x}_P = \varepsilon \boldsymbol{\omega}_P$. Then (omitting the subscript P),

$$\frac{d}{dt}(\boldsymbol{\delta}\mathbf{x}) = \boldsymbol{\delta}\mathbf{x} \cdot \nabla \mathbf{u}.$$

If we now apply the vorticity transport equation and neglect viscous diffusion,

$$\frac{d}{dt}(\boldsymbol{\delta}\mathbf{x} - \epsilon\boldsymbol{\omega}) = \boldsymbol{\delta}\mathbf{x} \cdot \nabla\mathbf{u} - \epsilon\boldsymbol{\omega} \cdot \nabla\mathbf{u} = 0. \tag{5.4}$$

So we see that a vortex line is convected in inviscid flow exactly as a material line. Thus the dynamics of vorticity are closely linked to the kinematics of the flow.

Replacing the element of a material line by an elemental tube of vortex lines with cross-sectional area A_P, mass conservation and the identity between material and vortex line transport imply $\omega_P A_P$ is constant.

As the flow moves along a conduit, variations in the velocity field will cause the elemental tube to be stretched or compressed, and since incompressibility requires the volume $|\boldsymbol{\delta}\mathbf{x}_P|A_P$ to remain constant, increases in $|\boldsymbol{\delta}\mathbf{x}_P|$ due to stretching reduce A_P in proportion and thus increase vorticity $\boldsymbol{\omega}_\mathbf{P}$. The overall impact of the vorticity distribution on the flow often depends to a large degree on its integrated value, as expressed by circulation:

$$\Gamma = \int_A \boldsymbol{\omega} \cdot \mathbf{n} dA.$$

The circulation remains constant in inviscid flow as shown by integrating the vorticity transport equation over a surface which cuts across (i.e is approximately orthogonal to) the vortex tube. Proceeding as we did to establish 5.4 it follows that

$$\frac{d\Gamma}{dt} = \nu \int_A \nabla^2\boldsymbol{\omega} \cdot \mathbf{n} dA.$$

Even at the rather modest Reynolds numbers of the larger arteries, (mean flow $Re_D \sim O(100)$ or above), the flow progresses several diameters before viscous diffusion from the wall penetrates to the interior. In some regions of the arterial vasculature, the flow structure thus comprises a largely inviscid core flow with a viscous wall layer. Provided the interaction between the core and wall layers is relatively weak, inviscid models can provide a good approximation of the flow dynamics. However this nicely compartmentalised flow picture breaks down when strong viscous-inviscid interactions develop, leading to eruption of the viscous layer into the main core, as we show when considering strongly curved model geometries.

5.2.3 Coherent structures/secondary flows

Swirling or rotating components of velocity often arise in arteries, and may be induced by rapid turning of the flow direction as arteries bend and branch along their length, or by flow separation. Although we generally associate a vortex with a swirling velocity, it is not always straightforward to detect such motions in a complex flow field. Despite being of considerable physiological significance, these components may appear relatively weak compared to the mean flow. Furthermore, although vorticity is related to rotational motion, examining isosurfaces of vorticity can be misleading, since where high strain co-exists with high vorticity, as at the wall, there is no net rotation of pathlines.

To identify vortical motions, Jeong and Hussain [245] propose that a vortex corresponds to a connected region where the second of the eigenvalues $(\lambda_1, \lambda_2, \lambda_3)$ of $(\mathbf{D}^2 + \boldsymbol{\Omega}^2)$ is negative, assuming they are ordered so that $\lambda_1 \geq \lambda_2 \geq \lambda_3$. This follows from the condition that for a local minimum of pressure, two eigenvalues of the Hessian should be positive. However in forming the pressure Hessian from the gradient of the momentum equations, both the unsteady strain term, $d\mathbf{S}/dt$, which can produce spurious pressure minima, and the viscous terms are neglected.

We can also relate the so-called λ_2 criterion to the local kinematics of the flow. Consider the relative motion of two points O and P and let $\mathbf{dx}(t) = \mathbf{OP}$ represent the instantaneous position of P relative to O as the points move with the flow. Referring to Fig. 5.3 with $\boldsymbol{\delta}\mathbf{x}$ replacing $\mathbf{x}_P$, the motion of P relative to axes translating with point O is a curve in space, unless the flow is everywhere uniform, in which case P appears fixed. The rate of change of the separation vector, $\dot{\boldsymbol{\delta}}\mathbf{x}$ is related by $\dot{\boldsymbol{\delta}}\mathbf{x} = \upsilon\mathbf{s}$ to the tangent $\mathbf{s}$, and to the speed of P along the curve, $\upsilon = \dot{s}$ as previously outlined. Differentiating, and again using the Frenet Serret relations,

$$\ddot{\boldsymbol{\delta}}\mathbf{x} = \upsilon^2\kappa\mathbf{n} + \dot{\upsilon}\mathbf{s} = \upsilon^2\kappa\mathbf{n} + \frac{\dot{\upsilon}}{\upsilon}\dot{\boldsymbol{\delta}}\mathbf{x}.$$

Now as described in Doorly et al. [128], to first order,

$$\dot{\boldsymbol{\delta}}\mathbf{x} = \frac{d}{dt}(\boldsymbol{\delta}\mathbf{x}) = \boldsymbol{\delta}\mathbf{x} \cdot \nabla\mathbf{u} = (\nabla\mathbf{u})^T \cdot \boldsymbol{\delta}\mathbf{x}$$
$$\ddot{\boldsymbol{\delta}}\mathbf{x} = \frac{d}{dt}(\boldsymbol{\delta}\mathbf{x}) \cdot \nabla\mathbf{u} + \boldsymbol{\delta}\mathbf{x} \cdot \frac{d}{dt}(\nabla\mathbf{u}).$$

Under the 'frozen' flow assumptions used to derive the λ_2 condition, we neglect the second term on the right above, and again approximate $\dot{\boldsymbol{\delta}}\mathbf{x}$ to first order in space, yielding an expression for the acceleration of P relative to O.

$$\ddot{\boldsymbol{\delta}}\mathbf{x} = \dot{\boldsymbol{\delta}}\mathbf{x} \cdot \nabla\mathbf{u} = (\nabla\mathbf{u})^T(\nabla\mathbf{u})^T \cdot \boldsymbol{\delta}\mathbf{x}.$$

The scalar product of the separation and acceleration vectors

$$\boldsymbol{\delta}\mathbf{x} \cdot \ddot{\boldsymbol{\delta}}\mathbf{x} = \boldsymbol{\delta}\mathbf{x} \cdot ((\nabla\mathbf{u})^T(\nabla\mathbf{u})^T \cdot \boldsymbol{\delta}\mathbf{x}) = (\mathbf{D}^2 + \boldsymbol{\Omega}^2) : \boldsymbol{\delta}\mathbf{x} \otimes \boldsymbol{\delta}\mathbf{x},$$

whereas from the geometry of the pathline,

$$\boldsymbol{\delta}\mathbf{x} \cdot \ddot{\boldsymbol{\delta}}\mathbf{x} = \upsilon^2\kappa\mathbf{n} \cdot \boldsymbol{\delta}\mathbf{x} + \frac{\dot{\upsilon}}{\upsilon}\dot{\boldsymbol{\delta}}\mathbf{x} \cdot \boldsymbol{\delta}\mathbf{x}.$$

Thus we can directly relate the local geometry of the pathline of any point P about another by projection onto an eigenplane of $(\mathbf{D}^2 + \boldsymbol{\Omega}^2)$. For a pure solid body rotation, the second term on the right is zero, and the magnitude of λ_2 is thus directly related to the strength of rotation. Thus although the λ_2 criterion is not a perfect indicator of the presence and strength of swirling flows (as revealed by the different terms in the equation above) it is a highly useful measure of vortical structure and intensity.

5.3 Flow in characteristic geometries

5.3.1 Bends and secondary flows

Viscous analysis

For a good introduction to the haemodynamics of flow in a bend, reference should be made to the text by Pedley [373]. Here we outline the essentials of different analytic treatments, contrasting the fully viscous approach which treats a specific geometry under restrictive assumptions, with the more general inviscid approach which is concerned with modelling the dynamics of flow along curved pathlines.

If a non-uniform flow is forced to turn, the balance of angular momentum will cause rotational or swirl components of velocity to develop. The rotational velocity components are called 'secondary flows' as they lie in a plane normal to the main or axial flow direction. In terms of vorticity, the curvature of the flow pathlines causes an exchange in the components of $\boldsymbol{\omega}$, and the development of a streamwise component, ω_s. Squire and Winter [475] first showed that secondary flows arise where the inlet flow contains a velocity gradient in a direction normal to the plane of the bend, even if the flow is inviscid. The original analysis of secondary flow in a circular pipe bend is however due to Dean, who assumed the radius of curvature of the pipe to be much greater than the pipe radius, and the pipe to be of infinite extent.

The section of toroidal pipe shown in Fig. 5.4 illustrates the form of geometry considered, where the plane of curvature is taken to be the $[yz]$ plane, and the centre of curvature is located at $y = -R_C$. In the limit of weak curvature ratio, $(D/2R_C \ll 1)$, Dean obtained a truncated series solution [113] for the axial velocity profile $u(r, \theta)$. The series expansion, valid for small Dean numbers, 5.1(b) is:

$$\frac{u(r,\theta)}{2U^*} = 1 - \left(\frac{2r}{D}\right)^2 + \left(\frac{De^*}{96}\right)^2 \left[\frac{19}{40}\left(\frac{2r}{D}\right) - \left(\frac{2r}{D}\right)^3 + \frac{3}{4}\left(\frac{2r}{D}\right)^5 - \frac{1}{4}\left(\frac{2r}{D}\right)^7 - \frac{1}{40}\left(\frac{2r}{D}\right)^9\right] \sin(\theta).$$

To be consistent with the original derivation by Dean, in the previous equation U^* should be interpreted as half the maximum velocity which would be

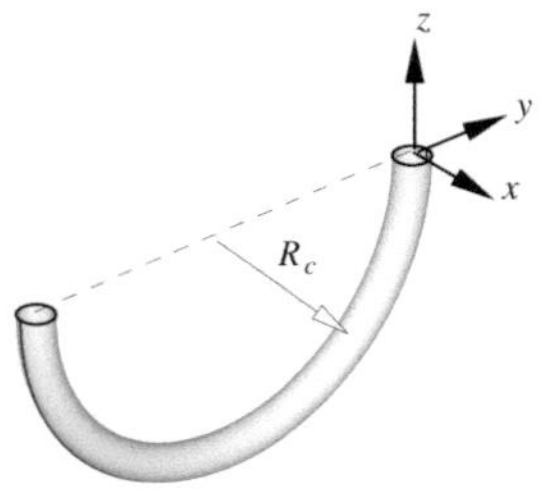

Fig. 5.4. Toroidal geometry for the definition of low Dean number flows

generated in a straight pipe by the pressure gradient applied along the curved pipe. In the limit of zero Dean number this means that U^* would be half the peak velocity of the parabolic Poiseuille flow which is exactly the mean flow definition we have used previously. De* is defined analogously to the Dean number introduced in section 5.1 but based upon U^* rather than U.

The axial flow profiles for De = 0,100 and 200 are shown in Fig. 5.5. The expansion is only valid for low $De < 96$[1] and so the case of $De = 200$ is not strictly valid. Nevertheless the bulk flow displacement is characteristic of the exact flow profile of a curved pipe and is therefore a useful equation to illustrate the role of upstream curvature on the flow profile. For comparison purposes the axial flow profile from a numerical solution of the full Navier Stokes equations after a quarter turn at $De = 200$ is also shown in this figure;

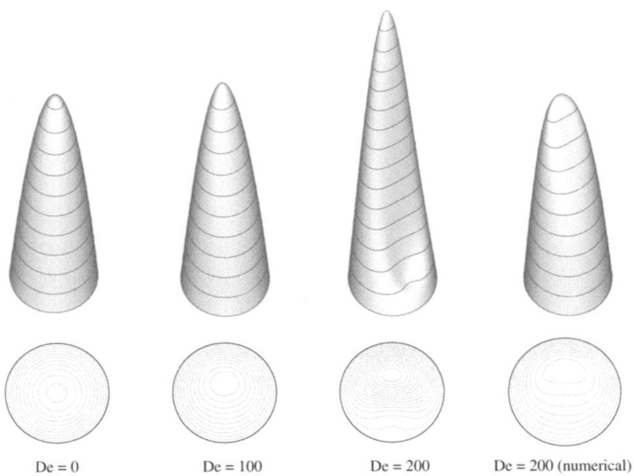

Fig. 5.5. Asymptotic Dean flow patterns at $D_e = 0$ (Poiseuille flow) and $De = 100, 200$. For comparison purposes the numerical evaluation of a $De = 200$ flow when from a configuration with a normalised radius of curvature of $R_C/D = 6.25$

[1] Strictly speaking it is only valid for $De^* < 96$; however the differences of using U rather than U^* in the definition of De appear negligible for this regime.

where the calculation is for a geometry with $R_C/D = 6.25$ and $Re_D = 125$. We see that the peak flow at this Dean number is much lower but the crescent shape of the iso-levels of velocity is still present.

For $De = 0$, the standard Hagen–Poiseuille flow in a straight pipe is obtained and this is plotted to scale so that it has a unit mean. If we consider the case where we fix the Reynolds number to $Re_D = 125$ then Dean numbers of $De = 100$ and 200 correspond to a radius of curvature normalised by diameter of $R_C/D = 25$ and 6.25 respectively. As we can see from Fig. 5.5 the introduction of the curvature and corresponding increase in the Dean number and centripetal forces causes the peak velocity to increase and to be displaced away from the centre of curvature.

Since the work of Dean, an extensive literature has developed on the theoretical analysis of flow in curved tubes, see Smith [469] for example. The analysis of Dean is limited not only in terms of flow (steady and relatively low Re_D) but in geometry to a planar bend of large radius of curvature, and low curvature ratio. Removing these limitations introduces additional similarity parameters; we can account for finite curvature ratio by taking $\delta_C = D/2R_C$ as an independent similarity parameter or to incorporate torsion, we require the Germano number Gn and potentially additional parameters.

In reality the curvature ratio of arteries cannot generally be taken as low enough to warrant its neglect, for example $\delta_C = D/2R_c \sim 1/4$ for the aortic arch, nor can arterial curvature be assumed to be planar, [63]. Physically we expect $\delta = D/R_c$ to emerge as an independent similarity parameter once the bend radius becomes small enough for the variation across the pipe in the possible turning radii of the flow pathlines to become significant. The study by Siggers and Waters [464] shows that incorporating finite curvature does not change the qualitative features of the flow, but that quantitative features, such as the variation in azimuthal distribution of wall shear stress are significantly altered. In particular, finite curvature is found to reduce the azimuthal variation in wall shear stress from inside to outside of the bend.

Referring again to the distinction between *global* and more *local* geometric characteristics, the Dean number can be considered as the global parameter of primary significance for the flow in curved pipes. Non-planarity associated with the introduction of torsion significantly influences the flow; it breaks the symmetry of the Dean vortex pair, either by making one vortex more dominant or completely obliterating the second vortex, depending on De and Gn parameter values [460, 554].

Describing more complex bend or bend-like configurations (such as multiple non-planar bends in sequence and end-to-side anastomoses) using coordinate transformation is difficult. The formulation of the equations becomes complex, rendering theoretical analysis rather intractable. Whilst it is necessary to resort to direct computation of the Navier Stokes equations for accurate solutions, as we will see below, we can apply inviscid approximations and analyses to provide understanding to complement the computational approach.

5.3.2 Inviscid secondary flow dynamics

Using the concept of vorticity and vortex models let us first explore the origin of secondary flow in a bend. We begin with a lumped vortex model for Poiseuille flow in a straight tube, which defines the bend inflow. At any point along the tube, the vorticity is purely azimuthal is distributed linearly over the cross-section $\boldsymbol{\omega} = (0, \omega_\theta, 0)$ with a maximum at the walls, falling to zero along the pipe axis (Fig. 5.6). The continuous ω distribution can be represented as a series of discrete concentric rings, which can then be approximated as a single lumped ring with circulation $\Gamma_0 = \int \omega dA \cdot \mathbf{dx} = -2\overline{\mathbf{u}} \cdot \mathbf{dx}$, where as we discussed above, the circulation is a measure of the effective strength of the vorticity. The choice of radius for the lumped ring approximation depends on whether we wish to match the linear or angular impulse of the distribution, [442]; as discussed in [128], $r = \frac{1}{\sqrt{2}}$ matches the linear impulse or $r = (2/5)^{1/3}$ matches the angular impulse. The difference is not significant within the accuracy of the idealisation and we thus idealise flow in a straight pipe as a series of vortex rings at $r = \frac{1}{\sqrt{2}}$ which are convected by a constant mean flow.

Once the flow is forced to turn, the rings will become distorted by gradients in velocity. By the Helmholtz relation (5.4), tracking a series of such rings reveals the vortex dynamics of the flow. The length over which this model effectively captures the vorticity dynamics is limited by the growth of errors in the lumped treatment of the stretching/tilting term, and in the neglect of diffusion. At the walls, changes in the core flow are resisted by the generation of new vorticity which diffuses into the flow. The diffusive penetration depth grows as $Re_D^{-\frac{1}{2}}$, and we therefore might expect a limited effect at higher Reynolds numbers. However, the vorticity generated at the wall may erupt and be swept rapidly into the main flow, so the validity of this form of modelling is often confined to the initial portion of a bend.

The method works well to visualise the dynamics of flow at the distal anastomosis (i.e. where flow from the graft rejoins the host artery) of an end-to-side bypass graft. The sketch on the left in Fig. 5.7 is based on computations

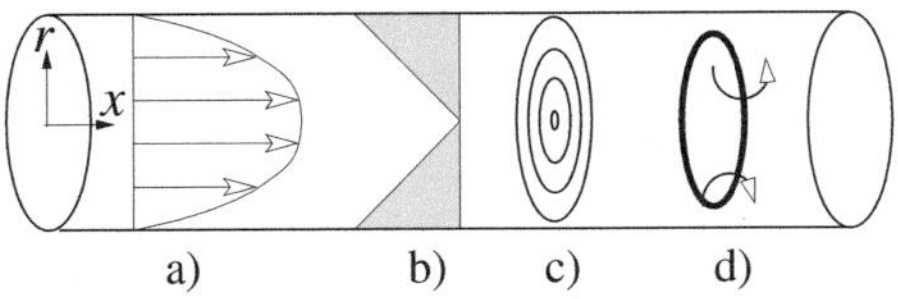

Fig. 5.6. Interpretation of Poiseuille flow in a straight pipe. a) In linear momentum terms the Poiseuille solution is a parabolic flow within the pipe, b) the parabolic velocity profile gives rise to a linear variation of vorticity across the pipe, c) an alternative local rotational momentum (vorticity) interpretation of the flow is a series of ring of varying circulation, d) from a modelling point of view we can consider an isolated ring with a lumped vorticity

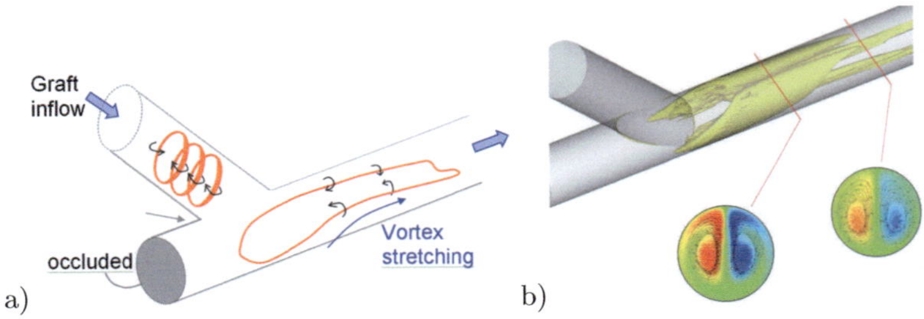

Fig. 5.7. (a) Vortex ring model of development of Dean vortex pair in graft outflow. Poiseuille inflow vorticity is represented as a sequence of lumped rings which impact on floor or bed of host artery. Tilting and stretching at sides of impacting rings intensifies streamwise vorticity and generates Dean pair. (b) Computation of graft flow at $Re_D = 500$ with zero wall shear stress. Without wall vorticity generation, flow development is predominantly inviscid, and roll-up of the inflow vorticity is as described qualitatively in part (a)

of the evolution of a series of rings placed at $r = \frac{1}{\sqrt{2}}$ which pass from a Poiseuille inflow to an equi-diameter host at an angle of 45 deg.

The tilting and stretching of the inflow vortex rings as they are forced to turn by the graft demonstrates the essentially inviscid nature of the Dean vortex creation [128], given a rotational inflow. Note however that the total deflection angle of the flow in this example is relatively low, (45°). As we will see later the viscous interactions, which we have neglected, turn out to be relatively weak for low deflections.

For comparison, the right hand of Fig. 5.7 (see [171]) shows the results of a computation for $Re_D = 500$, but with wall shear stress set to zero, to prevent generation of fresh vorticity at the wall. (The computation approximates an inviscid realisation of the flow, with the remaining interior viscosity preventing Euler instabilities). The gradual roll-up of the continuous inflow vorticity distribution is well illustrated by comparing the inset plots of axial vorticity at successive downstream stations, showing that the Dean vortexes are still formed for a rotational inflow even when surface vorticity generation (i.e. wall shear stress) is absent in the flow turning region. In this case the λ_2 criterion is not needed to reveal the core structure, owing to the lack of vorticity generation at the wall, and which would otherwise obscure the core.

A key question we may ask is:

how is the strength of the cross-flow related to the bend geometry?

We can partly answer this using inviscid modelling, and in some cases even derive approximate estimates. Referring again to Fig.5.7, the vorticity transport equation can be expressed along a pathline (or streamline, if steady) of the flow. To do so, we employ a local system of co-ordinates, known as intrinsic co-ordinates, in which the reference axes comprise the unit vectors $(\mathbf{s}, \mathbf{n}, \mathbf{b})$ of the Frenet frame. Following [267], we write the velocity as $\mathbf{u} = q\mathbf{s}$, in intrinsic co-ordinates the gradient operator is given by $\nabla = \mathbf{s}\frac{\partial}{\partial s} + \mathbf{n}\frac{\partial}{\partial n} + \mathbf{b}\frac{\partial}{\partial b}$.

The vorticity components $(\omega_s, \omega_n, \omega_b)$ are:

$$\nabla \times \boldsymbol{\omega} = q\sigma \mathbf{s} + \frac{\partial q}{\partial b}\mathbf{n} + (\frac{q}{R_c} - \frac{\partial q}{\partial n})\mathbf{b},$$

where $\sigma = \mathbf{s} \cdot \nabla \times \mathbf{s}$ is independent of the magnitude of q and depends only on the geometry of the pathlines. Assuming steady flow, the streamwise component in the transport equation for vorticity (5.3) reduces to a balance between convective,

$$\mathbf{s} \cdot (\mathbf{u} \cdot \nabla)\boldsymbol{\omega} = q\frac{\partial}{\partial s}(\mathbf{s} \cdot \boldsymbol{\omega}) - q\boldsymbol{\omega} \cdot \frac{\partial \mathbf{s}}{\partial s} = q\frac{\partial \omega_s}{\partial s} - q\frac{\omega_n}{R_c} \tag{5.5}$$

and vortex stretching/tilting terms

$$\mathbf{s} \cdot (\boldsymbol{\omega} \cdot \nabla)\mathbf{u} = \omega_s\frac{\partial q}{\partial s} + \omega_n\frac{\partial q}{\partial n} + \omega_b\frac{\partial q}{\partial b} = \omega_s\frac{\partial q}{\partial s} + \frac{q\omega_n}{R_c}. \tag{5.6}$$

Equating equations (5.5) and (5.6)), we find:

$$\frac{\partial}{\partial s}(\frac{\omega_s}{q}) = \frac{2\omega_n}{qR_c}.$$

The positive sign on the right hand side of the equation (5.6) assumes the normal vector points towards the centre of curvature. It is more common in the secondary flow literature to take the normal vector to point outwards, and a negative sign then precede the term on the left hand side of the equation.

Where flow is deflected through a total angle of θ, assuming torsion $\tau = 0$ and flow speed q remains constant, integrating the above yields the estimate

$$\omega_s = 2\omega_n\theta, \tag{5.7}$$

predicting linear growth with deflection angle, and noting again the difference in sign of the right hand side from that in common usage. This expression reveals the conversion of the vorticity component in to the bend's radial direction to streamwise vorticity. The above simple estimate can be improved to account for the deflection of the streamlines by the secondary flow associated with the developing streamwise vorticity. Assuming weak secondary flows, Rowe [433] adopted a marching procedure to solve for the streamfunction in the cross-sectional $(\mathbf{b}, \mathbf{n})$ plane at successive stations around the bend, allowing the incremental changes in streamwise vorticity to be appropriately corrected.

More general relations between all the components of secondary flow in a bend can be derived by considering the balance of angular momentum applied to a simple model of inviscid flows. As shown by Kitoh, [259] who investigated swirling flow in a bend, the angular momentum fluxes $(\boldsymbol{\Omega}, \boldsymbol{\Lambda}, \boldsymbol{\Xi})$ about the streamwise direction $\mathbf{s}$, radial component, $\hat{\mathbf{r}} = -\mathbf{n}$ and binormal axes $\mathbf{b}$ can be shown to be related by three coupled ordinary differential equations, the first of which

$$\frac{d\mathbf{\Omega}}{d\theta} = -\mathbf{\Lambda}$$

reduces to the Squire and Winter result for a simple model flow.

5.4 Flow in bends

5.4.1 Single bend

The bends which occur in arteries are generally less intense than the 180 degree turning of the aortic arch, yet even shallow bends significantly alter the flow. To show this, we first consider flow in a single toroidal 45 degree arc segment with $R_C = 2D$ ($\delta_C = 1/4$) at $Re_D = 250$, from which $De \simeq 700$, and apply the spectral h/p finite element method [253] to obtain numerical solution of the Navier Stokes equations.

In Fig. 5.8 on the left, we plot the evolution of a series of rings, where the colour shading represents the axial component of vortex stretching/tilting. The plot shows the intensification of vorticity as the rings become distorted in turning around the bend. The right-hand image, taken from Pitt [390] shows the streamwise (axial) velocity component (top) and streamwise vorticity (bottom) at slice locations corresponding to: (1) halfway through the bend, i.e. deflection $\theta = \pi/8$, (2): bend exit, and (3): at $3\pi/8D$ downstream of the end of the bend. The rapid development of the characteristic crescent-shaped axial velocity profile and the growth of streamwise vorticity are both evident, so that the entrance length required to establish the Dean type flow for these values of δ_C and Re_D are clearly far lower than those predicted by Yao and Berger [547]. In particular it can be seen that the streamwise vorticity in the core rapidly becomes comparable in magnitude to the peak value

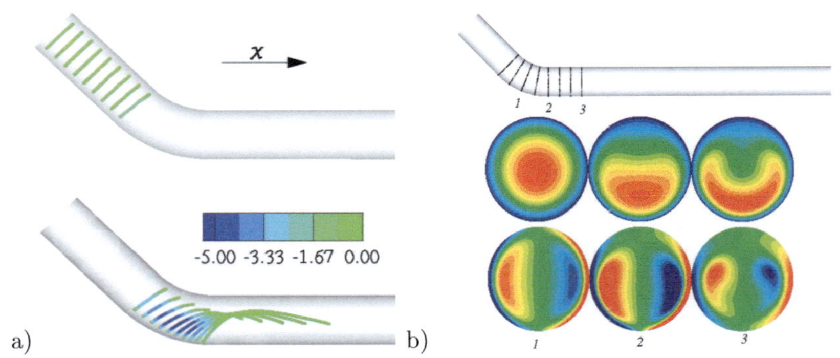

Fig. 5.8. Dean vortex generation in a single bend. (a) Ring transport and x-component vorticity stretching. (b) Sectional axial flow profile (top) and vorticity (bottom) and salient locations along the bend and exit

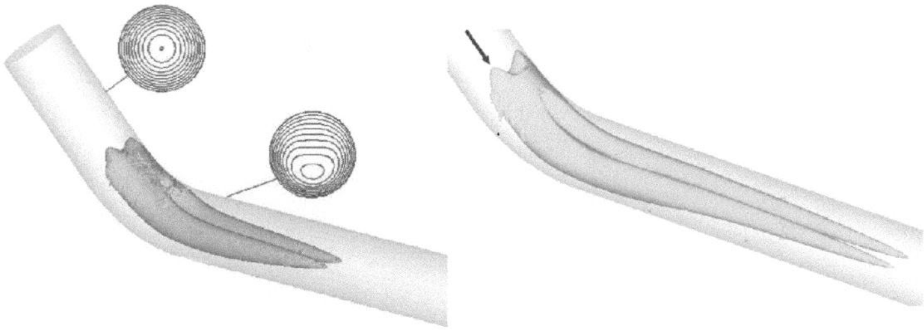

Fig. 5.9. Visualisation of the Dean vortex cores in flow through a $\pi/4$ arc bend with $R_C/D = 2$ for Re_D =125 left, and for Re_D =250 right

of 4 for the azimuthal vorticity of the Poiseuille inflow, normalised for unit values of mean velocity and pipe diameter.

The results also show that the growth of streamwise vorticity in the core is counteracted by the generation of oppositely signed streamwise vorticity at the wall. The core vortex pair shows significant decay even after one diameter, as viscous diffusion promotes annihilation both through transport of opposing vorticity from the wall, and to a lesser extent through self-cancellation.

The λ_2 criterion is required to reveal the core structure, due to the masking effect that the wall vorticity would have on isosurfaces of vorticity. Figure 5.9 clearly shows the rapid emergence and relatively rapid decay of the Dean vortex pair at $Re_D = 125$, compared with the greater persistence of the vortex pair at $Re_D = 250$.

5.4.2 Series of Bends

45 degree bends

As arteries are constantly turning and branching along their length, it is generally necessary to consider the influence of the upstream geometry on the flow in any given section. First we examine flow through two consecutive shallow (45°) toroidal bends, with a straight pipe inflow and outflow regions. The bends have $R_C = 2D$ ($\delta_C = 1/4$), with their central axes co-planar, but have curvature of opposite sense, so that the outflow and inflow axes are parallel. The radius of curvature gives a curve centre-line length of $1.57D$ for each toroidal section.

The development of the flow in the first bend follows that for the single bend considered previously. Initially the streamwise vorticity grows approximately linearly as we observe from equation (5.7). Integrating the vorticity across each half section of the pipe yields the circulation of each core, and as shown in Fig. 5.10(a), the growth in circulation approaches the theoretical estimate more closely as Re_D increases.

In Fig. 5.10(b) from the results of [390], the axial vorticity component is shown in contour plots at three sections, for $Re_D = 125$ (top three plots) and

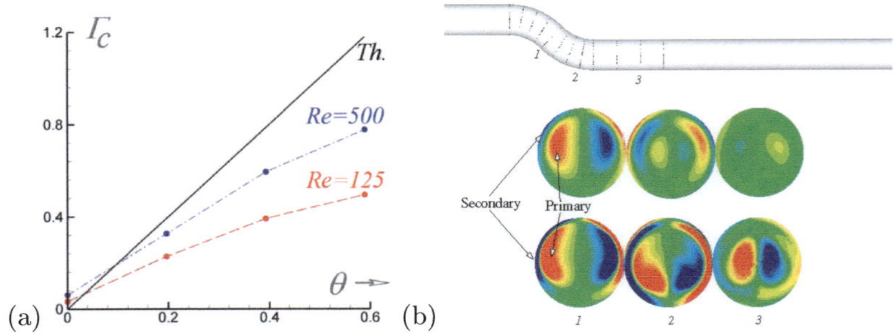

Fig. 5.10. (a) Growth of streamwise core vortex circulation in initial portion of first bend in double 45° bend geometry. (b) Contours of streamwise vorticity in double 45° bend geometry, at (1) outlet of first bend, (2) outlet of second bend, (3) $3\pi/8D$ downstream. Upper three plots correspond to $Re_D = 125$, lower three plots are for $Re_D = 500$. Note how opposite signed vorticity is generated at wall to oppose primary Dean vortex pair

for $Re_D = 250$, lower three plots. Section 1 corresponds to the outflow from the first 45° bend, section 2 is near the exit of the second bend, and section 3 is at two diameters downstream of the second bend.

Referring to section numbers in parentheses, we see the characteristic Dean vortex pair at the outflow of the first bend, (1). At the higher Re_D, the wall reaction to the Dean flow is much stronger, with vortex sheets of opposite sign evident. By the outlet of the second bend, (2), at the lower Re_D, the primary vortex pair has been much weakened due to viscous diffusion; the vorticity generated at the wall in the first bend (often referred to as 'secondary vorticity') has detached and is rolling up to form a new dominant Dean pair. Nearest the wall new vorticity to oppose the newly detached sheets is generated, and is of the same sign as the primary vortex pair. At the higher Re_D however the original Dean pair are still strong at the end of the second bend, and the penetration of the wall generated vorticity is lower, due to the weaker viscous transport. Also the second bend vorticity appears to be only partly detached from the wall. Finally at two diameters downstream, (3), at the lower Re_D, all that remains is the weak vortex pair remnant from the second bend, the primary cores having been totally annihilated. By contrast, at the higher Reynolds number, the initial bend pair is still dominant at this stage, and it is the turn of the secondary vorticity to be annihilated through cancellation with its wall generated opposite.

In Fig. 5.11, the vortical structures for $Re_D = 125, 250$ and at $Re_D = 500$ are visualised using isosurfaces of λ_2, non-dimensionalised by $(U/D)^2$.

The plots clearly show the effect of more rapid viscous transport and decay at the lower Reynolds number, where the initial bend structure is rapidly subsumed by the second bend, and the ensuing cores soon dissipate. The persistence of the first bend vortex cores is particularly striking at the highest Reynolds numbers, extending far downstream of the bend.

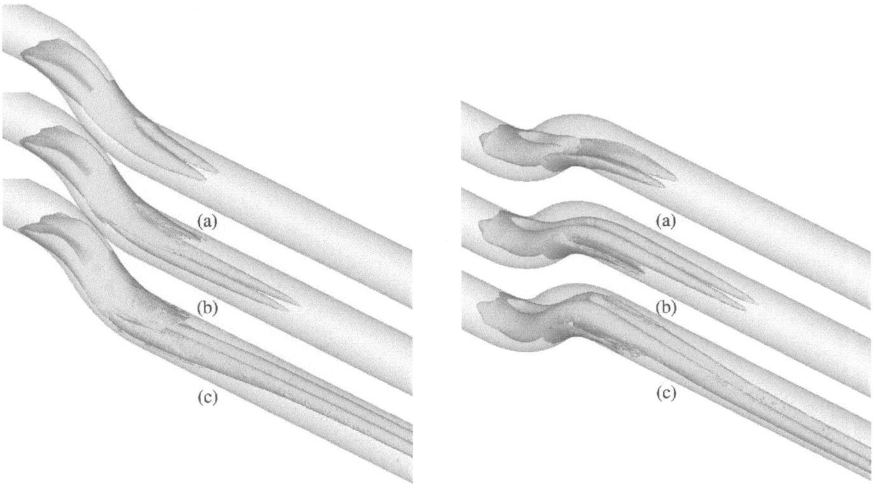

Fig. 5.11. Vortical structures in the double bend visualised using the $\lambda_2 D^2/U^2 = -0.3$ iso-contour and viewed from above (left) and below (right): (a) $Re_D = 125$, (b) $Re_D = 250$, and (c) $Re_D = 500$

90 degree bends

Lee [274, 275] has considered flow through a sequence of planar and non-planar 90° bends. Five configurations were studied, with the downstream bend rotated in 45° increments with respect to the plane of the first bend; in the 0° configuration the second bend outflow is in the same direction as the inflow. Compared to the shallow bends, the greater turning of the flow and so the geometry is similar to the previous 45° bend. in the sequence of 90° bends produces more intense interactions between the core and wall vorticity, significantly altering the flow, particularly at higher Re_D.

Separation of the wall boundary layers is possible, in which case the penetration of vorticity generated at the wall into the interior is not limited by viscous diffusion and merging. An illustration of the phenomenon is shown in Fig. 5.12 for the 180° degree bend at $Re_D = 500$. As shown from the upper plot, the eruption of the wall layers into the core alters the roll up of the primary vortex pair and introduces new vortical structures. The cross-flow streamlines (lower plot) show multiple centres of rotation corresponding to the dramatic modification of the vortical structures.

In a non-planar configuration, the rotation of the second bend out of the plane causes a realignment of the core vorticity, the positions of which are rotated and displaced within the cross section. This realignment can alter the flow in two new ways. Firstly a core vortex on one side can merge with the erupted wall or secondary vorticity layer generated by the opposite core. One core may become dominant through re-enforcement by such vortex merging. Secondly, and in contrast, the realignment may cause part of the core vortex

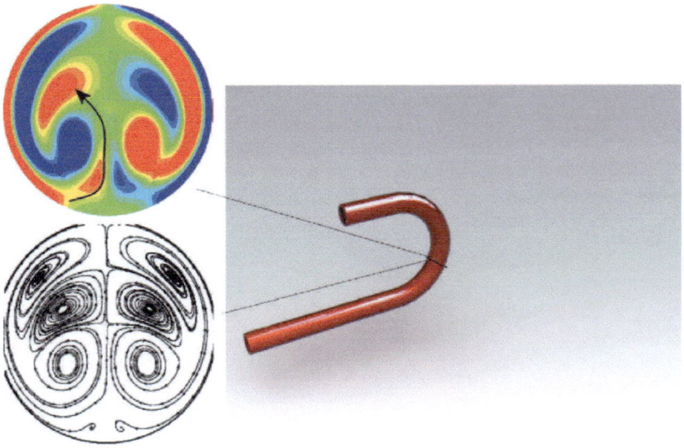

Fig. 5.12. Eruption of wall layer (secondary) vorticity into core flow at Re_D 500 in 180° bend. Top left: streamwise vorticity, bottom left: cross-flow streamlines. Location of cross-section indicated on right hand figure. As flow progresses through the bend, the wall layer vorticity is swept into the interior forming a new pair of secondary vortex cores, partly enfolded by the primary vortex cores, as indicated for left half of section by arrow. At the bottom of the cross-section (inside of the bend), another weak pair of vortices are just becoming detached from the wall. The sequence of vorticity eruptions produces the multiple recirculation regions shown in the lower left plot

on one side to become totally encircled by opposing vorticity and thus more rapidly annihilated.

These phenomena are illustrated in the sequence of streamwise vorticity and cross-flow velocity plots for the 135° non-planar bend shown in Fig. 5.13. From left to right, we can observe the encirclement of the left-hand primary vortex core (large arrow pointing to blue circular region) and its annihilation through cancellation in the interior. By contrast, the primary vortex on the

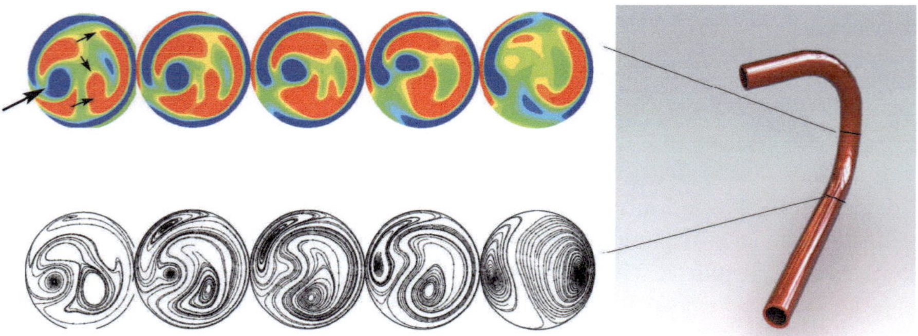

Fig. 5.13. Vortex merging and cancellation in non-planar 135° sequence of bends at Re_D=500

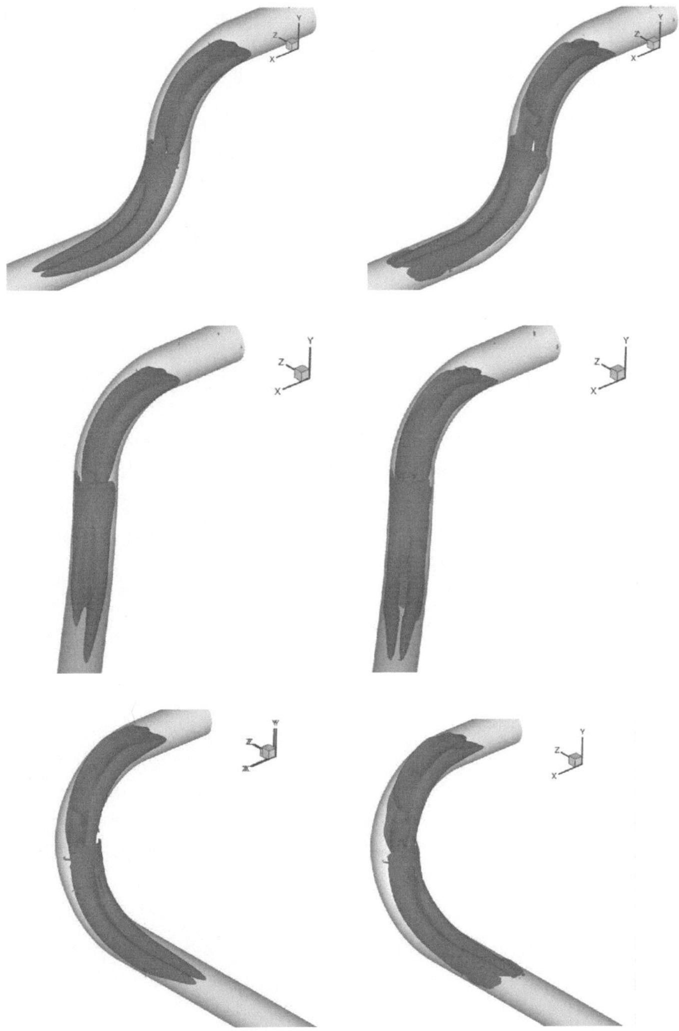

Fig. 5.14. Three 90 degree bend sequence configurations in steady flow at $Re_D =$ 125 left, and $Re_D = 500$ right. Top pair: S bend or zero degree configuration. Middle pair: 45 degree configuration. Bottom: 90 degree configuration

right-hand section is reinforced by merging with the erupted wall vorticity on the opposite side, as indicated by the three small arrows within the section. At the outlet of the second bend in the 135° double bend configuration, an asymmetric cross flow results, with the right-hand vortex core dominating the flow.

For a qualitative comparison of the effects of Reynolds number and bend planarity on the flow, we can examine the vortical flow structures, as shown in Fig. 5.14 from [274]. Not all the vortical structures can be visualised as some become enfolded and thus hidden as discussed above, but the dominant features are mostly visible. The top pair of images in Fig. 5.14 compare the vortical structures in an “S” or zero degree configuration of 90 degree bends, for $Re_D = 125$ left and $Re_D = 500$ right. Note that unlike the case of the 45 degree bend sequence, the initial core structure does not survive the passage through the second bend, due to the much stronger interaction between the core and the wall flow regions. Nevertheless, the core structure at the second bend outflow shows some alteration due to the presence of the upstream bend. The middle pair of images contrast the flow for the same two Reynolds numbers in a sequence of 90 degree bends where the second bend is rotated by 45 degrees from the plane of the first bend. In this case, at the lower Reynolds number, there is re-enforcement of one of the second bend vortices, resulting in an asymmetric outflow. At the higher Reynolds number however, the strong viscous-inviscid interaction does not preserve the coherence of the initial core features, and a nearly symmetric outflow results. Finally for the configuration where the second bend is rotated 90 degrees out of the plane of the first bend, we note the high degree of re-orientation of the vortical structures within the cross-section, which we would expect to enhance mixing. At the outlet, we again see a symmetric flow structure in both cases.

In classifying the geometry, it is clear that for the lower Reynolds number, the first bend has little impact on the flow in the second bend outlet. This suggests that viewed globally, each bend is approximately independent, and from a modelling perspective, it suggests that the flow quickly forgets upstream influences, i.e. we do not need to worry too much about the inflow condition after the flow has passed through one or two bends at modest Reynolds numbers. However we must not overlook two facts. Firstly, the flow is noticeably asymmetric for the 45 degree configuration, and secondly, the re-arrangement of vortical structures from one bend to the next will have significant consequences for mixing.

For flow at the higher Reynolds numbers, it is only for the 135 degree configuration [274] that pronounced asymmetry in the outflow results. Nevertheless the influence of the first bend strongly affects the flow character, even if the structure appears superficially similar to that of a single bend. The most striking feature is the less compact vortex cores at the second bend outflow, which are associated with a blunter streamwise velocity distribution than for a single bend.

5.4.3 Branches/anastomoses

In Fig. 5.15 we show the coherent structures, using the λ_2 criterion and the particle ring transport coloured by streamwise component vorticity stretching for a series of equal diameter pipe junctions for a Reynolds number of 125. In Fig. 5.15(a)–(c) we see three cases where there is no proximal flow in the downstream vessel and the junction angle is changed from 45 to 90 and 135 degrees, respectively. The inset plot in these figures shows the cross plane streamlines in a plane 0.25D distal (downstream) of the middle of the junction.

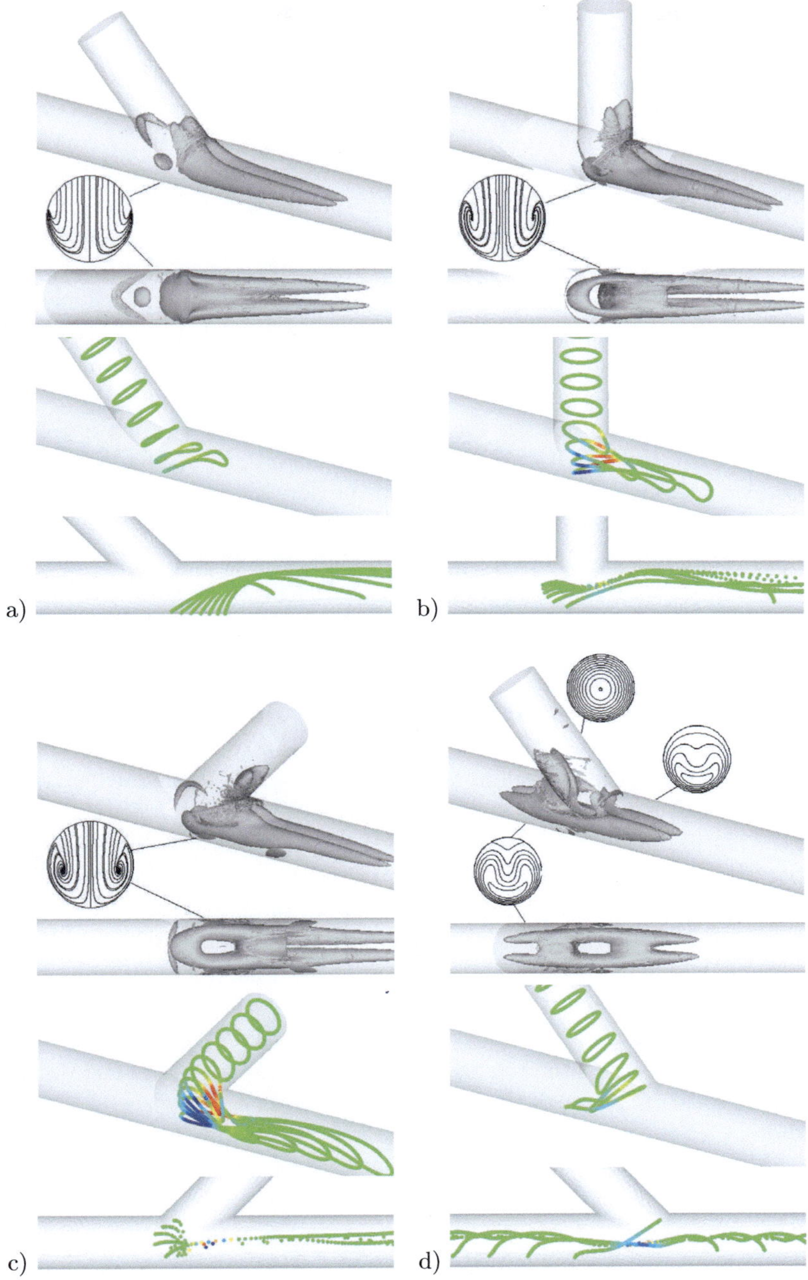

Fig. 5.15. Coherent structure identified (using the λ_2 criterion) and particle ring transport/streamwise vorticity stretching in (a) 45° graft (no flow split), (b) 90° graft (no flow split), (c) 135° graft (no flow split) and (d) 45° graft (50 – 50 flow split). Inset plots show secondary flow in (a)–(c) and axial flow in (d)

In general a surgically generated branches, for example due to bypass grafts, or even a natural vessel bifurcations have a flow split in the downstream vessel. Therefore in Fig. 5.15 we have considered a 45 degrees branch with a $50 - 50$ proximal-distal flow split. A more detailed investigation of the flows discussed in this section can be found in [458].

We observe that the two Dean vortexes are generated in all cases and appear to have a similar form to the single bend case. although the branch angle has a significant effect on the vortex strength. In the bottom half of the plots we observe the particle/vorticity ring transport within the branch coloured by x-component stretching and tilting (x is aligned to the centre of the downstream pipe). Similar to the single bend model, we observe that the rings transport up to the point of impact on the branch or anastomosis floor. The lower part of each particle ring plot then highlights how the particles transport after the impact on the floor at time intervals which are twice as large as the upper plots. Considering the transport of the ring before impact we observe that when the ring has reached the floor there is a greater distortion of the ring into the distal host vessel in the grafts with larger branch angles. This can be directly related to the stretching in the axial direction of the downstream vessel and the establishment of the Dean vortices.

From Fig. 5.15 we also observe that as the branching angle is increased there is a more notable particle recirculation in the occluded region after the ring impacts on the anastomosis floor. The stronger recirculation is also related to the looping structure evident just above the floor coherent structure plots of Figs. 5.15(a)–(c). In the occluded region of the 45 degrees anastomosis a vortical structure is evident when the recirculation is sufficiently strong to distinguish the particle motion from the rotational action of the boundary layers. This is not the case at either side of the structure as the impact of the particles on the floor does not generate a sufficiently strong recirculation in these regions. When we increase the branch angle however the impact of the particles is sufficiently strong to generate a vortical structure not only in the occluded region but also at the sides of the anastomoses leading to the looping structures. This process is analogous to a vortex ring impacting on a solid curved surface. The trajectories of the particles within the cross flow plane at 0.25D distal to the centre of the junction are shown in the inset plots of figs 5.15(a)-(c). From these streamline patterns we observe that there is no evidence of a vortex in the secondary flow pattern of the 45 degrees anastomosis. The secondary flow pattern of the 90 and 135 degrees anastomoses however clearly show the vortex curves which connect to the downstream Dean vortices.

We have previously explained in Section 5.3.2 that the generation of the Dean vortexes can be modelled as the azimuthal vorticity, generated in the graft, is realigned and stretched as it is transported through the anastomosis. This stretching and tilting mechanism is clearly shown in lower plots of Fig. 5.15 for the transport of the ring at $r/D = 1/\sqrt{8}$. Along these particle paths the peak stretching and tilting normalised by mean velocity over diameter squared was 8.5, 27.7 and 36.5 in Fig. 5.15, respectively. The corresponding peak axial vorticity at $x = 2D$, also normalised by mean velocity over diameter was 2.8, 4.4 and 7.0 for the 45, 90 and 135 degrees anastomoses respectively. This is in accord with the conservation of local angular momentum since as the stretching increases the vortex core diminishes and higher and higher values of vorticity are expected. From the perspective of vortex stretching however, it is perhaps more immediately obvious that the increase in intensity of the Dean like flow vortexes should be directly related to the degree of turning imposed on the flow by the anastomosis angle.

We see from Fig. 5.15(d) that as the flow enters the anastomosis it is stretched in both the proximal and distal directions. This is consistent with the combined effects of the fully distal and proximal flow cases shown in Fig. 5.15(a) and (c). We also note that the stretching is more pronounced in the proximal direction where the flow sees a larger branch angle. We note the coherent structures in the distal direction are smaller in the $50 - 50$ proximal-distal flow split implying that the flow recovers more rapidly, this is consistent with the lower Reynolds number of the distal and proximal graft. However a significantly larger vorticity stretching arises at the branch.

Consideration of the axial flow profiles shown by the inset plots of 5.15(d) demonstrates that the amount of axial flow distortion from the Hagen-Poiseuille flow profile is far greater in the $50 - 50$ proximal-distal flow split configuration when compared to the fully occluded configuration 5.15(a). This axial flow distortion is directly associated with a stronger secondary flow as also indicated by the larger stretching which also has a significant effect on the peak wall shear stress magnitude [458].

5.4.4 Pulsatile flow

In Section 5.1 we introduced the idea of using a non-dimensional time parameter based on a reduced velocity rather than the classical use of the Womersley number. In this section we provide some examples where the reduced velocity is useful in providing a physical insight into different pulsatile flow regimes. The motivation for consideration of an alternative time parameter to the Womersley number arises from the interpretation of Womersley number as the ratio of two length-scales within a given cross section (one of which is related to time). This parameter is therefore helpful if different flow dynamics arise within a specific cross section of a vessel. However if a change in flow dynamics is related to length scales which are not purely related to a given cross section alternative parameters are likely to be more physically relevant. An alternatively time related parameter is the reduced velocity $U_{red} = \bar{U}T/D$ which we recall is the ratio of the length that the mean sectional velocity $\bar{U}$ propagates over a time period T to the vessel diameter D. The potential for this type of parameter to help understand pulsatile idealised flows is highlighted in the following two examples.

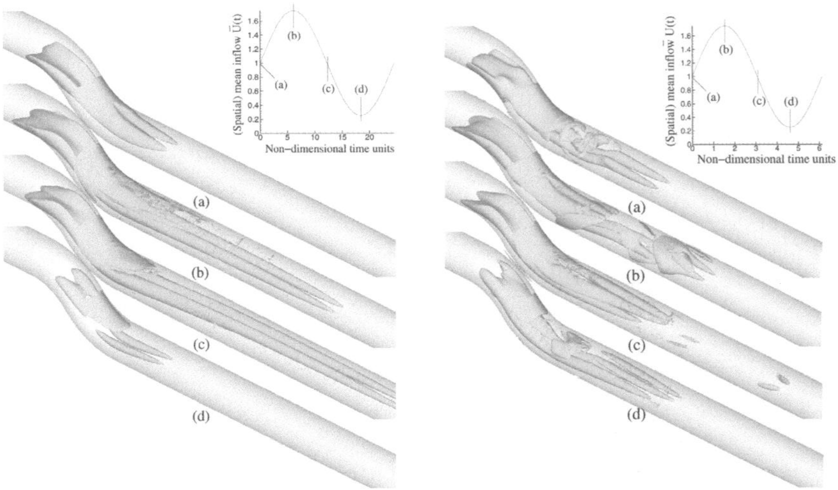

Fig. 5.16. Vortical structure in unsteady flow at $Re_D = 250$, $Wo = 4$, ($U_{red} = 24.5$) (left) and $Re_D = 250$, $Wo = 8$, ($U_{red} = 6.13$) (right), visualised using the $\lambda_2 D^2/U^2 = -0.3$ isocontour.

In Fig. 5.16 we consider the geometry of a 45° double bend previously discussed in Section 5.4.2. In this example, taken from [390], the flow is driven by a sinusoidally varying pulsatile flow with a peak to mean velocity of 1.75. In the left series of plots in Fig. 5.16 we consider the vortex cores at four time instances under the physiologically realistic parameters of a Womersley number $Wo = 4$ and a mean Reynolds number of $Re_D = 250$. At these values of Reynolds number and Womersley number we can determine from equation (5.2) that the reduced velocity is $U_{red} = 24.5$. Comparison of the vortex structures with Fig. 5.11 highlight the quasi-steady nature of the flow thereby having a similar flow structure and also supported by the large value of the reduced velocity.

We next consider a pulsatile flow under similar conditions but at four times the frequency which corresponds to doubling the Womersley number to $Wo = 8$. These conditions relate to a reduced velocity of $U_{red} = 6.13$ and as shown in the right set of plots in Fig. 5.16 we see a significantly different flow structure appearing throughout the pulsatile cycle. The reduced velocity tells us that the mean velocity only travels approximately 6 diameters throughout the pulsatile cycle. Therefore the flow structures generated during one cycle are unable to propagate through the entire double bend before the next pulsatile cycle begins. The reduced velocity therefore indicates that interactions of flow structures between each cycle is likely leading to the differing vortex structures in the downstream (distal) portion of the pipe [390].

Another example of how pulsatility can change the flow dynamics is highlighted in Fig. 5.18. In this figure we observe the transitional flow in the distal region behind an axi-symmetric stenosis as detailed in [39, 456]. During each

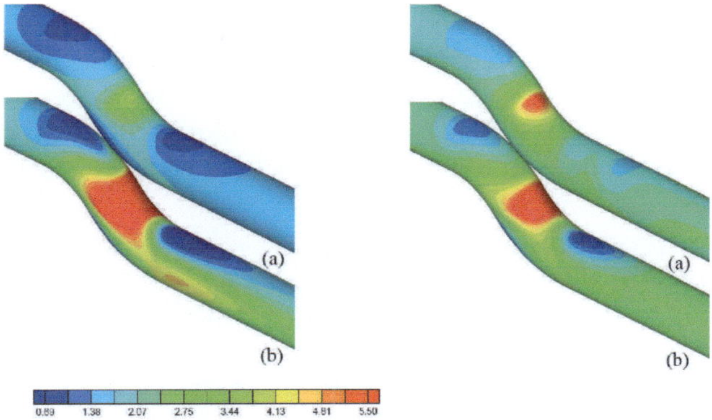

Fig. 5.17. Comparison of wall shear stress at instants (a),(b) in unsteady flow cycle for double bend flow: $Re_D = 250$, $Wo = 4$, $(U_{red} = 24.5)$ (left) and $Re_D = 250$, $Wo = 8$, $(U_{red} = 6.13)$ (right)

pulsatile cycle a jet is generated from the 75 % stenosis on the front of which a vortex ring is generated. Depending on the frequency of the pulsatility and the separation of the vortex rings (and therefore the reduced velocity) we observe a different types of transition to turbulence. In Figs. 5.18(a) and (b) we observe the flow at $Re_D = 400$ and $U_{red} = 2.5$ where, as in the previous example, a sinusoidal pulsatile waveform with a peak to mean ratio of 1.75 is imposed. Under these conditions the flow transitions due to a *tilting* mechanism where each vortex ring ejected from the stenosis tilts and subsequently stretches and breaks down into a turbulence cloud. In the above figure the vortex ring is

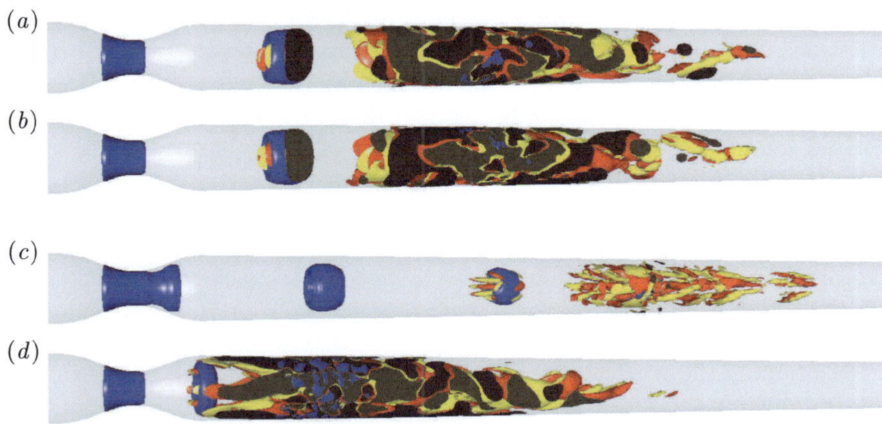

Fig. 5.18. Breakdown of pulsatile flow through a stenosis. (a), (b): $Ured = 2.5$ leads to breakdown via period doubling instability. (c), (d): $Ured = 1$ leads to breakdown through wavy instability of the vortex rings. At non-linear saturation the transition occurs close to the stenosis as shown in Fig. (a),(b) and (d)

indicated by an isocontour of the velocity gradient tensor discriminant in blue and the turbulent cloud is highlighted by isocontours of positive and negative axial vorticity in red and yellow. The axi-symmetrical nature of the stenotic geometry leads to a period doubling type instability where the tilting of the vortex ring during one period is in the opposite direction to the tilting of the vortex ring generated in the next cycle.

In Fig. 5.18(c) and (d), we consider the transition to turbulence under similar conditions but at a higher frequency corresponding to a reduced velocity of $U_{red} = 1$ and Reynolds number of $Re_D = 350$. At this reduced velocity the flow transitions by the vortex ring ejected during each cycle breaking down through a wavy type instability on the ring similar to the isolated vortex breakdown investigated by Widnall [544]. Although the wavy ring vortex (and the previous vortex tilting breakdown) initiates relatively far downstream from the stenosis, after many pulsatile cycles the breakdown region moves towards the stenosis as highlighted by Fig. 5.18(d).

5.5 Anatomically realistic geometries

5.5.1 Curved artery modelling

The preceding examples demonstrate that a vortical flow structure is rapidly established in a single bend; in a series of bends, the structure of the flow may be altered in several ways: (i) in a sequence of weak (short) bends, the initial vortical structure may carry through or be annihilated depending on Re_D, (ii) non-planar sequences of bends can lead to asymmetric or helical type outflows, (iii) strong (90 degree) bends at higher Reynolds numbers produce eruptions of wall vorticity which appear to effectively destroy the coherence of any structures remaining from the first bend.

For comparison, we now consider the flow in a real arterial geometry, derived from a cast of the right coronary artery of a pig obtained under conditions representative of diastole, [273]. The geometry is tortuous and we ignore side branches; hence there is an artificial acceleration of the flow as the lumen tapers along its length. For comparison we consider a slightly idealised geometry in which a constant diameter tube is fitted to the same centreline curve. On the right of Fig. 5.19 the wall shear stress distribution shows considerable variation as the artery twists and turns.

Examining the vortical flow structures however shows high degree of similarity between the vortical structures in the real and idealised geometries. Cross-plane velocity vectors in Fig. 5.19 (a1,b1) likewise show a high degree of similarity, with an asymmetric vortex pair in both realisations. As reported in [273], if the wall shear stress values for the real model are re-scaled to remove the effect of taper, there is very good correlation between the spatial distributions in the real and idealised geometries.

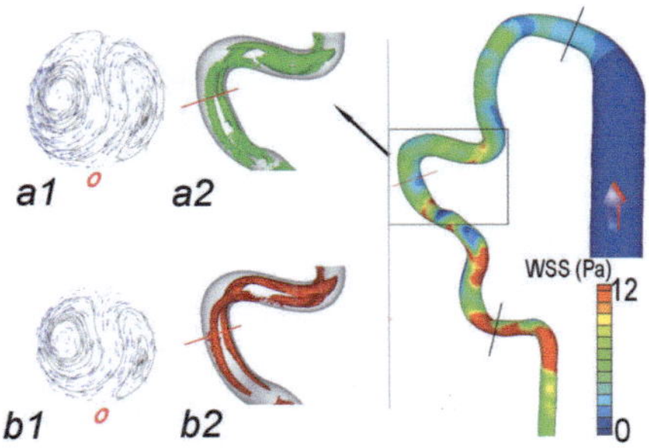

Fig. 5.19. Right: Dimensional distribution of wall shear stress in tortuous porcine coronary artery in steady flow at $Re_D = 286$. Left: cross-flow velocities and vortical structures after third bend. Top pair corresponds to real geometry on right, lower pair is for model with same centreline geometry but constant circular cross-section

5.5.2 Bypass graft models

Finally we present two examples of more complex, realistic geometries which illustrate many of the features we have discussed. The first example, Fig. 5.20, is that of the distal anastomosis of a femoro-tibial bypass graft. The geometry of the anastomosis shortly after surgery, together with contour plots of the streamwise velocity at the three indicated sections are shown in parts (a) and (b) of the figure. Cross-flow streamlines indicated on the velocity contour plot of the graft flow, (uppermost plot in part (a)), show a Dean-like vortex pair resulting from the curvature of the graft as it approaches the anastomosis.

The bias of the graft flow towards the outer wall of the bend is shown in the middle contour plot, and is also evident in the 20 cm/s isosurface of velocity

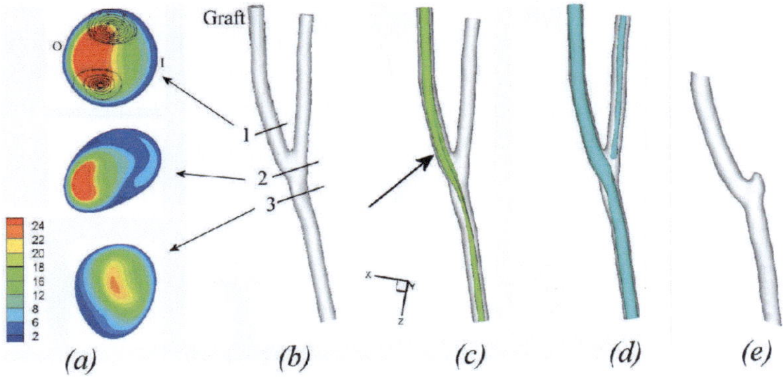

Fig. 5.20. Computed flow in femoro-tibial bypass graft geometry derived from *in vivo* imaging shortly after surgery. (a), velocity contours, (b) geometry and slice location, (c) 20 cm/s velocity isosurface – note bias towards outer wall as for bend, (d) 10 cm/s velocity isosurface showing low proximal outflow, (e) geometry after six months

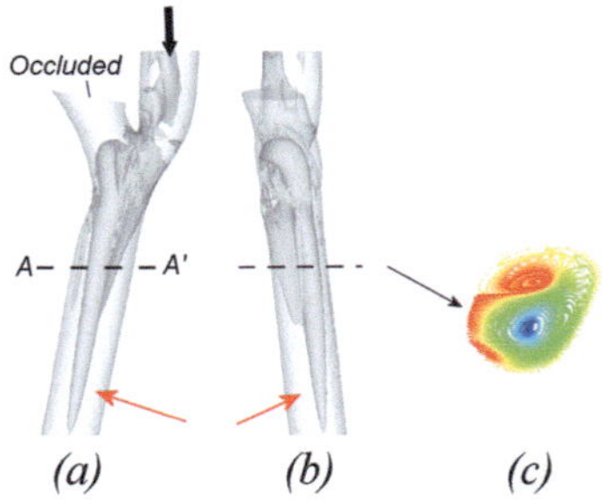

Fig. 5.21. Left: Vortical flow structures at distal anastomosis of aorto-coronary graft. Although the global geometry is that of a shallow S-bend, localised constriction produces highly asymmetric flow shown by dominant vortex core. Right: Distribution of particles (coded by distance from centreline radius at inflow) at indicated section AA'

shown in part (c). Most of the graft flow carries on to the distal artery, though with some retrograde flow to the proximal artery as shown in the 10 cm/s isosurface of velocity (d). Consequently the wall shear stress distribution (not shown) is uniformly low in the proximal outflow portion. Finally part (e) shows the graft geometry six months post operatively. Remodelling of the arterial lumen is evident in the region of the anastomosis, and there is no longer any measurable flow to the proximal artery.

Next we consider flow in a the vicinity of the distal anastomosis of an aorto-coronary bypass graft. The model geometry was again derived by casting a porcine heart *ex vivo*,as described in [370]. Here the geometry of the graft centreline is similar to that of the 45 degree model double bend configuration, and we would thus expect to find a relatively symmetric pair of Dean type vortices in the host artery outflow. As shown in Fig. 5.21 however, the outflow vortical structure is highly asymmetric, with a dominant swirl component. In this case a highly localised asymmetric narrowing of the graft at the anastomosis produces a strongly biased inflow, overriding the influence of the global geometry.

5.6 Conclusions

In this chapter we have examined how the flow in the large arteries is influenced by their geometric form. We provided a brief outline of the mathematical tools and some concepts used to identify essential features and the mechanisms leading to the development of secondary flows. The physical basis of dimensionless similarity parameters was discussed and their use in characterising flow regimes emphasised. Summarising:

- Reynolds number, Re_D, is overall the pre-eminent parameter, both in determining the stability of a flow and the persistence of geometric influences downstream of a bend or other disturbance;
- the reduced velocity, U_{red} is a more appropriate parameter than the Womersley number for unsteady flows where there are significant streamwise flow variations;
- the Dean number De is the dominant parameter used to characterise flow in bends; in tightly curved or helical bends other parameters in addition to De may be required.

A major focus of the discussion centred on the flow in bends and sequences of bends. In particular we demonstrated that:

- In sequences of bends, the flow response to bends with high deflection (90°) was significantly different from that with modest (45°) deflection, due to the generally less intense interaction between the core and the wall layers.
- In non-planar sequences of high deflection bends, re-orientation of the core vortical structures is accompanied by merging and cancellation with the wall vortical layers. This is likely to provide enhanced mixing. Symmetric or asymmetric outflows may occur, depending on the degree of vortex reorientation and the interactions between the core of the flow and wall.
- In pulsatile flow, if the mean flow propagation distance over one cycle is long (many diameters or greater than the immediate geometry) the flow character is quasi-steady, though not necessarily its impact for example on mixing. If the mean flow propagation distance is relatively short, new shedding-like structures arise which are not seen in steady flow.

Finally we chose a few examples of flow in anatomically realistic geometries.

- The first case comprised a tortuous artery at a modest Reynolds number appropriate to the coronaries. There it was found that an idealised model of the same centreline geometry but of circular cross-section captured the essential dynamics well.
- In the second example of a bypass-graft flow, we observed characteristic non-uniform velocity distributions and vortical structures introduced by the global graft curvature. Post-operative evolution of the geometry emphasises the potential for the vasculature to re-model, with profound changes in topology.
- In the third example, again of a bypass graft configuration, we found a very different flow pattern from that expected by consideration of the global vascular geometry. A localised narrowing at the anastomosis produced a strongly biased inflow and led to a highly asymmetric outflow.

In conclusion, the modelling of arterial flow in anatomically realistic geometries calls for an understanding of the delicate balance between global and local anatomical features.

6

Rheological models for blood

Anne M. Robertson, Adélia Sequeira, and Robert G. Owens

Rheology is the science of the deformation and flow of materials. It deals with the theoretical concepts of kinematics, conservation laws and constitutive relations, describing the interrelation between force, deformation and flow. The experimental determination of the rheological behaviour of materials is called *rheometry.* The object of haemorheology is the application of rheology to the study of flow properties of blood and its formed elements, and the coupling of blood and the blood vessels in living organisms. This field involves the investigation of the macroscopic behaviour of blood determined in rheometric experiments, its microscopic properties *in vitro* and *in vivo* and studies of the interactions among blood cellular components and between these components and the endothelial cells that line blood vessels.

Advances in the field of haemorheology have contributed in particular to the fundamental understanding of the changes in the rheological properties of blood and its components due to pathological disturbances, and are based on the evidence that they might be the primary cause of many cardiovascular diseases. Haemorheological aberrations can easily be considered as a result (or an indicator) of insufficient circulatory function. Alternatively, deviations in haemorheological parameters may affect tissue perfusion and be manifested as circulatory problems. Basically, pathologies with haematological origin like leukemia, haemolytic anemia, thalassemia or pathologies associated with the risk factors of thrombosis and atherosclerosis like myocardial infarction, hypertension, strokes or diabetes are mainly related to disturbances of local homeostasis. Therefore, the mathematical and numerical study of powerful, yet simple, constitutive models that can capture the rheological response of blood over a range of flow conditions is ultimately recognised as an important tool for clinical diagnosis and therapeutic planning (see e.g. [127, 302]).

The aim of this chapter is to present the rheological properties of blood, including its non-Newtonian characteristics, and review some of the macroscopic mathematical models that have been proposed in the literature to model these features.

Formaggia L, Quarteroni A, Veneziani A (Eds.): Cardiovascular Mathematics. Modeling and simulation of the circulatory system

6.1 Physical mechanisms behind the mechanical properties of blood

As already discussed in Chapter 1 whole blood is a concentrated suspension of formed cellular elements that includes red blood cells (RBCs) or erythrocytes, white blood cells (WBCs) or leukocytes and platelets or thrombocytes. These cellular elements are suspended in an aqueous polymer solution, the plasma, containing electrolytes and organic molecules such as metabolites, hormones, enzymes, antibodies and other proteins. Erythrocytes have been shown to exert the most significant influence on the mechanical properties of blood, mainly due to their presence in very high concentration compared to the other formed elements (approximately $4\text{–}6 \times 10^6$ RBCs/mm^3), comprising about 40 to 45 % of its volume in healthy individuals (haematocrit, Ht).

While plasma is nearly Newtonian in behaviour, whole blood exhibits marked non-Newtonian characteristics, particularly at low shear rates. The non-Newtonian behaviour of blood is mainly explained by three phenomena: the erythrocytes' tendency to form a three-dimensional microstructure at low shear rates, their deformability and their tendency to align with the flow field at high shear rates [86, 449].

As will be elaborated on below, the formation and breakup of this 3D microstructure, as well as the elongation and recovery of red blood cells, contribute to blood's shear thinning, viscoelastic and thixotropic behaviour[1]. Aggregation and deformation of erythrocytes are complex dynamic processes in which cellular and plasma components of blood contribute as essential factors. Experimental data under various flow conditions, particularly physiologically relevant flows, are required to develop meaningful models of these complex processes (see [466, 468]).

In this section we briefly discuss the physical behaviour of erythrocytes that have the strongest influence on the non-Newtonian behaviour of whole flowing blood at low shear rates.

6.1.1 Low shear rate behaviour: aggregation and disaggregation of erythrocytes

In the presence of fibrinogen and globulins (two plasma proteins), erythrocytes have the ability to form a primary aggregate structure of rod shaped stacks of individual cells called *rouleaux*. At very low shear rates the rouleaux align themselves in an end-to-side and side-to-side fashion and form a secondary structure consisting of branched three-dimensional aggregates [450]

---

[1] While the definition of thixotropy varies greatly in the literature, here we refer to thixotropy as the dependence of the material properties on the time over which shear has been applied. This dependence is largely due to the finite time required for the three-dimensional structure of blood to form and break down. This issue will be elaborated on in Section 6.2.1.

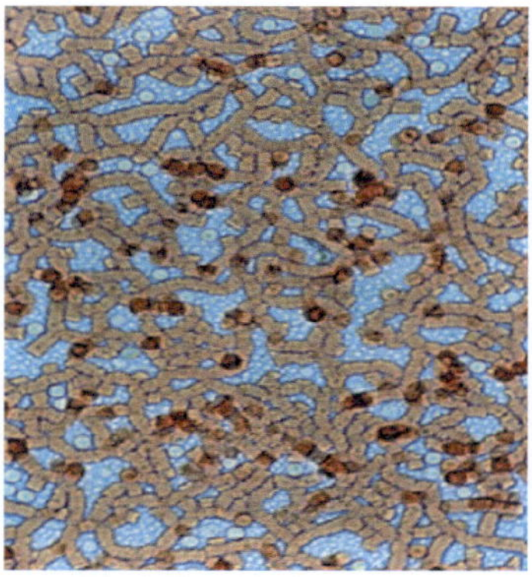

Fig. 6.1. Three-dimensional microstructure of RBC aggregates in human blood from a healthy donor. Rouleaux formed by rod shaped stacks of RBCs can be seen. The isolated darker circles on top of the rouleaux arise from rouleaux branching off these stacks, forming the three-dimensional microstructure of RBC aggregates. These branches are less transparent and therefore darker. The large light circles are white blood cells while the much smaller light circles are platelets. Magnification 100X, (courtesy of Prof. M.V. Kameneva, University of Pittsburgh, USA)

(see Fig. 6.1). The biochemical process of rouleaux formation is still unclear. It has been experimentally observed that these stacks will not form if the erythrocytes have been hardened or in the absence of fibrinogen and globulins.

For blood at rest, the three-dimensional structure formed by the RBCs appears solid-like, appearing to resist flow until a finite level of force is applied. The applied stress needed to initiate flow, e.g. in simple shear, is often referred to as the yield stress and, under normal conditions, is primarily a function of the haematocrit and the fibrinogen concentration of the plasma [322,324,448]. Additional factors such as the red cell shape, deformability and tendency to aggregate also influence the value of the yield stress parameter. As discussed below, the existence of a yield stress for fluids in general and treatment of this yield stress as a material parameter is a somewhat controversial issue (see, e.g., [27,338]).

When blood begins to flow, the solid-like structure breaks into three-dimensional networks of various sizes which appear to move as individual units and reach an equilibrium size for a fixed shear rate. Increases in shear rate lead to a reduction in equilibrium size and lower effective viscosity. In the studies of Schmid-Schönbein [450] at shear rates between 5.8 and $46\,\mathrm{s}^{-1}$, each doubling of the shear rate resulted in a decrease in average aggregate size of approximately 50 % (see also Section 3 of [429] for further discussion).

Once the chains are broken down to 4–10 cells, they are resistant to further shearing and, at high shear rates they roll, rotate and tumble as units along with individual cells. A critical shear rate $\dot{\gamma}_{\max}$ is defined as a constant shear rate at which, effectively there are no more aggregates (larger than $15\,\mu\mathrm{m}$). In whole blood from healthy humans, different values are reported for this critical shear rate, largely in the range of 5–100 s^{-1} (e.g. [127, 200]). Dintenfass [127] attributed this variation in reported values to the degree of aggregation of the original sample which, as discussed later, is consistent with the thixotropic nature of blood (see Section 6.2). In diseased states, the critical shear rate can increase substantially. For example, in blood samples from patients with acute myocardial infarctions, the critical shear rate for dispersion was found to be greater than approximately 250 s^{-1} and the average aggregate size was larger than in the controls for all shear rates [200, 450].

The process of disaggregation under increasing shear is reversible. When the shear rate is quasi-statically stepped down to lower values, the individual cells form shorter chains, then longer rouleaux and eventually a 3-D microstructure [200]. The finite time necessary for equilibrium of the structure to be reached (both during aggregation and disaggregation) is responsible for the thixotropic behaviour of blood at low shear rates (see, Section 6.2.1 and, for example, Section 6 of [428]). The associated time constants are a function of shear rate. The equilibria are found to be reached more rapidly at higher shear rates and more gradually with lower shear rates (e.g. [127]). For example, in a cone and plate viscometer, for shear rates between 0.01 and 1.0 s^{-1} the equilibrium distributions were found to be reached after time intervals of 20 to 200 seconds.

Accelerating flow has a marked effect on the structure of the aggregate. Under acceleration between fixed shear rates, significant elongation of rouleaux occurs which is not seen when the flow is held at a fixed shear rate. The elongation is particularly evident in rouleaux that bridge larger secondary structures and is found to arise from realignment of the individual cells (sliding of the cells from a parallel stack to a sheared stack) and deformation of individual cells (ellipsoidal deformation and eventually prolate deformation). As a result of these mechanisms, the aggregate length can increase up to three fold [450]. Under a sinusoidal variation of shear, elastic behaviour of the aggregates is observed [102, 449, 517]. While typical data for whole blood viscosity are obtained from quasi-static shear experiments, small amplitude oscillatory shear experiments are used to measure both viscous and elastic properties in the regime of small deformations from the rest history (Section 6.2).

6.1.2 High shear rate behaviour of whole blood: shear flow of dispersed erythrocytes

In a Couette rheometer, when blood is subjected to a constant shear rate slightly above $\dot{\gamma}_{\max}$, the cells can be seen to rotate. With increasing shear rate, they rotate less and for shear rates above 230 s^{-1}, they cease to rotate and remain aligned with the flow direction [450].

For shear rates above 400 s^{-1}, the RBCs lose their biconcave shape, become fully elongated and are transformed into flat outstretched ellipsoids with major axes parallel to the flow direction. At this stage the collision of red cells only occurs when a more rapidly moving cell touches a slower one but there are no further interactions between the cells. Close observation suggests that the changing cells contours are consistent with a tank-treading motion of the cells membranes about their interior, similar to a fluid drop deformation, [83, 154, 449]. The high deformability of erythrocytes is due to the absence of a nucleus, to the elastic and viscous properties of its membrane and also to geometric factors such as the shape, volume and membrane surface area.

6.1.3 Further comments on the role of erythrocyte deformability

It has been shown experimentally that at a haematocrit above 30 % and at a shear rate of $230\,\mathrm{s}^{-1}$ the viscosity of a suspension of hardened red cells in saline solution is much higher than that of a suspension of normal cells [450]. This increase in viscosity is also observed in blood of sickle cell anemia parents (see, e.g. [46, 133, 372]). This is a congenital pathology in which the loss of deformability of the red cells causes ischemic manifestations in the capillary bed. RBCs become sickle-shaped and less flexible, and have difficulty passing through small blood vessels. Chien et al. [85] found that the viscosity of blood containing irreversible sickled cells exceeds that of normal blood under all experimental conditions and it can be of the order of fifty times greater. On the basis of the rheological changes, a mechanism has been suggested to explain the amplification of the clinical symptoms: oxygen is decreased, cells change into the sickled form, blood viscosity increases, capillary flow decreases, fragility of the sickle cells is decreased, blood flow slows down, more oxygen is taken from the red cells to the tissues and thrombosis and haemolysis may result. Other clinical applications of blood rheology can be found, for example, in [302, 485].

6.2 Measurements of the mechanical properties of blood

Measurements of the mechanical properties of whole blood are technically challenging, particularly at low to medium shear rates where denatured protein films, sedimentation and phase separation can lead to erroneous results. At high shear rates, inertial effects can be problematic. As a result, measuring the mechanical properties of blood over a wide range of shear rates (e.g. 0.01–500 s^{-1}), can require the use of more than one rheometer. Therefore, before discussing rheological data for whole blood, we first turn attention to the measurements of the mechanical properties of whole blood including a brief discussion of material functions which are measured, an overview of typical blood rheometers and a discusion of some of the challenges which are particular to blood rheometry.

6.2.1 Material functions

In this section, we provide an overview of typical material functions used to quantify the rheological behaviour of blood. Many of the continuum models for blood are examples of a large category of constitutive models called incompressible simple fluids. As defined in [100],

> ... an *incompressible simple material* ... is a substance whose mass density never changes and for which the stress is determined, to within a pressure, by the history of strain. ... We then define an *incompressible simple fluid* as an incompressible simple material with the property that all of its local configurations are intrinsically equivalent in response, with all observable differences in response being due to definite differences in history.

The material functions used to quantify the viscous and viscoelastic properties of blood have precise meaning within the context of simple fluid theory.

Viscometric functions

The mechanical response of incompressible Newtonian fluids in shear is completely determined by one material constant: the viscosity μ. The response of general fluids is much more complicated and can include behaviours not displayed by Newtonian fluids such as rod climbing, shear thinning and memory. Remarkably, the behaviour of an arbitrary simple fluid in a broad class of flows called *viscometric flows* only requires knowledge of three material functions for that fluid. Appropriately, these three functions are called *viscometric material functions* and are intrinsic properties of the fluid.

For brevity we do not introduce the kinematics necessary to rigorously define viscometric flows, but just recall that these are a special type of constant stretch history flow which, from the point of view of the fluid element, are indistinguishable from a steady simple shear flow described in terms of suitably chosen local Cartesian coordinates (see [15, 100] for a more detailed discussion). Some examples of viscometric flows are steady flow between parallel plates driven by the motion of one or both of the plates (simple shear flow) and steady, fully developed flows in channels and pipes of constant cross section. The three viscometric material functions are easily defined relative to simple shear flow (expressed in a Cartesian frame $(\boldsymbol{e}_1, \boldsymbol{e}_2, \boldsymbol{e}_3)$) with velocity field $\boldsymbol{u} = \dot{\gamma}_0 x_2 \boldsymbol{e}_1$ where the shear rate $\dot{\gamma}_0$ is a positive constant,

$$\begin{aligned} &\text{Viscosity or Shear Viscosity} && \mu(\dot{\gamma}_0) \equiv \sigma_{12}/\dot{\gamma}_0 \\ &\text{First normal stress coefficient:} && \psi_1(\dot{\gamma}_0) \equiv (\sigma_{11} - \sigma_{22})/\dot{\gamma}_0^2 \\ &\text{Second normal stress coefficient:} && \psi_2(\dot{\gamma}_0) \equiv (\sigma_{22} - \sigma_{33})/\dot{\gamma}_0^2, \end{aligned} \tag{6.1}$$

and σ_{ij} are the rectangular components of the Cauchy stress tensor defined in Chapter 3 [2]. For Newtonian and generalised Newtonian fluids ψ_1 and ψ_2 will be zero.

[2] Note that alternative definitions of the first and second normal stress definitions are sometimes used, though they can be formed from linear combinations of these given here.

In short, if rheologists measure the functions $\mu(\dot{\gamma}), \psi_1(\dot{\gamma}), \psi_2(\dot{\gamma})$ in one viscometric flow, they can predict the behaviour of this material in all other viscometric flows. In addition, any incompressible simple fluid can undergo all viscometric flows. The three functions are shown to be material functions that have meaning without selecting a particular constitutive model for a fluid. It is therefore not surprising, that all three of the commonly used rheometers discussed below are designed to generate flows that are approximations of viscometric flows.

Linear viscoelastic properties

The magnitudes of viscoelastic effects in blood are small. In fact, to date, measurements of the first and second normal stress differences for blood have not been reported. Instead, the majority of viscoelastic studies on blood are directed at obtaining the *linear viscoelastic* properties of blood. For linear viscoelastic theory to be valid, the general kinematics of a simple fluid are restricted to motions in which the norm of the strain relative to the rest history is small (see, e.g. [100]). All nonlinear effects are treated as negligible. These linear viscoelastic properties are often determined by subjecting the fluids to periodic flows in the limit of small deformations.

A commonly reported linearly viscoelastic property is the complex modulus G^*. The real and imaginary parts of $G^* = G' + iG''$ are referred to as the storage modulus and loss modulus, respectively, where G' and G'' are both real numbers. The role of these parameters is easily seen for infinitesimal oscillatory shear flows. For convenience, as for the discussion of simple shear flow, we use a Cartesian frame with the plates parallel to $\boldsymbol{e}_1$. In particular, consider flow of blood between two parallel plates generated by the motion of the upper plate when it is subjected to a oscillatory displacement $\gamma_0 h \sin \omega t \boldsymbol{e}_1$. The corresponding plate velocity is then $\gamma_0 \omega h \cos \omega t \boldsymbol{e}_1$. In the limit of infinitesimal linear viscoelasticity, the shear stress can be written as (e.g. Section 7.2.1 of [428]),

$$\sigma_{12} = \gamma_0 \left(G' \sin \omega t + G'' \cos \omega t \right). \tag{6.2}$$

For purely elastic materials, the shear stress and displacement are in phase, in which case G'' is zero and G' plays the role of an elastic shear modulus. For purely viscous materials, the shear stress is in phase with the velocity gradient, requiring G' to be zero. Hence, G'' is the quantity associated with viscous losses in the material. It is for this reason that G' and G'' are referred to as the storage and loss moduli, respectively. A related quantity is the loss tangent, $\tan \delta$ defined as,

$$\tan \delta = G''/G'. \tag{6.3}$$

It follows from (6.3), that δ will be zero for a purely elastic material and $\pi/2$ for a purely viscous material.

Another quantity which is often reported in the literature on linear viscoelasticity is the complex viscosity μ^*,

$$\mu^* = \mu' - i\mu'', \tag{6.4}$$

where μ' and μ'' are real. The shear stress in small amplitude oscillatory shear can be written in terms of these linear viscoelastic parameters (e.g. Sec. 7.2.1 of [428]) through

$$\sigma_{12} = \gamma_0\, \omega\, (\mu' \cos \omega t + \mu'' \sin \omega t)\,. \tag{6.5}$$

Following similar arguments as used to determine the roles of G' and G'', we see that μ' is zero for elastic materials and μ'' is zero for viscous materials. It is for this reason that μ'' and μ' are referred to as the elastic and viscous components of the complex viscosity, respectively.

The relationships between the complex viscosity and the complex modulus as well as their components are

$$\mu^* = G^*/i\omega, \qquad \mu' = G''/\omega, \qquad \mu'' = G'/\omega. \tag{6.6}$$

In typical experiments, the material moduli of linear viscoelasticity are given as a function of frequency ω.

Thixotropic response

The formation of the three-dimensional microstructure and the alignment of the RBC are not instantaneous, which gives blood its thixotropic behaviour. As emphasised by Barnes [26], there is a tremendous variation in published definitions for thixotropy. Outside of industrial applications, these definitions largely focus on the time dependence of rheological properties under fixed shear rate (e.g. viscosity, normal stress effects) arising from the finite time required for the breakdown and buildup in microstructure such as that just described for blood. Bauer and Collins [31] provide the following representative definition,

> *Thixotropy*: When a reduction in magnitude of rheological properties of a system, such as elastic modulus, yield stress, and viscosity, for example, occurs reversibly and isothermally with a distinct time dependence on application of shear strain, the system is described as *thixotropic*.

Many theories for thixotropy introduce a metric of the level of microstructure denoted by λ. It is helpful to use this concept in the following discussion of blood thixotropy. For simplicity, λ is normalised such that $\lambda \in [0, 1]$ and $\lambda = 0$ refers to the absence of structure (e.g. only individual RBCs remain) and $\lambda = 1$ refers to the largest level of structure possible under the given physical conditions. An evolution equation is then introduced to describe the rate of change of λ as result of competing effects driving build up or breakdown in microstructure. To complete the theory, an expression for the functional dependence of viscosity and viscoelastic parameters on the level microstructure λ is given.

Unsteady shear flows are often used to probe the thixotropic material response. In this section, we consider two such flows. Once again, flow between two parallel plates is considered, driven by the motion of the upper plate. Here, we consider the upper plate to move with unsteady, non-periodic velocity of the form $\boldsymbol{u} = v(x_2, t)\boldsymbol{e}_1$. The magnitude of either of the two equal non-zero components of the symmetric part of the velocity gradient is denoted by $\dot{\gamma}(t)$ and referred to as the shear rate, (also defined below, see (6.19), Section 6.4.1). The applied shear stress is denoted by σ_{12}.

Shown in Fig. 6.2(a), is $\dot{\gamma}(t)$ for one such flow. Here, the plate is subjected to a step increase in shear rate at time t_0 from zero to $\dot{\gamma} = \dot{\gamma}_a$. This is followed by a step decrease at $t = t_1$ to a constant value $\dot{\gamma}_b < \dot{\gamma}_a$. For experiments on thixotropic fluids, it is necessary to know the state of the material structure at the beginning of the experiment. Here, we assume the material has maximum structure at $t = t_0$. For times larger than t_1, the shear rate is held constant at $\dot{\gamma}_b$. The response of a representative thixotropic material to this loading regime is seen in Fig. 6.2(b). After the step increase in load, the structure begins to diminish, resulting in a decrease in the viscosity and hence the applied shear stress. A finite amount of time is required for the material to approach the equilibrium structure (and hence viscosity) for the applied shear rate $\dot{\gamma}_a$. This is reflected in the finite amount of time it takes for the applied shear stress to approach σ_a. Just before the abrupt drop in shear rate, the level of the microstructure has nearly reached the equilibrium value for $\dot{\gamma}_a$. Immediately after the drop in shear rate, the level of the microstructure falls below that of the equilibrium value for the new shear rate $\dot{\gamma}_b$. With increasing time at this lower shear rate, the structure builds back up, tending towards the equilibrium value for $\dot{\gamma}_b$. The viscosity increases due to this increasing structure, requiring increased applied shear stress to maintain the shear rate $\dot{\gamma}_b$.

Shown in Fig. 6.3(a) is a loading regime for a second experiment used to test thixotropic materials. It consists of a linear increase in shear rate followed

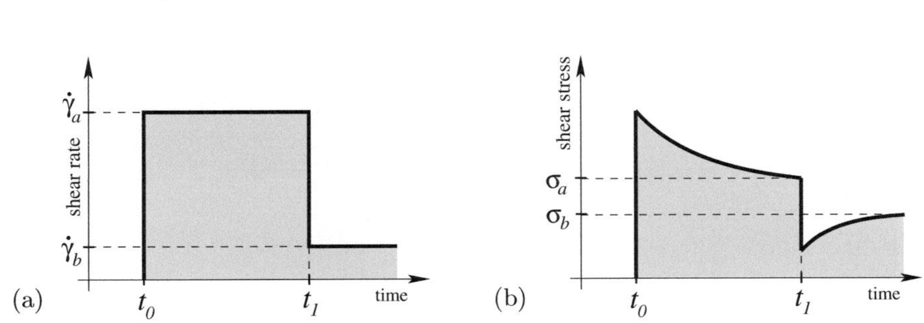

Fig. 6.2. Qualitative behaviour of a thixotropic fluid undergoing a step increase then decrease in shear rate: (a) imposed shear rate as a function of time (b) resulting shear stress as a function of time

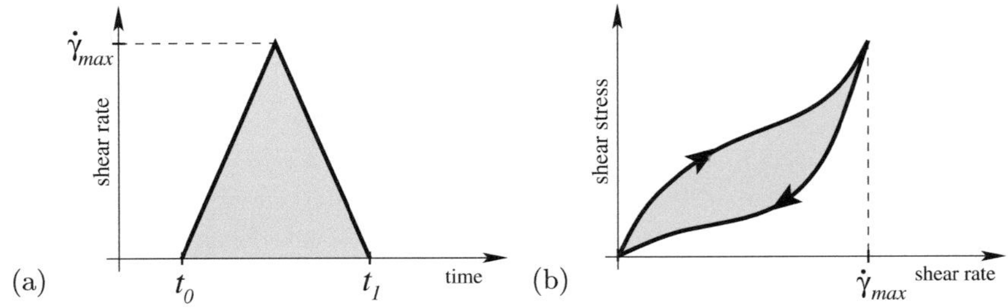

Fig. 6.3. Qualitative features of the dependence of shear stress on shear rate for a representative thixotropic fluid experiencing a linear increase in shear rate followed directly by a linear decrease: (a) imposed shear rate as a function of time; (b) resulting shear stress as a function of shear rate

directly by a linear decrease. The shear rate is constantly changing so that there is no possibility for the material structure to approach its equilibrium value. As a result, the response of the material to this loading is more complex than the step loading in Fig. 6.2. As before, we assume the material started out with the maximum microstructure. For simplicity, we consider thixotropic materials with no viscoelastic behaviour. The microstructure will break down as the shear rate is increased to $\dot{\gamma}_{\text{max}}$, Since there is not sufficient time for the structure to break down to its equilibrium value for the current shear rate, the viscosity and hence shear stress will be larger than the corresponding equilibrium values. As the shear rate is decreased from $\dot{\gamma}_{\text{max}}$, the structure level will begin to increase. Since this increase is not instantaneous, the structure level (and viscosity) will be lower than the values at the same shear rate during the first half of the loading regime. The corresponding shear stress is lower, resulting in the hysteresis loop seen in Fig. 6.3(b). The size of this loop is often used as a measure of thixotropy. In contrast, for fluids like water with no substantial change in microstructure, the curve traced out during increasing and decreasing shear rate would be identical.

It should be emphasised that, unfortunately, there are no thixotropic material functions analogous to the viscometric functions. These non-periodic time dependent flows can only provide information about material functions for specific thixotropic constitutive models or used as a probe of qualitative features of the thixotropic behaviour. Even this qualitative interpretation can be confounded by combined viscoelastic and thixotropic effects. This is in contrast to the viscometric and oscillatory flows discussed earlier which can be used to measure viscometric and viscoelastic material functions.

6.2.2 Overview of rheometers

The three most commonly used rheometers for blood are the concentric cylinder rheometer (Couette rheometer), the cone and plate rheometer and the

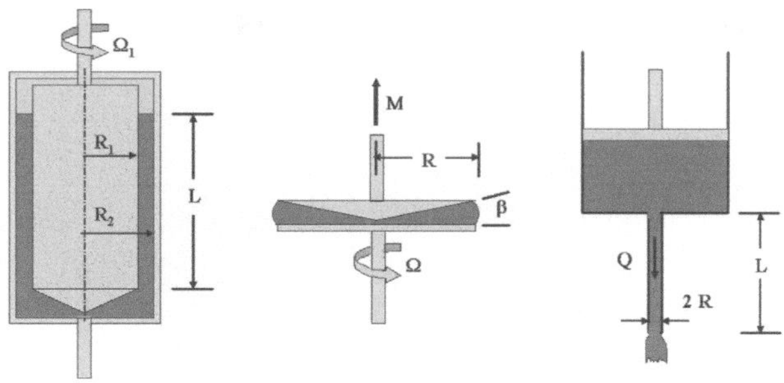

Fig. 6.4. Schematic of three rheometers commonly used for blood: (a) Couette, (b) cone and plate, and (c) capillary

capillary rheometer, Fig. 6.4. These rheometers can be used to approximate the viscometric, oscillatory and non-periodic unsteady flows discussed in the last section.

Couette rheometer

In a Couette rheometer, the test fluid is placed in the annulus between two concentric cylinders, Fig. 6.4(a). The inner and outer radii are denoted by R_1 and R_2 respectively and the length of the test regime by L. The fluid motion is generated by the rotation of one or both cylinders. We denote the difference in rotation rate between the outer and inner cylinders by $\Delta\Omega = |\Omega_2 - \Omega_1|$. Experimental values of the magnitude of the applied torque M necessary to maintain the relative rotation rate $\Delta\Omega$ can then used to obtain the viscosity (e.g [100]).

The Couette rheometer is often used under steady rotation to measure the viscosity of fluids μ. In many applications, the Couette geometry is designed such that the gap between the cylinders is narrow. In this case, there is a simple relationship between the viscosity and the measured quantities. For example, if the inner cylinder is rotated and the outer cylinder held fixed,

$$\mu = \frac{M}{4\pi R_1^2 L \, \Omega_1}(1 - \kappa^2), \tag{6.7}$$

where $\kappa = R_1/R_2$. It is recommended that the narrow gap approximation only be used for very small gaps ($\kappa \geq 0.99$ [306]). Significantly, this simple relationship can be used without a priori selection of a particular constitutive model.

However, as elaborated on below, problems can arise when using a narrow gap rheometer for blood, particularly in situations when the size of the 3D microstructure is elevated. To address these problems, a finite gap Couette rheometer is used. However, when the gap is finite there is no longer an explicit solution for the relationship between viscosity and the experimental parameters for general simple fluids. Instead, it is necessary to select subclasses of theoretical models. For example, for constant viscosity fluids, we have

$$\mu = \frac{M(R_2^2 - R_1^2)}{4\pi L R_2^2 R_1^2 \Delta\Omega}. \tag{6.8}$$

The difficulty in obtaining explicit expressions of this kind arises because the shear rate is not constant across the finite gap, in contrast to the solution for the narrow gap rheometer. Therefore, the viscosity will vary across the gap in flows of fluids with shear rate dependent viscosity. The corresponding equations governing this flow are then more complex, and typically do not have explicit solutions. In practice, blood viscosity is sometimes reported using (6.8), even though the blood displays non-constant viscosity.

In obtaining (6.7) and (6.8), the fluid is assumed to travel in a purely circular path. This assumption can be violated by the onset of a secondary motion due to an inertial instability. In addition, deviations from the idealised purely circumferential flow can arise due to wall slip and end effects [306].

Couette rheometers are also used to measure linear viscoelastic properties and to evaluate the thixotropic behaviour discussed in Section 6.2.1.

Cone and plate rheometer

A schematic of a cone and plate rheometer is shown in Fig. 6.4(b). The test fluid is loaded between the cone and flat plate and driven by the rotation of the cone. The pathlines of the flow are assumed to be purely circumferential, in planes parallel to the flat plate, which is reasonable when inertial effects are negligible. Additionally, the free surface is assumed to be spherical, which also limits the shear rates that can be tested. Corrections for the influence of secondary motions are available (see, e.g. [306], p. 209–213). The angle between the cone and plate β is small, typically less than 0.10 radians. Under these assumptions, the stress and shear rate within the fluid are approximately constant and the fluid viscosity is related to the applied torque M and rotation rate Ω through,

$$\mu = \frac{3M}{2\pi R^3}\frac{\beta}{\Omega}, \tag{6.9}$$

where R is the cone radius. Viscoelastic fluids can generate a force normal to the plate. If this force is measured, the first normal stress coefficient ψ_1 can be determined (e.g. [28]),

$$\psi_1 = \frac{2F}{\pi R^2}\frac{\beta^2}{\Omega^2}, \tag{6.10}$$

where F is the resultant force upward on the cone. A detailed discussion of other limitations involved in the use of this rheometer can be found in [306], p. 205–217.

Capillary rheometer

The test region of a capillary rheometer consists of a cylindrical rigid tube of radius R and length L, Fig. 6.4(c). The test fluid is driven through this cavity by gravity, compressed gas, or a piston from a reservoir. Measurements of viscosity are often made by applying a steady pressure drop ΔP across the test region in order to generate a flow with constant volumetric flow rate Q. For constant viscosity fluids, the viscosity can be related to measured quantities through,

$$\mu = \frac{\pi R^4 \Delta P}{8QL}, \tag{6.11}$$

where in writing (6.11), it has been assumed the flow is approximately unidirectional, fully developed and steady.

Even for steady flow of a constant viscosity fluid, the shear rate is not constant across the gap. For fluids with shear rate dependent viscosity, the viscosity will therefore vary over the cross section. As a result, an explicit relationship between viscosity and the measurable parameters of the apparatus only exists for a small number of cases, constant viscosity and power-law fluids being the most obvious examples.

The Weissenberg-Rabinowitsch relationship provides a means of obtaining the viscosity function from measurements of Q and ΔP without choosing a form of the viscosity function a priori ([339,416], see also, for example, p. 238–242 of Macosko [306]),

$$\mu = \frac{\pi R^4 \Delta P}{8QL}\left(\frac{4n'}{3n'+1}\right) \quad \text{where} \quad \frac{1}{n'} = \frac{d\ln Q}{d\ln \Delta P}. \tag{6.12}$$

However, (6.12) is typically not used in blood rheology. Rather, only an approximation to the viscosity is calculated using the expression for constant viscosity fluids rather than the more precise results (6.12). Alternatively, the true viscosity can be calculated by assuming a form of the constitutive equation, such as the power-law model, a priori. This constitutive equation will be discussed in more detail in Section 6.4. Error in using the capillary rheometer can arise from end effects due to increased pressure losses at the entrance and exit of the test region. Correction factors have been introduced for these end effects (e.g. [306]).

The capillary rheometer is frequently used to measure linear viscoelastic properties of blood (e.g. Section 8 of [429] and references cited therein).

6.2.3 General challenges in measuring rheological properties of blood

We first consider difficulties in rheological studies of blood which are common to all three devices. A classic reference on this subject is that by Merrill, [321]. At the basis of most applications of these rheometers is the assumption that blood is a single phase, homogeneous medium. One requirement for this assumption to be reasonable is that the smallest length scale of the device is large compared to the largest length scale of the RBC (or the characteristic length of the three-dimensional microstructure when the shear rate is low enough). However, like other suspensions, this is not a guarantee of homogeneity. The cells themselves may be non-uniformly distributed due to geometric and fluid dynamical mechanisms.

Particle migration and phase separation near boundaries can lead to a non-homogeneous distribution of red blood cells in all three rheometers. These effects are exacerbated at low shear rates, where blood microstructure increases the characteristic length scale from that of the RBC diameter to the length of microstructure formed by the RBCs. The walls of the cylinders in Couette rheometers are sometimes roughened to diminish this effect [321].

Sedimentation in rheometers limits the time over which meaningful results can be obtained without remixing the blood. The specific gravity of an RBC is 1.10 and that of plasma is 1.03, resulting in sedimentation rates for individual RBC on the order of a few mm/hr [57]. However, the sedimentation rates in blood increase with RBC aggregation, limiting the shear rates over which viscosity can be measured. As discussed above, in some disease states the size of the microstructure can be dramatically elevated over the normal level. In these cases, sedimentation is even more rapid [200]. At low rotation rates, the sedimentation of the red blood cells in cone and plate rheometers can lead to a cell free layer adjacent to the upper plate [321], invalidating the assumption of fluid homogeneity inherent in obtaining (6.9). As noted as early as the work of Fåhraeus and Lindqvist [140], sedimentation is also a problem in the reservoir chambers of capillary rheometers. The coaxial cylinder viscometer is less sensitive to sedimentation [306].

Outside the body, blood has a tendency to coagulate after a few minutes. Various additives are effective at preventing coagulation, though at the expense of altering the blood from its native state. Merrill and co-workers found the rheological properties of blood to be similar between native blood and blood with heparin added, as long as the tests were performed within eight hours of withdrawal. Similarly, Copley et al. [101] found the viscosity to be insensitive to the addition of two different anti-coagulants: heparin and EDTA over a wide range of shear rates (0.0009–$1000\,\mathrm{s}^{-1}$).

When viscoelastic effects are of interest, the cone and plate rheometer has the major advantage of being able to directly measure normal stress effects for finite viscoelasticity, though to date this has not been done for blood. All three rheometers can be used to measure blood properties for the linear viscoelastic regime, though it should be emphasised that measurements made for small deformations from the rest state cannot be used to predict the behaviour of blood in a nonlinear regime of deformation.

Another consideration is whether the viscosity can be measured directly without a priori selection of a constitutive equation. The shear rate is constant throughout the fluid domain in Couette rheometers as well as cone and plate rheometers, under the assumptions of small gap and small cone angle, respectively. In contrast, in capillary rheometers and large gap Couette rheometers, an elaborate data reduction process is required to obtain the true viscosity function unless a prior selection of a constitutive model for blood is made. It is for this reason that blood rheologists often report only an approximate viscosity of blood from capillary and large gap Couette rheometers (Section 6.3.1). This is not an issue at higher shear rates where the viscosity of blood is approximately constant.

At low shear rates, extended periods of time are required before meaningful measurements can be made, due to the time needed for the blood microstruture to reach a state of equilibrium. For example, at shear rates of $0.01\,\mathrm{s}^{-1}$, approximately three minutes are required for the shear stress to reach equilibrium in a Couette viscometer (Ht = 70 %) [387]. The lack of a constant shear rate in these rheometers can also lead to erroneous results when the thixotropy of blood is important

Another consideration is sample size, particularly for cases where the supply of whole blood is limited, such as in small animal studies. An advantage of the cone and plate rheometer is the relatively small sample size.

In practice, commercial capillary rheometers are used to measure the approximately constant viscosity plateau of blood (shear rates above 200–300 s^{-1}). Relatively standard Couette or cone and plate rheometers are used at low to medium shear rates of 1 to 200–300$\,\mathrm{s}^{-1}$. Low shear rate Couette viscometers have been developed for shear rates much below $1\,\mathrm{s}^{-1}$.

6.2.4 Challenges in thixotropy measurements

One of the greatest obstacles in evaluating the thixotropic properties of a material is the lack of a clearly defined state at the initiation of the experiment (see discussion in [325]). This point is often overlooked and is in fact difficult to achieve if the material has been mixed or pumped prior to running the experiment. Even the seemingly benign task of loading fluid in the rheometer may affect the structure of the material at the time the experiment is initiated [26]. In the example above (Section 6.2.1) it was given that $\lambda = 1$ at the initiation of the experiment. This might be achieved for example by holding the sample in a quiescent state for a known recovery period after loading the rheometer. Thixotropy is particularly difficult to measure in blood due to the increase in sedimentation rate as the microstructure increases in size [26]. Blood is frequently highly sheared prior to thixotropic experiments in an effort to resuspend the RBCs (e.g. [54, 247, 431]). A period of minutes is then typically allowed with the assumption that this is sufficient time for nearly maximal microstructure to be reached without significant sedimentation. Measurements have been reported to be quite sensitive to this procedure [54].

An additional difficulty for blood rheology is interpretation of the hysteresis loops due to the concurrent viscoelastic and thixotropic responses of blood during the experiments [26]. When thixotropic data is used to develop a constitutive model, it is imperative that the initial state be clearly defined in the experiment and included in the modelling.

6.3 Mechanical properties of blood

In this section, we discuss representative experimental data for the mechanical properties of blood.

6.3.1 Viscosity of blood

Before discussing the viscosity of blood, it is helpful to comment on some nomenclature for viscosity in the literature which appears to have been given different meanings by different authors. We will refer to the viscosity function defined in (6.1) as the viscosity or sometimes as the *material viscosity* to emphasise that it is a material property. The measured value of this quantity should be independent of the choice of rheometer, assuming the rheometer is used in an appropriate test regime. In some works, this viscosity is called the *apparent viscosity* (e.g. [98]). A second viscosity which is sometimes reported is an approximate viscosity based on using shear rates that would be found if the fluid in the rheometer had a constant viscosity (Section 6.2). For example, in the discussion above on capillary rheometers, the viscosity is calculated using (6.11) rather than (6.12), even for shear rates where the viscosity is shear rate dependent. A number of authors refer to this viscosity as the *apparent viscosity* (e.g. Fung [179, Chapter 5]) and others refer to this as the *effective viscosity* (e.g. [98]). At high shear rates, where the blood viscosity is nearly constant, the apparent viscosity will be the same as the actual viscosity. A third viscosity is the viscosity of blood (actual or approximate) relative to the viscosity of either plasma or water at the same temperature, which is typically referred to as the *relative viscosity.*

Figure 6.5 displays the shear thinning behaviour of whole blood as experimentally observed by Chien [82]. Each of these data points represents an equilibrium value obtained at a fixed shear rate. While most constitutive models for viscosity predict that $\mu(\dot{\gamma})$ will reach an approximately constant value denoted as μ_o as the shear rate tends to zero, in fact it is commonly believed that blood displays a yield stress, corresponding to an infinite viscosity at zero shear rate. The proper method for measuring yield stress and even the existence of a yield stress for blood are controversial, complicated by the difficulties in measuring blood properties at low shear rates. We therefore delay a discussion of blood yield stress until Section 6.3.4. As the shear rate is increased, there is a steep decrease in viscosity until a plateau in viscosity μ_∞ is reached.

As discussed earlier in this chapter, the mechanical properties of blood are dominated by the 3D microstructure formed by the RBCs and general distribution of RBCs in the flowing plasma. At lower shear rates, the behaviour

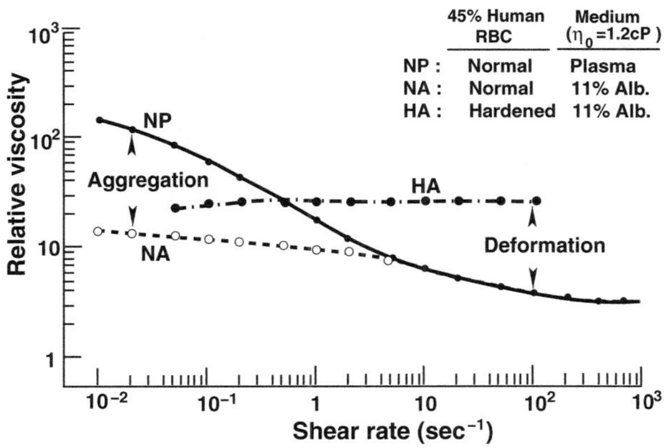

Fig. 6.5. Variation of the relative viscosity as a function of the shear rate for normal RBC in heparinised plasma (NP), normal RBC in albumin-Ringer solution (NA) and hardened RBCs in albumin-Ringer solution (HA) at a temperature of 37 °C, haematocrit Ht = 45 %, using a Couette viscometer (From S. Chien, Shear dependence of effective cell volume as a determinant of blood viscosity. Science, 168:977–979, 1970. Reprinted with permission from the American Association for the Advancement of Science [86])

is controlled by the effect of the 3D RBC formations on the flow and the ability of these formations to deform and store energy. At moderate to high shear rates, these cells are dispersed in the plasma and the properties of the blood are then influenced by their tendency to align and form layers in the flow, as well as by their deformation [506]. The importance of RBC aggregation on blood viscosity at low shear rates was clearly demonstrated by Chien who compared the viscosity of RBCs suspended in heparinised plasma and albumin-Ringer solution (Alb) [85]. The normal RBC aggregation found in plasma does not occur in Alb. Though the viscosity of plasma and Alb were both the same, the viscosity of the RBC solution was greatly increased at low shear rates by RBC aggregation (less than approximately $5\,\mathrm{s}^{-1}$) but unaffected at larger shear rates, Fig. 6.5. The effect of RBC deformability on viscosity of suspensions of these cells was also clearly shown in [85]. Chien compared the viscosity of normal RBCs in Alb and that of hardened RBCs in Alb (presumably hardened at zero shear rate). The ability of normal RBCs to deform (change shape and stretch) significantly decreased the viscosity over all shear rates tested.

In addition to shear rate, the aggregate size is a function of cell shape, plasma composition and haematocrit. This is reflected in the dependence of viscosity on these same variables. We do not address quantitative results for these variables here, but refer the reader to references such as [127] and [543].

The viscosity of whole blood is strongly dependent on temperature and care must be taken in noting the temperature at which the data was obtained when comparing data from different sources. For example, the reported blood viscosity at a haematocrit Ht = 40 %, and temperatures of 20 °C and 37 °C for two representative shear rates are [418]:

μ	20 °C	37 °C
$\mu\,(6\,\mathrm{s}^{-1})$	11.1 mPa s	5.8 mPa s
$\mu\,(212\,\mathrm{s}^{-1})$	6.3 mPa s	3.8 mPa s

(6.13)

Merrill et al. [324] found the dependence of blood viscosity on temperature to be similar to that of water for temperatures ranging from 10 ° to 40 °C and shear rates from 1 to $100\,\mathrm{s}^{-1}$. The variation of plasma viscosity with temperature is also known to approximately follow that of water [76]. For these reasons, blood viscosity is often reported relative to the viscosity of plasma or water at the same temperature.

6.3.2 Viscoelasticity of blood

The viscoelastic properties of blood are attributed primarily to reversible deformation of the 3D microstructure of RBCs, e.g. [484, 508], (see also, Section 8 of [429]). However, these properties are of relatively small magnitude and to date have generally only been measured in the context of *linear* viscoelasticity, (e.g. references cited in [508]). The value of μ'' (see (6.6)) in whole blood from healthy patients decreases monotonically with increasing shear rate [508]. In an experiment involving both steady and small amplitude oscillatory tube flow, Thurston [507] showed that at shear rates of the order of $10\mathrm{s}^{-1}$ rms the elastic nature of the blood sample became negligible, as evidenced by a merging of the oscillatory and steady flow viscosities. The reader is referred to [508] for a review of the dependence of blood viscoelasticity on factors such as temperature, haematocrit and RBC properties.

While the linear viscoelastic functions are relatively straightforward to obtain in the rheometers described above, it should be emphasised that blood flow in the circulatory system is rarely in the regime applicable for linear viscoelasticity theory. The linear elastic material constants are indicative of aspects of the microstructure and therefore can be used as a method of quantifying blood properties. However, ultimately, there is a need to consider the finite viscoelastic behaviour of blood, if viscoelastic constitutive equations are going to be used to model blood behaviour in the circulatory system.

6.3.3 Thixotropy of blood

The thixotropic properties of blood are believed to arise from the finite time required for the formation and breakup of the 3D microstructure, elongation and recovery of red blood cell microstructure, and the formation and breakdown of layers of aligned RBCs, as already mentioned in Section 6.2.

Bureau et al. [54] employed a Couette rheometer to expose blood to the second type of non-periodic unsteady flows discussed in Section 6.2.1. In Fig. 6.6 (A) and (B) we reproduce shear stress hysteresis curves for normal human

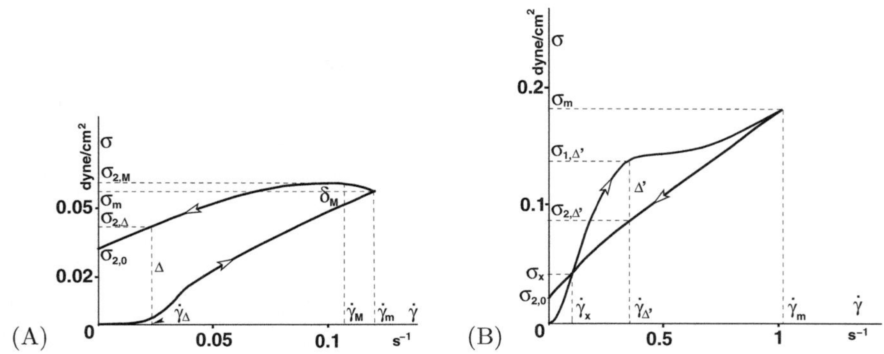

Fig. 6.6. Data from Bureau et al. [54] plotted in dynes/cm^2. (Reprinted from Biorheology, 17, M. Bureau, J. C. Healy, D. Bourgoin and M. Joly, Rheological hysteresis of blood at low shear rates, pages 191–203, Copyright (1980), with permission from IOS Press). (A) $\dot{\gamma} = 0.0185t$ for $0 \leq t \leq 6.5$s and $\dot{\gamma} = 0.0185(13-t)$ for $6.5s \leq t \leq 13$s. Dispersion: 5.5×10^{-2} dynes/cm^2 $\leq \sigma_{r\theta}(t_0) \leq 8.5 \times 10^{-2}$ dynes/cm^2, 3.2×10^{-2} dynes/cm^2 $\leq \sigma_{r\theta}(2t_0) \leq 3.8 \times 10^{-2}$ dynes/cm^2; (B) $\dot{\gamma} = 0.043$t for $0 \leq t \leq 23.8$s and $\dot{\gamma} = 0.043(47.6-t)$ for 23.8s $\leq t \leq 47.6$s. Dispersion: 1.9×10^{-1} dynes/cm^2 $\leq \sigma_{r\theta}(t_0) \leq 2.5 \times 10^{-1}$ dynes/cm^2, 1.7×10^{-2} dynes/cm^2 $\leq \sigma_{r\theta}(2t_0) \leq 4.1 \times 10^{-2}$ dynes/cm^2

blood from [54] where these correspond, respectively to $\dot{\gamma}_{\max} = 0.12025\,\mathrm{s}^{-1}$, $t_0 = 6.5\,\mathrm{s}$ (experiment (A)) and $\dot{\gamma}_{\max} = 1.0234\,\mathrm{s}^{-1}$, $t_0 = 23.8\,\mathrm{s}$ (experiment (B)). In both cases a residual non-zero shear stress may be seen at the end of the cycle, indicating that blood is viscoelastic and that the stress depends on the entire deformation history and not just the instantaneous rate of deformation, as would be the case for a Newtonian or generalised Newtonian fluid. That the two branches of the stress curve, cross in experiment (B), is a manifestation of thixotropic behaviour. So sensitive is this flow to the rheological properties of blood that Bureau et al. encountered significant dispersion in the results they obtained for different samples of normal blood. A measure of this dispersion for $\sigma_{r\theta}(t_0)$ and $\sigma_{r\theta}(2t_0)$ is supplied in the captions of Fig. 6.6.

For experiment (A) the stress response is, as may be expected for a low shear rate experiment, mainly viscoelastic. In experiment (B) the maximum shear rate attained is higher and thixotropic effects are much more important, as anticipated.

6.3.4 Yield stress of blood

The behaviour of a number of fluids at low shear stress, including blood, has led researchers to believe in the existence of a critical value of stress below which the fluid will not flow. This critical stress level, called the yield value or yield stress (see also Section 6.1.1), is typically treated as a material property (constant) of the fluid.[3] An extensive description of methods for measuring yield stress is given in [349]. Briefly, there are two categories of methods: indirect methods and direct methods. In indirect methods, the shear stress versus shear rate curve is back extrapolated to zero, possibly using a specific constitutive model or simple linear approximation. Sometimes the yield stress is set to the lowest measured shear stress [388]. In direct methods, an attempt is made to directly measure the shear stress at which the fluid begins to flow.

Reported values for the yield stress of blood vary greatly ranging from 0.002 to 0.40 dynes/cm^2 (see, e.g. [127]). This variation in reported values has been attributed to artifacts arising from interactions between the RBCs and surfaces of the rheometer [76] as well as the experimental method used to measure the yield stress. The large range seen for blood is consistent with results for other fluids where this spread is attributed to the experimental methodology, the criterion used to define the yield stress, and the length of time over which the experiment is run [349]. A true material constant should be independent of these factors. These results have called into serious question the treatment of the yield stress as a material parameter [27, 29, 338, 349]. Dintenfass appears to have been the first to question the appropriateness of such a material constant for blood (see, e.g. [127], p. 82). He suggested that rather than treating the yield stress as a constant, it should be considered as a function of time. A time dependence was also noted in [80] and is consistent with the link between yield stress and thixotropy proposed years later by other researchers [338].

6.4 Constitutive models for blood

As discussed earlier in this chapter, the presence of the formed elements in blood leads to some significant and fascinating changes in its rheological properties. In this section, we will discuss constitutive models introduced to capture one or more of these properties. We will assume that all macroscopic length and time scales are sufficiently large compared to time and length scales at the level of the individual erythrocyte that the continuum hypothesis holds. Thus the models presented in the pages that follow would not be appropriate in the capillary network, for example, and for an overview of haemorheology in the microcirculation we refer the reader to the review articles of Popel and Johnson [393] and Pries and Secomb [394].

Since both the shear thinning and viscoelastic properties diminish rapidly as the 3D microstructure of RBCs breaks down, it is important to consider in which flow regimes and clinical situations the non-Newtonian properties of

[3] While it is not discussed in the blood literature, it should be understood that this material parameter must be a true scalar, independent of the system of coordinates used. In most discussions, the yield stress is considered for approximations of simple shear flows and the yield stress is just the corresponding applied shear stress at which flow begins, (see also [429]).

blood will be important. The Blood would need to be subjected to shear rates below $1\,\mathrm{s}^{-1}$ per period sufficient for these structures to form and alter the flow. Schmid-Schönbein and co-workers found the half-time for aggregate formation to be 3–5 seconds for normal blood and 0.5–1.5 seconds for pathological blood samples [452]. In their experiments, the time for aggregation was measured after samples were exposed to an abrupt drop in shear rate from $460\,\mathrm{s}^{-1}$ to approximately zero. Thurston estimated an aggregation time on the order of a minute after the abrupt stoppage of oscillatory shear with shear rate of $500\,\mathrm{s}^{-1}$ and shear strain of 1.77 (*rms*) [182].

The blood circulation time for humans is on the order of minutes, so for normal blood, the RBC structure will be broken down in the majority of the arterial system and only exist in regions of the circulation where there are stable recirculation zones with shear rates significantly below $1\,\mathrm{s}^{-1}$ (see, Sects. 6.3 and 8.3 of [429] for a more in depth discussion of this issue). Possible locations where the non-Newtonian behaviour will be significant include segments of the venous system and stable vortices downstream of some stenoses and in the sacs of some aneurysms. For various pathologies, the 3D microstructure formed by the RBCs is substantially stronger than for normal blood. For these patients, it is possible the 3D microstructure will exist in more widespread regions of the circulatory system. Increased RBC aggregation has been observed for patients with infections, trauma, burns, diabetes mellitus, AIDS and other diseases [302].

The quantification of the mechanical response of blood (shear thinning, viscoelasticity) can also be important for patient diagnosis. For example, η'' has been shown to be very sensitive to myocardial infarction, peripheral vascular disease and diabetes [508].

As a first step towards the macroscopic modelling of blood flow we recall the equations for the balance of linear momentum and conservation of mass (or incompressibility condition) for isothermal flow (see Chapter 2)

$$\begin{aligned} \rho\frac{D\boldsymbol{u}}{Dt} &= -\boldsymbol{\nabla}P + \mathbf{div}\boldsymbol{\tau}, \\ \operatorname{div}\boldsymbol{u} &= 0. \end{aligned} \tag{6.14}$$

Here, $\boldsymbol{\tau}$ denotes the extra-stress tensor accounting for differences in behaviour from a purely inviscid, incompressible fluid. To close the system of equations, we require an equation relating the state of stress to the kinematic variables such as rate of deformation of fluid elements. These *constitutive equations* and the elaboration of macroscopic constitutive models suitable for blood flow under certain flow conditions are the primary subjects of this section.

6.4.1 Generalised Newtonian and yield stress models

The simplest viscous fluid model is that due to Newton. On the assumption that the components of the extra-stress tensor are each linear isotropic functions of the components of the velocity gradient $\nabla\boldsymbol{u}$, it may be shown (see, for example, [368, Chapter 2]) that for an incompressible fluid

$$\boldsymbol{\tau} = 2\,\mu\,\boldsymbol{D}(\boldsymbol{u}), \tag{6.15}$$

where μ is a (constant) viscosity and $\boldsymbol{D}(\boldsymbol{u})$ is the rate of deformation tensor, defined in Chapter 2. The substitution for $\boldsymbol{\tau}$ in (6.14) from (6.15) leads to the well-known Navier-Stokes equations for an incompressible viscous fluid (see Chapter 3). This set of equations is commonly used with some justification to describe blood flow in the heart and healthy arteries (see, e.g. [263]). Blood is nonetheless non-Newtonian and in the previous sections evidence has been presented to show that under certain experimental or physiological conditions (6.15) is inadequate as a constitutive relation for blood. In this subsection, we first discuss representative rheologically admissible constitutive equations with shear thinning viscosity, and then introduce the Casson model, a representative yield stress fluid.

Without loss of generality (e.g. [15]), the most general incompressible constitutive model of the form $\boldsymbol{\tau} = \boldsymbol{\tau}(\boldsymbol{\nabla u})$ that respects invariance requirements can be written in the form

$$\boldsymbol{\tau} = \phi_1(I_2, I_3)\boldsymbol{D}(\boldsymbol{u}) + \phi_2(I_2, I_3)\boldsymbol{D}(\boldsymbol{u})^2 \tag{6.16}$$

where I_2 and I_3 are the second and third principal invariants of the rate of deformation tensor,

$$I_2 = \frac{1}{2}\left((\mathrm{tr}\boldsymbol{D}(\boldsymbol{u}))^2 - \mathrm{tr}\boldsymbol{D}(\boldsymbol{u})^2\right), \quad I_3 = \det(\boldsymbol{D}(\boldsymbol{u})), \tag{6.17}$$

and $\mathrm{tr}\boldsymbol{D}(\boldsymbol{u})$ is identically zero for divergence free velocity fields essential for incompressible fluids (isochoric motions). Incompressible fluids of the form (6.16) are typically called *Reiner-Rivlin fluids.* The behaviour of Reiner-Rivlin fluids with non-zero values of ϕ_2 in simple shear does not match experimental results on real fluids [15]. In addition, the dependence on the value of I_3 is often considered negligible [15]. For this reason, attention is typically confined to a special class of Reiner-Rivlin fluids called *generalised Newtonian fluids.*

$$\boldsymbol{\tau} = 2\,\mu(I_2)\,\boldsymbol{D}(\boldsymbol{u}), \tag{6.18}$$

where μ is the same viscosity (a viscometric function) defined in (6.1). In viscometric flows, I_3 is identically zero and it is not necessary to explicitly assume the dependence of μ on I_3 is negligible. The quantity I_2 is not a positive quantity, so it is useful to introduce a metric of the rate of deformation, denoted by $\dot\gamma$,

$$\dot\gamma \equiv \sqrt{2\,tr\,(\boldsymbol{D}(\boldsymbol{u})^2)} = \sqrt{-4I_2}. \tag{6.19}$$

Using (6.19), the generalised Newtonian model (6.18) takes the useful form,

$$\boldsymbol{\tau} = 2\,\mu(\dot\gamma)\,\boldsymbol{D}(\boldsymbol{u}). \tag{6.20}$$

For example in simple shear flow, the metric (6.19) coincides with the shear rate $\dot{\gamma}_0$ introduced in (6.1). It should be emphasised that the use of the representation (6.20) does not restrict attention to simple shear or other viscometric flows.

Power-law type models

A simple example of a generalised Newtonian fluid is that of the power-law fluid, which has viscosity function given by

$$\mu = k\dot{\gamma}^{(n-1)}, \tag{6.21}$$

k being a positive constant and n a constant chosen to have a maximum value 1, leading to a monotonic decreasing function of shear rate (shear thinning fluid) when $n < 1$ and a constant viscosity (Newtonian) fluid when $n = 1$. One of the major advantages of this model is that it is possible to obtain numerous analytical solutions to the governing equations. Two major drawbacks of the power-law model for the shear thinning case are that the zero shear rate viscosity is unbounded and the asymptotic limit as $\dot{\gamma} \to \infty$ is zero. Both these behaviours are unphysical and limit the range of shear rates over which the power-law model is reasonable for blood.

One of the more successful viscosity laws for blood is an extension of the power-law model due to Walburn and Schneck [534]. In addition to the shear rate, they considered the dependence of the viscosity on the haematocrit (Ht) and total protein minus albumin (TPMA) content through the parameter k and n in (6.21). Using a nonlinear regression analysis they found that shear rate and haematocrit were the two most important factors in decreasing order of importance. Based on these two factors, they formulated the following expressions for k and n,

$$k = C_1 \exp(C_2 Ht), \qquad n = 1 - C_3 Ht. \tag{6.22}$$

They found an R-squared statistical increase from 62 % to 88 % when Ht was included in the power-law model in addition to shear rate. The statistical significance rose to nearly 91 % when TPMA was also added. Walburn and Schneck attribute the two parameter model (6.21) to Sacks [441].

Quemada model

In 1978 Quemada [412] used a semi-phenomenological approach to develop a constitutive law suitable for concentrated disperse systems (such as blood) that had an apparent viscosity μ determined from

$$\mu = \mu_F \left(1 - \frac{1}{2}\frac{k_0 + k_\infty\sqrt{\dot{\gamma}/\dot{\gamma}_c}}{1 + \sqrt{\dot{\gamma}/\dot{\gamma}_c}}\varphi\right)^{-2}, \tag{6.23}$$

where μ_F, φ and $\dot{\gamma}_c$ are the viscosity of the suspending fluid, the volume concentration of the dispersed phase and a critical shear rate, respectively. Quemada showed that calculating the absolute value of the shear stress τ_{12} in simple shear flow from the generalised Newtonian constitutive relation

$$|\tau_{12}| = \mu\dot{\gamma}, \tag{6.24}$$

led to an expansion for $\sqrt{|\tau_{12}|}$ valid for $\dot{\gamma} \gg \dot{\gamma}_c$ of the form

$$\sqrt{|\tau_{12}|} = \frac{\sqrt{\mu_F\dot{\gamma}}}{1-\frac{1}{2}k_\infty\varphi} + \sqrt{\mu_F\dot{\gamma}_c}\frac{\varphi}{2}\frac{k_0-k_\infty}{(1-k_\infty\varphi/2)^2} + O(\sqrt{\dot{\gamma}_c/\dot{\gamma}}). \tag{6.25}$$

Equation (6.25) is, to order $\sqrt{\dot{\gamma}_c/\dot{\gamma}}$ of the form

$$\sqrt{|\tau_{12}|} = \sqrt{K}\sqrt{\dot{\gamma}} + \sqrt{|\tau_0|}, \tag{6.26}$$

where

$$K = \mu_F\left(1-\tfrac{1}{2}k_\infty\varphi\right)^{-2} = \lim_{\dot{\gamma}\to\infty}\mu(\dot{\gamma}) = \mu_\infty,$$

$$\tau_0 = \frac{1}{4}\mu_F\dot{\gamma}_c(k_0-k_\infty)^2\frac{\varphi^2}{(1-k_\infty\varphi/2)^4} + O(\sqrt{\dot{\gamma}_c/\dot{\gamma}}).$$

Equation (6.26) is *Casson's equation* [69] for the absolute value of the shear stress τ_{12} as a function of the shear rate when the magnitude of the shear stress exceeds that of a *yield stress* τ_0.

The controversy over the existence of a yield stress and the use of it as a material parameter were introduced in Section 6.3.4. Here, we briefly summarise some of the results obtained for these measurements, but caution that measurements of the yield stress are expected to be quite sensitive to the microstructure of the blood prior to yielding, which is in turn expected to be sensitive to both the shear rate history as well as time [338].

Merrill et al. [323], obtained data supporting the existence of a yield stress using both a rotational viscometer and pressure-flow in capillaries. His data was well fitted using Casson's equation. Their results corroborated what had been previously seen by researchers such as Cokelet et al. [99] and Merrill et al. [324] and confirmed the importance of the presence of fibrinogen for the magnitude of the yield stress. Also haematocrit levels had to exceed a critical threshold (typically between 0.05 and 0.08) for there to be a measurable yield stress. Results in the literature for the yield stress of blood show it to be very small, however: Neofytou [348] tabulated measurements made by different research groups at temperatures varying between 22 °C and 37 °C and haematocrits between 0.42 and 0.46 and the maximum reported value of the yield stress was 25.6 mPa. More recent measurements of the yield stress in human blood using a Couette rheometer have been performed by Picart et al. [388] and their Fig. 7 supplies an interesting synthesis of yield stress data in the literature as a function of haematocrit. Picart et al. used the shear stress measured at a shear rate of $1 \times 10^{-3}\,\mathrm{s}^{-1}$ as an approximation for the yield stress.

Material parameters for blood in generalised Newtonian and Casson models

Commonly used values used in the literature for blood density ρ and μ_o and μ_∞ at 37 °C are ([88])[4],

$$\rho = 1056\text{kg/m}^3, \qquad \mu_o = 0.056\text{Pa s}, \qquad \mu_\infty = 0.00345\text{Pa s}, \tag{6.27}$$

where μ_0 and μ_∞ are the asymptotic viscosities at zero and infinite shear rates, i.e.

$$\mu_0 = \lim_{\dot\gamma \to 0} \mu(\dot\gamma), \quad \mu_\infty = \lim_{\dot\gamma \to \infty} \mu(\dot\gamma).$$

Note that these definitions are only meaningful in the context of theoretical constitutive models. In practice, the lower limit in shear rate at which viscosity can be measured is limited by the experimental challenges discussed in Section 6.2.3. The high shear rate limit has no real physical meaning since the cells will lyse at sufficiently high shear rates. In practice, it is taken as the high shear plateau value.

As discussed earlier in this chapter, the material parameters of blood are quite sensitive to the state of blood constituents as well as temperature. The dependence on temperature has been found to be similar to water.

The dependence on haematocrit is included in material parameters for the power-law model that were obtained for human blood, Table 6.1. The corresponding viscosity functions are shown in Fig. 6.7. The viscosity functions obtained from [258] and [534] for Ht = 40 % are quite close. In contrast, those in [288] and [534] for Ht = 45 % are substantially different, likely due to the lower temperature used in [288] compared to those in [534].

Table 6.2 summarises some of the most common generalised Newtonian models that have been considered in the literature for the shear dependent viscosity of whole human blood. Values for the material constants obtained by Cho and Kensey [88] for a compilation of human and canine blood are also given in this table. Table 6.3 provides material parameters for the Quemada and Casson models for blood used in [348].

6.4.2 Viscoelastic and thixotropic models

Experimental *in vitro* evidence for the viscoelastic behaviour of human blood and discussion of its connection with the storage and dissipation of energy during the distortion of the 3D microstrucure formed by the RBC at low shear rates abounds in the literature: see, for example [84,303,503,504,532]. A word of caution is in order at this point, however. A study of blood in sinusoidal flow

[4] The values for μ_o and μ_∞ presented by Cho and Kensey [88] were obtained from a compilation of data including both human and canine blood and for haematocrits ranging from 33–45 %.

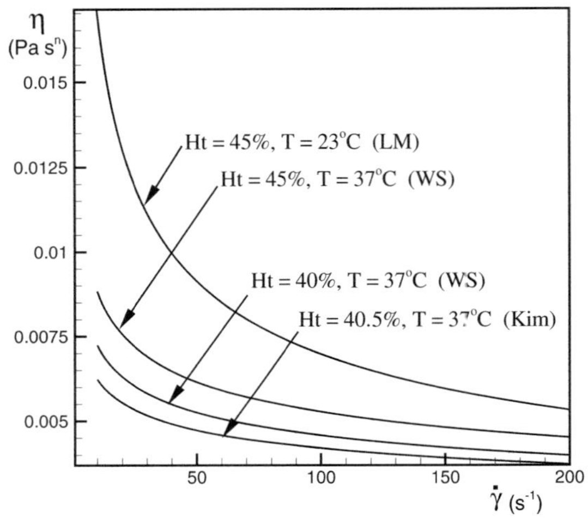

Fig. 6.7. Comparison of viscosity functions $\mu(\dot{\gamma})$ for the power-law model (6.21) using material constants provided by Kim et al. [258] (Kim) and Liepsch and Moravec [288] (LM) for human blood. Also shown are representative viscosity curves for the Walburn-Schneck model (WS) [534] that includes a dependence on haematocrit (6.22). Values for the material constants n and k are given in Table 6.1

Table 6.1. Material constants for power-law model obtained by various researchers using fit of (6.21) to human blood data at different haematocrits. For comparison, results predicted from the Walburn-Schneck model (6.22) are shown

Ht (%)	n	k (Pa s^n)	*Background*
40.5	0.828	0.00927	From Kim et al. [258] for unadulterated human blood at 37° using a rotating viscometer for $\dot{\gamma} \in [30, 375]\,\text{s}^{-1}$ and scanning capillary viscometer for $\dot{\gamma} \in [1, 375]\,\text{s}^{-1}$.
35 40 45	0.825 0.800 0.775	0.00888 0.0115 0.0148	From Walburn and Schneck [534] for anticoagulated blood at 37° using a cone and plate viscometer for $\dot{\gamma} \in [23.28, 232.80]\,\text{s}^{-1}$ with $C_1 = 0.00148\,\text{Pa s}^n$, $C_2 = 0.0512$, $C_3 = 0.00499$.
45	0.61	0.042	From Liepsch and Moravec [288] for human blood at 23 °C using a rotational rheometer for $\dot{\gamma} \in [0.2, 400]\,\text{s}^{-1}$.

in glass tubes by Federspiel and Cokelet in 1984 [143] using tube diameters, flow rate amplitudes and oscillation frequencies that attempted to mimic those in small arteries indicated that blood elasticity was effectively negligible in this flow regime. Differences with measurements made earlier by Thurston [503] were attributed to the larger shear rates in Federspiel and Cokelet's work, and Thurston's work was suggested as being more applicable to venous flows

Table 6.2. Material constants for various generalised Newtonian models for blood with $\mu_0 = 0.056\,\text{Pa s}$, $\mu_\infty = 0.00345\,\text{Pa s}$

Model	$\dfrac{\mu(\dot\gamma) - \mu_\infty}{\mu_0 - \mu_\infty}$	*Material constants for blood*
Powell-Eyring	$\dfrac{\sinh^{-1}(\lambda\dot\gamma)}{\lambda\dot\gamma}$	$\lambda = 5.383\,\text{s}$
Cross	$\dfrac{1}{1 + (\lambda\dot\gamma)^m}$	$\lambda = 1.007\,\text{s},\ m = 1.028$
Modified Cross	$\dfrac{1}{(1 + (\lambda\dot\gamma)^m)^a}$	$\lambda = 3.736\,\text{s},\ m = 2.406,\ a = 0.254$
Carreau	$(1 + (\lambda\dot\gamma)^2)^{(n-1)/2}$	$\lambda = 3.313\,\text{s},\ n = 0.3568$
Carreau-Yasuda	$(1 + (\lambda\dot\gamma)^a)^{(n-1)/a}$	$\lambda = 1.902\,\text{s},\ n = 0.22,\ a = 1.25$

Table 6.3. Material constants for Quemada (6.23) and Casson (6.25) models. The Quemada parameters were chosen to fit the data of Schmid-Schönbein et al. [451] and are for Ht = 45 %. The Casson parameters are drawn from the experimental papers of Charm et al. [77] and Charm and Kurland [78] and correspond to Ht = 45 % and a temperature of 37° C

Model	*Equation*	*Material constants for blood*
Quemada	(6.23)	$\mu_F = 1.2\,\text{mPa s}$ $k_\infty = 2.07$ $k_0 = 4.33$ $\dot\gamma_c = 1.88\,\text{s}^{-1}$ $\varphi = 0.45$
Casson	(6.26)	$\mu_\infty = 3.1\,\text{mPa s}$ $\sigma_0 = 10.86\,\text{mPa}$

or pathological low-flow rate flows than arterial flows. In addition to being a viscoelastic fluid, the fact that red cell aggregates neither form nor break up instantaneously leads to blood being thixotropic (see, Section 6.3.3) and the reader is also referred to [215, 231, 505], for example, for further discussion.

None of the models in Section 6.4.1 accounts for either the viscoelasticity or the thixotropy of blood. Happily, a number of non-linear viscoelastic constitutive models for blood are now available but because of their complexity we will avoid presenting the mathematical details here, providing instead a summary of the relevant literature. Viscoelastic constitutive models of differential type, suitable for describing blood, have been proposed recently by Yeleswarapu [548, 549] and by Anand and Rajagopal [10] (the latter being developed in the context of the general thermodynamic framework of Rajagopal and Srinivasa [417]).

An alternative approach to modelling blood rheology for time-dependent flows has been made by authors such as Quemada [413–415], Williams et al. [545] and De Kee and co-workers [112, 490]. The common outcome of the modelling done by all these authors is a generalised Maxwell-type equation for the stress due to the size and position distributions of the rouleaux. Both viscosity and relaxation time are functions of a structure variable which, in the papers cited above, is either the number fraction of red blood cells in aggregates (more generally, aggregated particles) [413–415, 490] or of aggregated cell faces [545].

The obvious analogy that exists between polymer network theories, in which macromolecules form a network of temporary junctions, and the (reversible) aggregation of erythrocytes into a network of rouleaux at very low shear rates, has been exploited by a number of authors in order to develop nonlinear constitutive equations for blood. Stoltz and Lucius [484], for example, drawing inspiration from the earlier work of Carreau and De Kee [68, 111], provided a constitutive model for blood in which the extra-stress tensor $\boldsymbol{\tau}$ of (6.14) included a memory function dependent on the second invariant of the rate of strain tensor $\boldsymbol{D}(\boldsymbol{u})$.

In 2006 Owens [141, 367] followed ideas drawn from the classical theory of network models for viscoelastic fluids to derive a relatively simple single-mode structure-dependent generalised Maxwell model for the contribution $\boldsymbol{\tau}$ of the erythrocytes to the total Cauchy stress. In the model developed in [141, 367] the erythrocytes were represented in their capacity to be transported, stretched and orientated in a flow by Hookean dumbbells, thus limiting the model to low shear rate flows. The extra-stress tensor $\boldsymbol{\tau}$ in Eq. (6.14) may be written as the sum of a Newtonian viscous stress tensor and an elastic stress tensor $\boldsymbol{\tau}_E$:

$$\boldsymbol{\tau} = 2\,\mu_N\,\boldsymbol{D}(\boldsymbol{u}) + \boldsymbol{\tau}_E, \tag{6.28}$$

where μ_N is the (Newtonian) plasma viscosity and $\boldsymbol{\tau}_E$ represents the contribution to the extra-stress due to the erythrocytes.

The constitutive equation for $\boldsymbol{\tau}_E$ derived in [141] assumed the form

$$\boldsymbol{\tau}_E + \xi\left(\frac{D\boldsymbol{\tau}_E}{Dt} - \nabla\boldsymbol{u}\cdot\boldsymbol{\tau}_E - \boldsymbol{\tau}_E\cdot\nabla\boldsymbol{u}^T\right) = 2N_0 k_B T\xi\boldsymbol{D}(\boldsymbol{u}), \tag{6.29}$$

where ξ is a relaxation time, dependent upon the local shear rate, time and average aggregate size n. N_0 in (6.29) denotes the number density of red blood cells and is thus related to the haematocrit Ht by $N_0 = Ht/V$, where V is the volume of a single erythrocyte (approximately $92\mu\text{m}^3$). The average aggregate size n was shown to evolve according to

$$\frac{Dn}{Dt} = \frac{1}{2}a(\dot{\gamma})N_0 - \frac{1}{2}b(\dot{\gamma})n^2 + \frac{1}{2}b(\dot{\gamma})n, \tag{6.30}$$

where $a(\dot{\gamma})$ and $b(\dot{\gamma})$ are (shear rate dependent) aggregation and fragmentation rates. In the special case of homogeneous flow ($\nabla\boldsymbol{u}$ is a constant) the number density N_0 is a constant and it may be shown that (6.30) becomes

$$\frac{dn}{dt} = -\frac{1}{2}b(\dot{\gamma})(n - n_{st})(n + n_{st} - 1), \tag{6.31}$$

where n_{st} is the steady-state value of n.

6.5 Comparison of predictions of constitutive models with experimental data

6.5.1 Viscosity functions

In a study in 1980 by Easthope and Brooks [130] an attempt was made to fit the measured steady shear stress data obtained from a Couette device from thirty one different samples at shear rates ranging from $0.031\,\mathrm{s}^{-1}$ to $120\,\mathrm{s}^{-1}$ using eleven different explicit constitutive models for viscosity. The model of Walburn and Schneck resulted in the closest fit. The predictions of the Walburn and Schneck model have been compared with those of a Newtonian fluid, Casson model and Bingham model for laminar flow through a straight tube under flow conditions bearing some similarity to those that exist in the femoral artery by Rodkiewicz et al. [430]. The Walburn and Schneck model was seen to give markedly different results from the other models in pulsatile flow and these were stated as being in conformity with some experimental results [289]. The authors noted that the constitutive model of Walburn and Schneck was developed for low shear rates, however, and was not valid for certain shear rate regimes seen in their pulsatile flow simulations.

Details of a recent comparison between a Newtonian, Casson, power-law and Quemada [412] model are to be found in the paper of Neofytou [348]. The author considered the case of channel flow where part of one of the channel walls was forced to oscillate laterally, this being claimed to reproduce some flow phenomena seen under realistic arterial conditions. The Casson and Quemada models were seen to agree well in their predictions and were preferred over the power-law model which has an unbounded viscosity at zero shear rate, as discussed in Section 6.4.1.

6.5.2 Comparison of theory with triangular step shear rate experiments

The triangular step shear rate experiment performed by Bureau et al. has proved to be a popular one against which to test constitutive models and some examples may be found in papers by Huang and Horng [230], Quemada [413], Stoltz and Lucius [484], Williams et al. [545] and Owens [367].

Excellent agreement with the the stress hysteresis data of Bureau et al. was found both for the model of Stoltz and Lucius [484] as well as that of Owens [367]. Agreement was close between the experimental and theoretical predictions for the shear stress growth when the shear rate $\dot{\gamma}$ in the time-dependent simple shear flow passed from zero to $0.05\,\mathrm{s}^{-1}$ and from zero to $0.1\,\mathrm{s}^{-1}$. As evidence of thixotropic behaviour, Stoltz and Lucius noted a shear stress overshoot in the experiment with the larger step increase in shear rate.

6.5.3 Pulsatile flow in a straight tube

Although sophisticated experimental techniques such as 3D phase contrast magnetic resonance imaging (see, for example [479, 493]) now exist for the imaging of velocity fields *in vivo*, information about the rheology and consequent flow behaviour of blood, useful for developing constitutive models, may be gleaned from controlled experiments of pulsatile blood flow in a straight, rigid-walled tube. Reference has been made already in Secs. 6.4.1 and 6.4.2 to the experiments of Merrill et al. [323] and Federspiel and Cokelet [143] in glass tubes, where the magnitude of the yield stress and elastic character of blood were evaluated, and their dependence on haematocrit, fibrinogen levels and shear rate quantified.

A full description of all the comparisons that have been performed with the model of Owens may be found in [141]. Other viscoelastic models have already been used with some success for the simulation of this flow. For example, the pressure field predictions of the viscoelastic model of Anand and Rajagopal [10] were in reasonable agreement with the data of Thurston [504] for oscillatory tube flow and comparisons were also made between the experimental data and the results from a model of Yeleswarapu [548,549] and generalised Oldroyd-B and Maxwell models. Neither of the generalised models was found to give satisfactory results for oscillatory flows, however.

6.6 Conclusions

In this chapter we have attempted to elucidate the manner in which the material properties of flowing human blood, and in particular its shear viscosity, elasticity and thixotropy may be explained in terms of the complex evolving microstructure, and especially that of the deforming and migrating red blood cells in their different states of aggregation. We would suggest, therefore, that the most promising rheological models to date are those developed from an underlying microstructure similar to that of blood (albeit necessarily simplified). The retention of sufficient detail at the microscopic level may be hoped to translate into faithful reproduction of some of the complex characteristics of blood, particularly those associated with its thixotropic nature.

It seems to us that at least three significant challenges face those who will develop the next generation of rheological models and use them in large-scale numerical simulations. First, attention has been drawn to the particular difficulties associated with the measurement of some of the basic macroscopic rheological properties of blood, and especially in flow regimes where non-Newtonian effects are most likely to be observed. There is a pressing need for further experimental data to validate the current microstructural rheological models and provide a rational basis for the further development of these models. Experiments are needed both at the scale of the RBC as well as that of the blood vessels. For example, data on the inhomogeneous spatial distribution of the RBCs and the time constants associated with the formation and break up of RBC aggregates in representative flow regimes and geometries would be of tremendous value. Moreover the availability of reliable measurements of quantities such as the velocity, wall shear stress and pressure in well characterised (and hence reproducible) physiological flows (*in vivo*) is essential if numerical simulations are going to have anything really useful to say about blood flow in the cardiovascular system. Such *in vivo* measurements are only now starting to make an appearance in the literature (see [83, 87]). Secondly, when we write of the desirability of sufficient detail at the microstructural level being retained in rheological models we mean *just* sufficient. Although we want to be able to successfully predict non-Newtonian effects in, say, an aneurysm we would like any reasonable model to collapse to the Navier-Stokes equations (with some suitable apparent viscosity) in bulk arterial flow, for example. A model that is unnecessarily complicated or costly, may have a sound rheological foundation but has little chance of attracting the attention of the medical community and therefore of being implemented in practical situations. Thirdly, and finally, the development of stable, accurate and affordable numerical methods tailored to the new set of constitutive equations for blood is of the utmost importance. For example, proper account must be taken of the mathematical type of the system of equations, and the possible addition of elastic stress variables make the use of parallelisable algorithms even more crucial than they are in present day CFD Newtonian solvers. Faster large-scale computing platforms are opening up new possibilities in simulation and visualisation.

7

Mathematical models of mass transfer in the vascular walls

Karl Perktold, Martin Prosi, and Paolo Zunino

As illustrated in detail in chapters 1 and 2, the arterial wall is a heterogeneous structure consisting of several layers which strongly differ in their thickness and in their biological and physical properties, that we briefly recall here for the sake of clarity. The layers constituting the wall are the *endothelium*, the *intima*, the *internal elastic lamina or lamella* (IEL), the *media* and the *adventitia*, see Fig. 7.1 for a simplified sketch. The endothelium is a type of epithelium composed of a single layer of smooth, thin cells that lines the heart, blood vessels, lymphatics, and serous cavities. It forms a continuous lining on blood contacting surfaces in the vascular system, providing the principal barrier against the entry of cholesterol and blood cells into the wall and inhibiting platelet adherence to the vessel walls. Endothelial cells create chemicals and control the transport of mass into and out of the wall. The sub-endothelial layer is an extra-cellular matrix of randomly distributed fibres, mainly collagenous bundles and proteoglycans (glycoproteins which have a very high polysaccharide content). This layer is surrounded by the IEL, which is composed by elastic fibres. Under normal physiological loading, the fibres form an approximately circular band. Together with the sub-endothelial layer it helps the wall to withstand haemodynamic stresses. Outside the IEL there is the media, which is made of smooth muscle cells and is the primary regulator of vessel diameter. The outer layer is the adventitia, which is a complex structure that merges into the surrounding tissue. It tethers arteries in place and it carries nutrients to and wastes away from smooth muscle cells in the media. Moreover, it provides resistance to overextension and rupture. Sometimes, what we call *intima* is denoted with *sub-endothelial layer*. In this case, the term *intima* is used for the group of endothelium, sub-endothelial layer and IEL. However, we do not follow this nomenclature.

The behaviour and the interaction of these layers are regulated by a complex set of chemical and mechanical phenomena. There is evidence (see [287] for a general introduction or [169] for a more specific analysis) that these mechanisms depend also on fluid dynamics and mass transport phenomena in the blood stream and in the wall. The role of fluid dynamics and mass trans-

Formaggia L, Quarteroni A, Veneziani A (Eds.): Cardiovascular Mathematics. Modeling and simulation of the circulatory system

port processes in the physiological and patho-physiological functions of the vascular system are of great interest. As discussed in Chapter 1, arteriosclerotic disease consists in degenerative changes in the arteries, characterised by thickening of the vessel walls and accumulation of calcium with consequent loss of elasticity and lessened blood flow. Atherosclerosis, in particular, is a common form of arteriosclerosis in which fatty substances form a deposit of plaque on the inner lining of arterial walls. Based on the knowledge that abnormal accumulation of macromolecules such as low density lipoprotein (LDL) or other atherogens in the arterial wall is an important component of the atherosclerotic disease processes, the quantification of the transport phenomena is required. It is world-wide accepted that an improved understanding of vascular mass transport phenomena and the influence of fluid dynamics will have a significant impact on public health.

Atherosclerosis tends to be localised in zones of artery bifurcations and bends where the shearing forces imposed by the flowing blood are disturbed compared with the straight tube patterns ([174, 264]). It has been observed that LDL accumulation in the intima occurring at zones of low and oscillating wall shear stress (in flow separation regions) is associated with the tendency to intimal thickening ([64, 65]). A powerful tool to analyse and quantify the relevant phemomena is computational modelling which provides detailed description of transport features, see [136].

The goals of vascular mass transport studies are to correlate mass transfer in anatomic geometries with the localisation of atherosclerotic lesions and to determine the influence of disturbed flow patterns on the local concentration distribution of substances in the blood stream and in the vessel wall layers. Vascular mass transport analysis requires the development of appropriate mathematical and numerical models. Because of the extreme complexity, the biological problem can be cast with difficulty into a formal physical framework, and simplifications with respect to the real biological situation are unavoidable. Basically the presented analysis is restricted to the dynamics of solutes in large and medium sized arteries. As a consequence, for the specific study of mass transfer blood can be idealised as a *Newtonian fluid* (see for instance [406], [383]). For a more detailed discussion of this assumption, we refer to Chapter 2. Furthermore, rigid arterial walls are assumed, with the justification that for the mass transfer study of large molecules (LDL) from blood to arterial walls accounting for wall displacement is not crucially important. However, for small molecules (oxygen), the wall compliance affects the flux into the wall significantly, see [399]. The application of mass and momentum conservation laws under these assumptions comes up to the incompressible *Navier-Stokes equations* (see Chapter 2). According to the fact that blood plasma filtrates from the inner to the outer part of the arterial walls under the action of blood pressure, it will be necessary to model the fluid flow in the wall layers, considered to be homogeneous porous media. In this case the conservation laws describing the plasma filtration lead to the *Darcy or Darcy-Brinkman equation.* Moreover, recent experiences show that intra-cellular transport also plays a role in the mass transfer through the arterial walls ([491] and references therein). Regarding the solute dynamics the limitation to consider the presence of just one solute is applied. Moreover, according to physical evidence, the concentration of chemicals dissolved in blood is small; consequently the blood motion is not influenced by chemicals. Then, by virtue of the mass conservation principle, the concentration of the considered solute is governed by a classical *advection-diffusion equation.*

Several mathematical models have been developed recently for the study of the transport of macromolecules (such as LDL) in arteries e.g., [249, 397, 476, 533, 563]). Essentially, the models can be classified in three categories corresponding to the level of description of the arterial wall.

For the simplest model, the *wall-free* model, the arterial wall is described by means of an appropriate boundary condition at the inner surface of the artery (lumen-endothelial boundary). The appropriate boundary conditions depend on the considered molecules. The transfer of *dissolved gases* (small molecules, e.g., oxygen) to and into the wall is diffusion boundary layer controlled, because of the fact that the endothelium is not an essential barrier to these molecules. The assumption of a constant concentration at this boundary is justified. Originally, this model was applied for the study of arterial oxygen concentration by [20, 132, 421]. The main resistance to the transfer of *macromolecules* from lumenal blood into the arterial wall is the endothelial layer. The flux across the endothelium into the inner layers of the arterial wall is determined by the endothelial permeability and by the concentration differential across the layer. Therefore, the permeability boundary condition (which is of Robin type) can be applied. The model requires the prescription of the concentration in the sub-endothelial intima. This model needs a relatively small number of parameters, the diffusivity, the overall mass transfer coefficient of the wall and the filtration velocity. The model was applied to analyse the local concentration of potentially atherogenetic molecules by [305] (ATP), by [533] (LDL). The model cannot provide any information on the concentration of solute within the wall, however, concentration polarisation effects in the blood phase directly at the wall can be addressed accurately.

Improved developments, the *fluid-wall* models, account for the arterial wall, where the mass transport in blood and in the wall are described applying physically appropriate laws to model the interaction between the blood flow and the biochemical transport. In the first stage of improvement the complex physiologic heterogeneous wall structure is approximated by one homogeneous porous layer representing the media. This layer is separated from the lumen by a membrane, which corresponds to the three physiologic layers endothelium, intima and IEL. The transport processes in the blood stream (lumen) and in the wall are coupled applying appropriate membrane equations. This model is well suited to describe the dynamics of solutes in healthy arteries, where the intima is a very thin layer, and the endothelium represents the main resistance to the solid. The most complex arterial transport model proposed so far is the *multilayer* model, which takes into account for the several heterogeneous layers, endothelium, intima, IEL and media (see [175, 176] for its definition; [58,563] for the analysis of existence and uniqueness of solutions; [249,251] for the analysis of a finite element scheme applied to this case). The multilayer model provides the most realistic information on the dynamics of chemicals (macromolecules) in the wall. The physical behaviour of the different layers are approximated with the laws of mass transport in homogeneous porous media (intima and media) and through plasma-permeable membranes (endothelium and IEL).

7.1 Governing equations for mass transfer in the cardiovascular system

The mathematical modelling for mass transfer in the cardiovascular system originated from the study of microcirculation with the aim to provide models for the mass transfer through the capillaries. Basic references are Friedman [173], Katchalsky and Curran [254] and for the specific application to the vascular system we mention Curry [106]. These works mainly neglect the space dependence of the quantities of interest because of the geometrical complexity of the capillary network. According to this tendency, we start our work with the study of two solutions of one single chemical whose concentration is small and uniform and we address in this setting the basic principles of transport processes. Then, we present the general lines to set up a mathematical model for mass transfer through the arterial walls. This procedure applies either to the wall-free, fluid-wall and multilayer model. Finally, we focus our attention on the multilayer model, which deserves a detailed discussion because of its complexity.

7.1.1 Principles of transport processes

We consider two solutions that are separated by a porous thin membrane that allows the flux of both solvent and solute from one compartment to the other. The membrane is not totally transparent with respect to the transport of mass, and makes a selection between the molecules that can pass through its interstices and those that can not. Membranes featuring this behaviour are called *selective permeable membranes*. As it will be made clear in the following paragraphs, these phenomena typically happen between the lumen and the wall or between the different layers of the wall.

Given a semipermeable membrane separating two solutions of concentration c in a suitable solvent, we denote with J_v the filtration velocity of the solvent across the membrane and with J_s the mass flux of the chemical per unit surface. Let L_p and $\mathcal{P}$ the hydraulic conductivity and the permeability of the membrane. The sieving coefficient, denoted with s, determines the ratio of molecules that can sieve across the membrane. In what follows we will also use the reflection coefficient that is the complementary of s with respect to the unity. We denote the reflection coefficient with $\sigma = 1 - s$. We will consider two different kind of reflection and sieving coefficients, the osmotic one (also called solvent drag sieving coefficient), denoted with $\sigma_d = 1 - s_d$ and the frictional one $\sigma_f = 1 - s_f$. Finally, the index $i = 1, 2$ denotes here the two compartments separated by the semipermeable membrane.

A well accepted mathematical model for the fluxes of solvent and the solute is given by the following set of equations, called *Kedem-Katchalsky* equations (see for example [254, 255]).

$$J_v = L_p(\delta p - \sigma_d \delta\pi) \tag{7.1}$$

$$J_s = \mathcal{P}\delta c + J_v(1 - \sigma_f)\overline{c}, \tag{7.2}$$

where $\overline{c}$ is the mean concentration inside the membrane and $\delta c = c_1 - c_2$, $\delta p = p_1 - p_2$, while

$$\delta\pi = RT\delta c, \tag{7.3}$$

where R, T are the gas constant and the absolute temperature. Equation (7.1) is called Starling's law of filtration and states that the solvent flux across the membrane is proportional to the pressure jump between the two compartments. The pressure jump is, on the other hand, split in two parts, the jump of static pressure δp and the jump of osmotic pressure $\delta\pi$. The latter depends on the solute concentration on the two sides of the membrane, according to the Van't Hoff's law (7.3). On the other hand, the solute flux, defined by equation (7.2), can be interpreted as the sum of a diffusive term (depending on the jump of concentration across the membrane) and a transport term (defined as the product of effective solvent flux and the mean concentration within the membrane). From another point of view, system (7.1,7.2) can be interpreted as the description of the influence of the driving forces acting through a membrane, namely δp and δc on the physical quantities J_v, J_s. The parameters $L_p, \mathcal{P}$ are the coefficients that govern this dependence and are called *phenomenological coefficients.*

A very delicate parameter appearing in the Kedem-Katchalsky equations is the average concentration within the membrane ($\overline{c}$). In fact, several models can be considered to estimate this quantity starting from physical considerations.

Let us assume that the dynamics of solute within the membrane are governed by diffusion and transport. Precisely, the concentration within the membrane satisfies the following boundary-value problem,

$$\begin{aligned} &-ac''(x) + bc'(x) = 0, \quad x \in (0, l) \\ &c(0) = c_1, \quad c(l) = c_2, \end{aligned} \tag{7.4}$$

where the cross-section of the membrane is represented by the interval $(0, l)$ while the coefficients $a := \mathcal{P}$ and $b := L_p(1 - \sigma_f)(p_1 - p_2)$ take into account the diffusion and the transport respectively. Finally c_1 and c_2 represent the concentration on the sides of the membrane. The solution of problem (7.4) is,

$$c(x) = \frac{1}{1 - \exp(Pe)}\left[c_2 - \exp(Pe)c_1 + (c_1 - c_2)\exp\left(\frac{bx}{a}\right)\right], \quad x \in (0, l),$$

where we have introduced the *global Péclet number* associated with problem (7.4), $Pe := bl/a$. Then the average concentration within the membrane, defined as $\overline{c} := (1/l) \int_0^l c(x)dx$ becomes,

$$\overline{c} = f_w(c_1, c_2) = w_1 c_1 + w_2 c_2$$

$$w_1 = \frac{\exp(Pe)}{\exp(Pe) - 1} - \frac{1}{Pe}, \quad w_2 = \frac{1}{Pe} - \frac{1}{\exp(Pe) - 1}.$$

In what follows, we call $f_w(c_1, c_2)$ the weighted arithmetic average. For example, let us consider this average for a membrane representing the endothelium. Thus, we set $l = 10^{-4}$cm, $\mathcal{P} = 10^{-7}$cm/s, $a = 10^{-11}$cm^2/s and $b = 10^{-6}$cm/s (the latter provides a reasonable approximation for the filtration velocity in the wall). The solute dynamics in the endothelium are in this case transport dominated (indeed, the Péclet number is high, $Pe = 100$) and we obtain $w_1 = 0.99, w_2 = 0.01$. This choice of the average concentration $\overline{c}$ is appropriate for membranes whose thickness is considerable with respect to the characteristic size of the molecules that filtrate through them.

An alternative approach to determine the average concentration within the membrane makes use of irreversible thermodynamics, the Kedem-Katchalsky equations can be theoretically derived from the general Onsager's phenomenological equations (see for example [254] Chapter 8), by applying them to the study of mass transport through membranes. For this matter the interested reader is referred to [173, 254, 255]. In this framework, the average concentration within the membrane can be defined starting from the Nerst-Planck equation for equilibrium of chemical potentials and it becomes $\overline{c} = f_l(c_1, c_2) = (c_1 - c_2)/\ln(c_1/c_2)$, which we call logarithmic average. Physical experience suggests that this model is suitable for extremely thin selective permeable membranes.

It is straightforward to verify that these models lead to different values of the average concentration. For example, in the common case of highly resistant membranes and of solute exchange dominated by transport, one has $c_1/c_2 \gg 1$ as well as $Pe \gg 1$, which leads to $f_w(c_1, c_2) \simeq c_1$ while $f_l(c_1, c_2) \simeq 0$. On the other hand, we observe that if the solute dynamics within the membrane is dominated by diffusion and the membrane is very permeable, one has $c_1/c_2 \simeq 1$ and $Pe \simeq 1$, which leads to $f_l(c_1, c_2) \simeq f_w(c_1, c_2) \simeq 1/2(c_1 + c_2)$. Finally, we observe that in the general case, the concentration within the membrane will be denoted as $\overline{c} = f(c_1, c_2)$.

7.1.2 Set up of the multilayer model

The starting point of this section is the description of the blood flow into the arterial lumen. It is governed by the Navier-Stokes equations, which are extensively discussed in Chapter 3 (see in particular equations (3.32) and (3.40)).

Concerning the arterial wall, we remind that in any biological tissue flow may take place through a complex network of interconnected pores, or openings. However, when dealing with such flow, we overlook the microscopic flow patterns inside individual pores and we consider some fictitious average which takes place in the porous medium comprising the tissue. By doing so, we are employing the concept of a continuum, which is common in most branches of physics. The obvious reason for employing the continuum approach in flow through a porous medium, is that it is practically impossible to describe in any exact mathematical manner the complicated geometry that bounds the flowing fluid. In order to set up the mathematical models for flow in porous media based on the continuum approach, we introduce the porosity of the tissue, $0 < \epsilon < 1$, and its hydraulic permeability (or Darcy permeability), K_D, which is assumed here to be a constant scalar quantity. In the case of a free fluid we set $\epsilon = 1$. We denote with $\boldsymbol{u}$ the volume averaged velocity and with $\tilde{\boldsymbol{u}}$ the velocity of the fluid phase. Similar notations, c and $\tilde{c}$, are adopted for the concentration of chemical dissolved in the solution permeating the tissue. We notice that the ratio between volume averaged value of a physical quantity and the value of the corresponding quantity in the fluid phase is given by $\epsilon = \boldsymbol{u}/\tilde{\boldsymbol{u}} = c/\tilde{c}$.

Under the assumption that blood plasma completely fills the void space of the porous medium, we consider two options to describe the average fluid flow into the tissue, the Darcy's model and the Brinkman's model. Both the Darcy's and the Brinkman's equations can be derived by means of homogeneisation techniques starting from the Stokes flow through an array of particles (for a detailed discussion we refer for example to [283]). Moreover, the Brinkman's model can be regarded as a correction of the Darcy's one featuring a viscous term inspired from the Stokes equations. The Darcy's model reads as follows,

$$\boldsymbol{u} = -\frac{K_D}{\mu}\boldsymbol{\nabla} p \quad \text{with} \quad \mathbf{div}\boldsymbol{u} = 0,$$

while the Brinkman's model is given by,

$$\boldsymbol{u} = -\frac{K_D}{\mu}[\boldsymbol{\nabla} p - \mu'(\nabla \boldsymbol{u} + \nabla \boldsymbol{u}^T)], \quad \mathbf{div}\boldsymbol{u} = 0,$$

where μ' is called the Brinkman's modified viscosity. Finally, the dynamics of chemicals is governed by a system of advection-diffusion equations. Precisely, applying the mass conservation principle on a generic control volume, we obtain the following equation

$$\partial_t c + \mathbf{div}(-D\boldsymbol{\nabla} c + \gamma \boldsymbol{u} c/\epsilon) = 0. \tag{7.5}$$

We observe that collisions of large molecules with the structure of the porous tissue layer result in a reduced convective transport. This phenomenon is taken into account by using a hindrance coefficient $0 < \gamma \leq 1$ in the mathematical model (see below).

In the wall-free model the fluid dynamics and the mass transport in the arterial lumen are described by the Navier-Stokes equations and the advection-diffusion equations. At the boundary between the lumen and the arterial wall appropriate conditions for the volume flux (J_v) and the mass flux (J_s) are assumed,

$$\boldsymbol{u}_l \cdot \boldsymbol{n}_l = J_v \quad \text{on} \quad \Gamma$$
$$(-D_l \nabla c_l + \boldsymbol{u}_l c_l) \cdot \boldsymbol{n}_l = J_s \quad \text{on} \quad \Gamma.$$

In this case the values of J_v and J_s are provided by experimental data in [49, 492, 513, 533]. In the case of the fluid-wall model and the multilayer model we need suitable matching conditions between the governing equations in different media. These conditions are provided by the Kedem-Katchalsky equations (7.1)–(7.2) and their application will be presented in detail for the multilayer model in what follows.

To set up the multilayer model, first of all we recall that the arterial wall consists of the endothelium (whose thickness is of the order of 2 µm), intima (thickness $\simeq$ 10 µm), internal elastic lamina (IEL, thickness $\simeq$ 2 µm), media (thickness $\simeq$ 300 µm) and adventitia. In the latter layer, pressure and the concentration are supposed to be known from measurements. In order to reduce the complexity of the resulting numerical problem, some simplifications are in order. An approach, proposed and discussed in [411, 420, 421], consist of treating the thinner layers as membranes through the Kedem-Katchalsky equations, see e.g. (7.1,7.2). Consequently the problem that we address here features three coupled domains: the lumen, the intima, the media, separated by interfaces, representing the endothelium and the IEL. A representation of the domains is given in Fig. 7.1. In order to set up the equations of the model,

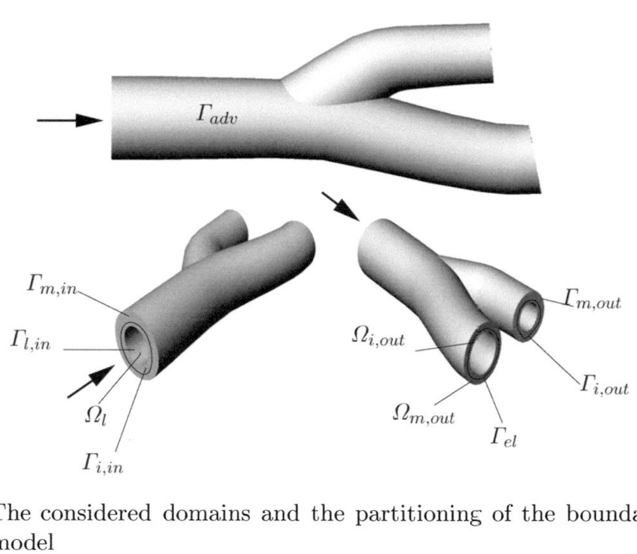

Fig. 7.1. The considered domains and the partitioning of the boundaries for the multilayer model

we will denote with the subscripts l, i, m the physical quantities related with the lumen, the intima and the media respectively. Moreover, we will apply the subscripts *end* and *iel* for the endothelium and the internal elastic lamina.

Fluid dynamics models

In order to find out whether the Darcy's or the Brinkman's model is more suited to our purpose, we focus on the interface conditions between the lumen and the wall, corresponding to the endothelial layer denoted with Γ_{end}. We notice that on the lumenal side we consider the interface as a non-slip surface that only allows normal flow. On the other hand, since the Darcy model does not allow any control on the tangential velocity on the boundary, there might be a discontinuity of it across Γ_{end}. Although, this is not likely to happen because the flow in the wall is driven by the pressure jump $p_l - p_{adv}$ and is mainly radial, the Darcy-Brinkman model is able to override this drawback. In fact it can be supplemented by conditions enforcing the continuity of the velocity across interfaces, since it features a viscous term. In general these conditions seem to be more realistic than the ones imposed in the Darcy case. However, we observe that the tangential velocity on the lumen-wall interface rapidly goes to zero into the wall. A rough estimation of the boundary layer thickness can be computed as in [445]. Assuming that the wall is characterised by the following parameters

- diameter of the pores, $D_p = 30\text{nm} = 30 \cdot 10^{-9}\text{m}$;
- porosity of the wall, $\epsilon = 0.96$;
- channel thickness, $H = 1\text{cm}$;
- permeability of the wall $K_i = [D_p^2 \epsilon^3]/[150(1-\epsilon)^2] = 0.33 \cdot 10^{-14}\text{m}^2$,

the boundary layer thickness δ is then,

$$\delta = K_i^{1/2} \log \left[50(h/K_i^{1/2} - 1) \right] = 9.2 \cdot 10^{-7}\text{m} \simeq 1\,\mu\text{m}.$$

We observe that the thickness of the boundary layer is half the thickness of the endothelium (about $2\,\mu$m). Furthermore, we point out that in the multilayer model the endothelium and the internal elastic lamina are treated as membranes, due to their extremely small thickness. Consequently, the Darcy-Brinkman model does not look fully consistent with the multilayer model since, in order to be correctly applied, it could require us to resolve details on a scale that is smaller than the thickness of the endothelium or the internal elastic lamina. Hence the Navier-Stokes/Darcy coupling looks more suitable in our case. Then, the system including the Navier-Stokes and the Darcy's equations (where we use the previously introduced notation) reads as flows.

$$J_{v,end} = L_{p,end}(p_l - p_i) - L_{p,end}\sigma_d RT(c_l - c_i) \text{ on } \Gamma_{end}, \tag{7.6}$$

$$J_{v,iel} = L_{p,iel}(p_i - p_m) - L_{p,iel}\sigma_d RT(c_i - c_m) \text{ on } \Gamma_{iel}. \tag{7.7}$$

Problem 7.1.1 Find the velocities and pressures in the lumen, intima and media $\boldsymbol{u}_l, p_l$, $\boldsymbol{u}_i, p_i$, $\boldsymbol{u}_m, p_m$, respectively, such that

$$
\begin{aligned}
&(a)\ \frac{\partial \boldsymbol{u}_l}{\partial t} + (\boldsymbol{u}_l \cdot \nabla)\boldsymbol{u}_l - \mathbf{div}\boldsymbol{\sigma}_l/\rho = \mathbf{0} \quad \text{in } \Omega_l, \quad t > 0\\
&(b)\ \mathbf{div}\boldsymbol{u}_l = 0 \quad \text{in } \Omega_l, \quad t > 0\\
&(c)\ \boldsymbol{u}_l = \boldsymbol{u}_{l,in} \quad \text{on } \Gamma_{l,in}, \quad t > 0\\
&(d)\ \boldsymbol{\sigma}_l \boldsymbol{n}_l = p_{out}\boldsymbol{n}_l \quad \text{on } \Gamma_{l,out}, \quad t > 0\\
&(e)\ \boldsymbol{u}_l \times \boldsymbol{n}_l = \mathbf{0}, \quad \boldsymbol{u}_l \cdot \boldsymbol{n}_l = \boldsymbol{u}_i \cdot \boldsymbol{n}_l \quad \text{on } \Gamma, \quad t > 0\\
&(f)\ \boldsymbol{u}_l = \boldsymbol{u}_0 \quad \text{with} \quad \mathbf{div}\boldsymbol{u}_0 = 0 \quad \text{in } \Omega_l,
\end{aligned}
\tag{7.8}
$$

(where $\boldsymbol{\sigma}_l$ is the Cauchy stress tensor defined in equation (3.33). Condition (7.8_e) states that Γ is a no-slip boundary that allows for filtration in the normal direction. Moreover, we require the normal velocity component across Γ to be continuous)

$$
\begin{aligned}
&(a)\ \boldsymbol{u}_i + \tfrac{K_i}{\mu_i}\boldsymbol{\nabla} p_i = 0 \quad \text{in } \Omega_i, \quad t > 0,\\
&(b)\ \mathbf{div}\boldsymbol{u}_i = 0 \quad \text{in } \Omega_i, \quad t > 0,\\
&(c)\ \boldsymbol{u}_i \cdot \boldsymbol{n}_i = 0 \quad \text{on } \Gamma_{i,in} \cup \Gamma_{i,out}, \quad t > 0,\\
&(d)\ \boldsymbol{u}_i \cdot \boldsymbol{n}_i = -J_{v,end} \quad \text{on } \Gamma_{end}, \quad t > 0,\\
&(e)\ \boldsymbol{u}_i \cdot \boldsymbol{n}_i = J_{v,iel} \quad \text{on } \Gamma_{iel}, \quad t > 0,
\end{aligned}
\tag{7.9}
$$

(equation (7.9_a) is the Darcy's law of filtration with a constant and scalar Darcy's permeability, K_i. Equation (7.9_b) accounts for the conservation of mass. Boundary condition (7.9_c) enforces the filtration velocity to be tangential to the distal and proximal sections of the wall. Conditions ($7.9_{d,e}$) determine the value of the filtration velocity into the endothelium and the IEL according to the Kedem-Katchalsky equations (7.1),(7.2))

$$
\begin{aligned}
&(a)\ \boldsymbol{u}_m + \tfrac{K_m}{\mu_m}\boldsymbol{\nabla} p_m = 0 \quad \text{in } \Omega_m, \quad t > 0,\\
&(b)\ \mathbf{div}\boldsymbol{u}_m = 0 \quad \text{in } \Omega_m, \quad t > 0,\\
&(c)\ \boldsymbol{u}_m \cdot \boldsymbol{n}_m = 0 \quad \text{on } \Gamma_{m,in} \cup \Gamma_{m,out}, \quad t > 0,\\
&(d)\ \boldsymbol{u}_m \cdot \boldsymbol{n}_m = -J_{v,iel} \quad \text{on } \Gamma_{iel}, \quad t > 0,\\
&(e)\ p_m = p_{adv} \quad \text{on } \Gamma_{adv}, \quad t > 0,
\end{aligned}
\tag{7.10}
$$

(equations ($7.10_{a,b}$) and conditions ($7.10_{c,d}$) are analogous to the ones set for the intima. Condition (7.10_e) fixes the pressure value on the adventitia to a known value p_{adv}). □

Finally, we point out that it is still possible account for the shear phenomena in the tangential direction on the fluid-wall interface. This is achieved by a special matching condition applied to the fluid side, proposed at first by Beavers and Joseph and generalised by Jones (see [445]). This condition reads as follows,

$$\frac{K_i^{1/2}}{\mu_i}\left[(\boldsymbol{\sigma}_l \boldsymbol{n}_l) \times \boldsymbol{n}_l\right] = \left(\frac{\mu_i'}{\mu_i}\right)^{1/2} \left[\boldsymbol{u}_l \times \boldsymbol{n}_l - \boldsymbol{u}_i \times \boldsymbol{n}_l\right] \quad \text{on } \Gamma. \tag{7.11}$$

Indeed, (7.11) states that the shear stress on the fluid-wall interface induces a jump on the tangential velocity across the interface. This boundary condition looks particularly suitable in our case, since it takes into account the variation of the tangential velocity across the endothelium, still represented as a membrane.

Solute dynamics models

First of all, we remind that because of friction phenomena on the motion of molecules, the actual transport velocity in the wall is smaller than the filtration velocity obtained from Problem 7.1.1. Consequently, we denote the transport field in equations (7.15,7.16) as an *effective* velocity, given by $(\gamma_\lambda/\epsilon_\lambda)\boldsymbol{u}_\lambda), \lambda = i, m$, where γ_λ is a constant called *friction or hindrance coefficient*, as in equation (7.5). For a more detailed discussion of this issue, we refer to [138, 249, 251]. Furthermore, we rewrite equation (7.2) with a general mean concentration within the membrane that we denote with $f(\cdot,\cdot)$:

$$J_{s,end} = \mathcal{P}_{end}(c_l - c_i) + L_{p,end}(1-\sigma_f)(p_l - p_i) f(c_l, c_i) - \\ L_{p,end}(1-\sigma_f)\sigma_d RT f(c_l, c_i)(c_l - c_i), \tag{7.12}$$

$$J_{s,iel} = \mathcal{P}_{iel}(c_i - c_m) + L_{p,iel}(1-\sigma_f)(p_i - p_m) f(c_i, c_m) - \\ L_{p,iel}(1-\sigma_f)\sigma_d RT f(c_i, c_m)(c_i - c_m). \tag{7.13}$$

Then, making use of these definitions, we propose the following problem for the solute dynamics.

Problem 7.1.2 Find the concentrations in the lumen, intima and media c_l, c_i, c_m respectively such that,

$$\begin{aligned} &\frac{\partial c_l}{\partial t} + \mathbf{div}(-D_l \boldsymbol{\nabla} c_l + \boldsymbol{u}_l c_l) = f_l,\ t>0,\ c_l(0) = c_{l,0} \text{ in } \Omega_l, \\ &(a) \quad c_l = c_{l,in} \text{ on } \Gamma_{l,in},\ t>0 \\ &(b) \quad \boldsymbol{\nabla} c_l \cdot \boldsymbol{n}_l = 0 \text{ on } \Gamma_{l,out},\ t>0 \\ &(c) \quad -D_l \boldsymbol{\nabla} c_l \cdot \boldsymbol{n}_l + \boldsymbol{u}_l \cdot \boldsymbol{n}_l c_l = J_{s,end} \text{ on } \Gamma_{end},\ t>0, \end{aligned} \tag{7.14}$$

(condition (7.14_c) that determines the solute flux across Γ_{end} according to theKedem-Katchalsky equations. Moreover, we refer to Fig. 7.1 for the definitions concerning the boundary partition)

$$\begin{aligned}
&\frac{\partial c_i}{\partial t} + \mathbf{div}(-D_i \boldsymbol{\nabla} c_i + \frac{\gamma_i}{\epsilon_i} \boldsymbol{u}_i c_i) + r_i c_i = f_i,\ t > 0, c_i(0) = c_{i,0} \text{ in } \Omega_i,\\
&(a)\quad \boldsymbol{\nabla} c_i \cdot \boldsymbol{n}_i = 0 \text{ on } \Gamma_{i,in} \cup \Gamma_{i,out},\ t > 0,\\
&(b)\quad -D_i \boldsymbol{\nabla} c_i \cdot \boldsymbol{n}_i + \tfrac{\gamma_i}{\epsilon_i} \boldsymbol{u}_i \cdot \boldsymbol{n}_i c_i = -J_{s,end} \text{ on } \Gamma_{end},\ t > 0,\\
&(c)\quad -D_i \boldsymbol{\nabla} c_i \cdot \boldsymbol{n}_i + \tfrac{\gamma_i}{\epsilon_i} \boldsymbol{u}_i \cdot \boldsymbol{n}_i c_i = J_{s,iel} \text{ on } \Gamma_{iel},\ t > 0,
\end{aligned} \tag{7.15}$$

(we introduced into the governing equations the term $r_i c_i$ accounting for consumption of chemicals by the tissues constituting the intima. Condition (7.15_a) enforces a null diffusive flux on the proximal and distal section of the intima. Condition ($7.15_{b,c}$) enforce on Γ_{end} and Γ_{iel} the flux prescribed by the Kedem-Katchalsky equations)

$$\begin{aligned}
&\frac{\partial c_m}{\partial t} + \mathbf{div}(-D_m \boldsymbol{\nabla} c_m + \frac{\gamma_m}{\epsilon_m} \boldsymbol{u}_m c_m) + r_m c_m = f_m,\ t > 0\ c_m(0) = c_{m,0} \text{ in } \Omega_i,\\
&(a)\quad c_m = c_{adventitia} \text{ or } \boldsymbol{\nabla} c_m \cdot \boldsymbol{n}_m = 0 \text{ on } \Gamma_{adv},\ t > 0,\\
&(b)\quad \boldsymbol{\nabla} c_m \cdot \boldsymbol{n}_m = 0 \text{ on } \Gamma_{m,in} \cup \Gamma_{m,out},\ t > 0\\
&(c)\quad -D_m \boldsymbol{\nabla} c_m \cdot \boldsymbol{n}_m + \tfrac{\gamma_m}{\epsilon_m} \boldsymbol{u}_m \cdot \boldsymbol{n}_m c_m = -J_{s,iel} \text{ on } \Gamma_{iel},\ t > 0.
\end{aligned} \tag{7.16}$$

(the governing equation and the boundary conditions for the media are analogous to the ones prescribed for the intima). □

In conclusion, Problems 7.1.1 and 7.1.2 represent the multilayer model for mass transfer across the arterial wall. Besides its technical complexity, its definition presents some intrinsic difficulties that appear both in the mathematical analysis of the well posedness of the problem and in its numerical approximation.

On one hand, we observe that Problems 7.1.1 and 7.1.2 are coupled by the interface conditions based on the fluxes $J_{v,end}$, $J_{v,iel}$ and $J_{s,end}$, $J_{s,iel}$ that contain terms involving both the pressure and the concentration. We want to simplify this situation. Since our aim is to study the absorption of macromolecules in the arterial wall, we avoid any simplification on the solute dynamics model, rather we make some assumptions on the equations concerning the blood flow. We obtain a simplification dropping in equations (7.6, 7.7) the term depending on the concentration. More precisely, by taking $J_{v,end} = L_{p,end}(p_l - p_i)$ on Γ_{end} and $J_{v,iel} = L_{p,iel}(p_i - p_m)$ on Γ_{iel}, as *reduced solvent fluxes*, equations (7.9,7.10) do not depend on the concentration, so they can be rewritten with the pressure as an unknown. On the other hand, the coupling between subequations of problems 7.1.1 and 7.1.2 will be approached in Section 7.3 in the framework of the numerical approximation of the multilayer model.

These difficulties also make the mathematical analysis of the coupled Problems 7.1.1 and 7.1.2 an extremely challenging task. Indeed, this is still an open issue. Indeed, we observe that the expressions of $J_{s,end}$, $J_{s,iel}$ are nonlinear functions of the concentrations. This is a major difficulty in the analysis of the well posedness and of the mathematical properties of the model 7.1.2, even when it is split from 7.1.1. We will not dwell here with a complete treatment of these topics, but we point out that the relevance of the analytical study with respect to the aim of this work is twofold. On one side, existence and uniqueness of a solution are the basic properties that have to be satisfied by mathematical models representing physical phenomena. These properties make also possible to consider the numerical approximation of the problem and to compute its solution by numerical methods. In addition to this, if the solution of the original problem is regular enough, the analysis of accuracy of the numerical method can be pursued (see for example Section 7.3). On the other side, the analysis of other specific mathematical properties, as for instance the maximum principle, allows us to characterise more precisely the behaviour of the solution. To sum up, the mathematical analysis provides a synthetic description of the multilayer model that turns out to be very useful in the applications, for example for the interpretation of the numerical results.

Remark 7.1.1 (Mathematical analysis) *Properties as existence, uniqueness and maximum principles have been widely investigated for standard elliptic operators, see e.g. [192], and in the parabolic case, in particular for advection diffusion problems in [398] or [471]. However, we point out that the multilayer model can not be casted into the classical framework, because of the non standard, non linear boundary or matching conditions on the interface between lumen and wall. In the linear case, the analysis of the model has been pursued in [411]. In the non linear case, existence and uniqueness results have been obtained in [58]. However, many analytical issues are still open. For instance, the solution of the multilayer problem may blow up in finite time. The study of blow up is a peculiar topic in analysis of partial differential equations for which we refer to [24] and [87] for a general introduction and to [152, 153, 280, 281] for analytical results that fit our case.*

7.2 Characterisation of physiological data

The physiological correct set up of the mathematical model for the lumenal and transmural fluid and solute dynamics needs appropriate transport parameters. These parameters describe the transport properties of the domains considered in the model (lumen, endothelium, intima, IEL and media). Many of these parameters can not be gained directly by experimental measurements. In this chapter we will discuss two possible mathematical methodologies developed to obtain a complete set of parameters for the different kinds of wall layers (membranes and fibre layers). The first part focuses on the estimation by using the pore theory that bases on the assumption that the wall layers are porous structures whose physical properties can be identified by their geometrical structure. This kind of method has been proposed in [11, 106, 233, 234, 270]. The majority of this part has been take from [251] where these models have been applied to obtain all parameters of the heterogenous wall structure. The second part describes a different kind of approach by a simplified inverse model based on an electrical analogy for the transport processes. The derivation of the electrical analogies for membranes and porous structers and their application to the arterial wall has been described in detail in [397].

7.2.1 Pore theory

Mass transport in the porous intima and media

The healthy subendothelial intima and the media generally consist of an extracellular matrix of randomly distributed proteoglycan and collagen fibres. In the media, as well as in the thickened intima smooth muscle cells occur in addition to the fibrous fluid phase. The transport processes in these arterial wall layers only occur in the fluid phase.

The fibre matrix is characterised by the wall layer thickness H, the fibre radius r_f and by the total length of the fibres l_f within the unit volume. Hence the fractional void volume of the fibre matrix results from,

$$\epsilon_f = 1 - \pi r_f^2 l_f.$$

The Darcy permeability $K_{D,f}$ of the porous tissue is given as,

$$K_{D,f} = \frac{r_f^2 \epsilon_f^3}{4G(1-\epsilon_f)^2}, \tag{7.17}$$

where G is the Kozeny constant, [232]. The restricted diffusivity of the solid of interest with a mean molecular radius r_{mol} in the extracellular matrix is calculated from the equation,

$$D_f = D \cdot \exp\left(-(1-\epsilon_f)^{1/2}\left(1 + \frac{r_{mol}}{r_f}\right)\right), \tag{7.18}$$

where D is the solute diffusivity in water and D_f is the restricted diffusion in the fiber matrix. According to [235] the hindrance coefficient for convective transport in the fibre matrix can be obtained from,

$$\gamma_f = 2 - \Phi_f. \tag{7.19}$$

The reduction coefficient Φ_f represents the relation between the space available to the solute relative to the space available to water,

$$\Phi_f = \exp\left[-(1-\epsilon_f)\left(\frac{2r_{mol}}{r_f} + \frac{r_{mol}^2}{r_f^2}\right)\right]$$

As discussed in Chapter 1, the media is formed by layers of smooth muscle cells. The presence of such cells is also observed in the case of a thickened intima. The contribution of smooth muscle cells is included in the model by means of an additional volume fraction ϵ_{SMC} that reduces the total porosity of the wall layer $\epsilon_{eff} = \epsilon_f(1-\epsilon_{SMC})$. In this case the transport parameters (diffusivity, Darcy permeability and lag coefficient) have to be transformed into effective parameters, see [235]. Without smooth muscle cells the parameters calculated from the equations (7.17)–(7.19) represent the effective parameters.

Example 7.2.1 (Intima) The mean radius of the fibres building up the extracellular matrix of the intima is $r_f = 3.22\,\text{nm}$ [235]. By assuming an average spacing of 5 nm and an average ratio between fibre length and intima thickness of 1.5 [232] we get a total length of the fibres within the unit volume of $l_f = 1.225 \cdot 10 - 3\,\text{nm}^{-2}$ and therewith a fractional void volume of $\epsilon_f = 0.96$ and a Darcy permeability of $K_{D,f} = 8.7 \cdot 10^{-13}\,\text{cm2}/(\text{s} \cdot \text{dyne})$. For LDL with a mean molecule radius $r_{mol} = 11\,\text{nm}$ we get a restricted diffusivity of $D_f = 1.2 \cdot 10^{-7}\,\text{cm2/s}$ and a reduction coefficient of $\Phi_f = 0.47$.

Example 7.2.2 (Media) The fractional void volume of the fibres in the media is $\epsilon_f = 0.43$ and the fraction of the smooth muscle cells is $\epsilon_{SMC} = 0.4$ which results in an effective values of $\epsilon_{eff} = 0.258$, $K_{D,eff} = 7.75 \cdot 10^{-16}\,\text{cm2}/(\text{s} \cdot \text{dyne})$, $\Phi_{eff} = 6.8 \cdot 10^{-6}$, $D_{eff} = 8.14 \cdot 10^{-9}\,\text{cm2/s}$.

Transport across the endothelium and internal elastic lamina

The endothelium and the internal elastic lamina (IEL) are treated as selective permeable membranes. They are assumed to be layers of constant thickness H. Exchange of water and solutes across the endothelium takes place through clefts (pores) which occur between the endothelial cells. The pores can be divided into normal endothelial clefts which are modelled as cylindrical pores and leaky junctions which are approximated as pores with a ringlike cross-section surrounding the leaky cells (cells which are either dying or in mitosis). The IEL contains fenestral pores through which transport between the intima and the media takes place. According to [232] the fenestrae can be approximated as cylindrical pores. The transport of molecules which is small in relation to the pore size across such porous membranes can be basically described using the convection-diffusion-reaction equation. The only effect of the porous membrane on the transport is the reduction of the space available to the solution. The transport of large molecules through these membranes is highly restricted by the pore structure. It is assumed that for entrance into the pore a molecule must pass through the opening without striking the edge [270]. This restriction causes the reflection and sieving of large molecules at the surface of membranes with relatively small pores. During the transport through the pores the molecules collide with the pore walls. These interactions between the molecules and the pore walls causes a loss in the kinetic energy of the molecules which results in a restricted transport within the pores.

We subdivide the pores on the endothelium and IEL into cylindrical pores and pores with ring-like cross section. The hydraulic conductivity of a cylindrical pore is,

$$L_p = \frac{\rho_{pore} \pi R^4}{8\mu L},$$

where ρ_{pore} is the average density of the pores, R is the radius and L the length of the pore. The restricted diffusivity coefficient in the pore D_p is defined as

$$D_p = DF(\alpha),$$

where $\alpha = r_{mol}/R$ is the ratio between the molecule radius and the radius of the pores and $F(\alpha)$ is, from [106],

$$F(\alpha) = \left[2(1-\alpha)^2 - (1-\alpha)^4\right]\left[1 - 2.1\alpha + 2.09\alpha^3 - 0.95\alpha^5\right].$$

Then, the permeability of the pore can be calculated by

$$\mathcal{P}_p = \Phi D_p / L, \tag{7.20}$$

where $\Phi = (1-\alpha)^2$ considers the reduction of pore cross section that is available to the solute. Fig. 7.2 (left) shows the relation of the free and the restricted pore diffusivity as function of α. The osmotic reflection coefficient is calculated by following the equation, which is obtained in [11],

$$\sigma_{d,p} = (1 - \Phi)^2$$

and the solvent drag reflection coefficient is given according to [106] by,

$$\sigma_{f,p} = \frac{16}{3}\alpha^2 - \frac{20}{3}\alpha^3 + \frac{7}{3}\alpha^4.$$

The functions the reflection coefficients are depicted in Fig. 7.2 (right).

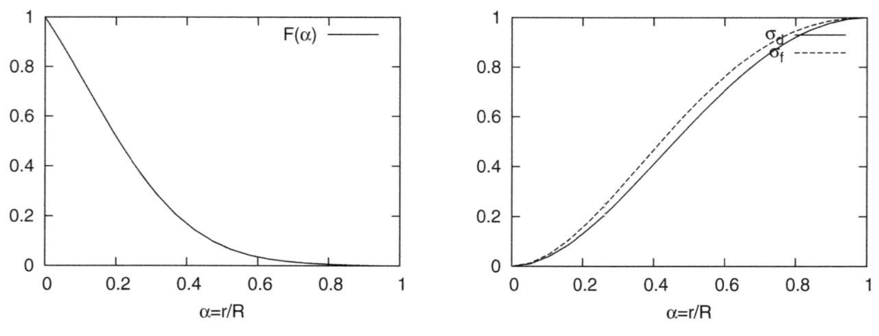

Fig. 7.2. Relation between the pore diffusivity and the free diffusivity (left), the osmotic reflection coefficient and the solvent drag reflection coefficient (right) as functions of the relation between the molecule and the pore radius, α

A pore with a ringlike cross-section is treated in the same way like a infinite long slit with constant width $2b$ as proposed by [106]. Hence the hydraulic conductivity of a ringlike pore is given by,

$$L_s = \frac{b^2}{3\mu L}. \tag{7.21}$$

The restricted diffusivity coefficient in the pore D_s is defined as,

$$D_s = DF_s(\alpha_s),$$

where $\alpha_s = r_{mol}/b$ is the ratio of the molecule radius to the half pore width size. The function of the restricted pore diffusivity [105] is,

$$F_s(\alpha_s) = (1 - \alpha_s)\left(1 - 1.004\alpha_s + 0.418\alpha_s^3 - 0.169\alpha_s^5\right).$$

The permeability of the pore is calculated in the same way like the circular pore (7.20), where $\Phi_s = 1 - \alpha_s$ accounts for the reduction of pore cross section that is available to the solute. The osmotic reflection coefficient follows form the model of [11],

$$\sigma_{d,s} = (1 - \Phi_s)^2 = \alpha_s^2$$

and the solvent drag coefficient [105] equals to

$$\sigma_{f,s} = 1 - \left(1 - \frac{3}{2}\alpha_s^2 + \frac{1}{2}\alpha_s^3\right)\left(1 - \frac{1}{3}\alpha_s^2\right).$$

The functions the reflection coefficients are depicted in Fig. 7.3.

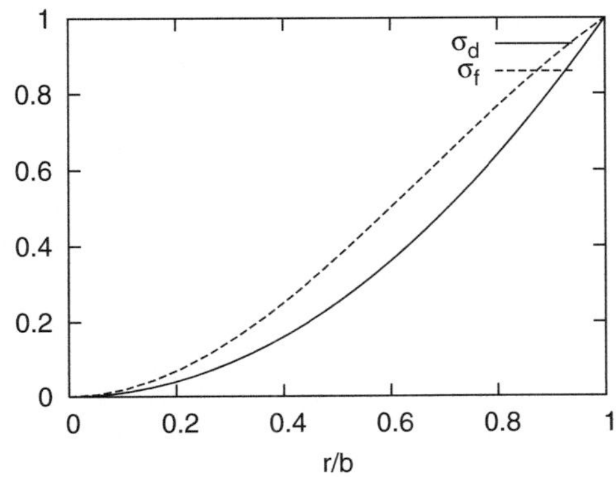

Fig. 7.3. Osmotic reflection coefficient and solvent drag reflection coefficient as functions of the ratio between molecule and half width size of the pore

Example 7.2.3 (Endothelium) The transport parameters of the leaky clefts ($L_{p,lj}$, $\mathcal{P}_{lj}$, Φ_{lj}, $\sigma_{f,lj}$, $\sigma_{d,lj}$) and the normal junctions($L_{p,nj}$, $\mathcal{P}_{nj}$, $\sigma_{f,nj}$, $\sigma_{d,nj}$) are calculated by equations described above. According to [232], the values of the hydraulic conductivity, permeability and reflection coefficients of the endothelium containing normal clefts and leaky clefts are

$$L_{p,end} = L_{p,nj} + L_{p,lj}\epsilon_{lj}$$

$$\mathcal{P}_{end} = \mathcal{P}_{nj} + \mathcal{P}_{lj}\epsilon_{lj}\Phi_{lj}$$

$$\sigma = \frac{L_{p,nj}\sigma_{nj} + L_{p,lj}\epsilon_{lj}\sigma_{lj}}{L_{p,e}},$$

where ϵ_{lj} is the area of leaky clefts per unit area of the endothelial surface. The average fraction of leaky cells for a healthy endothelium is 0.05 %. Their cell radius is 15 μm and the width is 20 nm–25 nm. The normal junctions have a radius of 5.5 nm and an average distance of 2.5 μm [232]. The resulting hydraulic conductivity is $L_{p,end} = 3 \cdot 10^{-11}$ cm3/(s · dyne). For LDL the permeability is $\mathcal{P}_{end} = 1.07 \cdot 10^{-11}$ cm/s and the reflection coefficients are $\sigma_{d,end} = 0.996$ and $\sigma_{f,end} = 0.997$.

Example 7.2.4 (Internal elastic lamina) The average radius of the fenestral pores of the IEL is 0.15 μm [278] and their average density is $2210/mm2$ [235]. The resulting hydraulic conductivity is $L_{p,IEL} = 3.05 \cdot 10^{-9}$ cm3/(s · dyne). For LDL the permeability is $\mathcal{P}_{IEL} = 1.59 \cdot 10^{-7}$ cm/s and the reflection coefficients are $\sigma_{d,IEL} = 1.99 \cdot 10^{-2}$ and $\sigma_{f,IEL} = 1.93 \cdot 10^{-2}$.

7.2.2 Electrical analogy

Although the idea of applying an electrical analogy to set up reduced models for transport phenomena, including fluid flows, will be introduced in Chapter 10, we address here for the first time its application to mass transfer, more precisely to convection and diffusion processes.

The models to calculate the transport parameters described in the previous section are based on the assumption that the transport of the considered molecules occurs only in the fluid phase of the different layers. The transcellular transport, representing an essential part of the complete solid dynamics for very large molecules [355], cannot be considered in this kind of models. Therefore the help of experimental measurements is needed to make the theoretical estimations successful in the specific applications.

In this section a short overview of a methodology is presented that allows to estimate the physical parameters of the wall layers starting from a set of data that can be easily determined by experimental measurements like LDL concentration profiles in the arterial wall (see [49, 129, 326, 492]). A simplified problem is used to define the relationship between the set of physical parameters characterizing the wall (formally denoted with the vector $\mathbf{p}$) and the concentration profiles of LDL the wall (described as a collection of concentration samples stored in the vector $\mathbf{c}$). The mathematical relationship between $\mathbf{p}$ and $\mathbf{c}$ will be denoted with $\mathbf{c} = F(\mathbf{p})$. We search for an analytical expression of F, which could be easily inverted leading to an explicit solution of the inverse problem $\mathbf{p} = F^{-1}(\mathbf{c})$. For this reason, an electrical analogy is applied to describe the mass transfer phenomena through the arterial walls. The derivation of the electrical analogy and its application to the transport through the wall layers is described in detail in [397].

Fluid dynamics

The electrical analog of the arterial wall with respect to fluid dynamics can be represented as a sequence of four resistances in series, corresponding to each single layer constituting the wall, as shown in Fig. 7.4.

The electrical representation of each layer is derived by a simplification of the governing equations for the fluid dynamics (first Kedem-Katchalsky equation and Darcy's law). The pressure drop is the driving force resulting in a volume flux representing the flux of the electrical analogy.

Using the transport parameters obtained from pore theory results in a filtration velocity of $J_v = 4.25 \cdot 10^{-7}\,\text{cm/s}$ by applying a pressure drop of 70 mmHg. This value does not correspond to the measurements reported in [326]. Therefore the electric analog is used to rescale the parameters from pore theory to obtain the measured flux of $J_v = \boldsymbol{u} \cdot \boldsymbol{n} = 1.78 \cdot 10^{-6}\,\text{cm/s}$. The updated transport parameters for the fluid dynamics are $L_{p,end} = 1.20 \cdot 10^{-10}\,\text{cm}^3/(\text{s} \cdot \text{dyne})$, $K_{D,i} = 3.64 \cdot 10^{-12}\,\text{cm}^2/(\text{s} \cdot \text{dyne})$, $L_{p,IEL} = 1.28 \cdot 10^{-8}\,\text{cm}^3/(\text{s} \cdot \text{dyne})$ and $K_{D,m} = 3.24 \cdot 10^{15}\,\text{cm}^3/(\text{s} \cdot \text{dyne})$.

Dynamics of chemicals

The simplification of the equations describing the solid dynamics in membranes and porous media (second Kedem-Katchalsky and advection-diffusion-reaction equation) ends up with an electrical analogy of two parallel resistances for each layer. These resistances represent the convective and the diffusive solid transport.

The electrical analog of the system featuring the different wall layers with respect to the transfer of molecules is represented in Fig. 7.5. The first two

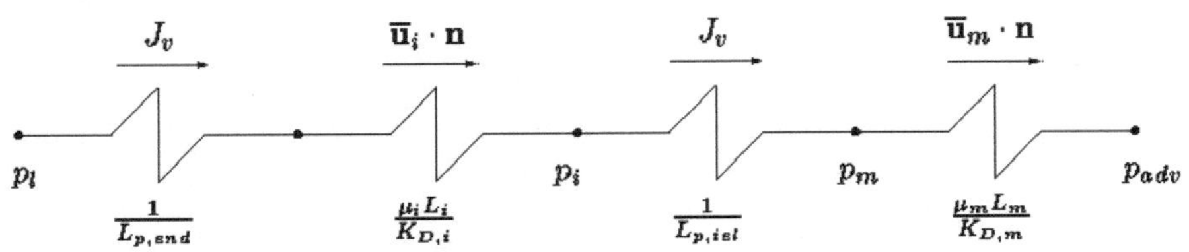

Fig. 7.4. Electrical analog-on for the plasma filtration inside the arterial wall

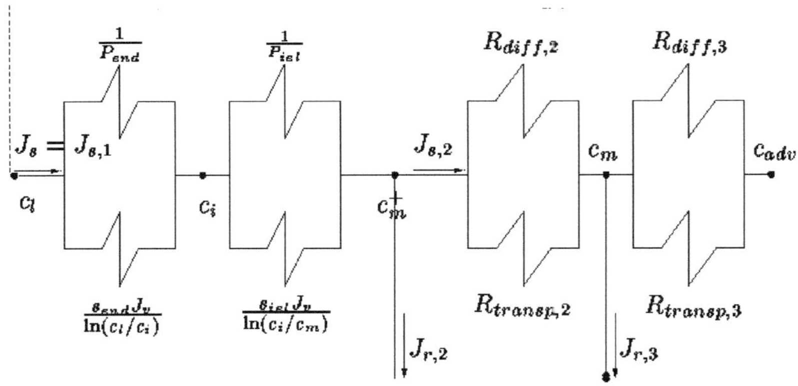

Fig. 7.5. Electrical analogon for the dynamics of chemicals of the arterial wall

modules represent the endothelium and the IEL, the remaining ones represent the media. Since the media is the thickest layer it is split in two parts, as this makes easier to take into account of the degradation of solute due to chemical reactions. Furthermore, physical experience suggests that the intima is the less resistant layer to diffusion transport. Consequently, to simplify our model, it is assumed that the concentration drop across the intima is negligible.

By fixing the value of the parameters that are experimentally determined with reasonable accuracy, precisely the wall thickness $L = 200\,\mu\text{m}$, the solute diffusivity inside the media, $D_m = 8 \cdot 10^{-9}$, and the porosity of the media, $\epsilon_m = 0.15$ we are able to cacluate the missing set of parameters starting from a number of experimentally measured concentration values. For instance we consider $\bar{c}_m^+ = 10^{-2}, \bar{c}_m = 2.5 \cdot 10^{-3}, \bar{c}_m^- = 10^{-2}$, given by [326]. The concentration in the intima is considered as unknown that will be determined by means of the equation arising from the electrical analogy. A detailed description of the complete procedure can be found in [397]. As a result of that, we determine the missing set of transport parameters that are given by $\mathcal{P}_{end} = 2 \cdot 10^{-8}\,\text{cm/s}$, $\mathcal{P}_{IEL} = 3.18 \cdot 10^{-4}\,\text{cm/s}$, $\sigma_{end} = 0.998$, $\sigma_{IEL} = 0.983$, $\gamma_i = 0.17$, $\gamma_m = 0.117$ and $r_m = 3.197 \cdot 10^{-4}\,\text{s}^{-1}$.

7.3 Computer simulation

This section is devoted to the numerical approximation of the mathematical models which have been introduced in Section 7.1. First of all, we point out that a self contained treatment of the topics involved in the numerical approximation of partial differential equations would be rather extensive and complex, and consequently it goes beyond the scope of this chapter and of this book. For this reason, the aim of this section is to provide a survey on numerical approximation of PDEs and computational fluid dynamics that is specifically adapted to the problems involved on the mass transfer in the cardiovascular system. We will enter into details only for those topics that are peculiar to this matter. Furthermore, we will provide at first an overview and the main references to build up the numercal discretisation of the multilayer model. Then, we will consider a simplified model where the arterial walls are assumed to be an homogeneous layer. In this context, we will address those topics that are peculiar to the treatment of mass transfer in the arterial walls.

As already seen, the multilayer model involves the coupling of the flow equations for blood and plasma, with an advection-diffusion-reaction problem (see Problems 7.1.1 and 7.1.2 respectively). In these models, the advection-diffusion-reaction equations depend on the fluid dynamics through the advective field. Hence the fluid dynamics problem is solved at a first step, and then we solve the advection-diffusion-reaction problem.

For the space discretisation of the space-dependent partial differential operators, we apply the finite element method. In particular, for what concerns the Navier–Stokes equations, in order to satisfy the compatibility *inf-sup* condition, we have adopted a linear approximation based on the so-called $\mathbb{P}^1 iso\mathbb{P}^2 - \mathbb{P}^1$ element, while the backward Euler time discretisation has been coupled with a semi-implicit treatment of the nonlinear term. Finally, a splitting of the velocity and pressure problem based on the so-called *Yosida method* is carried out. For more details about these techniques, the interested reader is referred to [404, 405, 407].

For the discretisation of the Darcy problem we consider a mixed-hybrid finite element formulation based on Raviart-Thomas elements, for which we refer to [79]. By means of this method we approximate $\boldsymbol{u}_i, p_i$ and $\boldsymbol{u}_m, p_m$ by means of $\mathbb{RT}^0 - \mathbb{P}^0$ elements. Then, the discrete velocities are projected by means of the standard L^2 inner product on the space of vector valued linear finite elements in order to be more easily exploited in the discretisation of the solute dynamics problem.

Concerning the advection-diffusion equations, we observe that the multilayer problem is characterised by very low diffusivity coefficients. In other terms, this problem is dominated by the advection effects. Indeed, if h denotes the space discretisation step (which in our simulations is in the range of 10^{-2}cm), $|\boldsymbol{u}|$ is a representative value of the blood velocity, for instance equal to 10cm/s, and the diffusivity of LDL is about $D = 10^{-7}\text{cm}^2/\text{s}$, we have an indicative value of the *local Péclet number*, $Pe = h|\boldsymbol{u}|D^{-1}$, (which weighs the convection effects with respect to the diffusive ones) of 10^6. As it is well known, finite element techniques (and in general Galerkin methods) could be inaccurate when facing convection dominated problems and resorting to a stabilisation technique becomes mandatory. Different strategies can be pursued in this regard: the interested reader is referred to [236] and [407]. In our simulations, streamline-upwind/Petrov–Galerkin (SUPG) has been successfully adopted and will be addressed later on.

A further difficulty is related to the fact that we consider phenomena that take place both into blood and into the arterial tissues. By consequence, from the point of view of either fluid dynamics or solute dynamics, we notice that the multilayer problem, as well as its simplified variants, can not be reformulated as problems governed by a unique differential operator on a single domain. For this reason, we focus our attention on *iterative substructuring methods* to split the multilayer problem into subproblems. For the treatment of this topic, we will focus on the solute dynamics model, namely Problem 7.1.2, which consists mainly in a system of advection-diffusion equations on adjacent domains coupled by suitable matching conditions. A general theory, discussed for instance by Quarteroni and Valli in [408], is available for this matter in the case of linear symmetric problems, for example diffusion dominated processes, but the presence of a non negligible advection term makes the multilayer problem to be governed by strongly unsymmetric operators. Furthermore, the specific matching conditions that we apply between blood and the arterial walls are definitely non-standard and in particular they are nonlinear. Consequently, the general framework of [408] does not apply to our case. Thus, in this section we will discuss in detail the convergence properties of the iterative substructuring methods suitable for the multilayer problem.

7.3.1 Numerical approximation of the solute dynamics

As already mentioned, in order to concentrate on the main ideas and to simplify at most the notation and the technical aspects of this subject, we do not consider here the complete multilayer problem 7.1.2. Instead of the multilayer model we consider an instance of the fluid-wall models, where the complex heterogeneous structure of the arterial walls is approximated by a simple homogeneous layer. Such model, proposed in [137, 138] to study the concentration of oxygen and LDL within the arterial walls, reads as follows:

Problem 7.3.1 Find the concentrations c_l, defined on $\Omega_l \times [0,T]$, and c_w, defined on $\Omega_w \times [0,T]$, such that

$$\begin{aligned}
&\frac{\partial c_l}{\partial t} + \mathbf{div}(-D_l \nabla c_l + \boldsymbol{u}_l c_l) = f_l, \quad \text{in } \Omega_l,\ t>0\\
&c_l = c_{l,in} \quad \text{on } \Gamma_{l,in},\ t>0\\
&D_l \nabla c_l \cdot \boldsymbol{n}_l = 0 \quad \text{on } \Gamma_{l,out}, \quad t>0\\
&c_l(0) = c_{l,0} \quad \text{in } \Omega_l, \quad t=0,
\end{aligned} \tag{7.22}$$

$$\begin{aligned}
&\frac{\partial c_w}{\partial t} - \mathbf{div}(D_w \nabla c_w) = f_w \quad \text{in } \Omega_w, \quad t>0\\
&c_w = c_{w,ext} \quad \text{on } \Gamma_{w,ext}, \quad t>0\\
&D_w \nabla c_w \cdot \boldsymbol{n}_w = 0, \quad \text{on } \Gamma_{w,in} \cup \Gamma_{w,out},\ t>0,\\
&c_w(0) = c_{w,0} \quad \text{in } \Omega_w,\ t=0,
\end{aligned} \tag{7.23}$$

with the following matching conditions at the interface,

$$D_w \nabla c_w \cdot \boldsymbol{n}_w = -D_l \nabla c_l \cdot \boldsymbol{n}_l \quad \text{on } \Gamma, \quad t > 0, \tag{7.24}$$

$$-D_l \nabla c_l \cdot \boldsymbol{n}_l = \mathcal{P}(c_l - c_w) \quad \text{on } \Gamma, \quad t > 0, \tag{7.25}$$

where the notation of Section 7.1 has been mantained.

In order to define the numerical discretisation of Problem 7.3.1 we introduce $\mathcal{T}_{h,l}, \mathcal{T}_{h,w}$ admissible triangulations of $\overline{\Omega}_l, \overline{\Omega}_w$ respectively. Moreover, we assume that $\mathcal{T}_{h,l}, \mathcal{T}_{h,w}$ are conforming triangulations on Γ. In other words we require that $\mathcal{T}_h = \mathcal{T}_{h,l} \cup \mathcal{T}_{h,w}$ is an admissible triangulation for $\overline{\Omega}_l \cup \overline{\Omega}_w$. Then, we are in position to define the finite element spaces,

$$V_{h,l} = \{v_{h,l} \in C^0(\overline{\Omega}_l) \mid v_{h,l} \in \mathbb{P}_k, \ \forall K \in \mathcal{T}_{h,l}, \ v_{h,l}|_{\Gamma_{l,in}} = 0\}$$
$$V_{h,w} = \{v_{h,w} \in C^0(\overline{\Omega}_w) \mid v_{h,w} \in \mathbb{P}_k, \ \forall K \in \mathcal{T}_{h,w}, \ v_{h,w}|_{\Gamma_{w,ext}}, \ v_{h,m}|_{\Gamma_{adv}} = 0\}.$$

Moreover, let Λ_h be the finite dimensional space defined by the traces on Γ of functions in $V_{h,l}$ or $V_{h,w}$. To introduce the time discretisation we subdivide the time interval $[0, T]$ in N time steps $t^n = n\Delta t$ with $\Delta t > 0$ and $n = 1, \ldots, N$, and use backward Euler finite difference schemes. In order to simplify our notation, let us introduce the following time discrete bilinear forms,

$$a_l^n(w, v) = \frac{1}{\Delta t}(w, v) + (D_l \nabla w, \nabla v) + \left(\boldsymbol{u}_{h,l}^n \cdot \nabla w, v\right), \tag{7.26}$$

$$a_w^n(w, v) = \frac{1}{\Delta t}(w, v) + (D_w \nabla w, \nabla v), \tag{7.27}$$

and the corresponding right hand side terms, $\mathcal{F}_\lambda^{n-1} = f_\lambda + \frac{1}{\Delta t} c_\lambda^{n-1}$ for $\lambda = l, w$. The fully discrete counterpart of the fluid-wall model reads as follows:

Problem 7.3.2 For all $n = 1, \ldots, N$, given $[c_{h,l}^0, c_{h,w}^0] \in V_{h,l} \times V_{h,w}$, find $c_{h,l}^n \in V_l, c_{h,w}^n \in V_{h,w}$ such that

$$a_l^n\left(c_{h,l}^n, v_{h,l}\right) + \left(c_{h,l}^n, v_{h,l}\right)_{\mathcal{P}} = \left(c_{h,w}^n, v_{h,l}\right)_{\mathcal{P}} + \left(\mathcal{F}_l^{n-1}, v_{h,l}\right) \quad \forall v_{h,l} \in V_{h,l}$$

$$a_w^n\left(c_{h,w}^n, v_{h,w}\right) + \left(c_{h,w}^n, v_{h,w}\right)_{\mathcal{P}} = \left(c_{h,l}^n, v_{h,w}\right)_{\mathcal{P}} + \left(\mathcal{F}_w^{n-1}, v_{h,w}\right) \quad \forall v_{h,w} \in V_{h,w}. \tag{7.28}$$

Let us now introduce the algebraic counterpart of Problem 7.3.2. To this aim, let us denote with $\mathbf{c}_\lambda^n \in \mathbb{R}^{N_\lambda}$, $\lambda = l, w$ the vectors of the degrees of freedom of the discrete approximation of the concentration on $\mathcal{T}_{h,\lambda}$. The application of Lagrangian finite elements leads to systems of algebraic equations for the unknowns $\mathbf{c}_\lambda^n$. More precisely, at every time step t^n, Problem 7.3.2 leads to the system of linear equations,

$$A^n \mathbf{c}^n = \mathbf{b}^n \quad \Leftrightarrow \quad \begin{bmatrix} A_{ll}^n & A_{lw}^n \\ A_{wl}^n & A_{ww}^n \end{bmatrix} \cdot \begin{bmatrix} \mathbf{c}_l^n \\ \mathbf{c}_w^n \end{bmatrix} = \begin{bmatrix} \mathbf{b}_l^n \\ \mathbf{b}_w^n \end{bmatrix} \tag{7.29}$$

Denoting with $\{\psi_{i,l}\}, i = 1,\ldots,N_l$ and $\{\psi_{i,w}\}, i = 1,\ldots,N_w$ the set of linear finite element shape functions of $V_{h,l}, V_{h,w}$ respectively, the matrices $A^n_{ll}, A^n_{lw}, A^n_{wl}, A^n_{ww}$ are defined as follows.

$$[A^n_{ll}]_{i,j} = a^n_l\left(\psi_{j,l},\psi_{i,l}\right) + (\psi_{j,l},\psi_{i,l})_{\mathcal{P}} \quad i=1,\ldots,N_l,\ j=1,\ldots,N_l,$$

$$[A^n_{lw}]_{i,j} = -\left(\psi_{j,w},\psi_{i,l}\right)_{\mathcal{P}} \quad i=1,\ldots,N_l,\ j=1,\ldots,N_w,$$

$$[A^n_{wl}]_{i,j} = -\left(\psi_{j,l},\psi_{i,w}\right)_{\mathcal{P}} \quad i=1,\ldots,N_w,\ j=1,\ldots,N_l,$$

$$[A^n_{ww}]_{i,j} = a^n_w\left(\psi_{j,w},\psi_{i,w}\right) + (\psi_{j,w},\psi_{i,w})_{\mathcal{P}} \quad i=1,\ldots,N_w,\ j=1,\ldots,N_w.$$

Moreover, the right hand sides $\mathbf{b}^n_l, \mathbf{b}^n_w$ are given by, $[\mathbf{b}^n_\lambda]_i = \left(\mathcal{F}^{n-1}_\lambda, \psi_{\lambda,i}\right)$ with $i = 1,\ldots,N_\lambda,\ \lambda = l, w$. The obvious strategy to solve system (7.29) consists of applying either direct or iterative methods to the global problem $A^n\mathbf{c}^n = \mathbf{b}^n$. An approach more specific to our case consists of splitting (7.29) into subsystems associated to the finite element discretisation on $\mathcal{T}_{h,l}, \mathcal{T}_{h,w}$ separately. The latter strategy seems more attractive, because it makes easier to handle a discontinuous concentration across the interface. Indeed, in the finite element framework, the concentration on the nodes laying on Γ has two different values, one associated to the lumen and one to the wall. Moreover, as we will see later, the analysis of iterative techniques to split Problems 7.3.2, suggests the way to build efficient preconditioners for the global system $A^n\mathbf{c}^n = \mathbf{b}^n$. The splitting technique gives even more advantages in the nonlinear case. In fact, an explicit treatment of the nonlinear term, allows us to reduce the solution of the multilayer problem to a sequence of linear subproblems.

7.3.2 Iterative substructuring methods for the solute dynamics

Since all the relevant equations deal only with unknowns evaluated at the time step t^n, for notational convenience from now on, we drop the index n. The time index will be explicitly indicated only when referring to a time step different than t^n. Moreover, since the results presented in this section hold true also in the infinite dimensional case with respect to space dependence, we drop the index h denoting the space discrete functions.

To split Problem 7.3.2 into subproblems, we introduce an iterative procedure where the concentration at the wall, in the advection diffusion equation in the lumen, is evaluated at the previous iterative step. This leads to the following iterative procedure:

$$\begin{aligned}
&\tfrac{1}{\Delta t}c_l^k + \mathbf{div}(-D_l\boldsymbol{\nabla} c_l^k + \boldsymbol{u}_l c_l^k) = f_l + \tfrac{1}{\Delta t}c_l^{n-1} \quad \text{in } \Omega_l,\\
&c_l^k = c_{D,l}, \quad \text{on } \Gamma_{D,l},\\
&\boldsymbol{\nabla} c_l^k \cdot \boldsymbol{n}_l = 0 \text{ on } \Gamma_{N,l},\\
&-D_l\boldsymbol{\nabla} c_l^k \cdot \boldsymbol{n}_l = \mathcal{P}(c_l^k - c_w^{k-1}), \quad \text{on } \Gamma,
\end{aligned}$$

$$\frac{1}{\Delta t}c_w^k + \mathbf{div}(-D_w \boldsymbol{\nabla} c_w^k + \boldsymbol{u}_w c_w^k) = f_w + \frac{1}{\Delta t}c_w^{n-1} \text{ in } \Omega_w,$$
$$c_w^k = c_{D,w}, \quad \text{on } \Gamma_{D,w},$$
$$\boldsymbol{\nabla} c_w^k \cdot \boldsymbol{n}_w = 0 \text{ on } \Gamma_{N,w},$$
$$-D_w \boldsymbol{\nabla} c_w^k \cdot \boldsymbol{n}_w = \mathcal{P}(c_w^k - c_l^k), \quad \text{on } \Gamma.$$

Reinterpreting this iterative method in the variational form, we obtain the following problem.

Problem 7.3.3 For all $n = 1, \dots, N$, given an initial guess c_w^0 and a tolerance ϵ, for $k = 1, 2, \dots$ find a sequence $[c_l^k, c_w^k]$ such that,

$$\begin{aligned} a_l^n\left(c_l^k, v_l\right) + \left(c_l^k, v_l\right)_{\mathcal{P}} &= \langle \mathcal{F}_l^{n-1}, v_l\rangle + \left(c_w^{k-1}, v_l\right)_{\mathcal{P}} \quad \forall v_l \in V_l \\ a_w^n\left(c_w^k, v_w\right) + \left(c_w^k, v_w\right)_{\mathcal{P}} &= \langle \mathcal{F}_w^{n-1}, v_w\rangle + \left(c_l^k, v_w\right)_{\mathcal{P}} \quad \forall v_w \in V_w, \end{aligned} \tag{7.30}$$

until the stopping criterion,

$$\frac{\|c_l^k - c_l^{k-1}\|_0}{\|c_l^k\|_0} + \frac{\|c_w^k - c_w^{k-1}\|_0}{\|c_w^k\|_0} < \epsilon \tag{7.31}$$

is satisfied.

Of course the stopping criterion can be modified. Such method is often referred as *Robin-Robin* iterative method, because the interaction between the subdomains is achieved by Robin matching conditions.

At this stage, the issue of major importance is to understand whether the iterative method presented in Problem 7.3.3 is convergent, or in other words to prove that the sequence $[c_l^k, c_w^k]$ converges in a suitable norm to the solution of Problem 7.3.2. Because of the lack of continuity between c_l and c_w at the interface Γ, the analysis of convergence for this splitting method does not straightforwardly follows from available convergence results, namely the Dirichlet-Neumann, the Neumann-Neumann or the Robin-Robin methods arising from domain decomposition techniques, for which we refer to [408]. We need thus to develop a specific analysis. First of all we introduce the *splitting error*, namely

$$e_{h,l}^{n,k} = c_{h,l}^n - c_{h,l}^{n,k}, \quad e_{h,w}^{n,k} = c_{h,w}^n - c_{h,w}^{n,k}$$

where $[c_{h,l}^n, c_{h,w}^n]$ is the solution of problem 7.3.2. As stated before, in the sequel we will use the abridged notation e_l^k, e_w^k. Now, if we subtract equations (7.30) from (7.28), we obtain the following equations for $[e_l^k, e_w^k]$, that we call the splitting error equations,

$$a_l^n\left(e_l^k, v_l\right) + \left(e_l^k, v_l\right)_{\mathcal{P}} = \left(e_w^{k-1}, v_l\right)_{\mathcal{P}} \quad \forall v_l \in V_l \tag{7.32}$$
$$a_w^n\left(e_w^k, v_w\right) + \left(e_w^k, v_w\right)_{\mathcal{P}} = \left(e_l^k, v_w\right)_{\mathcal{P}} \quad \forall v_w \in V_w. \tag{7.33}$$

We resume the convergence property of Problem 7.3.3 in the theorem below.

Property 7.3.1 *The iterative method defined in problem 7.3.3 is convergent (for both the Galerkin and the stabilised SUPG or GaLS discretisations). More precisely we have* $\lim_{k\to\infty} \|e_l^k\|_1 + \|e_w^k\|_1 = 0$. *The convergence rate may depend on the physical data but not on the mesh size h.*

Remark 7.3.1 (Advanced topics) *In the framework of the mathematical analysis of iterative substructuring methods, a more advanced approach consists in rewriting the the fluid-wall problem for an unknown living on the interface between the lumen and the wall. In this case, special Steklov-Poincaré operators, see [408] and [410], are necessary to consider the non standard Robin-Robin matching conditions. This reinterpretation leads to a detailed characterisation of the convergence properties of the iterative scheme of Problem 7.3.3, where a parameter that accelerates the convergence is introduced. This study, which is addressed in detail in [410], also suggests that the scheme of Problem 7.3.3 can be seen as an* optimal *preconditioner for the original coupled Problem 7.3.2. This observation give rise to the discussion of efficient computational techniques to solve the fluid-wall problem. In particular, the application of the* flexible preconditioned GMRES *method, proposed by Saad in [439] leads to a very efficient numerical scheme for the problems at hand.*

Furthermore, the introduction of mesh adaptive techniques would be an extremely useful goal useful goal to approximate accurately the mass transfer from the blood to the arterial walls. Some preliminary applications of anisotropic mesh adaptivity techniques to these problems have been presented in [161].

7.4 Numerical results and discussion

In this section we apply the models and methods developped so far to two study cases. To this aim we apply a common paradigm. First of all we introduce the geometrical model and then we discuss the lumeanl and transmural transport processes. In the first study we will analyse the effect of disturbed flow patterns (flow separation, stagnation and recirculation) inside an axisymetric stenosed artery, while in the second case we consider a realistic 3D bifurcation. These results are discussed with further details in [395].

In the case of the stenosed axisymetric arterial segment we will focus our attention on the influence of local flow recirculation and separation downstream the stenosis on the LDL transport. Additionally the impact of the different wall models (fluid-wall model and multilayer model) on the concentration distribution inside the wall will be addressed. Due to the low diffusivity of the substances of interest (LDL) the lumenal transport is highly convection dominated and therefore strongly influenced by the flow patterns. The water-permeable nature of the arterial wall and the related transmural plasma filtration determine a local accumulation of LDL at the blood/wall interface.

In the case of the realistic human carotid bifurcation geometry only the fluid-wall model is applied to simulate the coupled lumenal and transmural transport process. In this case the influence of the resulting complex inplane flow patterns on the LDL transport will be discussed.

In both cases the blood flow in the arterial lumen has a mean velocity of $U_0 = 15.7\,\text{cm/s}$, the reference length (lumenal inflow diameter) is $L_0 = 0.67\,\text{cm}$. Blood is modelled as Newtonian fluid with the apparent viscosity $\mu = 0.035$ Poise and the constant fluid density $\rho = 1.05\,\text{g/cm}^3$ leading to a Reynolds number $Re = 300$. The viscosity of plasma in the arterial wall is $\mu_p = 0.7210^{-2}\,\text{cm}^2/\text{s}$ and a constant pressure drop of $p_l - p_{adv} = 70\,\text{mmHg}$ across the arterial wall is assumed. The studies only focus on the stationary flow because in the case of macromolecules (LDL) and constant transport parameters of the wall layers the influence of pulsatility on the LDL distribution is very small.

7.4.1 LDL transport in a stenosed axisymetric artery

Geometrical model

The influence of flow separation onto the LDL transport processes is analysed in a simplified geometrical model of an axisymetric stenosed arterial segment (Fig. 7.6). The computational domain has a total length of $70L_0$, where L_0 is the arterial diameter. The length of the stenotic region is $1.5L_0$. The upstream and downstream lengths with respect to the stenotic region are $18.75L_0$ and $49.75L_0$, respectively. The minimal section is equal to the 25 % of the inflow one. The thickness of the arterial wall in the fluid-wall model and of the media in the multilayer model is 200 µm ($0.03L_0$). The thickness of the intima in the multilayer wall case is 10 µm ($0.0015L_0$). The wall thickness is uniform along the artery.

The finite element meshes consist of 50082 velocity/pressure elements for the lumen, 14730 velocity/pressure elements for the wall (media) and additionally 4910 velocity/pressure elements for the discretisation of the intima in the multilayer model. For the calculation of the concentration field each velocity/pressure element was subdivided into 16 concentration elements resulting in 801312 elements in the lumen, 235680 elements in the wall (media) and 78560 concentration elements in the intima.

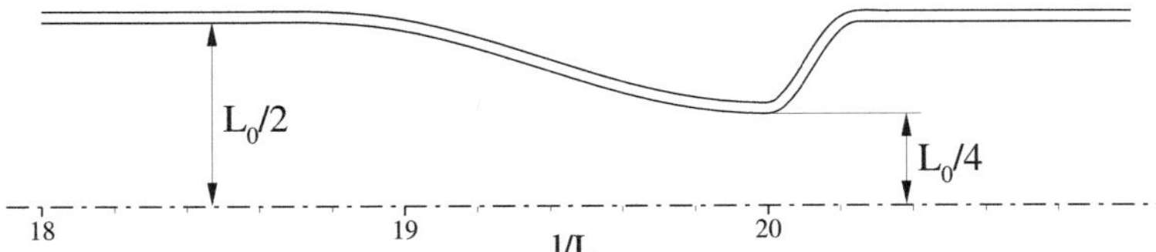

Fig. 7.6. Geometrical model of the stenosed tube

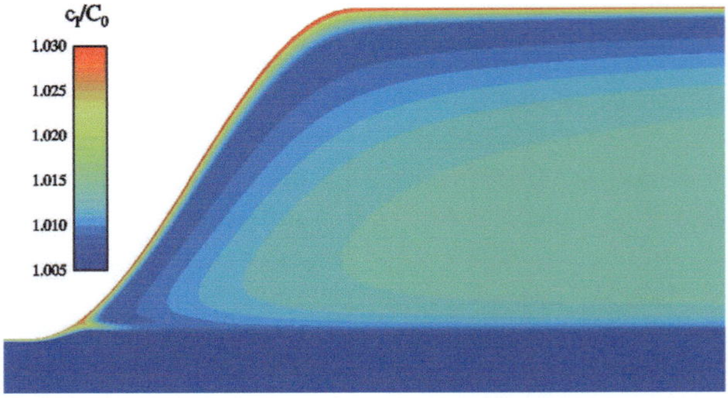

Fig. 7.7. Concentration contours near the stenosis

Lumenal LDL distribution

The development of lumenal surface concentration and the effect of flow separation on the local mass transfer to and into the wall in the downstream region of the stenosis is demonstrated in Fig. 7.7. The figure shows LDL accumulation near the tube wall. The equilibrium concentration at the fluid-endothelium boundary is higher than the concentration in the bulk stream. This polarisation effect at the surface occurs due to the plasma-permeability of the wall. The figure displays the steep concentration gradient across the separating streamline and a concentration increase of about one percent in the separation region compared to the bulk concentration. At the wall region directly downstream the stenosis a decrease of surface concentration polarisation can be observed.

The results of the mass transport study support the conclusion that the filtration process at the wall causes a lumenal surface concentration of LDL which is a dominant effect of mass transport processes including plasma-permeable walls. Flow separation downstream the axisymmetric stenosis influences the concentration boundary layer resulting in a decrease of surface concentration. The equilibrium concentration at the lumenal surface depends on the local convective transport near the surface in the lumen, on the filtration velocity of plasma into the wall and on the diffusive processes of the molecules.

Transmural transport processes

Fig. 7.8 shows the normal velocity contours in the media (panel a) and the velocity vectors in the media and in the intima (panel b) for the multilayer model in the expanding region. The magnitude of the normal velocity is uniform and mainly determined by the pressure gradient across the arterial wall. However, small but non negligible velocity gradients can be related to the geometrical shape of the arterial wall. More precisely, due to the convex curvature at $l/L_0 = 20$ we observe a decreasing cross-sectional area in radial direction. As a result of that, the wall velocity increases at the outer region of the arterial

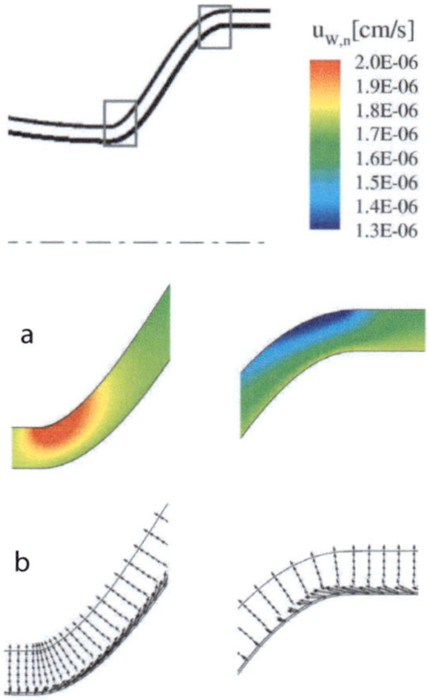

Fig. 7.8. Normal velocity contours in the media (panel a) and the velocity vectors in the media and in the intima (panel b) for the multilayer wall model in the expanding region

wall. On the other hand, because of the concave wall shape at $l/L_0 = 20.25$, the increasing cross-sectional area causes a decreasing wall velocity in radial direction. However, we observe that the normal velocity at the endothelium is only slightly affected by these geometrical properties and its value is about $J_v = 1.76 \cdot 10^{-6}$ cm/s in the expansion region, in very good agreement with the available measurements. The multilayer model also provides the flow field in the intima. The pressure drop across this layer is very low compared to the pressure drop across the whole arterial wall, while we observe high pressure gradients in the expanding region of the lumen. As a result of this, a high axial wall velocity occurs within the intima (Fig. 7.8 panel b). On the other hand, in the media the dominating driving force is the pressure gradient in the normal direction and consequently the axial flow is of minor importance.

These irregularities in the flow field across the arterial wall influence the concentration distribution within the wall. Figure 7.9 display the concentration contours in the wall of the two different wall models at selected locations in the expanding region of the stenosis. We observe that the perturbations in the velocity field in the intima and the media affect the concentrations as well. For example in the media, the concentration in the region of high filtration velocities is slightly higher than the average value, while it is lower than the average in correspondence of low filtration velocities. This is also clearly put into evidence by Fig. 7.10 that provides a quantitative comparison of the profiles of c_l, c_m^+, c_m and c_m^- plotted along the axial coordinate.

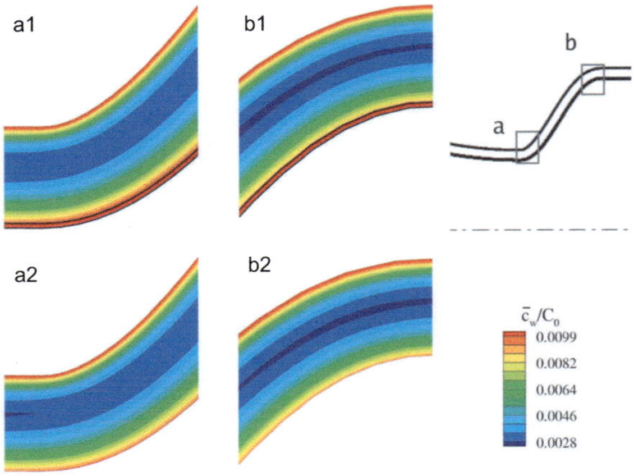

Fig. 7.9. Concentration contours provided by the fluid-wall model (bottom) and the multilayer model (top). In the latter case, the presence of the intima is put into evidence

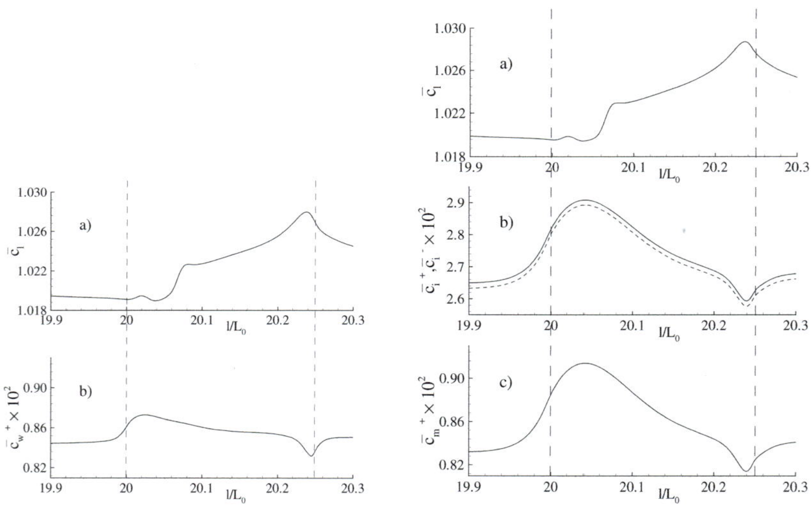

Fig. 7.10. Concentration values at the lumen-membrane boundary (panel a, left), the membrane-wall boundary (panel b, left) provided by the fluid-wall model. Concentration values at the lumen-endothelium boundary (panel a, right), the endothelium-intima boundary ((panel b, right), solid line), the intima-IEL boundary ((panel b, right), dashed line), the IEL-media boundary (panel c, right) computed with the multilayer model.

Focusing on Fig. 7.10 it can be seen that the lumenal concentration at the arterial wall is neither influenced by the concentration field in the arterial wall nor by the different wall models. The concentration polarisation mainly depends on the velocity field in the lumen. In particular, the polarisation effect is negligible where the blood flow is attached to the wall and the axial component is dominating. On the other hand, the filtration velocity normal to the wall surface sensibly influence the concentration field in the regions of blood recirculation where the axial flow next to the wall is highly reduced. Indeed, the maximal polarisation occurs at the expanding region of the stenosis where the recirculation zone has the largest extent (Fig. 7.10 panel a, left, and panel a, right). The behaviour of the wall concentration of the fluid-wall model (Fig 7.10 panel b, left) is qualitatively similar to the one observed with the multilayer model. However, the results provided by the two models differ from the quantitative point of view. We analyse the total variation of concentration reported for both the fluid-wall model and the multilayer model in Fig. 7.10 (on the left and on the right, respectively). We observe that for the fluid-wall model the increase in the concentration level due to the bending of the arterial wall results in about $0.26 \cdot 10^{-3}$ that corresponds to $3\,\%$ of the average concentration value on the membrane-wall interface. Conversely, for the multilayer model we obtain a similar profile but the increase in concentration in correspondence of the geometrical perturbation is equivalent to $0.8 \cdot 10^{-3}$, namely $9.5\,\%$ of the average concentration value. Consequently, we point out that the two models react very differently to the geometrical perturbation represented by the bending of the arterial wall. Indeed the ratio of the aforementioned figures is of order 3. The larger variations in the multilayer wall model can be explained by the additional presence of plasma filtration with high axial components in the intima, that can not be captured by the simpler fluid-wall model. In this examination the variations of concentration in the wall layers are within a few percent, but this values might change under different conditions (e.g. a damaged endothelium). Moreover, the peak in the multilayer case is located downstream with respect to the fluid-wall case. This could be explained by observing that in the multilayer model the axial velocity in the intima transports and accumulates molecules in the centre of the expansion region (identified by $20 < x/L_0 < 20.2$, see Fig. 7.8).

7.4.2 LDL transport in realistic model of a 3D carotid artery bifurcation

Geometrical model

An anatomically realistic computational model of a human carotid artery bifurcation has been developed by K. Perktold and his research group at the Graz University of Technology on the basis of an experimental lumenal cast prepared and digitalised by D. Liepsch, FH Munich, see [250,379]. To develop the computational model surface measured surface data were smoothed using

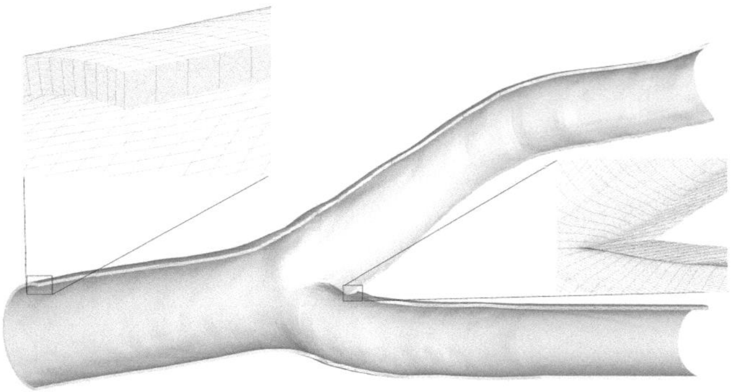

Fig. 7.11. Anatomically realistic computational model surface of the human carotid artery bifurcation

weighted least squares B-splines. This surface corresponds to the lumen/wall interface of the geometrical model. The arterial wall was created by the extension of the this surface in normal direction. A constant wall thickness of 200 μm (beside the region of the flow divider tip) was assumed (Fig. 7.11).

The finite element grid of the arterial lumen was generated applying a mesh generator based on local optimisation of geometric properties such as smoothness and orthogonality of the grid [380]. The finite element discretisation of the arterial wall was created by the extension of the lumenal grid at the lumen/wall surface in normal direction. The discretisation employs eight node isoparametric brick elements with tri-quadratic velocity and tri-linear pressure approximation. The subdivision yields 49 536 brick elements for the arterial lumen (resulting in 420 081 nodes for each velocity component and 55 601 nodes for the pressure) and 76 272 brick elements for the arterial wall (resulting in 656 265 nodes for each velocity component and 87 832 nodes for the pressure). For the solution of the mass transport problem each velocity element is subdivided into 32 subelements. The approximation of the transport problem applies tri-linear interpolation functions for the concentration resulting in 1 675 857 concentration nodes in the lumen and 2 537 587 concentration nodes in the arterial wall.

Lumenal transport processes

To illustrate the influence of the arterial geometry on the lumenal convective transport and the correlated LDL concentration distribution near the wall, Fig. 7.12 displays the wall shear stress and the concentration distribution at the interface lumen/membrane. The graphic demonstrates an accumulation of macromolecules at the lumen side of the membrane (Fig. 7.12 panel b). It is most pronounced in regions of low flow (indicated by low shear stress) occurring in the bifurcation region. At the flow divider walls of the bifurcation (high shear region) no accumulation of macromolecules occurs.

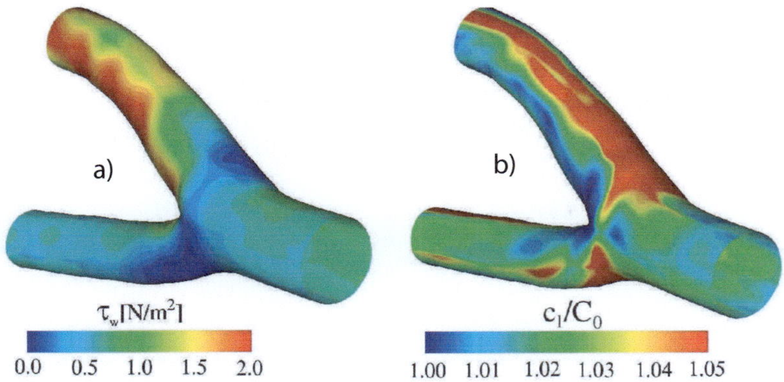

Fig. 7.12. Wall shear contours (panel a) and LDL concentration distribution (panel b) at the lumen-membrane interface

Fig. 7.13 displays the lumenal LDL concentration distribution and the inplane velocity component at different cross-sections in and downstream the bifurcation region. Downstream near the bifurcation (cross-section B), two symmetric vortices occur. This typical Dean flow is superposed further downstream by secondary motion caused by the nonplanarities of the vessel. It can be seen that at the sites of stagnating inplane motion at the outer wall of the vessel high polarisation occurs also downstream the bifurcation (level B,C and D). This points out a strong correlation between concentration polarisation and inplane motion. Indeed the inplane motion can be interpreted as additional convective effect which transports the accumulated macromolecules back to the bulk flow and reduces the polarisation of LDL near the arterial wall.

Transmural transport processes

The plasma flow field at the interface membrane/wall is shown in Fig. 7.14. Due to the high pressure gradient across the wall (70 mmHg) the velocity field vectors are mainly oriented in normal direction (Fig. 7.14 panel a). The low pressure drop along the vessel segment results in a small axial component of the plasma field in the range of 10^{-8} cm/s. This axial component is about 100 times lower than the average value of the filtration velocity in normal direction of 1.7610^{-6} cm/s. A 0.7 % variation of the filtration velocity occurs due to the non-constant pressure distribution at the lumenal side that results from the superposition of hydrostatic and hydrodynamic pressure (Fig. 7.14 panel b).

Figure 7.15 shows the concentration profile across the wall at selected points. The small variations of the plasma velocity field and the constant transport parameters of the wall layers result in a relatively uniform concentration distribution of LDL in the arterial wall. The typically U-shaped

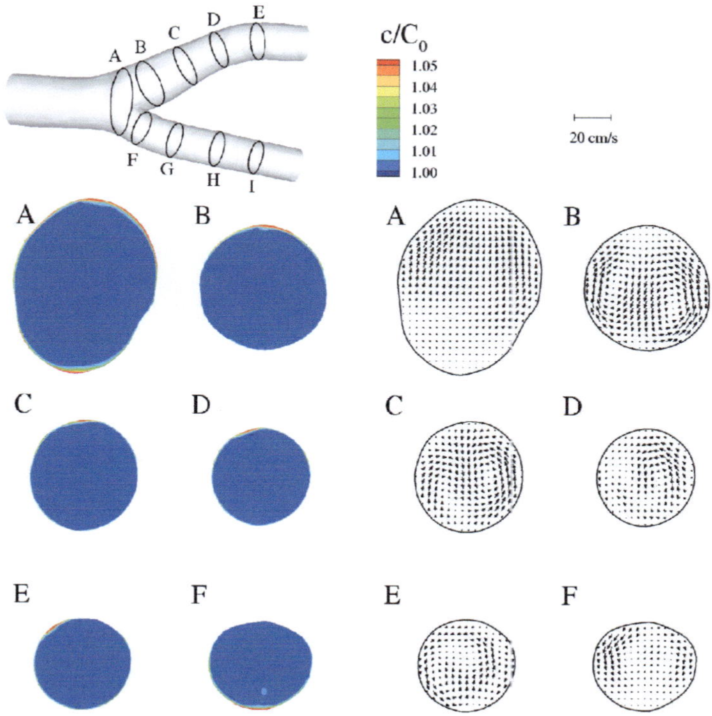

Fig. 7.13. Concentration contours of the LDL distribution and inplane motion in the arterial lumen at selected cross-sections in and downstream the bifurcation region

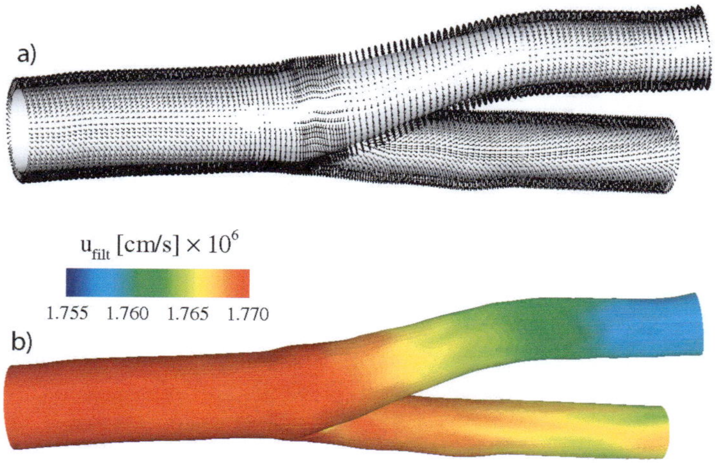

Fig. 7.14. Plasma filtration velocity field in the arterial wall at the interface membrane-wall, represented by means of vectors (a) and magnitude contours (b)

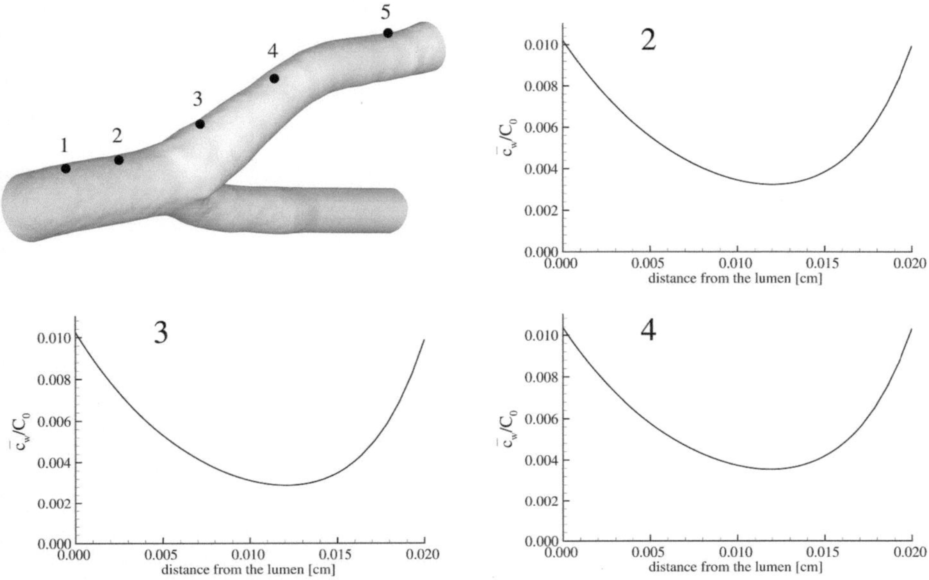

Fig. 7.15. Concentration profiles of the LDL-distribution at selected locations through the arterial wall

profiles are in good agreement with measured data of [49], [326] and suggest that the estimation method proposed in [397] provide suitable values of the transport parameters of the wall. Only small variation of LDL concentration at the membrane/wall side occurs due to the increased convective and diffusive transport in regions of high polarisation (point 3). This variation is small compared to the changes of concentration in normal direction caused by reaction of LDL with the wall tissue.

7.4.3 Numerical simulations of drug release from stents

A novel application of the mathematical models of mass transfer in the vascular walls is promoted by the introduction of drug eluting stents for the treatment of stenotic coronary arteries. Drug eluting stents (DES) are apparently simple medical implanted devices used to restore blood flow perfusion into stenotic arteries. Such structures are coated with a micro-film containing a drug that is locally released into the arterial walls for healing purposes. However, the design of such devices is a very complex task, because their performance in widening the arterial lumen and preventing further restenosis is influenced by many factors such as the geometrical design of the stent, the mechanical properties of the material and the chemical properties of the drug that is released. All these topics are relevant for an effective stent design. In this framework, numerical simulation techniques play a relevant role in understanding what are the most appropriate choices for the optimal design of DES. These topics will be addressed in detail in Chapter 12.

7.5 Conclusions

In this chapter we have proposed a possible way to set up suitable mathematical models with the aim to study the transfer of molecules, such as oxygen, macromolecules or drugs, through the arterial walls. A few recipes for their numerical discretisation have been considered. By means of these tools, we have addressed several applications and discussed their results in order to put into evidence the role of mass transfer in the physiological functions of the vascular system.

8

Analysis of coupled models for fluid-structure interaction of internal flows

Yvon Maday

The modelling of the behaviour of blood flows in (large or small) arteries has to reflect two types of phenomenon that coexist: the blood flow – with any suitable model to represent its behaviour – and the artery wall displacement – with or without the tissues or muscles that surround the wall. This feature relative to the coupling of different phenomena is a new one as regards the mathematical analysis of the system of equations involved in the model and it is present independently of the complexity and the accuracy of the models chosen to represent each individual phenomenon. In addition to the theory required for analyzing each individual model, the analysis of the coupling or interaction raises new and specific difficulties. Mathematically speaking, the resulting equations are nonlinear, firstly because any realistic model for the fluid is nonlinear (cf. equation (2.1)), but also because the interaction involves a nonlinearity in addition to any anterior nonlinearity of the primitive independent model.

This chapter aims to shed some light on the mathematical tools that have been adapted or originally proposed to understand if the equations stemming from the model designer provide a mathematically well posed problem. There are many reasons to justify this type of analysis, not including the fact that from the beginning this subject has provided more than 20 research papers, most of them in good journals (some of them being referred to in this chapter). But the main reason is that the various numerical problems that appear at the discretisation level for the simulation of such strongly coupled problems are better hinted at and even sometimes better understood from the theoretical analysis synthesised in this chapter. Another side effect is to guide the intuition on what should be modified if one wants to change the fluid model or the structure model at the level of the interface where the exchange of information takes place.

In this contribution we consider mainly the case where either the whole external fluid boundary is composed of an elastic structure or only part of it is and the remaining part is solid or fixed. This means that we shall not integrate in this chapter the many contributions dealing with the interaction

Formaggia L, Quarteroni A, Veneziani A (Eds.): Cardiovascular Mathematics. Modeling and simulation of the circulatory system

of elastic structure floating within a fluid flow itself placed in a rigid container since this is outside the scope of this book dealing with flow in elastic vessels.

8.1 A simplified model with half of the interaction

The first model we consider dates from almost 40 years ago and can be found in a book by Jacques-Louis Lions [291]. It takes only one aspect of the interaction into account since both the interface and the fluid domain are assumed to be fixed. This simplifies the analysis quite a lot, but it is still not immediate. This model could represent the fluid structure interaction in the case where the motion of the interface is neglected. The following analysis is directly extracted from [291] and serves as an introduction to the methods that will be used later in the context of the full interaction problem.

8.1.1 A transmission parabolic-hyperbolic problem

Two domains of $\mathbb{R}^n$ are involved: Ω_f where the fluid flows and Ω^s representing the elastic envelop as described in Fig. 8.1.

Here we do not indicate the time dependency or the "*hat*" of the reference configuration, since, in this model, these domains are fixed. The transmission problem involves a velocity $\boldsymbol{u}_f = (u_1, u_2, u_3)$ and a pressure P defined over $\Omega_f \times (0,T)$ such that

$$\frac{\partial \boldsymbol{u}_f}{\partial t} - 2\mathbf{div}(\nu \boldsymbol{D}\boldsymbol{u}_f) + (\boldsymbol{u} \cdot \boldsymbol{\nabla})\boldsymbol{u}_f + \nabla P = \boldsymbol{f}, \quad \text{in } \Omega_f \times (0,T) \tag{8.1}$$

$$\mathbf{div}\boldsymbol{u}_f = 0, \quad \text{in } \Omega_f \times (0,T), \tag{8.2}$$

and a displacement $\boldsymbol{\eta}$ over $\Omega_s \times (0,T)$ such that

$$\frac{\partial^2 \boldsymbol{\eta}}{\partial t^2} - \Delta \boldsymbol{\eta} = g, \quad \text{in } \Omega_s \times (0,T). \tag{8.3}$$

Equations (8.1) and (8.2) are the Navier-Stokes equations already derived in Chapter 3 (see (3.42)) that we report here for the reader's convenience.

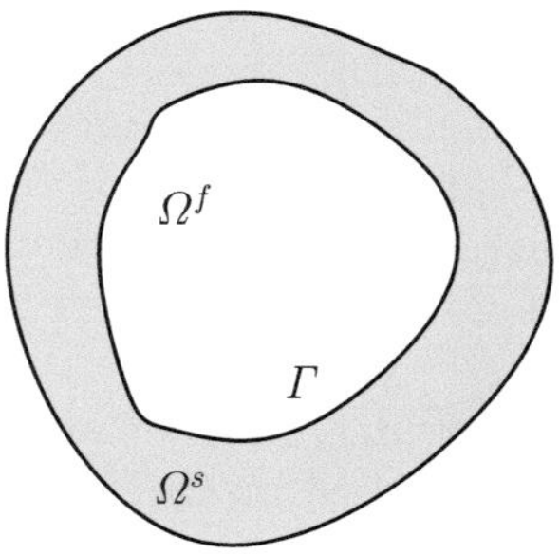

Fig. 8.1. The two domains for fluid-structure transmission

These equations are complemented with the transmission conditions over the interface $\varGamma$ between $\varOmega_f$ and $\varOmega_s$, namely

$$\boldsymbol{u}_f = \frac{\partial \boldsymbol{\eta}}{\partial t}, \qquad \text{over } \varGamma \times (0,T), \tag{8.4}$$

and

$$2\nu \boldsymbol{D}\boldsymbol{u}_f.\boldsymbol{n} - P\boldsymbol{n} - \frac{1}{2}\Big(\sum_{j=1}^{n} u_j \cos n_j\Big)\boldsymbol{u}_f = \frac{\partial \boldsymbol{\eta}}{\partial \boldsymbol{n}}, \qquad \text{over } \varGamma \times (0,T), \tag{8.5}$$

together with the boundary condition over the remaining boundary of $\varOmega^s$

$$\boldsymbol{\eta} = 0, \qquad \text{over } [\partial\varOmega^s \setminus \varGamma] \times (0,T), \tag{8.6}$$

and the initial conditions

$$\begin{aligned} \boldsymbol{u}_f(0) &= \boldsymbol{u}_{f\,0} & & \text{over } \varOmega_f, \\ \boldsymbol{\eta}(0) &= \boldsymbol{\eta}_0, \qquad \tfrac{\partial \boldsymbol{\eta}}{\partial t}(0) = \boldsymbol{\eta}_1 & & \text{over } \varOmega_s. \end{aligned} \tag{8.7}$$

It should be noted that the interface between the fluid and the structure does not follow the motion of the structure represented by $\boldsymbol{\eta}$; this represents a major simplification but corresponds fairly well to situations where the displacements we expect are very small and are thus neglected in the modelling of the fluid behaviour. Note that this simplification imposes that in (8.5) a nonlinear contribution needs to be added to the normal stress equilibrium (see Section 8.2.3 for a further comment in the full interaction case). In spite of this simplification, the coupling is still a strong one since neither the fluid flow nor the elastic displacement can be evaluated without considering the other. In what follows, we shall present the mathematical analysis of this problem resulting in the following theorem

Theorem 8.1. *There exists a solution $(\boldsymbol{u}_f, P, \boldsymbol{\eta})$ to the transmission problem. Moreover, this solution is unique in the two-dimensional case.*

8.1.2 Frame setting for the analysis of the transmission problem

The analysis starts by introducing the structure velocity $\varPhi = \frac{\partial \eta}{\partial t}$ which, from (8.3), satisfies

$$\frac{\partial \varPhi}{\partial t} - \Delta\Big(\int_0^t \varPhi(s)ds\Big) = g + \Delta\boldsymbol{\eta}_0, \quad \in \varOmega_s. \tag{8.8}$$

Then we formulate the problem in an equivalent variational setting. Let us first define the two spaces V_f and V_s as follows

$$\begin{aligned} V_f &= \{\boldsymbol{v}_f | \boldsymbol{v}_f \in [H^1(\varOmega_f)]^n, \operatorname{div} \boldsymbol{v}_f = 0\}, \\ V_s &= \{\varphi | \varphi \in [H^1(\varOmega^s)]^n, \varphi = 0 \text{ over } \partial\varOmega_s\}. \end{aligned} \tag{8.9}$$

Then, for any Banach space Z, and any real number p, $p \in [0, \infty]$, we define the functional space $L^p(0,T;Z)$ as follows

$$L^p(0,T;Z) = \{f | f : [0,T] \to Z \text{ measurable },\\ \int_0^T \|f\|_Z^p < \infty, \text{ if } p < \infty,\\ \sup_{t\in[0,T]} \|f(t)\|_Z < \infty, \text{ if } p = \infty,$$

The variational problem is: find $(\boldsymbol{u}_f, \Phi)$ with

$$\boldsymbol{u}_f \in L^2(0,T;V_f) \cap L^\infty(0,T;[L^2(\Omega_f)]^n),\\ \Phi \in L^\infty(0,T;[L^2(\Omega^s)]^n), \int_0^t \Phi(s)ds \in L^\infty(0,T;V_s),\\ \boldsymbol{u}_f = \Phi \text{ over } \Gamma \times (0,T),$$

such that, $\forall \boldsymbol{v}_f \in V_F, \forall \varphi \in V_s$, with $\boldsymbol{v}_f = \varphi$ over Γ,

$$\int_{\Omega_f} \frac{\partial \boldsymbol{u}_f}{\partial t} \boldsymbol{v}_f d\boldsymbol{x} + \int_{\Omega^s} \frac{\partial \Phi}{\partial t} \varphi d\boldsymbol{x} + \nu a_f(\boldsymbol{u}_f, \boldsymbol{v}_f) + a_s(\int_0^t \Phi(s)ds, \varphi)\\ + b_f(\boldsymbol{u}_f, \boldsymbol{u}_f; \boldsymbol{v}_f) - \frac{1}{2} \sum_{i,j=1}^n \int_\Gamma u_i u_j v_j \cos n_i d\gamma \qquad (8.10)\\ = \int_{\Omega_f} f \boldsymbol{v}_f + \int_{\Omega^s} g\varphi + a_s(\boldsymbol{\eta}_0, \varphi).$$

where

$$a_f(\boldsymbol{u}_f, \boldsymbol{v}_f) = 2 \int_{\Omega_f} \boldsymbol{D}\boldsymbol{u}_f : \boldsymbol{D}\boldsymbol{v}_f, \qquad (8.11)$$

$$b_f(\boldsymbol{u}_f, \boldsymbol{v}_f, \boldsymbol{w}_f) = \sum_{i,j=1}^n \int_{\Omega_f} u_i \frac{\partial v_j}{\partial x_i} w_j, \qquad (8.12)$$

$$a_s(\boldsymbol{u}_f, \boldsymbol{v}_f) = \sum_{i,j=1}^n \int_{\Omega^s} \frac{\partial u_i}{\partial x_j} \frac{\partial v_i}{\partial x_j}. \qquad (8.13)$$

These equations are complemented with the initial conditions (8.7).

In order to check the equivalence of the two formulations (the strong one: (8.1)–(8.7) and the weak one (8.10)), we first notice that the direction strong $\to$ weak is obvious by integration by parts. Then, assuming that (8.10) holds, we choose in (8.10) $\boldsymbol{v}_f$ with compact support into Ω_f together with $\varphi = 0$, which leads to equation (8.1) in the sense of distributions. Then we choose in (8.10) φ with compact support into Ω^s together with $\boldsymbol{v}_f = \boldsymbol{0}$ and we get equation (8.8) again in the sense of the distributions. Multiplying now the two equations (8.1) and (8.8) that we have just derived by $\boldsymbol{v}_f$ and φ, integrating and taking into account that $\boldsymbol{v}_f = \varphi$ over Γ, we get $\forall \boldsymbol{v}_f \in V_F, \forall \varphi \in V_s$

$$\int_{\Omega_f} \frac{\partial \boldsymbol{u}_f}{\partial t} \boldsymbol{v}_f d\boldsymbol{x} + \int_{\Omega^s} \frac{\partial \Phi}{\partial t} \varphi d\boldsymbol{x} + \nu a_f(\boldsymbol{u}_f, \boldsymbol{v}_f) + a_s(\int_0^t \Phi(s) ds, \varphi)$$
$$+ b_f(\boldsymbol{u}_f, \boldsymbol{u}_f; \boldsymbol{v}_f) + \int_\Gamma \Big(-2\nu \boldsymbol{D}\boldsymbol{u}_f.\boldsymbol{n} + P\boldsymbol{n} + \frac{\partial}{\partial \boldsymbol{n}} (\int_0^t \Phi(s) ds) \Big) \boldsymbol{v}_f d\Gamma$$
$$= \int_{\Omega_f} f \boldsymbol{v}_f + \int_{\Omega^s} g\varphi + a_s(\boldsymbol{\eta}_0, \varphi) - \int_\Gamma \frac{\partial \boldsymbol{\eta}_0}{\partial \boldsymbol{n}} \varphi d\Gamma,$$

so that recalling (8.10), we derive $\forall \boldsymbol{v}_f \in V_F$

$$\int_\Gamma \Big(-2\nu \boldsymbol{D}\boldsymbol{u}_f.\boldsymbol{n} + P\boldsymbol{n} + \frac{\partial}{\partial \boldsymbol{n}} (\int_0^t \Phi(s) ds + \boldsymbol{\eta}_0) + \frac{1}{2} (\sum_{j=1}^n u_j . \cos n_j) \boldsymbol{u}_f \Big) \boldsymbol{v}_f d\Gamma = 0 \tag{8.14}$$

Since $\operatorname{div} \boldsymbol{v}_f = 0$, we notice $\int_\gamma \boldsymbol{v}_f.\boldsymbol{n} d\gamma = 0$, and reciprocally, to any $\boldsymbol{v}_{f*} \in (H^{1/2}(\Gamma))^n$ with $\int_\gamma \boldsymbol{v}_{f*}.\boldsymbol{n} d\gamma = 0$ we can associate a $\boldsymbol{v}_f \in V_f$ with $\boldsymbol{v}_{f|\Gamma} = \boldsymbol{v}_{f*}$, hence (8.14) is equivalent to (we refer to [294] for the introduction of the trace space $H^{1/2}(\Gamma)$))

$$-2\nu \boldsymbol{D}\boldsymbol{u}_f.\boldsymbol{n} + P\boldsymbol{n} + \frac{\partial}{\partial \boldsymbol{n}} (\int_0^t \Phi(s) ds + \boldsymbol{\eta}_0) + \frac{1}{2} (\sum_{j=1}^n u_j . \cos n_j) \boldsymbol{u}_f = \lambda \boldsymbol{n},$$

with $\lambda \in \mathbb{R}$. Finally, by changing P into $P - \lambda$ we get (8.5).

8.1.3 Analysis of the transmission problem

Approximated solutions

We turn now to the proof of Theorem 8.1. The classical tool that will be introduced here and used over and over in the following sections is known as the Faedo Galerkin method where, by restricting the trial and test functional spaces to a sequence of finite dimensional subspaces, we define a series of systems of differential equations for which the existence of a discrete solution follows from Cauchy Lipschitz's theorem. Different *a priori* estimates are then derived and provide uniform bounds on the sequences of solutions. This is the corner stone of the proof, as it allows us to state that there exists a subsequence of discrete solutions that converges to a solution of (8.10) when the dimension of the finite dimensional subspaces tends to infinity.

To be more precise, let us introduce a "special basis" of eigenfunctions for the following space

$$W^\sigma = \{\boldsymbol{v} | \boldsymbol{v} \in (H_0^\sigma(\Omega))^n, \Omega = \overline{\Omega}_f \cup \Omega^s, \operatorname{div} \boldsymbol{v} = 0 \text{ over } \Omega_f\}$$

with $\sigma = n/2$ and scalar product $(.,.)_\sigma$. These are solutions of the following problem

$$(\boldsymbol{w}_j, \boldsymbol{v})_{W^\sigma} = \lambda_j(\boldsymbol{w}_j, \boldsymbol{v}) = \lambda_j \int_\Omega \boldsymbol{w}_j \boldsymbol{v} d\boldsymbol{x}, \tag{8.15}$$

where $(.,.)_{W^\sigma}$ is any preferred choice of scalar product over W^σ. This spectral problem possesses a sequence of eigensolutions corresponding to an increasing sequence of positive eigenvalues λ_i; they constitute a complete set of orthogonal functions in both $L^2(\Omega)$ and W^σ. With these eigenfunctions, we define the basis $(\boldsymbol{v}_j, \varphi_j)_j$ with $\boldsymbol{v}_j = \boldsymbol{w}_{j|\Omega_f}$ and $\varphi_j = \boldsymbol{w}_{j|\Omega^s}$ and we introduce, for any positive integer N, the discrete subspaces of $V_f \times V_s$

$$X_N = \operatorname{span}\{(\boldsymbol{v}_j, \varphi_j), j = 1, \ldots, N\},$$

and, for any m, we then define the discrete solutions $(\boldsymbol{u}_{f_m}, \Phi_m) \in X_m$ of

$$\begin{aligned}
&\int_{\Omega_f} \frac{\partial \boldsymbol{u}_{f_m}}{\partial t} \boldsymbol{v}_f d\boldsymbol{x} + \int_{\Omega^s} \frac{\partial \Phi_m}{\partial t} \varphi d\boldsymbol{x} + \nu a_f(\boldsymbol{u}_{f_m}, \boldsymbol{v}_f) + a_s\Big(\int_0^t \Phi_m(s) ds, \varphi\Big) \\
&\quad + b_f(\boldsymbol{u}_{f_m}, \boldsymbol{u}_{f_m}; \boldsymbol{v}_f) - \frac{1}{2} \sum_{i,j=1}^n \int_\Gamma u_{m,i} u_{m,j} v_{m,j} \cos n_i d\gamma \qquad (8.16)\\
&= \int_{\Omega_f} f \boldsymbol{v}_f + \int_{\Omega^s} g\varphi + a_s(\boldsymbol{\eta}_0, \varphi), \quad \forall (\boldsymbol{v}_f, \varphi) \in X_m
\end{aligned}$$

supplemented again with the initial conditions

$$\boldsymbol{u}_{f_m}(0) = \boldsymbol{u}_{m0} \to \boldsymbol{u}_0 \text{ and } \Phi_m(0) = \boldsymbol{\eta}_{1m} \to \boldsymbol{\eta}_1 \text{ when } m \to \infty,$$

these last convergences being in the L^2 sense.

By choosing alternatively $(\boldsymbol{v}_f, \varphi) = (\boldsymbol{v}_j, \varphi_j), j = 1, \ldots, m$, the previous set of equations yields a system of nonlinear differential equations in the components $g_{jm}(t)$ with $(\boldsymbol{u}_{f_m}, \Phi_m) = \sum_{j=1}^m g_{jm}(t)(\boldsymbol{v}_j, \varphi_j)$, which possesses a unique solution at least over a time interval $(0, t_m)$, for a suitable time t_m depending on m.

Derivation of *a priori* estimates

We choose now $(\boldsymbol{v}_f, \varphi) = (\boldsymbol{u}_{f_m}, \Phi_m)$ in (8.16) which yields

$$\begin{aligned}
&\frac{\partial}{\partial t} \int_{\Omega_f} |\boldsymbol{u}_{f_m}(.,t)|^2 d\boldsymbol{x} + \frac{\partial}{\partial t} \int_{\Omega^s} |\Phi_m(.,t)|^2 d\boldsymbol{x} + 2\nu a_f(\boldsymbol{u}_{f_m}, \boldsymbol{u}_{f_m}) \\
&\quad + \frac{\partial}{\partial t} a_s\Big(\int_0^t \Phi_m(.,s) ds, \int_0^t \Phi_m(.,s) ds\Big) + 2b_f(\boldsymbol{u}_{f_m}, \boldsymbol{u}_{f_m}; \boldsymbol{u}_{f_m}) \qquad (8.17)\\
&\quad - \sum_{i,j=1}^n \int_\Gamma u_{m,i} u_{m,j}^2 \cos n_i d\gamma = 2 \int_{\Omega_f} f \boldsymbol{u}_{f_m} + 2 \int_{\Omega^s} g \Phi_m + 2a_s(\boldsymbol{\eta}_0, \Phi_m).
\end{aligned}$$

Since $\boldsymbol{u}_f$ is divergence free, using integration by parts gives

$$2b_f(\boldsymbol{u}_{f_m}, \boldsymbol{u}_{f_m}; \boldsymbol{u}_{f_m}) = \sum_{i,j=1}^{n} \int_{\Gamma} u_{m,i} u_{m,j}^2 \cos n_i d\gamma.$$

Hence from applying the Cauchy Schwarz inequality to the right-hand side of (8.17) we deduce

$$\begin{aligned} &\frac{\partial}{\partial t} \int_{\Omega_f} |\boldsymbol{u}_{f_m}(.,t)|^2 d\boldsymbol{x} + \frac{\partial}{\partial t} \int_{\Omega^s} |\Phi_m(.,t)|^2 d\boldsymbol{x} + \nu a_f(\boldsymbol{u}_{f_m}, \boldsymbol{u}_{f_m}) \\ &+ \frac{\partial}{\partial t} a_s\left(\int_0^t \Phi_m(.,s) ds, \int_0^t \Phi_m(.,s) ds \right) \\ &\leq C \left[\int_{\Omega_f} f^2 + \int_{\Omega^s} g^2 + a_s(\boldsymbol{\eta}_0, \boldsymbol{\eta}_0) \right]. \end{aligned} \tag{8.18}$$

Integrating in time, we first deduce that actually we can choose $t_m = T$ and moreover

$$\begin{aligned} \boldsymbol{u}_{f_m} &\text{ is a bounded sequence in } L^2(0,T;V_f) \cap L^\infty(0,T;(L^2(\Omega_f))^n), \\ \Phi_m &\text{ is a bounded sequence in } L^\infty(0,T;L^2(\Omega^s))^n), \\ \textstyle\int_0^t \Phi_m(.,s) ds &\text{ is a bounded sequence in } L^\infty(0,T;V^s). \end{aligned} \tag{8.19}$$

In order to be allowed to pass to the limit in the nonlinear term, we need further bounds for derivatives in time. Let P_m denote the projection operator from $L^2(\Omega)$ onto X_m. This operator is self-adjoint and bounded with norm equal to 1 in $L^2(\Omega)$ but also in W^σ due to the use of the special basis. It results, by transposition, that

$$\|P_m\|_{\mathcal{L}((W^\sigma)',(W^\sigma)')} \leq 1,$$

where $(W^\sigma)'$ is the dual space of W^σ. We now propose another way of writing (8.16) through operators:

$$\frac{\partial}{\partial t}(\boldsymbol{u}_{f_m}, \Phi_m) = -P_m[A(\boldsymbol{u}_{f_m}, \Phi_m)] - P_m[G(\boldsymbol{u}_{f_m}, \Phi_m)] - P_m[F] \tag{8.20}$$

where $\forall(\boldsymbol{v}_f, \varphi) \in W^\sigma$,

$$\begin{aligned} \langle A(\boldsymbol{u}_{f_m}, \Phi_m), (\boldsymbol{v}_f, \varphi)\rangle &= \nu a_f(\boldsymbol{u}_{f_m}, \boldsymbol{v}_f) + a_s\left(\int_0^t \Phi_m(s) ds, \varphi \right) \\ \langle G(\boldsymbol{u}_{f_m}, \Phi_m), (\boldsymbol{v}_f, \varphi)\rangle &= b_f(\boldsymbol{u}_{f_m}, \boldsymbol{u}_{f_m}; \boldsymbol{v}_f) \\ &\quad - \frac{1}{2} \sum_{i,j=1}^{n} \int_{\Gamma} u_{m,i} u_{m,j} v_j \cos n_i d\gamma \\ \langle F(\boldsymbol{v}_f, \varphi)\rangle &= \int_{\Omega_f} f \boldsymbol{v}_f + \int_{\Omega^s} g\varphi + a_s(\boldsymbol{\eta}_0, \varphi). \end{aligned} \tag{8.21}$$

It is straightforward to note that A is bounded in $\mathcal{L}(W^\sigma,(W^\sigma)')$, that F belongs to $(W^\sigma)'$ and the following lemma states that G is continuous from W^σ into $(W^\sigma)'$:

Lemma 8.1. *There exists a positive constant c such that for any $\boldsymbol{v}_f \in H^\sigma(\Omega_f)$*

$$|b_f(\boldsymbol{u}_{f\,m},\boldsymbol{u}_{f\,m};\boldsymbol{v}_f)| \leq c\|\boldsymbol{u}_{f\,m}\|^{1/2}_{L^2(\Omega_f)}\|\boldsymbol{u}_{f\,m}\|^{3/2}_{H^1(\Omega_f)}\|\boldsymbol{v}_f\|_{H^\sigma(\Omega_f)}$$

$$|\sum_{i,j=1}^{n}\int_\Gamma u_{m,i}u_{m,j}v_j\cos n_i d\gamma| \leq c\|\boldsymbol{u}_{f\,m}\|^{1/2}_{L^2(\Omega_f)}\|\boldsymbol{u}_{f\,m}\|^{3/2}_{H^1(\Omega_f)}\|\boldsymbol{v}_f\|_{H^\sigma(\Omega_f)}$$

that follows from the equality

$$\sum_{i,j=1}^{n}\int_\Gamma u_{m,i}u_{m,j}v_j\cos n_i d\gamma = b_f(\boldsymbol{u}_{f\,m},\boldsymbol{u}_{f\,m};\boldsymbol{v}_f) + b_f(\boldsymbol{u}_{f\,m},\boldsymbol{v}_f;\boldsymbol{u}_{f\,m})$$

and the bound

$$\|v\|^2_{L^4(\Omega_f)} \leq c\|v\|_{L^2(\Omega_f)}\|v\|_{H^1(\Omega_f)}$$

valid in 2D and

$$\|v\|^2_{L^3(\Omega_f)} \leq c\|v\|_{L^2(\Omega_f)}\|v\|_{H^1(\Omega_f)}$$

valid in 3D, together with the imbedding of $H^\sigma(\Omega_f)$ into any $L^p(\Omega_f)$ (choose $p=4$ if $n=2$ and $p=6$ if $n=3$). We deduce from (8.20), (8.21) and Lemma 8.1 that

$$\left(\frac{\partial \boldsymbol{u}_{f\,m}}{\partial t},\frac{\partial \Phi_m}{\partial t}\right) \text{ is a bounded sequence in } L^{4/3}(0,T;(W^\sigma)'). \tag{8.22}$$

Passing to the limit

From the boundedness of the sequences $(\boldsymbol{u}_{f\,m},\Phi_m)$ we know we can extract a subsequence (still indexed by m) that converges weakly

$$\begin{cases} \boldsymbol{u}_{f\,m} \rightharpoonup \boldsymbol{u}_f \text{ in } L^2(0,T;V_f)\cap L^\infty(0,T;(L^2(\Omega_f))^n), \\ \Phi_m \rightharpoonup \Phi \text{ in } L^\infty(0,T;L^2(\Omega^s))^n), \\ \int_0^t \Phi_m(.,s)ds \rightharpoonup \int_0^t \Phi(.,s)ds \text{ in } L^\infty(0,T;V^s) \\ \left(\frac{\partial \boldsymbol{u}_{f\,m}}{\partial t},\frac{\partial \Phi_m}{\partial t}\right) \rightharpoonup \left(\frac{\partial \boldsymbol{u}_f}{\partial t},\frac{\partial \Phi}{\partial t}\right) \text{ in } L^{4/3}(0,T;(W^\sigma)'). \end{cases} \tag{8.23}$$

These weak limits allow us already to pass to the limit in the linear terms, for any $(\boldsymbol{v}_f,\varphi)\in \cup_{n\in\mathbb{N}}X_n$,

$$\langle A((\boldsymbol{u}_{f\,m},\Phi_m),(\boldsymbol{v}_f,\varphi)\rangle \to \langle A((\boldsymbol{u}_f,\Phi),(\boldsymbol{v}_f,\varphi)\rangle$$

as $n \to \infty$, and

$$\int_{\Omega_f} \frac{\partial \boldsymbol{u}_{f_m}}{\partial t} \boldsymbol{v}_f d\boldsymbol{x} + \int_{\Omega^s} \frac{\partial \Phi_m}{\partial t} \varphi d\boldsymbol{x} \to \int_{\Omega_f} \frac{\partial \boldsymbol{u}_f}{\partial t} \boldsymbol{v}_f d\boldsymbol{x} + \int_{\Omega^s} \frac{\partial \Phi}{\partial t} \varphi d\boldsymbol{x}.$$

The remaining nonlinear terms require the fundamental lemma: let B_0, B and B_1 be three reflexive Banach spaces with

$$B_0 \hookrightarrow B \hookrightarrow B_1 \text{ with continuous imbeddings}$$
$$\text{the imbedding } B_0 \hookrightarrow B \text{ is compact.}$$

Let then

$$Z = \{v | v \in L^{p_0}(0,T;B_0), \quad \frac{\partial v}{\partial t} \in L^{p_1}(0,T;B_1) \tag{8.24}$$

with $1 < p_0, p_1 < \infty$. Then

Lemma 8.2. *Under the previous hypotheses, the imbedding of Z in $L^{p_0}(0,T;B)$ is compact.*

We now use this compactness theorem in the following situation : $p_i = 2$, $B_0 = V^f \times [L^2(\Omega^s)]^n$, $B_1 = (W^\sigma)'$ and we choose $B = \{\boldsymbol{v} \in [H^{1-\varepsilon}(\Omega_f)]^n$, $\operatorname{div} \boldsymbol{v} = 0\} \times [H^{-\varepsilon}(\Omega^s)]^n$ for $0 < \varepsilon < 1/2$. Let us remember (see e.g., [293]) that the imbedding $H^1(\Omega_f) \hookrightarrow H^{1-\varepsilon}(\Omega_f)$ is compact for any $\varepsilon > 0$ and so is the imbedding $L^2(\Omega^s) \hookrightarrow H^{-\varepsilon}(\Omega^s)$; thus there exists a convergent subsequence

$$\boldsymbol{u}_{f_\mu} \to \boldsymbol{u}_f, \quad \text{in } L^2(0,T;(H^{1-\varepsilon}(\Omega_f))^n), \tag{8.25}$$

where the convergence is strong. In addition, for any $\varepsilon < \frac{1}{2}$, the trace operator

$$\boldsymbol{v} \mapsto \boldsymbol{v}_{|\Gamma}$$

is continuous from $H^{1-\varepsilon}(\Omega_f) \to L^2(\Gamma)$, hence the convergence

$$\boldsymbol{u}_{f_{m|\Gamma}} \to \boldsymbol{u}_{f|\Gamma}, \quad \text{is strong in } L^2(0,T;(L^2(\Gamma))^n). \tag{8.26}$$

These two strong convergences allow us to prove that

$$\langle G((\boldsymbol{u}_{f_m}, \Phi_m), (\boldsymbol{v}_f, \varphi)\rangle \to \langle G((\boldsymbol{u}_f, \Phi), (\boldsymbol{v}_f, \varphi)\rangle, \tag{8.27}$$

which guarantees that the limit $(\boldsymbol{u}_f, \Phi)$ is a solution to this first transmission problem.

8.2 Some preliminary basic considerations on the full interaction system

One of the ingredients in the analysis of the interaction problem that has been illustrated in the previous section is the derivation of *a priori* estimates on the solution of the problem or on the solutions of its approximated versions. These estimates constitute the fundamental argument for the analysis of the coupled nonlinear problem since they allow bounds on the finite dimensional approximate solutions that lead to convergence in weak norms. This is the first step to pass to the limit in most of the linear terms of the problem. Then, combined with some further *a priori* estimates, compactness results allow us to claim the existence of the solution to the coupled problem. In this section we want to make clear the link between the model of the exchange of informations between the fluid and the structure and the derivation of some *a priori* estimates. This analysis is actually quite simple to derive in the general setting. Unfortunately the following steps are much more difficult to perform and currently the general analysis in this context is not complete.

8.2.1 A general setting of the problem

We denote by $\hat{\Omega}_s$ the reference configuration of a structure surrounding a fluid. For each time $t \in (0,T)$, we denote by $\Omega_f(t)$ the fluid domain delimited by the deformed elastic structure. The structure is modelled by the behaviour of the displacement $\boldsymbol{\eta}_s$ such that the structure at time t is the range of $\hat{\Omega}_s$ through deformation $\phi(t,.) = Id + \boldsymbol{\eta}_s(t,.)$. The outside boundary of $\hat{\Omega}_s$ is assumed to be fixed (just for the sake of simplicity); the inner boundary, denoted as $\hat{\Gamma}$, is assumed to constitute the boundary of the fluid domain. We are thus looking for the displacement $\boldsymbol{\eta}_s$ over $\hat{\Omega}_s$, a divergence-free velocity field $\boldsymbol{u}_f(t,.)$ and a pressure $P(t,.)$ defined over $\Omega_f(t)$ such that, in addition to (8.1), (8.2) valid with $\Omega_f = \Omega_f(t)$, we have the following interface conditions (see Section 3.5 of Chapter 3, with slight modifications of the notations since we choose here to state the interface conditions over $\hat{\Gamma}$)

$$\begin{aligned} \boldsymbol{u}_f(t,\phi(t,\hat{\boldsymbol{x}})) &= \frac{\partial \boldsymbol{\eta}_s}{\partial t}(t,\hat{\boldsymbol{x}}), & \forall \hat{\boldsymbol{x}} \in \hat{\Gamma} \\ \big[2\nu \boldsymbol{D}\boldsymbol{u}_f.\boldsymbol{n} - P\boldsymbol{n}\big](t,\phi(t,\hat{\boldsymbol{x}}))\frac{\partial \boldsymbol{\eta}_s}{\partial \hat{x}} &= \big[t_{elastic}(\boldsymbol{\eta}_s)\big](t,\hat{\boldsymbol{x}}), & \forall \hat{\boldsymbol{x}} \in \hat{\Gamma} \end{aligned} \tag{8.28}$$

where the traction vector $t_{elastic}(\boldsymbol{\eta}_s)$ is the normal stress to the structure, the expression of which varies according to the definition of the structural energy. For example, going back to the model

$$\hat{\rho}_{s,0}\frac{\partial^2 \boldsymbol{\eta}_s}{\partial t^2} - \mathbf{div}_{\hat{\boldsymbol{x}}}(\hat{\boldsymbol{F}}_s\hat{\boldsymbol{\Sigma}}) = 0 \quad \text{in } \hat{\Omega}_s \tag{8.29}$$

the traction would be equal to

$$t_{elastic}(\boldsymbol{\eta}_s)(t,\hat{\boldsymbol{x}}) = [\hat{\boldsymbol{F}}_s\hat{\boldsymbol{\Sigma}}](t,\hat{\boldsymbol{x}}).\hat{\boldsymbol{n}}(\hat{\boldsymbol{x}}), \tag{8.30}$$

where $\hat{\boldsymbol{n}}$ denotes the outside normal to $\hat{\Omega}_s$. These equations are then complemented with the necessary initial conditions on the displacement and the fluid velocity.

8.2.2 A basic set of *a priori* estimates

Assuming that this coupled problem possesses a solution, then, by multiplying equation (8.1) by $\boldsymbol{u}_f$, and integrating has formally over $\Omega_f(t)$ we get

$$\int_{\Omega_f(t)} \frac{\partial \boldsymbol{u}_f}{\partial t}\boldsymbol{u}_f - \int_{\Omega_f(t)} [2\mathbf{div}(\nu \boldsymbol{D}\boldsymbol{u}_f) + (\boldsymbol{u}\cdot\boldsymbol{\nabla})\boldsymbol{u}_f + \nabla P]\boldsymbol{u}_f = \int_{\Omega_f(t)} \boldsymbol{f}\boldsymbol{u}_f. \tag{8.31}$$

Integrating by parts in the fourth term, with (8.2) yields

$$\int_{\Omega_f(t)} \nabla P\boldsymbol{u}_f = \int_{\Gamma(t)} P\boldsymbol{n}.\boldsymbol{u}_f,$$

while integrating by parts in the second term yields

$$-\int_{\Omega_f(t)} 2\mathbf{div}(\nu \boldsymbol{D}\boldsymbol{u}_f)\boldsymbol{u}_f = 2\nu\int_{\Omega_f(t)} [\boldsymbol{D}\boldsymbol{u}_f]^2 - \int_{\Gamma(t)} 2\nu \boldsymbol{D}\boldsymbol{u}_f.\boldsymbol{n}.\boldsymbol{u}_f.$$

Similarly, by multiplying (8.29) by $\frac{\partial \boldsymbol{\eta}_s}{\partial t}$, integrating over $\hat{\Omega}_s$ and formally integrating by parts, we get

$$\int_{\hat{\Omega}_s} \hat{\rho}_{s,0}\frac{\partial^2 \boldsymbol{\eta}_s}{\partial t^2}\frac{\partial \boldsymbol{\eta}_s}{\partial t} + \int_{\hat{\Omega}_s} (\hat{\boldsymbol{F}}_s\hat{\boldsymbol{\Sigma}})\nabla[\frac{\partial \boldsymbol{\eta}_s}{\partial t}] - \int_{\hat{\Gamma}} [\hat{\boldsymbol{F}}_s\hat{\boldsymbol{\Sigma}}](t,.).\hat{\boldsymbol{n}}\frac{\partial \boldsymbol{\eta}_s}{\partial t} = 0. \tag{8.32}$$

From (8.28) we now recognise that

$$2\nu\int_{\Omega(t)} [\boldsymbol{D}\boldsymbol{u}_f]^2 - \int_{\Gamma(t)} 2\nu \boldsymbol{D}\boldsymbol{u}_f.\boldsymbol{n}.\boldsymbol{u}_f - \int_{\Gamma(t)} P\boldsymbol{n}.\boldsymbol{u}_f = \int_{\hat{\Gamma}} [\hat{\boldsymbol{F}}_s\hat{\boldsymbol{\Sigma}}](t,.).\hat{\boldsymbol{n}}\frac{\partial \boldsymbol{\eta}_s}{\partial t} \tag{8.33}$$

so that by adding (8.31) and (8.32), we get

$$\begin{aligned}\int_{\Omega_f(t)} \frac{\partial \boldsymbol{u}_f}{\partial t}\boldsymbol{u}_f &+ \textstyle\int_{\Omega_f(t)} (\boldsymbol{u}\cdot\boldsymbol{\nabla})\boldsymbol{u}_f\boldsymbol{u}_f + 2\nu\int_{\Omega(t)}[\boldsymbol{D}\boldsymbol{u}_f]^2 \\ &+ \int_{\hat{\Omega}_s} \hat{\rho}_{s,0}\frac{\partial^2 \boldsymbol{\eta}_s}{\partial t^2}\frac{\partial \boldsymbol{\eta}_s}{\partial t} + \int_{\hat{\Omega}_s} (\hat{\boldsymbol{F}}_s\hat{\boldsymbol{\Sigma}})\nabla[\frac{\partial \boldsymbol{\eta}_s}{\partial t}] \\ &= \int_{\Omega_f(t)} \boldsymbol{f}\boldsymbol{u}_f.\end{aligned} \tag{8.34}$$

The first remark is now

$$\int_{\hat{\Omega}_s} \hat{\rho}_{s,0}\frac{\partial^2 \boldsymbol{\eta}_s}{\partial t^2}\frac{\partial \boldsymbol{\eta}_s}{\partial t} = \frac{1}{2}\frac{\partial}{\partial t}\int_{\hat{\Omega}_s} \hat{\rho}_{s,0}[\frac{\partial \boldsymbol{\eta}_s}{\partial t}]^2;$$

next, depending on the definition of $\boldsymbol{F}$ and $\boldsymbol{\Sigma}$ we get

$$\int_{\hat{\Omega}_s} (\hat{\boldsymbol{F}}_s\hat{\boldsymbol{\Sigma}})\nabla[\frac{\partial \boldsymbol{\eta}_s}{\partial t}] = \frac{\partial}{\partial t}\mathcal{E}(\boldsymbol{\eta}_s)(t,.),$$

where $\mathcal{E}$ is some mechanical energy related to the displacement and is assumed to be positive. The only terms that do not seem to have an appropriate sign are the two first ones in (8.34). From the Reynolds theorem, nevertheless, we derive

$$\int_{\Omega_f(t)} \frac{\partial \boldsymbol{u}_f}{\partial t} \boldsymbol{u}_f = \frac{1}{2} \frac{\partial}{\partial t} \int_{\Omega_f(t)} |\boldsymbol{u}_f|^2 - \frac{1}{2} \int_{\Gamma(t)} |\boldsymbol{u}_f|^2 \boldsymbol{u}_f.\boldsymbol{n}; \tag{8.35}$$

on the other hand, from the divergence-free condition (8.2), we get

$$\int_{\Omega_f(t)} (\boldsymbol{u}_f \cdot \boldsymbol{\nabla}) \boldsymbol{u}_f \boldsymbol{u}_f = \frac{1}{2} \int_{\Omega_f(t)} (\boldsymbol{u}_f \cdot \boldsymbol{\nabla}) |\boldsymbol{u}_f|^2 = -\frac{1}{2} \int_{\Gamma(t)} |\boldsymbol{u}_f|^2 \boldsymbol{u}_f.\boldsymbol{n}; \tag{8.36}$$

hence, by summing up

$$\frac{1}{2} \frac{\partial}{\partial t} \int_{\Omega_f(t)} |\boldsymbol{u}_f|^2 + 2\nu \int_{\Omega(t)} [\boldsymbol{D}\boldsymbol{u}_f]^2 + \frac{1}{2} \frac{\partial}{\partial t} \int_{\hat{\Omega}_s} \hat{\rho}_{s,0} [\frac{\partial \boldsymbol{\eta}_s}{\partial t}]^2 + \frac{\partial}{\partial t} \mathcal{E}(\boldsymbol{\eta}_s)(t,.)$$
$$= \int_{\Omega_f(t)} \boldsymbol{f} \boldsymbol{u}_f. \tag{8.37}$$

After integration in time we obtain at any time t

$$\int_{\Omega_f(t)} {\boldsymbol{u}_f}^2 + 4\nu \int_0^t \int_{\Omega(s)} [\boldsymbol{D}\boldsymbol{u}_f]^2 ds + \int_{\hat{\Omega}_s} \hat{\rho}_{s,0} [\frac{\partial \boldsymbol{\eta}_s}{\partial t}(t)]^2 + 2\mathcal{E}(\boldsymbol{\eta}_s)(t,.)$$
$$= \int_0^t \int_{\Omega_f(s)} \boldsymbol{f} \boldsymbol{u}_f ds + \int_{\Omega_f(0)} {\boldsymbol{u}_f}^2 + \int_{\hat{\Omega}_s} \hat{\rho}_{s,0} [\frac{\partial \boldsymbol{\eta}_s}{\partial t}(0)]^2 + 2\mathcal{E}(\boldsymbol{\eta}_s)(0,.), \tag{8.38}$$

from which we derive that, should it exist, the solution $(\boldsymbol{u}_f, \boldsymbol{\eta}_s)$ of the coupled problem would be stable in the following sense :

$$\begin{aligned} \boldsymbol{u}_f &\text{ is uniformely bounded in } L^\infty(0,T; L^2(\Omega(t)), \\ \boldsymbol{D}\boldsymbol{u}_f &\text{ is uniformely bounded in } L^2(0,T; L^2(\Omega(t)), \\ \frac{\partial \boldsymbol{\eta}_s}{\partial t}(t) &\text{ is uniformely bounded in } L^\infty(0,T; L^2(\hat{\Omega}_s), \\ \mathcal{E}(\boldsymbol{\eta}_s) &\text{ is uniformely bounded in } L^\infty(0,T). \end{aligned} \tag{8.39}$$

Note that in order to derive some uniform $L^2(0,T;H^1(\Omega(t))$ bound for $\boldsymbol{u}_f$, we need to make use of a Korn-type inequality that may be true only according to some hypotheses on the shape of $\Omega(t)$, in particular the regularity of its boundary, which is, unfortunately, one of the unknowns of the problem! This is just a preliminary illustration of the difficulties that have still to be faced.

8.2.3 Some general remarks

One interesting feature of the previous analysis is the different types of balance in the energies. The first one holds between the fluid and the structure, as is illustrated in (8.33) and as might be expected. It allows us to rationally check that the interface conditions that have been proposed are coherent with the model. The second one, ehich is less obvious, states that the motion of the interface, i.e., the fluid domain boundary, is balanced by the convection term (see (8.35, 8.36)). Actually this is not so surprising since, in Lagrangian form, this convection term enters in the total time derivative that commutes with the spacial integration over the original fluid domain.

The corollary is that if, for the sake of simplification, we want to drop some contribution (e.g., the interface motion, as we did in the first section, or the convective component in order to arrive at a linear Stokes problem) or if we want to add some effects (e.g., visco-elastic terms in the structure), then special care should be taken with the way the interface contribution is written up so that the previous balances are maintained. In particular, this is the reason for the insertion of the term $-\frac{1}{2}\left(\sum_{j=1}^{n} \boldsymbol{u}_{f\,j} \cos n_j\right)$ in (8.5), a consequence of the fact that the motion of the interface does not enter in the model, yielding in turn the commutation of the time derivative operator with the integration over Ω_f.

The second corollary is that, if the balance is not possible, the consequence of the lack of an *a priori* bound on the solution is not only revealed by the difficulty of obtaining a solution to the coupled problem but it may hurt also at the discretisation and simulation level since there may not be any stable scheme for the simulation of this incorrect fluid structure interaction model.

To the best of our knowledge, these stability issues were first presented in [135], together with an illustration of the (real versus numerical) instability arrived at by getting rid of the nonlinear contribution in the fluid model.

8.3 Weak solution for a full interaction problem with an elastic plate

Let us summarise here the results presented in [73] by Chambolle, Desjardins, Esteban and Grandmont that deal with a more general situation where the domain Ω_f depends on time. The proof of the well-posedness of this problem relies on the *a priori* estimates and compactness properties that are available thanks to the simple shape of the geometry of the fluid that follows from the assumption made on the structure that can be modelled as a plate.

8.3.1 Set up of the interaction problem

In this model, the fluid is assumed to fill a three-dimensional cavity and to interact with a thin elastic structure sitting on one of its sides $\Gamma(t)$. The remaining part of the boundary, denoted as $\gamma_0 = \partial\Omega_f(t) \setminus \Gamma(t)$, is rigid. For the sake of simplicity, it is assumed that, in the reference state, the elastic part of the fluid boundary is $\omega \times \{1\}$ where ω denotes a Lipshitz domain in

$\mathbb{R}^2$; the initial state of the fluid occupies the domain Ω_{f0} defined by

$$\Omega_{f0} = \{\boldsymbol{x} = (x, y, z) \in \omega \times \mathbb{R}, 0 < z < 1 + \eta_0(x, y)\},$$

where η_0 is a given initial displacement. The deformation of the elastic part of the boundary is modelled by a classical linear plate theory for transverse motions and the in-plane motions are neglected. The transversal displacement of the plate η ($\eta = \eta(t, x, y) \in \mathbb{R}$) is supposed to satisfy

$$\begin{aligned} &\partial_{tt}\eta + \Delta^2\eta + \mu\Delta^2\partial_t\eta = g + (\sigma_f)_3 && \text{in } \omega, \\ &\eta = \frac{\partial\eta}{\partial n} = 0 && \text{over } \partial\omega, \\ &\eta(0) = \eta_0 \quad \partial_t\eta(0) = \eta_1. \end{aligned} \tag{8.40}$$

Here again g is a given force and $\sigma_f = \boldsymbol{\sigma}_f \cdot \boldsymbol{n}$ is fluid normal stress applied on the surface of the structure. As usual, the domain occupied by the fluid at time t is denoted by $\Omega_f(t)$

$$\Omega_f(t) = \{(x, y, z) \in \omega \times \mathbb{R}, 0 < z < 1 + \eta(t, x, y)\},$$

the divergence-free velocity field $\boldsymbol{u}_f(t, .)$ and the pressure $P(t, .)$ defined over $\Omega_f(t)$ satisfy (8.1), (8.2) over $\Omega_f = \Omega_f(t)$, together with initial and boundary conditions

$$\begin{aligned} &\boldsymbol{u}_f(t, 0) = 0 && \text{over } \gamma_0, \\ &\boldsymbol{u}_f(0, .) = \boldsymbol{u}_{f0} && \text{in } \Omega_{f0}, \\ &\boldsymbol{u}_f(t, x, y, 1 + \eta(t, x, y)) = (0, 0, \partial_t\eta(t, x, y))^T, && (x, y) \in \omega. \end{aligned} \tag{8.41}$$

The expression of the surface tension can now be given; it is simpler to express it under a variational form, since the equilibrium of energy flows appears clearly. It takes the form, valid for any regular enough function $\boldsymbol{v}$ defined on the interface

$$\int_\omega \sigma_f(x, y)\overline{\boldsymbol{v}} = \int_{\Gamma(t)} (2\nu \boldsymbol{D}\boldsymbol{u}_f).\boldsymbol{n} + p\boldsymbol{n}).\boldsymbol{v},$$

where $\overline{\boldsymbol{v}}(t, x, y) = \boldsymbol{v}(t, x, y, \eta(t, x, y))$. Similarly to in the previous section, by multipling equation (8.1) by $\boldsymbol{u}_f$, equation (8.40) by $\partial_t\eta$, integrating by parts over the corresponding domains and taking into account (8.41) we derive stability on the solution $(\boldsymbol{u}_f, \eta)$ (assuming it exists) whenever the datum $\boldsymbol{f} \in L^2(0, T; L^2(\mathbb{R}^3))^3$, $g \in L^2(0, T; L^2(\omega))$, $\boldsymbol{u}_{f0} \in L^2(\Omega_{f0})^3$, $\eta_0 \in H_0^2(\omega)$ and $\eta_1 \in L^2(\omega)$. These stability results on $(\boldsymbol{u}_f, \eta)$ provide

$$\boldsymbol{u}_f \in L^\infty(0, T; L^2(\Omega_f(t))^3), \boldsymbol{D}(\boldsymbol{u}_f) \in L^2(0, T; L^2(\Omega_f(t))^3)$$

and

$$\eta \in W^{1,\infty}(0, T; L^2(\omega)) \cap H^1(0, T; H_0^2(\omega)).$$

It should be noted that the various integrations by parts and trace restriction for the relative boundary terms should be carefully defined since the boundary is an unknown and is evolving in time. This issue is carefully analysed in [73] (see their subsection 1.3, for full details) and everything is fine over the domain $\Omega_f(t)$ as soon as e.g., the boundary deformation $\eta \in \mathcal{C}^0([0,T];\mathcal{C}^0(\overline{\omega})\cap H^1(\overline{\omega}))$.

In addition to the *a priori* estimates, the analysis of the problem involves a fixed point procedure together with a regularisation process based on two stable regularisation operators, $\mathcal{R}_\varepsilon$ from $L^2(0,T;L^2(\omega\times(0,2M))$ onto $\mathcal{C}^\infty([0,T]\times(\overline{\omega}\times[0,2M]))$ and $\mathcal{N}_\varepsilon$ from $\mathcal{C}^0([0,T]\times\overline{\omega})$ into $\mathcal{C}^\infty([0,T]\times\overline{\omega})$, where M is some large enough real number.

8.3.2 A linearised/regularised version of the problem

Let us take $\delta \in H^1(0,T;\mathcal{C}^0(\overline{\omega})\cap H^1(\overline{\omega}))$, a predictor for the plate displacement, and let us regularise it by introducing $\delta^\star_\varepsilon = \mathcal{N}_\varepsilon(\delta)$. This allows the definition of a domain $\Omega_{\delta^\star_\varepsilon}$ as follows

$$\Omega_{\delta^\star_\varepsilon}(t) = \{(x,y,z)\in\omega\times\mathbb{R}, 0<z<1+\delta^\star_\varepsilon(t,x,y)\}, \tag{8.42}$$

provided that we assume, e.g., $2M \geq 1+\delta(t,x,y) \geq \alpha > 0$, $\forall(t,x,y)\in[0,T]\times\overline{\omega}$. Next, similarly to in (8.9), we introduce the space

$$V_{\delta^\star_\varepsilon}(t) = \{\boldsymbol{v}_f | \boldsymbol{v}_f \in [H^1(\Omega_{\delta^\star_\varepsilon}(t))]^n, \operatorname{div}\boldsymbol{v}_f = 0, \boldsymbol{v}_{f|\gamma_0} = \boldsymbol{0}\}.$$

Let us now take $\boldsymbol{v} \in L^2(0,T;L^2(\omega\times(0,2M))$, that is a predictor for the fluid convection velocity, and let us regularise it by introducing $\boldsymbol{v}^\star_\varepsilon = \mathcal{R}_\varepsilon(\boldsymbol{v})$.

The intermediate problem we consider reads as follows : Find $(\boldsymbol{u}_{f\,\varepsilon}, \eta_\varepsilon)$ such that

- $\boldsymbol{u}_{f\,\varepsilon} \in L^2(0,T;V_{\delta^\star_\varepsilon}(t)) \cap L^\infty(0,T;L^2(\Omega_{\delta^\star_\varepsilon}(t)))$;
- $\eta_\varepsilon \in W^{1,\infty}(0,T;L^2(\omega)) \cap H^1(0,T;H^2_0(\omega))$;
- $\boldsymbol{u}_{f\,\varepsilon}(t,x,y,1+\delta^\star_\varepsilon(t,x,y)) = (0,0,\partial_t\eta_\varepsilon(t,x,y))^T$ in ω;
- $\dfrac{\partial \boldsymbol{u}_{f\,\varepsilon}}{\partial t} \in L^2(0,T;L^2(\Omega_{\delta^\star_\varepsilon}(t)))$;
- $\dfrac{\partial^2\eta_\varepsilon}{\partial t^2} \in L^2(0,T;L^2(\omega))$ and
- $$\begin{aligned}\int_0^t\int_{\Omega_{\delta^\star_\varepsilon}(s)} \frac{\partial \boldsymbol{u}_{f\,\varepsilon}}{\partial t}\boldsymbol{\varphi}_\varepsilon + \nu\int_0^t\int_{\Omega_{\delta^\star_\varepsilon}(s)} \nabla\boldsymbol{u}_{f\,\varepsilon}\nabla\boldsymbol{\varphi}_\varepsilon + \frac{1}{2}\int_0^t\int_{\Omega_{\delta^\star_\varepsilon}(s)} (\boldsymbol{v}^\star_\varepsilon.\nabla)\boldsymbol{u}_{f\,\varepsilon}.\boldsymbol{\varphi}_\varepsilon \\ -\frac{1}{2}\int_0^t\int_{\Omega_{\delta^\star_\varepsilon}(s)} (\boldsymbol{v}^\star_\varepsilon.\nabla)\boldsymbol{\varphi}_\varepsilon.\boldsymbol{u}_{f\,\varepsilon} + \frac{1}{2}\int_0^t\int_\omega \frac{\partial\eta_\varepsilon}{\partial t}\frac{\partial\delta^\star_\varepsilon}{\partial t}b + \int_0^t\int_\omega\frac{\partial\eta_\varepsilon}{\partial t^2}b \\ +\int_0^t\int_\omega\frac{\partial\Delta\eta_\varepsilon}{\partial t}\Delta b + \int_0^t\int_\omega \Delta\eta_\varepsilon\Delta b = \int_0^t\int_{\Omega_{\delta^\star_\varepsilon}(s)}\boldsymbol{f}.\boldsymbol{\varphi}_\varepsilon \int_0^t\int_\omega gb\end{aligned} \tag{8.43}$$

$$\forall \varphi_\varepsilon \in L^2(0,T;V_{\delta^\star_\varepsilon}(t)), \forall b \in L^2(0,T;H^2_0(\omega)) \quad \text{such that}$$

$$\varphi_\varepsilon(t,x,y,1+\delta^\star_\varepsilon(t,x,y)) = (0,0,b(t,x,y))^T \text{ in } \omega, \tag{8.44}$$

and complemented with initial conditions over $\boldsymbol{u}_{f_\varepsilon}$, η_ε and $\frac{\eta_\varepsilon}{\partial t}$ that are regularised versions of $\boldsymbol{u}_{f_0}$, η_0 and η_1 respectively.

The regularity of the boundary of the domain $\Omega_{\delta^\star_\varepsilon}(t)$ allows the definition of a change of variable χ_ε from a reference domain $\mathcal{C} = \omega \times (0,1)$ onto the domains $\Omega_{\delta^\star_\varepsilon}(t)$. Let us denote by $\boldsymbol{w}_\varepsilon$ the time derivative of χ_ε; the problem (8.43) becomes

$$\int_0^t\int_{\mathcal{C}} \frac{\partial \underline{\boldsymbol{u}_{f}}_\varepsilon}{\partial t}\underline{\varphi_\varepsilon} J_\varepsilon + \nu\int_0^t\int_{\mathcal{C}} A_\varepsilon \nabla \underline{\boldsymbol{u}_f}_\varepsilon \nabla\underline{\varphi_\varepsilon} + \frac{1}{2}\int_0^t\int_{\mathcal{C}}(\underline{\boldsymbol{v}}^\star_\varepsilon.(B_\varepsilon\nabla))\underline{\boldsymbol{u}_f}_\varepsilon.\underline{\varphi_\varepsilon}$$

$$-\frac{1}{2}\int_0^t\int_{\mathcal{C}}(\underline{\boldsymbol{v}}^\star_\varepsilon.(B_\varepsilon\nabla))\underline{\varphi_\varepsilon}.\underline{\boldsymbol{u}_f}_\varepsilon + \frac{1}{2}\int_0^t\int_\omega \frac{\partial\eta_\varepsilon}{\partial t}\frac{\partial\delta^\star_\varepsilon}{\partial t}b - \int_0^t\int_{\mathcal{C}}(\underline{\boldsymbol{w}}_\varepsilon.(B_\varepsilon\nabla))\underline{\boldsymbol{u}_f}_\varepsilon.\underline{\varphi_\varepsilon}$$

$$+\int_0^t\int_\omega \frac{\partial^2\eta_\varepsilon}{\partial t^2}b + \int_0^t\int_\omega\frac{\partial\Delta\eta_\varepsilon}{\partial t}\Delta b + \int_0^t\int_\omega \Delta\eta_\varepsilon\Delta b = \int_0^t\int_{\mathcal{C}}\underline{\boldsymbol{f}}.\underline{\varphi_\varepsilon}J_\varepsilon + \int_0^t\int_\omega gb \tag{8.45}$$

$$\forall \underline{\varphi_\varepsilon} \in L^2(0,T;V_0), b \in L^2(0,T;H^2_0(\omega)) \quad \text{such that}$$

$$\underline{\varphi_\varepsilon}(t,x,y,1) = (0,0,b(t,x,y))^T \text{ in } \omega \tag{8.46}$$

where the notation $\underline{\boldsymbol{v}}$ denotes the transported function of $\boldsymbol{v}$ under the flow χ_ε, and J_ε, A_ε, B_ε are the proper geometric factors that result from the change of variables.

In order to prove that there exists a solution to problem (8.45), we introduce, as in equation (8.15), a Galerkin basis of eigenfunctions of the Stokes problem. Restricting the spaces of trial and test functions in (8.45) to the spaces spanned by the first eigenfunctions allows a set of finite dimensional coupled problems to be obtained, which reads as a system of coupled ordinary differential equations that can be shown to possess unique solutions. A similar *a priori* analysis to the one that was performed in the previous subsection allows us to state that the sequence of discrete solutions is uniformly bounded (uniformly with respect to the dimension of the discrete space together with ε). In order to get enough information to pass to the limit in the convection terms, regularity with respect to time derivatives, similarly to in (8.22), is obtained, and the boundedness of these terms is uniform with respect to the dimension of the discrete space but not with respect to ε. Nevertheless, this is enough to pass to the limit and possibly prove the existence of a solution $(\underline{\boldsymbol{u}_f}_\varepsilon, \eta_\varepsilon)$ to problem (8.45) for every given ε, hence a solution $(\boldsymbol{u}_{f_\varepsilon}, \eta_\varepsilon)$ to problem (8.43). This solution satisfies the following energy estimates

$$\begin{aligned}
&\|\boldsymbol{u}_{f_\varepsilon}\|_{L^\infty(0,T;L^2(\Omega_{\delta^\star_\varepsilon}(t)))} + \|\nabla \boldsymbol{u}_{f_\varepsilon}\|_{L^2(0,T;L^2(\Omega_{\delta^\star_\varepsilon}(t)))}\\
&+\|\frac{\partial \eta_\varepsilon}{\partial t}\|_{L^\infty(0,T;L^2(\omega))} + \|\Delta\eta_\varepsilon\|_{H^1(0,T;H^2_0(\omega))}\\
&\leq C(T, \|\boldsymbol{u}_{f0}\|_{L^2(\Omega_{\eta_0})}, \|\boldsymbol{f}\|_{L^2((0,T)\times\mathbb{R}^3)}, \|\boldsymbol{g}\|_{L^2((0,T)\times\mathbb{R}^3)}, \|\eta_0\|_{H^2_0(\omega)}, \|\eta_1\|_{L^2_0(\omega)},
\end{aligned}$$

and

$$\|\frac{\partial \boldsymbol{u}_{f_\varepsilon}}{\partial t}\|_{L^2(0,T;L^2(\mathcal{C}))} + \|\frac{\partial \eta_\varepsilon}{\partial t^2}\|_{L^2(0,T;L^2(\omega)} \leq C_{\varepsilon,M,\alpha}. \tag{8.47}$$

The fact that this deformation of the boundary is only vertical and regular enough allows us to get an easy extension of $\boldsymbol{u}_{f_\varepsilon}$ in $L^2(0,T;L^2(\omega\times(0,2M)))$, noted by $\overline{\boldsymbol{u}_{f_\varepsilon}}$

$$\overline{\boldsymbol{u}_{f_\varepsilon}} = \begin{cases} \boldsymbol{u}_{f_\varepsilon} & \text{in } \Omega_{\delta^\star_\varepsilon}(t)\\ (0,0,\partial_t\eta_\varepsilon)^T & \text{in } (0,2M)\times\omega\setminus\Omega_{\delta^\star_\varepsilon}(t). \end{cases} \tag{8.48}$$

It is important to note that $\overline{\boldsymbol{u}_{f_\varepsilon}}$ is divergence free. We can now define the mapping F_ε

$$F_\varepsilon : (\delta, \boldsymbol{v}) \mapsto (\eta_\varepsilon, \overline{\boldsymbol{u}_{f_\varepsilon}}). \tag{8.49}$$

The previous estimates allow first to get a set $\mathcal{B}^M_\varepsilon$ such that $F_\varepsilon(\mathcal{B}^M_\varepsilon) \subset \mathcal{B}^M_\varepsilon$ for M large enough. Then these estimates – in particular those involving the time derivatives (8.47) – allow us to prove that $F_\varepsilon(\mathcal{B}_\varepsilon)$ is relatively compact in $\mathcal{B}_\varepsilon$. The hypotheses of Schauder's fixed point theorem are fulfilled and there exists at least a fixed point to F_ε over a time interval such that $\min_{[0,T]\times\overline{\omega}}(1+\eta_\varepsilon) > 0$, hence a solution $(\overline{\boldsymbol{u}_{f_\varepsilon}}, \eta_\varepsilon)$ to the regularised nonlinear problem.

The final step is to get rid of the regularisation ingredient. In order to pass to the limit as ε tends to zero, further estimates should be derived since the present available bounds on the time derivatives depend on ε and thus may blow up as ε goes to zero. From the estimates already derived, $\overline{\boldsymbol{u}_{f_\varepsilon}}$ remains uniformely bounded in the $L^2(0,T;H^1)\cap L^\infty(0,T;L^2)$ norm, but this is not enough to pass to the limit in the nonlinear terms. As is often the case for the Navier-Stokes equations, uniform estimates do not seem to be available. We replace such a bound by bounds on the "half" derivative of $\overline{\boldsymbol{u}_{f_\varepsilon}}$, expressed in a weak sense as follows : for any $h > 0$

$$\begin{aligned}
&\int_0^T \int_{(0,2M)\times\omega} |\overline{\boldsymbol{u}_{f_\varepsilon}}(t,x) - \overline{\boldsymbol{u}_{f_\varepsilon}}(t+h,x)|^2 dt dx\\
&\qquad + \int_0^T \int_\omega (\frac{\partial \eta_\varepsilon}{\partial t}(t,x) - \frac{\partial \eta_\varepsilon}{\partial t}(t+h,x)|^2 dt dx \leq C\sqrt{h}
\end{aligned}$$

with a constant C uniform in ε.

These estimates allow first the relative compactness of the sequences to be proved, which, in turn, allows us to pass to the limit in the equation satisfied by $\boldsymbol{u}_{f_\varepsilon}$ and η_ε, written as follows

$$\int_{\Omega_{\eta^\star_\varepsilon}(t)} \boldsymbol{u}_{f_\varepsilon}(t).\Phi_\varepsilon(t) - \int_0^t \int_{\Omega_{\eta^\star_\varepsilon}(s)} \boldsymbol{u}_{f_\varepsilon}(s).\frac{\partial \Phi_\varepsilon}{\partial t}(s) + \nu \int_0^t \int_{\Omega_{\delta^\star_\varepsilon}(s)} \nabla \boldsymbol{u}_{f_\varepsilon} \nabla \boldsymbol{\varphi}_\varepsilon$$
$$+\frac{1}{2}\int_0^t \int_{\Omega_{\delta^\star_\varepsilon}(s)} (\boldsymbol{u}_{f_\varepsilon}^\star.\nabla)\boldsymbol{u}_{f_\varepsilon}.\boldsymbol{\varphi}_\varepsilon - \frac{1}{2}\int_0^t \int_{\Omega_{\delta^\star_\varepsilon}(s)} (\boldsymbol{u}_{f_\varepsilon}^\star.\nabla)\boldsymbol{\varphi}_\varepsilon.\boldsymbol{u}_{f_\varepsilon}$$
$$-\frac{1}{2}\int_0^t \int_\omega \frac{\partial \eta_\varepsilon}{\partial t}\frac{\partial \eta_\varepsilon^\star}{\partial t} b + \int_\omega \frac{\partial \eta_\varepsilon}{\partial t}(t) b(t) - \int_0^t \int_\omega \frac{\partial \eta_\varepsilon}{\partial t}\frac{\partial b}{\partial t} + \int_0^t \int_\omega \frac{\partial \Delta \eta_\varepsilon}{\partial t} \Delta b$$
$$+\int_0^t \int_\omega \Delta \eta_\varepsilon \Delta b = \int_0^t \int_{\Omega_{\delta^\star_\varepsilon}(s)} \boldsymbol{f}.\boldsymbol{\varphi}_\varepsilon + \int_0^t \int_\omega g b + \int_{\Omega_{\eta^\star_\varepsilon}(0)} \boldsymbol{u}_{f_\varepsilon}(0).\Phi_\varepsilon(0) + \int_\omega \eta_1^\varepsilon b(0)$$

after verifying that the time for existence of the solutions does not tend to zero as ε converges to zero. Note that this weak treatment of the time derivative, while it requires different test functions as they now depend on time, allows the convergence to be handled despite the lack of convergence results of $\frac{\partial \boldsymbol{u}_{f_\varepsilon}}{\partial t}$. This allows the main result of the paper to be stated [73]:

Theorem 8.2. *There exists $T^\star \in (0, \infty]$ and a weak solution $(\boldsymbol{u}_f, \eta)$ on $[0,T]$ to the fluid/plate interaction problem in the sense that, for any Φ and b,*

$$\int_{\Omega_{\eta^\star}(t)} \boldsymbol{u}_f(t).\Phi(t) - \int_0^t \int_{\Omega_{\eta^\star}(s)} \boldsymbol{u}_f(s).\frac{\partial \Phi}{\partial t}(s) + \nu \int_0^t \int_{\Omega_\delta(s)} \nabla \boldsymbol{u}_f \nabla \phi$$
$$+\int_0^t \int_{\Omega_\delta(s)} (\boldsymbol{u}_f.\nabla)\boldsymbol{u}_f.\phi - \int_0^t \int_\omega [\frac{\partial \eta}{\partial t}]^2 b + \int_\omega \frac{\partial \eta}{\partial t}(t) b(t)$$
$$-\int_0^t \int_\omega \frac{\partial \eta}{\partial t}\frac{\partial b}{\partial t} + \int_0^t \int_\omega \frac{\partial \Delta \eta}{\partial t}\Delta b + \int_0^t \int_\omega \Delta \eta \Delta b$$
$$= \int_0^t \int_{\Omega_\delta(s)} \boldsymbol{f}.\phi + \int_0^t \int_\omega g b + \int_{\Omega_{\eta^\star}(0)} \boldsymbol{u}_f(0).\Phi(0) + \int_\omega \eta_1 b(0).$$

In addition, this solution satisfies the a priori bounds stated at the beginning of this section.

8.4 A strong solution to a two-dimensional fluid-vessel interaction

The technique involved in the previous section has marginally used an ALE-type change of variable from the actual deformed shape of the fluid domain to a reference domain in one preliminary step of the proof; during all following steps, the fluid solution is considered in Eulerian form and the *a priori* bounds and the limit process are performed on the Eulerian velocity and pressure. In this section, we report on the paper of Beirao da Veiga [33], which presents a technique that allows both configurations to be considered at the same time: the Eulerian form and the Lagrangian one. The change of variable is thus done all through the analysis. This requires more regularity on the solutions and the verification of the equations can be stronger than in the previous analysis.

8.4.1 The fluid vessel coupling

The configuration here is simplified as a two-dimensional fluid interacting with a one-dimensional membrane. The fluid domain is delimited by a periodic curve, $\Gamma(t)$, $t \in [0,T]$ of equation

$$y = 1 + \eta(t,x), \quad x \in [0,L]. \tag{8.50}$$

Without loss of generality, we assume that the initial condition $\eta^0(x) = \eta(0,x)$ satisfies

$$\int_0^L \eta^0(x)dx = 0 \tag{8.51}$$

and $1+\eta_0 \geq 2\delta_0 > 0$. The evolution of these curves is assumed to be governed by the following generalised string model (see Section 3.4.4 and [406])

$$\begin{cases} \dfrac{\partial^2 \eta}{\partial t^2} - \beta \dfrac{\partial^2 \eta}{\partial x^2} - \gamma \dfrac{\partial^3 \eta}{\partial t \partial x^2} + \alpha \dfrac{\partial^4 \eta}{\partial x^4} + \sigma \eta = \Phi, & \text{over } (0,T) \times (0,L), \\ \eta(0,x) = \eta_0(x), \quad \partial_t \eta(0,x) = \eta_1(x). & \end{cases} \tag{8.52}$$

Here $\gamma > 0$, and α, β, σ are nonnegative. The fluid domain

$$\Omega_f(t) = \{(x,y) \in (0,L) \times \mathbb{R}, 0 < y < 1 + \eta(t,x)\}. \tag{8.53}$$

The function Φ on the right-hand side of (8.52) is defined as follows

$$\Phi[\eta, \boldsymbol{u}_f, P] = \Big(\rho_1 P \boldsymbol{n} - \rho_2 \nu [\boldsymbol{D}\boldsymbol{u}_f].\boldsymbol{n}\Big)_{|\Gamma(t)} \sqrt{1+\eta_x^2}\,\boldsymbol{e}_y$$

where $\boldsymbol{e}_y$ denotes the unit vector in the y-direction. Again the fluid is assumed to be governed by the Navier-Stokes equations (8.1), (8.2) complemented with the initial and boundary conditions

$$\begin{cases} \boldsymbol{u}_f(0,x,y) = \boldsymbol{u}_{f0}(x,y), \quad in\ \Omega_0^f \\ \boldsymbol{u}_f(t,x,1+\eta(t,x)) = \dfrac{\partial \eta}{\partial t}(t,x)\boldsymbol{n}_y, \quad in\ (0,T) \times (0,L) \\ \boldsymbol{u}_f(t,x,0) = 0, \quad in\ (0,T) \times (0,L) \end{cases}$$

and periodicity is assumed in the x direction. The following compatibility condition is required

$$\begin{cases} \nabla . \boldsymbol{u}_{f_0} = 0, & in\ \Omega_0^f \\ \boldsymbol{u}_{f_0}(x,0) = 0, & in\ (0,L) \\ \boldsymbol{u}_{f_0}(x, 1+\eta_0(x)) = \eta_1(x)\boldsymbol{e}_y, & in\ (0,L) \\ \displaystyle\int_0^L \eta_1(x)dx = 0. \end{cases}$$

8.4.2 The problem in an ALE form

This geometry allows the use of a simple change of variable

$$x = x, \quad z = \frac{y}{1+\eta(t,x)}, \tag{8.54}$$

which transforms the fluid domain $\Omega_f(t)$ into the reference domain $\mathcal{C} = (0,1) \times (0,L)$ and the transformed functions are, as in the previous section, represented as

$$\overline{f}(x,z) = f(x,(1+\eta(t,x))z).$$

Note that, of course, the notation of the transformed function $\overline{f}$ has nothing to do with the classical complex conjugate notation. The Navier-Stokes equations now read

$$\begin{cases} \dfrac{\partial \overline{\boldsymbol{u}_f}}{\partial t} - \nu \Delta \overline{\boldsymbol{u}_f} + \nabla \overline{P} = \overline{\boldsymbol{F}}[\eta, \overline{\boldsymbol{u}_f}, \nabla \overline{p}] \quad \text{in } \mathcal{C}, \\ \mathbf{div} \overline{\boldsymbol{u}_f} = \overline{\boldsymbol{g}}[\eta, \overline{\boldsymbol{u}_f}] \quad \text{in } \mathcal{C}, \\ \overline{\boldsymbol{u}_f}(0,x,z) = \overline{\boldsymbol{u}_f}^0(x,z) \quad \text{in } \mathcal{C}, \\ \overline{\boldsymbol{u}_f}(0,x,1) = \dfrac{\partial \eta}{\partial t}(t,x)\boldsymbol{e}_y \quad \text{for } x \in (0,1), \\ \overline{\boldsymbol{u}_f}(0,x,0) = 0 \quad \text{for } x \in (0,1) \end{cases} \tag{8.55}$$

where

$$\begin{aligned} \boldsymbol{F}[\eta, \overline{\boldsymbol{u}_f}, \nabla \overline{p}] = & -\eta \frac{\partial \overline{\boldsymbol{u}_f}}{\partial t} + \left[z\frac{\partial \eta}{\partial t} + \nu z \Big(\frac{2\frac{\partial \eta}{\partial x}^2}{1+\eta} - \frac{\partial^2 \eta}{\partial x^2} \Big) \right] \frac{\partial \overline{\boldsymbol{u}_f}}{\partial z} \\ & + \nu \left(-2z \frac{\partial \eta}{\partial x} \frac{\partial^2 \overline{\boldsymbol{u}_f}}{\partial x \partial z} + \eta \frac{\partial^2 \overline{\boldsymbol{u}_f}}{\partial x^2} + \left[\frac{z^2 \frac{\partial \eta}{\partial x}^2 - \eta}{1+\eta} \right] \frac{\partial^2 \overline{\boldsymbol{u}_f}}{\partial z^2} \right) \\ & + z \Big(\frac{\partial \eta}{\partial x} \frac{\partial \overline{P}}{\partial z} - \eta \frac{\partial \overline{P}}{\partial x} \Big) \boldsymbol{e}_x - (1+\eta) \overline{u}_{f,1} \frac{\partial \overline{\boldsymbol{u}_f}}{\partial x} \\ & + \Big(z \frac{\partial \eta}{\partial x} \overline{u}_{f,1} - \overline{u}_{f,2} \Big) \frac{\partial \overline{\boldsymbol{u}_f}}{\partial z} \end{aligned}$$

and

$$\overline{\boldsymbol{g}}[\eta, \overline{\boldsymbol{u}_f}] = -\eta \frac{\partial \overline{u}_{f,1}}{\partial x} + z \frac{\partial \eta}{\partial x} \frac{\partial \overline{u}_{f,1}}{\partial z}. \tag{8.56}$$

The string equation (8.52) now has, as a right-hand side, a function in the fluid variables

$$\left\{\begin{array}{l}\dfrac{\partial^2\eta}{\partial t^2}-\beta\dfrac{\partial^2\eta}{\partial x^2}-\gamma\dfrac{\partial^3\eta}{\partial t\partial x^2}+\alpha\dfrac{\partial^4\eta}{\partial x^4}+\sigma\eta=\overline{\Phi}[\eta,\overline{\boldsymbol{u}_f},\overline{P}_0]+\rho_1\overline{\phi}[\eta,\overline{\boldsymbol{u}_f}],\\ \hfill \text{over } (0,T)\times(0,L),\\ \qquad\eta(0,x)=\eta_0(x),\quad \partial_t\eta(0,x)=\eta_1(x)\end{array}\right. \tag{8.57}$$

with

$$\overline{\Phi}[\eta,\overline{\boldsymbol{v}},\overline{P}]=\rho_1\overline{P}+\nu\rho_2\left(\frac{1}{1+\eta}\frac{\partial\eta}{\partial x}\frac{\partial\overline{v}_1}{\partial z}+\frac{\partial\eta}{\partial x}\frac{\partial\overline{v}_2}{\partial x}-2\frac{2+(\partial\eta/\partial x)^2}{1+\eta}\frac{\partial\overline{v}_2}{\partial z}\right). \tag{8.58}$$

$\overline{P}_0$ is such that

$$\int_0^L\overline{P}_0(t,x,1)dx=0$$

and

$$\overline{\phi}(t)=\overline{\phi}[\eta,\overline{\boldsymbol{u}_f}]=\frac{\nu\rho_2}{L\rho_1}\int_0^L\left(\frac{1}{1+\eta}\frac{\partial\eta}{\partial x}\frac{\partial\overline{v}_1}{\partial z}+\frac{\partial\eta}{\partial x}\frac{\partial\overline{v}_2}{\partial x}-2\frac{2+(\partial\eta/\partial x)^2}{1+\eta}\frac{\partial\overline{v}_2}{\partial z}\right)dx \tag{8.59}$$

so that the pressure in (8.55) is given by

$$\overline{P}(t,x,z)=\overline{P}_0(t,x,z)+\overline{\phi}(t).$$

8.4.3 The linearised coupled problem

This problem is written in a form well suited to propose a linearised version of it, where the terms in the right-hand side are supposed to be given. We are thus faced with a couple of systems :

$$\left\{\begin{array}{l}\dfrac{\partial^2\tilde{\eta}}{\partial t^2}-\beta\dfrac{\partial^2\tilde{\eta}}{\partial x^2}-\gamma\dfrac{\partial^3\tilde{\eta}}{\partial t\partial x^2}+\alpha\dfrac{\partial^4\tilde{\eta}}{\partial x^4}+\sigma\eta=\overline{\Phi}[\hat{\eta},\hat{\boldsymbol{u}}_f,\hat{P}_0]+\rho_1\overline{\phi}[\hat{\eta},\hat{\boldsymbol{u}}_f],\\ \hfill \text{over } (0,T)\times(0,L),\\ \qquad\tilde{\eta}(0,x)=\eta_0(x),\quad \partial_t\tilde{\eta}(0,x)=\eta_1(x)\end{array}\right. \tag{8.60}$$

corresponding to the string equation, and

$$\left\{\begin{array}{l}\dfrac{\partial\tilde{\boldsymbol{u}}_f}{\partial t}-\nu\Delta\tilde{\boldsymbol{u}}_f+\nabla\tilde{P}=\overline{\boldsymbol{F}}[\hat{\eta},\hat{\boldsymbol{u}}_f,\nabla\hat{p}]\quad\text{in }\mathcal{C},\\ \qquad\qquad\mathbf{div}\tilde{\boldsymbol{u}}_f=\overline{\boldsymbol{g}}[\hat{\eta},\hat{\boldsymbol{u}}_f]\quad\text{in }\mathcal{C},\\ \qquad\tilde{\boldsymbol{u}}_f(0,x,z)=\hat{\boldsymbol{u}}_f{}^0(x,z)\quad\text{in }\mathcal{C},\\ \qquad\tilde{\boldsymbol{u}}_f(0,x,1)=\dfrac{\partial\hat{\eta}}{\partial t}(t,x)\boldsymbol{e}_y\quad\text{for } x\in(0,1),\\ \qquad\tilde{\boldsymbol{u}}_f(0,x,0)=0\quad\text{for } x\in(0,1)\end{array}\right. \tag{8.61}$$

for the fluid part.

Here the triplet $(\hat{\eta}, \hat{\boldsymbol{u}}_f, \nabla\hat{p})$ is assumed to be given, the solution $(\tilde{\eta}, \tilde{\boldsymbol{u}}_f, \nabla\tilde{p})$ follows and we shall seek a fixed point to the mapping $(\hat{\eta}, \hat{\boldsymbol{u}}_f, \nabla\hat{p}) \longrightarrow (\tilde{\eta}, \tilde{\boldsymbol{u}}_f, \nabla\tilde{p})$.

The set $\mathbb{K}$ in which the fixed point procedure will be performed is expressed in terms of the following regularities

- on the displacement

$$|||\eta|||^2 \equiv \|\eta\|^2_{L^\infty(0,T;H^{7/2})} + \|\frac{\partial \eta}{\partial t}\|^2_{L^\infty(0,T;H^{3/2})} + \|\frac{\partial \eta}{\partial t}\|^2_{L^2(0,T;H^{5/2})} < \infty \tag{8.62}$$

and

$$\|\frac{\partial^2 \eta}{\partial t^2}\||^2_{L^2(0,T;H^{-1/2})} < \infty;$$

- on the velocity and pressure

$$|||\boldsymbol{u}_f, P|||^2 = \|\boldsymbol{u}_f\|^2_{L^2(0,T;H^2(\Omega))} + \|\frac{\partial \boldsymbol{u}_f}{\partial t}\|^2_{L^2(0,T;L^2(\Omega))} + \|P\|^2_{L^2(0,T;L^2(\Omega))} < \infty$$

which are more restrictive, as anticipated, than those we have encountered up to now. The generic constants that will appear in the sequel, all denoted by c, may depend on $L, \delta_0, \nu, \alpha, \beta, \gamma$ and σ.

We start by analysing the linearised string equation (8.60), for which a solution is quite simple. By considering the equation satisfied by $\lambda = \frac{\partial \tilde{\eta}}{\partial x}$ we deduce, by multiplying by $\frac{\partial^2 \tilde{\eta}}{\partial x \partial t}$, the following stability results:

- $\tilde{\eta}$ is bounded in $L^\infty(0,T;H^1)$;
- $\dfrac{\partial \tilde{\eta}}{\partial t}$ is bounded in $L^\infty(0,T;H^1)$;
- $\dfrac{\partial^2 \tilde{\eta}}{\partial x^2}$ is bounded in $L^\infty(0,T;H^1)$;
- $\dfrac{\partial \tilde{\eta}}{\partial t}$ is bounded in $L^2(0,T;H^2)$;

in terms of $\|\eta_0\|_{H^3}$, $\|\eta_1\|_{H^1}$ and the $L^2(0,T;L^2)$-norm of the right-hand side in (8.60). By multiplying the equation satisfied by λ by $-\frac{\partial^3 \lambda}{\partial t \partial x^2}$, we get the following stability results :

- $\tilde{\eta}$ is bounded in $L^\infty(0,T;H^2)$;
- $\dfrac{\partial \tilde{\eta}}{\partial t}$ is bounded in $L^\infty(0,T;H^2)$;
- $\dfrac{\partial^2 \tilde{\eta}}{\partial x^2}$ is bounded in $L^\infty(0,T;H^2)$;
- $\dfrac{\partial \tilde{\eta}}{\partial t}$ is bounded in $L^2(0,T;H^3)$;

in terms of $\|\eta_0\|_{H^4}$, $\|\eta_1\|_{H^2}$ and the $L^2(0,T;H^1)$-norm of the right-hand side in (8.60).

The required stability for $\mathbb{K}$ is derived by interpolation from the two previous stability results that lead to

$$\|\tilde{\eta}\|^2_{L^\infty(0,T;H^{7/2})} + \|\frac{\partial \tilde{\eta}}{\partial t}\|^2_{L^\infty(0,T;H^{3/2})} + \|\frac{\partial \tilde{\eta}}{\partial t}\|^2_{L^2(0,T;H^{5/2})} \\ \leq c\Big(\|\eta_0\|^2_{H^{7/2}} + \|\eta_1\|^2_{H^{3/2}} + \|\overline{\Phi}[\hat{\eta}, \hat{\boldsymbol{u}}_f, \hat{P}_0] + \rho_1\overline{\phi}[\hat{\eta}, \hat{\boldsymbol{u}}_f]\|_{L^2(H^{1/2})}\Big). \tag{8.63}$$

We complement this analysis by noticing that

$$\|\overline{\Phi}[\hat{\eta}, \hat{\boldsymbol{u}}_f, \hat{P}_0] + \rho_1\overline{\phi}[\hat{\eta}, \hat{\boldsymbol{u}}_f]\|^2_{L^2(H^{1/2})} \\ \leq c\rho_1^2\|\nabla\hat{P}_0\|^2_{L^2} + c\rho_2^2\Big(1 + \|\eta_0\|^3_{H^{5/2}} + T^{3/2}\|\frac{\partial \hat{\eta}}{\partial t}\|^3_{L^2(H^{5/2})}\Big)^2 |||\hat{\boldsymbol{u}}_f|||^2 \tag{8.64}$$

where the norm $|||.|||$ has been defined in (8.62). Similarly, we can derive an estimate of $\frac{\partial^2 \tilde{\eta}}{\partial t^2}$

$$\|\frac{\partial^2 \hat{\eta}}{\partial t^2}\|_{L^2(0,T;H^{-1/2})} \leq c\rho_1\|\nabla\hat{P}_0\|_{L^2} \\ + c\rho_2 T^{1/8}\Big(1 + \|\eta_0\|^2_{L^\infty} + |||\hat{\eta}|||^2\Big)|||\hat{\boldsymbol{u}}_f||| + cT^{1/2}|||\hat{\eta}|||. \tag{8.65}$$

Let us now consider the linearised fluid problem (8.61) that takes the form of a non-homogeneous unsteady Stokes problem. In order to transform the problem into another one that is more classical, Beirao da Veiga proposes to lift the two data $\overline{\boldsymbol{g}}[\hat{\eta}, \hat{\boldsymbol{u}}_f]$ and $\hat{\boldsymbol{u}_f}^0(x,z)$. This is done through the definition of a vector field $\boldsymbol{v}$ such that

$$\begin{aligned} \mathbf{div}\boldsymbol{v} &= \overline{\boldsymbol{g}}[\hat{\eta}, \hat{\boldsymbol{u}}_f], \\ \boldsymbol{v}(0,x,z) &= \hat{\boldsymbol{u}_f}^0(x,z). \end{aligned} \tag{8.66}$$

The construction of such a vector field is rather intricate and involves the resolution of different Poisson problems from which the gradient of the solution is taken. A stability in the $L^2(0,T;H^2) \cap H^1(0,T;L^2)$ norm is natural and is achieved thanks to a careful analysis of the traces. This allows the transformation of the original problem (8.61) into another one, similar but where the boundary condition is homogeneous and the divergence is free. The regularity and stability of the solution of such a standard Stokes problem is a consequence of the regularity of the boundary of the domain $\mathcal{C}$ (remembering the periodic condition imposed in the x direction). The stability of the associated solution in the $|||.|||$-norm is governed by the $L^2(0,T;L^2)$ bound on the right-hand side that leads to the following statement: the solution $(\tilde{\boldsymbol{u}_f}, \nabla\tilde{p})$ is stable in the following sense

$$
\begin{aligned}
|||\tilde{\boldsymbol{u}_f}, \nabla\tilde{p}|||^2 \leq{} & c\|\hat{\boldsymbol{u}_f}^0\|^2_{H^1}\\
& + c\Big(\|\eta_0\|^2_{L^\infty} + \frac{\partial\eta_0}{\partial x}\|^2_{L^\infty} + \frac{\partial\eta_0}{\partial x}\|^4_{L^\infty} + T^{2/3}\|\eta_0\|^2_{H^{5/2}}\\
+T\|\frac{\partial\hat{\eta}}{\partial t}\|^2_{L^\infty(0,T;H^{3/2})} & + T\|\frac{\partial\hat{\eta}}{\partial t}\|^2_{L^2(0,T;H^{5/2})} + T^2\|\frac{\partial\hat{\eta}}{\partial t}\|^4_{L^\infty(0,T;H^{5/2})}\Big)|||\hat{\boldsymbol{u}}_f|||^2\\
& + c\Big(\|\eta_0\|^2_{L^\infty} + \frac{\partial\eta_0}{\partial x}\|^2_{L^\infty}\Big)\|\frac{\partial\hat{\boldsymbol{u}}_f}{\partial t}|||^2_{L^2(0,T;L^2)}\\
& + cT^{1/2}\Big(1 + \|\eta_0\|^2_{H^{5/2}} + \|\frac{\partial\hat{\eta}}{\partial t}\|^2_{L^2(0,T;H^{5/2})}\Big)|||\hat{\boldsymbol{u}}_f|||^4\\
& + c\Big(\|\eta_0\|^2_{L^\infty} + \frac{\partial\eta_0}{\partial x}\|^2_{L^\infty} + T\|\frac{\partial\hat{\eta}}{\partial t}\|^2_{L^2(0,T;H^{5/2})}\Big)\|\nabla\hat{P}_0\|^2_{L^2(0,T;L^2)}\\
& + c\Big(\|\frac{\partial\hat{\eta}}{\partial t}\|^2_{L^2(0,T;H^{3/2})} + \|\frac{\partial\hat{\eta}}{\partial t}\|^2_{H^{3/4}(0,T;L^2)} + \|\frac{\partial^2\hat{\eta}}{\partial t^2}\|^2_{L^2(0,T;H^{-1/2})}\Big).
\end{aligned}
\tag{8.67}
$$

8.4.4 The fixed point procedure

From the inequalities

$$
\|\frac{\partial\hat{\eta}}{\partial t}\|_{L^2(0,T;H^{3/2})} \leq cT^{1/2}\|\frac{\partial\hat{\eta}}{\partial t}\|_{L^\infty(0,T;H^{3/2})}
$$

and

$$
\|\frac{\partial\hat{\eta}}{\partial t}\|_{H^{3/4}(0,T;L^2)} \leq c\|\frac{\partial\hat{\eta}}{\partial t}\|^{1/4}_{H^{3/4}(0,T;L^2)}\|\frac{\partial\hat{\eta}}{\partial t}\|^{3/4}_{H^1(0,T;H^{-1/2})}
$$

we first derive that

$$
\begin{aligned}
&\|\frac{\partial\hat{\eta}}{\partial t}\|_{H^{3/4}(0,T;L^2)} \leq\\
&\qquad cT^{1/8}\Big(\|\hat{\eta}\|_{L^\infty(0,T;H^{3/2})} + \|\frac{\partial\hat{\eta}}{\partial t}\|^{1/4}_{L^\infty(0,T;H^{3/2})}\|\frac{\partial^2\hat{\eta}}{\partial t^2}\|^{3/4}_{L^2(0,T;H^{-1/2})}\Big).
\end{aligned}
$$

We have illustrated here the way to incorporate some dependency on T in the estimates similar as those that have been used to get e.g., (8.67). Summing up, we derive that for a small enough T, the mapping $\mathcal{T} : (\hat{\eta}, \hat{\boldsymbol{u}}_f, \nabla\hat{p}) \longrightarrow (\tilde{\eta}, \tilde{\boldsymbol{u}_f}, \nabla\tilde{p})$ maps $\mathbb{K}$ into itself, provided that we choose

$$
\mathbb{K} = \{(\hat{\eta}, \hat{\boldsymbol{u}_f}, \nabla\hat{p})|, |||\hat{\boldsymbol{u}_f}, \nabla\hat{p}||| \leq K_0, |||\hat{\eta}||| \leq K_1, \|\frac{\partial^2\eta}{\partial t^2}|||^2_{L^2(0,T;H^{-1/2})} \leq K_2\}
$$

with three constants K_0, K_1 and K_2 appropriately chosen. In addition $\mathbb{K}$ is a compact subset of $L^2(0,T;L^2) \times L^2(0,T;L^2) \times H^{-1}(0,T;L^2)$.

The Schauder theorem can be applied to get a fixed point of $\mathcal{T}$ once it is checked that $\mathcal{T}$ is continuous with respect to the $L^2(0,T;L^2) \times L^2(0,T;L^2) \times$

$H^{-1}(0,T;L^2)$-topology, which is done in detail in [33]. This proves the existence of the solution to the problem in the ALE form. The regularities on the solution are sufficient to turn back to the original variables (t,x,y). By using the inverse transform to (8.54), we obtain a solution $(\eta, \boldsymbol{u}_f, P)$ to the fluid vessel coupling problem.

As a final remark, it should be noted that in this section and in the previous one, the regular feature of the structure is a fundamental ingredient for the proof of the existence of a solution. Indeed in both of these analyses, the presence of a visco-elastic contribution leads to increased stability that gives enough compactness to the solutions. Independently of the theoretical question, which at this point remains unanswered, of whether the coupled problem with standard elasticity (i.e. with no visco-elastic contribution) is well posed or not, this rings a bell at the level of the numerical simulation since most of the time no such visco-elastic contribution is incorporated in the models. It is well known however that discretisation schemes classically add inherent viscosity contributions to the original model. First this could be the reason why such terms are not needed in the current simulations; second, if the visco-elastic terms are revealed to be mandatory at the continuous level, this might lead to some problems if the discretisation parameters tend to zero. Until now this question has remained unsolved in this conformation. Nevertheless, we refer to the papers of Coutand and Shkoller [103, 104] where the elastic body, floating *within* a fluid, is analysed and no such viscoelastic term is added. The new ingredient in that paper is the analysis of the fluid part in a hyperbolic-type functional framework that, at the price of increased compatibility assessments between the initial and boundary conditions, allows the increased regularisation of the elastic behaviour to be discarded. These results have not yet been extended to the configuration we are interested in, in this chapter, and that deals with a fluid inside an elastic envelop.

8.5 A full interaction problem with zero structural mass

The model we consider in this last section corresponds to a more complete analysis. This work, done by Cheng, Coutand and Shkoller [13], deals with the full fluid-structure interaction problem where the fluid, modelled by the viscous incompressible equations, is enclosed by a moving thin nonlinear elastic shell. The three-dimensional fluid interacts here with a structure represented by a two-dimensional quasilinear elastic model of Koiter shell type which is directly derived from the asymptotic expansion in the nonlinear three-dimensional Saint-Venant Kirchhoff equations when the thickness of the shell converges to zero. The motion of the structure is assumed to be inertia-free, nevertheless the main difficulty of the coupling is present since the shape of the fluid domain is nonstationary and unknown.

8.5.1 Navier-Stokes/Koiter coupling

We denote again by Ω_{f0} an open bounded domain in $\mathbb{R}^3$ with boundary $\Gamma_0 = \partial\Omega_{f0}$. For each time $t \in (0,T)$ we look for a volume-preserving transformation $\boldsymbol{\eta}(t,.)$: $\Omega_{f0} \longrightarrow \mathbb{R}^3$, a domain $\Omega_f(t) = \boldsymbol{\eta}(t,\Omega_{f0})$, a divergence-free velocity field $\boldsymbol{u}_f(t,.)$ and a pressure $P(t,.)$ defined over $\Omega_f(t,.)$ such that, in addition to (8.1), (8.2) valid with $\Omega_f = \Omega_f(t)$, we have

$$\boldsymbol{\eta}_t(t,x) = \boldsymbol{u}_f(t,\boldsymbol{\eta}(t,x)) \tag{8.68}$$

complemented with the interface conditions

$$2\nu \boldsymbol{D}\boldsymbol{u}_f.\boldsymbol{n} - P\boldsymbol{n} = t_{shell}, \qquad \text{over } \Gamma(t) = \boldsymbol{\eta}(t,\Gamma_0) \tag{8.69}$$

(where the traction vector t_{shell} will be detailed later) and subject to the initial conditions

$$\begin{cases} \boldsymbol{u}_f(0) = u_0, & \text{over } \Omega_{f0}, \\ \boldsymbol{\eta}(0,x) = x, & \forall x \in \Omega_{fC}. \end{cases} \tag{8.70}$$

In the widest generality, the traction vector t_{shell} is derived from the nonlinear Saint Venant-Kirchhoff constitutive law by cancelling out the first variation of the hyperelastic stored energy:

$$E_{shall} = \varepsilon E_{mem} + \varepsilon^3 E_{ben}$$

where ε stands for the thickness of the shell and where the membrane energy satisfies

$$E_{mem} = \int_{\gamma(t)} \Big[\frac{\mu}{4}\sum_{\alpha,\beta=1}^{2}(g_{\alpha\beta} - g_{0\alpha\beta})^2 + \frac{\mu\lambda}{4(2\mu+\lambda)}\Big(\sum_{\alpha=1}^{2}(g_{\alpha\alpha} - g_{0\alpha\alpha})\Big)^2\Big]ds$$

while the bending energy E_{ben} is given by

$$E_{ben} = \int_{\Gamma(t)} \big[(4\mu + 2\lambda)H^2 - 2\mu K\big]ds.$$

In the previous expression, g denotes the induced metric on the surface $\Gamma(t)$, H and K denote the mean and Gauss curvature on $\Gamma(t)$, and $\lambda/2$ and $\mu/2$ are the Lamé constants (see [95]).

Adopting a local coordinate system in a tubular neighborhood of Γ_0 composed of tangential coordinates y^1 and y^2 and a normal one, the bending traction has the form of a, possibly degenerate, fourth-order tangent derivative operator acting on the normal displacement h taking the form

$$\frac{1}{\sqrt{\det(g)}}\frac{\partial^2}{\partial y^\gamma \partial y^\delta}\Big[\sqrt{\det(g)}A^{\alpha\beta\gamma\delta}\frac{\partial^2 h}{\partial y^\alpha \partial y^\beta}\Big]$$

(where $A^{\alpha\beta\gamma\delta}$ is a fourth-rank tensor) plus some lower-order terms, whereas the membrane traction is a second-order derivative operator.

8.5.2 Lagrangian formulation of the problem

Following the strategy developed in two former papers by Coutand and Shkoller [103, 104], the analysis is performed on the Lagrangian formulation of the problem. Hence after introducing the Lagrangian velocity $\boldsymbol{v}_f = \boldsymbol{u}_f \circ \boldsymbol{\eta}$ and the Lagrangian pressure $q = P \circ \boldsymbol{\eta}$ and $F = f \circ \boldsymbol{\eta}$ the coupled system can be rewritten as

$$
\begin{array}{lll}
\boldsymbol{\eta}_t & = \boldsymbol{v}_f, & \text{in } (0,T) \times \Omega_{f0}, \\
{\boldsymbol{v}_f}^i_t - \nu(a^j_\ell D_{\boldsymbol{\eta}}(\boldsymbol{v}_f)^i_\ell)_{,j} & = -(a^k_i q)_{,k} + F^i & \text{in } (0,T) \times \Omega_{f0}, \\
a^k_i {\boldsymbol{v}_f}^i_{,k} & = 0 & \text{in } (0,T) \times \Omega_{f0}, \\
(\nu D_{\boldsymbol{\eta}}(\boldsymbol{v}_f)^i_\ell - q\delta^i_\ell) a^j_\ell \boldsymbol{n}_j & = \varepsilon t_{mem} + \varepsilon^3 t_{ben} & \text{on } (0,T) \times \Gamma_0, \\
h_t & = h_{,\alpha}(\boldsymbol{v}_f \circ \boldsymbol{\eta}^{-\tau})_\alpha + (\boldsymbol{v}_f \circ \boldsymbol{\eta}^{-\tau})_z & \text{on } (0,T) \times \Gamma_0, \\
\boldsymbol{v}_f & = \boldsymbol{u}_{f0} & \text{in } \Omega_{f0}, \\
h & = 0 & \text{on } \Gamma_0, \\
\boldsymbol{\eta}(0,x) & = x, & \forall x \in \Omega_{f0}.
\end{array}
\tag{8.71}
$$

As in the previous sections, the interest of this transformation is to work over a fixed domain so that standard imbedding, compactness and Korn or Poincaré type inequalities are available.

The analysis of this nonlinear problem involves, as in Section 8.3, regularisation operators, one for ensuring that the forcing terms and the initial data are smooth enough, and another one to regularise the right-hand side of the linearised version of the problem. An additional penalisation ingredient is incorporated to take care of the transformed incompressibility constraint. One of the simplest results proved in this paper deals with the case where the membrane contribution is neglected and reads

Theorem 8.3. *Assume the data $\boldsymbol{F}$ satisfies*

$$\boldsymbol{F} \in L^2(0,T; H^2(\Omega_{f0})) \cap H^1(0,T; L^2(\Omega_{f0})), \quad \boldsymbol{F}(0) \in H^1(\Omega_{f0})$$

and that the initial data $\boldsymbol{u}_{f_0} \in H^{5/2}(\Omega_{f0})$ and its trace $\boldsymbol{u}_{f_{0|\Gamma_0}} \in H^{9/2}(\Gamma_0)$, and that the tangential component of $\boldsymbol{D}\boldsymbol{u}_{f_0}.\boldsymbol{n}$ vanishes. Suppose in addition that the shell traction is composed only of bending contributions

$$t_{shell} = t_{ben}.$$

There exists a solution $(\boldsymbol{u}_f, P, h)$ to the full interaction problem in Lagrangian form. More precisely, $\boldsymbol{u}_f \in L^2(0,T, H^3(\Omega_{f0})) \cap H^1(0,T, H^1(\Omega_{f0}))$ and $h \in L^2(0,T; H^{11/2}(\Gamma_0)) \cap H^1(0,T; H^{5/2}(\Gamma_0)) \cap H^2(0,T; H^{1/2}(\Gamma_0)) \cap L^\infty(0,T; H^2(\Gamma_0))$. The solution is unique under appropriate compatibility conditions between initial and boundary data.

8.6 Conclusions

The goal of this chapter was to provide a few ideas on the analysis of the coupled problem of fluid and structure interaction in the framework that best fits the applications that are pursued in this book. The analysis deals with questions of existence of solution to the partial differential equations resulting from the model construction. This involves discussions on the best functional space and even the sense in which the equations are satisfied. As announced in the introduction of the chapter, the difficulty comes from the highly nonlinear features of the equations, the modelling of the interaction involving new nonlinearities to an already nonlinear problem. In addition to the existence of a solution, the derivation of properties of uniqueness and regularity is also of interest both for the analyst and for the numerical analysis who has to choose the most appropriate discretisation scheme and algorithm to get an approximation of the solution. Some of these results appear in the references quoted in this chapter but the situation is still unresolved and there is a need for further contributions to answer some open questions. One of the most intriguing is whether a visco-elastic assumption for the structure model is required.

9

Algorithms for fluid-structure interaction problems

Miguel A. Fernández and Jean-Frédéric Gerbeau

Fluid-structure coupled problems and their analysis have been addressed in the previous chapters (particularly in Chapter 3 and Chapter 8). In this chapter, we present some computational issues encountered in the resolution of these problems and propose efficient algorithms to solve them.

A fluid-structure problem is defined by the fluid equations, the structure equations and by the transmission conditions at the fluid-structure interface $\Gamma(t)$:

$$\boldsymbol{u}_f = \boldsymbol{u}_s, \tag{9.1}$$

$$\boldsymbol{\sigma}_f \cdot \boldsymbol{n}_f + \boldsymbol{\sigma}_s \cdot \boldsymbol{n}_s = 0. \tag{9.2}$$

We will show in Section 9.1 that these conditions are the key ingredients when deriving the energy equality of the continuous fluid-structure system. After discretisation, a straightforward way to satisfy the discrete counterpart of (9.1) and (9.2) is to simultaneously solve the fluid and the structure problems in a unique solver. This approach is usually referred to as a *monolithic* method. When relations (9.1) and (9.2) are satisfied after time discretisation, one says that the method is *strongly coupled.* A monolithic method is typically strongly coupled and, hopefully, is stable in the energy norm. However, this approach needs *ad hoc* software development and results in a global solver which is less modular than two distinct fluid and structure solvers. In particular it is difficult to devise efficient global preconditioners and to maintain state-of-the-art schemes in each solver. With the so-called *partitioned* procedures (sometimes called *segregated*), the fluid and the structure are solved with their own software. This increases the capabilities of evolution and optimisation of each code. Among the partitioned schemes, we have to distinguish the *weakly* coupled ones from the *strongly* coupled. A scheme is said to be *weakly* (or *loosely* or *explicit*) coupled when (9.1) and (9.2) are not exactly satisfied at each time step or, in other words, when a spurious numerical power appears on the fluid-structure interface. Let us emphasise that a *partitioned* scheme is not necessarily *weakly* coupled: when sub-iterations are performed

Formaggia L, Quarteroni A, Veneziani A (Eds.): Cardiovascular Mathematics. Modeling and simulation of the circulatory system

at each time step, the transmission conditions (9.1) and (9.2) can be enforced with a high accuracy even though two different solvers are used. Nevertheless, partitioned procedures are often used to implement weakly coupled schemes. Indeed, many fluid-structure interaction problems, in particular in aeroelasticity, can be solved in practice without enforcing exactly (9.1) and (9.2). We will show in Section 9.2 on a toy model why it may be very difficult to achieve stability in blood flows with loosely coupled algorithms. This is the reason why several strongly coupled schemes have been proposed in the literature. We will present some of them in Section 9.3. We will show in Section 9.4 that it is in fact possible to avoid strong coupling without compromising stability, even for blood flows. In Section 9.5, we give some hints to compute the load on the structure after space discretisation in various cases of interest.

9.1 The coupled fluid-structure problem

At this stage, we assume that the reader is familiar with the basic notions of kinematics and mechanics introduced in Chapter 3. As shown in Section 3.5, the interaction of an incompressible viscous fluid and a hyperelastic structure is governed by a system of partial differential equations, which we repeat here for the sake of convenience.

- Fluid sub-problem:

$$\left\{\begin{aligned} \rho_f \frac{\partial \boldsymbol{u}_f}{\partial t}_{|\widetilde{\mathcal{A}}} + \rho_f(\boldsymbol{u}_f - \boldsymbol{w}) \cdot \boldsymbol{\nabla} \boldsymbol{u}_f - \mathbf{div} \boldsymbol{\sigma}(\boldsymbol{u}_f, P) = \mathbf{0}, &\quad \text{in} \quad \Omega_f(t), \\ \operatorname{div} \boldsymbol{u}_f = 0, &\quad \text{in} \quad \Omega_f(t), \\ \boldsymbol{\sigma}(\boldsymbol{u}_f, P)\boldsymbol{n}_f = \boldsymbol{g}_{f,N}, &\quad \text{on} \quad \Gamma_{f,N}. \end{aligned}\right. \tag{9.3}$$

- Solid sub-problem:

$$\left\{\begin{aligned} \hat{\rho}_{s,0} \frac{\partial^2 \widehat{\boldsymbol{\eta}}_s}{\partial t^2} - \mathbf{div}_{\widehat{\boldsymbol{x}}} \big(\widehat{\boldsymbol{F}}_s \widehat{\boldsymbol{\Sigma}}\big) = \mathbf{0}, &\quad \text{in} \quad \widehat{\Omega_s}, \\ \widehat{\boldsymbol{\eta}}_s = \mathbf{0}, &\quad \text{on} \quad \widehat{\Gamma}_{s,D}, \\ \widehat{\boldsymbol{F}}_s \widehat{\boldsymbol{\Sigma}} \widehat{\boldsymbol{n}}_s = \mathbf{0}, &\quad \text{on} \quad \widehat{\Gamma}_{s,N}. \end{aligned}\right. \tag{9.4}$$

- Coupling conditions:

$$\left\{\begin{aligned} \widetilde{\boldsymbol{\eta}}_f = \operatorname{Ext}(\widehat{\boldsymbol{\eta}}_{s|\widehat{\Gamma}}), \quad \Omega_f(t) = \widetilde{\mathcal{A}}(\widehat{\Omega_f}, t), \quad \widehat{\boldsymbol{w}} = \frac{\partial \widetilde{\boldsymbol{\eta}}_f}{\partial t}, &\quad \text{in} \quad \widehat{\Omega_f}, \\ \boldsymbol{u}_f = \boldsymbol{w}, &\quad \text{on} \quad \Gamma(t), \\ \widehat{\boldsymbol{F}}_s \widehat{\boldsymbol{\Sigma}} \widehat{\boldsymbol{n}}_s + \widetilde{J}_{\widetilde{\mathcal{A}}} \widehat{\boldsymbol{\sigma}}(\boldsymbol{u}_f, P) \widetilde{\boldsymbol{F}}_{\widetilde{\mathcal{A}}}^{-T} \widehat{\boldsymbol{n}}_f = 0, &\quad \text{on} \quad \widehat{\Gamma}, \end{aligned}\right. \tag{9.5}$$

where the unknowns are: the fluid domain displacement $\widetilde{\boldsymbol{\eta}}_f : \widehat{\Omega_f} \times \mathbb{R}^+ \longrightarrow \mathbb{R}^3$, the fluid velocity $\widehat{\boldsymbol{u}}_f : \widehat{\Omega_f} \times \mathbb{R}^+ \longrightarrow \mathbb{R}^3$, the fluid pressure $\widehat{P} : \widehat{\Omega_f} \times \mathbb{R}^+ \longrightarrow \mathbb{R}$

and the structure displacement $\widehat{\boldsymbol{\eta}}_s : \widehat{\Omega_s} \times \mathbb{R}^+ \longrightarrow \mathbb{R}^3$. We recall that $\widetilde{\mathcal{A}}$ denotes the ALE application that maps the reference fluid configuration $\widehat{\Omega_f}$ onto the current fluid configuration $\Omega_f(t)$, $\boldsymbol{w}$ denotes the fluid domain velocity and, for any function $\widehat{q}$ defined on $\widehat{\Omega_f}$, its Eulerian counterpart q is defined by $q(x) = \widehat{q}(\widehat{x})$ for $x = \widetilde{\mathcal{A}}(\widehat{x}, t)$.

9.1.1 Energy balance

In this paragraph we extend the formal *a priori* energy analysis performed in Chapter 8 to the case of the general fluid-structure interaction problem (9.3)–(9.5). Note that, here, the fluid domain $\Omega_f(t)$ is not necessarily a material domain and the fluid equations (9.3) are written in ALE form. As expected, dissipation only comes from the fluid viscosity and the power exchanged by the fluid and the structure exactly balance at the interface. This balance is a direct consequence of the coupling conditions (9.5).

Proposition 9.1. *Assume that the coupled fluid-structure system is isolated, i.e.,* $\boldsymbol{u}_f = \boldsymbol{0}$ *on* $\partial\Omega_f(t)\backslash\Gamma(t)$, $\widehat{\boldsymbol{F}}_s\widehat{\boldsymbol{\Sigma}}\widehat{\boldsymbol{n}}_s = \boldsymbol{0}$ *on* $\partial\widehat{\Omega_s}\backslash\widehat{\Gamma}$, *then the following energy balance holds:*

$$\frac{\mathrm{d}}{\mathrm{d}t}\Bigg[\underbrace{\int_{\Omega_f(t)} \frac{\rho_f}{2}|\boldsymbol{u}_f|^2\,\mathrm{d}\boldsymbol{x} + \int_{\widehat{\Omega_s}} \frac{\hat{\rho}_{s,0}}{2}|\widehat{\boldsymbol{u}_s}|^2\,\mathrm{d}\hat{\boldsymbol{x}}}_{\textit{Kinetic energy}} + \underbrace{\int_{\widehat{\Omega_s}} W(\widehat{\boldsymbol{E}})\,\mathrm{d}\hat{\boldsymbol{x}}}_{\textit{Elastic potential energy}}\Bigg] + \underbrace{\int_{\Omega_f(t)} 2\mu|\boldsymbol{D}(\boldsymbol{u}_f)|^2\,\mathrm{d}\boldsymbol{x}}_{\textit{Dissipated viscous power}} = 0. \tag{9.6}$$

The density of elastic energy W has been defined in (3.55).

Proof. We multiply the fluid equation $(9.3)_1$ by $\boldsymbol{u}_f$ and the solid equation $(9.4)_1$ by $\widehat{\boldsymbol{u}_s}$; we integrate by parts and use the boundary conditions. Finally, we add the resulting expressions by noticing that the interface integral contributions cancel thanks to the coupling conditions.

For the mass term in the fluid, using the change of variables $x = \widetilde{\mathcal{A}}(\hat{x}, t)$ and (3.26), we have

$$\begin{aligned}
\int_{\Omega_f(t)} \rho_f \frac{\partial \boldsymbol{u}_f}{\partial t}_{|\widetilde{\mathcal{A}}} \cdot \boldsymbol{u}_f\,\mathrm{d}\boldsymbol{x} &= \int_{\widehat{\Omega_f}} \rho_f \widetilde{J}_{\widetilde{\mathcal{A}}} \frac{\partial \widehat{\boldsymbol{u}_f}}{\partial t} \cdot \widehat{\boldsymbol{u}_f}\,\mathrm{d}\hat{\boldsymbol{x}} \\
&= \int_{\widehat{\Omega_f}} \frac{\rho_f}{2} \frac{\partial\big(\widetilde{J}_{\widetilde{\mathcal{A}}}|\widehat{\boldsymbol{u}_f}|^2\big)}{\partial t}\,\mathrm{d}\hat{\boldsymbol{x}} - \int_{\widehat{\Omega_f}} \frac{\rho_f}{2} \widetilde{J}_{\widetilde{\mathcal{A}}} \widehat{\mathrm{div}\,\boldsymbol{w}}|\widehat{\boldsymbol{u}_f}|^2\,\mathrm{d}\hat{\boldsymbol{x}} \\
&= \frac{\mathrm{d}}{\mathrm{d}t}\left[\int_{\Omega_f(t)} \frac{\rho_f}{2}|\widehat{\boldsymbol{u}_f}|^2\,\mathrm{d}\boldsymbol{x}\right] - \int_{\Omega_f(t)} \frac{\rho_f}{2}\,\mathrm{div}\,\boldsymbol{w}|\boldsymbol{u}_f|^2\,\mathrm{d}\boldsymbol{x}.
\end{aligned}$$

For the convective term, since $\operatorname{div} \boldsymbol{u}_f = 0$, integrating by parts, using the boundary conditions and the equality $\boldsymbol{u}_f = \boldsymbol{w}$ on $\Gamma(t)$, we have

$$\int_{\Omega_f(t)} \rho_f (\boldsymbol{u}_f - \boldsymbol{w}) \cdot \boldsymbol{\nabla} \boldsymbol{u}_f \cdot \boldsymbol{u}_f \, \mathrm{d}\boldsymbol{x} = \int_{\Omega_f(t)} \frac{\rho_f}{2} (\boldsymbol{u}_f - \boldsymbol{w}) \cdot \boldsymbol{\nabla} |\boldsymbol{u}_f|^2 \, \mathrm{d}\boldsymbol{x}$$
$$= \int_{\Omega_f(t)} \frac{\rho_f}{2} \operatorname{div} \boldsymbol{w} |\boldsymbol{u}_f|^2 \, \mathrm{d}\boldsymbol{x}.$$

For the stress term, integrating by parts we have

$$\begin{aligned} - \int_{\Omega_f(t)} \mathbf{div} \boldsymbol{\sigma}_f(\boldsymbol{u}_f, P) \cdot \boldsymbol{u}_f \, \mathrm{d}\boldsymbol{x} &= \int_{\Omega_f(t)} \boldsymbol{\sigma}_f(\boldsymbol{u}_f, P) : \boldsymbol{\nabla} \boldsymbol{u}_f \, \mathrm{d}\boldsymbol{x} \\ &\quad - \int_{\partial \Omega_f(t)} \boldsymbol{\sigma}_f(\boldsymbol{u}_f, P) \boldsymbol{n}_f \cdot \boldsymbol{u}_f \, \mathrm{d}\gamma \\ &= \int_{\Omega_f(t)} 2\mu \boldsymbol{D}(\boldsymbol{u}_f) : \boldsymbol{D}(\boldsymbol{u}_f) \, \mathrm{d}\boldsymbol{x} \\ &\quad - \int_{\Gamma(t)} \boldsymbol{\sigma}_f(\boldsymbol{u}_f, P) \boldsymbol{n}_f \cdot \boldsymbol{u}_f \, \mathrm{d}\gamma. \end{aligned}$$

Therefore, by adding these three contributions we have the following energy balance in the fluid:

$$\frac{\mathrm{d}}{\mathrm{d}t} \left[\int_{\Omega_f(t)} \frac{\rho_f}{2} |\boldsymbol{u}_f|^2 \, \mathrm{d}\boldsymbol{x} \right] + \int_{\Omega_f(t)} 2\mu |\boldsymbol{D}(\boldsymbol{u}_f)|^2 \, \mathrm{d}\boldsymbol{x} - \int_{\Gamma(t)} \boldsymbol{\sigma}_f(\boldsymbol{u}_f, P) \boldsymbol{n}_f \cdot \boldsymbol{u}_f \, \mathrm{d}\gamma = 0. \tag{9.7}$$

For the mass terms in the solid, we readily obtain

$$\int_{\widehat{\Omega}_s} \hat{\rho}_{s,0} \frac{\partial^2 \widehat{\boldsymbol{\eta}}_s}{\partial t^2} \cdot \frac{\partial \widehat{\boldsymbol{\eta}}_s}{\partial t} \, \mathrm{d}\hat{\boldsymbol{x}} = \frac{\mathrm{d}}{\mathrm{d}t} \int_{\widehat{\Omega}_s} \frac{\hat{\rho}_{s,0}}{2} |\hat{\boldsymbol{u}}_s|^2 \, \mathrm{d}\hat{\boldsymbol{x}}. \tag{9.8}$$

For the stress term, integrating by parts and using the boundary conditions we have

$$- \int_{\widehat{\Omega}_s} \mathbf{div}_{\hat{\boldsymbol{x}}} (\widehat{\boldsymbol{F}}_s \widehat{\boldsymbol{\Sigma}}) \cdot \hat{\boldsymbol{u}}_s \, \mathrm{d}\hat{\boldsymbol{x}} = \int_{\widehat{\Omega}_s} \widehat{\boldsymbol{F}}_s \widehat{\boldsymbol{\Sigma}} : \boldsymbol{\nabla}_{\hat{\boldsymbol{x}}} \hat{\boldsymbol{u}}_s \, \mathrm{d}\hat{\boldsymbol{x}} - \int_{\widehat{\Gamma}} \widehat{\boldsymbol{F}}_s \widehat{\boldsymbol{\Sigma}} \widehat{\boldsymbol{n}}_s \cdot \hat{\boldsymbol{u}}_s \, \mathrm{d}\hat{\gamma}. \tag{9.9}$$

On the other hand, since $\widehat{\boldsymbol{\Sigma}}$ is symmetric and using (3.53), it follows that

$$\begin{aligned} \widehat{\boldsymbol{F}}_s \widehat{\boldsymbol{\Sigma}} : \boldsymbol{\nabla}_{\hat{\boldsymbol{x}}} \hat{\boldsymbol{u}}_s &= \widehat{\boldsymbol{F}}_s \widehat{\boldsymbol{\Sigma}} : \frac{\partial \widehat{\boldsymbol{F}}_s}{\partial t} = \frac{\partial \widehat{\boldsymbol{F}}_s}{\partial t} \widehat{\boldsymbol{F}}_s : \widehat{\boldsymbol{\Sigma}} \\ &= \frac{1}{2} \left(\frac{\partial \widehat{\boldsymbol{F}}_s^T}{\partial t} \widehat{\boldsymbol{F}}_s + \widehat{\boldsymbol{F}}_s^T \frac{\partial \widehat{\boldsymbol{F}}_s}{\partial t} \right) : \widehat{\boldsymbol{\Sigma}} = \frac{\partial \widehat{\boldsymbol{E}}}{\partial t} : \widehat{\boldsymbol{\Sigma}}. \end{aligned}$$

In addition, since the material is hyperelastic, we have

$$\widehat{\boldsymbol{F}}_s \widehat{\boldsymbol{\Sigma}} : \boldsymbol{\nabla}_{\hat{\boldsymbol{x}}} \hat{\boldsymbol{u}}_s = \frac{\partial \widehat{\boldsymbol{E}}}{\partial t} : \widehat{\boldsymbol{\Sigma}} = \frac{\partial \widehat{\boldsymbol{E}}}{\partial t} : \frac{\partial \widehat{W}}{\partial \widehat{\boldsymbol{E}}} (\widehat{\boldsymbol{E}}) = \frac{\partial W(\widehat{\boldsymbol{E}})}{\partial t},$$

and, therefore from (9.9),

$$\begin{aligned}\int_{\widehat{\Omega}_s} \widehat{\boldsymbol{F}}_s \widehat{\boldsymbol{\Sigma}} : \boldsymbol{\nabla}_{\hat{\boldsymbol{x}}} \hat{\boldsymbol{u}}_s \,\mathrm{d}\hat{\boldsymbol{x}} &= \int_{\widehat{\Omega}_s} \frac{\partial W(\widehat{\boldsymbol{E}})}{\partial t} \,\mathrm{d}\hat{\boldsymbol{x}} - \int_{\widehat{\Gamma}} \widehat{\boldsymbol{F}}_s \widehat{\boldsymbol{\Sigma}} \widehat{\boldsymbol{n}}_s \cdot \hat{\boldsymbol{u}}_s \,\mathrm{d}\hat{\gamma} \\ &= \frac{\mathrm{d}}{\mathrm{d}t} \int_{\widehat{\Omega}_s} W(\widehat{\boldsymbol{E}}) \,\mathrm{d}\hat{\boldsymbol{x}} - \int_{\widehat{\Gamma}} \widehat{\boldsymbol{F}}_s \widehat{\boldsymbol{\Sigma}} \widehat{\boldsymbol{n}}_s \cdot \hat{\boldsymbol{u}}_s \,\mathrm{d}\hat{\gamma}.\end{aligned}$$

Finally, by combining this last equality with (9.8), we get the following energy balance for the solid

$$\frac{\mathrm{d}}{\mathrm{d}t} \int_{\widehat{\Omega}_s} \frac{\hat{\rho}_{s,0}}{2} |\hat{\boldsymbol{u}}_s|^2 \,\mathrm{d}\hat{\boldsymbol{x}} + \frac{\mathrm{d}}{\mathrm{d}t} \int_{\widehat{\Omega}_s} W(\widehat{\boldsymbol{E}}) \,\mathrm{d}\hat{\boldsymbol{x}} - \int_{\widehat{\Gamma}} \widehat{\boldsymbol{F}}_s \widehat{\boldsymbol{\Sigma}} \widehat{\boldsymbol{n}}_s \cdot \hat{\boldsymbol{u}}_s \,\mathrm{d}\hat{\gamma} = 0.$$

We then conclude the proof by adding this equality to (9.7) and using the interface coupling conditions (9.1) and (9.2).

9.1.2 Variational formulation

Problem (9.3)–(9.5) can be reformulated in a weak variational form using appropriate test functions, performing integrations by parts and taking into account the boundary and interface conditions.

Let $\hat{\boldsymbol{v}}_f : \widehat{\Omega_f} \longrightarrow \mathbb{R}^3$ and $\widehat{q} : \widehat{\Omega_f} \longrightarrow \mathbb{R}$ be time-independent smooth functions. We will take as test functions their Eulerian counterparts defined by

$$\boldsymbol{v}_f(\boldsymbol{x}, t) = \hat{\boldsymbol{v}}_f(\widetilde{\mathcal{A}}_t^{-1}(\boldsymbol{x})), \quad q(\boldsymbol{x}, t) = \widehat{q}(\widetilde{\mathcal{A}}_t^{-1}(\boldsymbol{x})),$$

for all $\boldsymbol{x} \in \Omega_f(t)$. Notice that, in contrast to test functions on fixed domains, these functions are time-dependent. However, since $\hat{\boldsymbol{v}}_f$ is independent of t, $\boldsymbol{v}_f$ has zero ALE time-derivative

$$\frac{\partial \boldsymbol{v}_f}{\partial t}_{|\widetilde{\mathcal{A}}} = \mathbf{0}. \tag{9.10}$$

The same property holds for q.

By multiplying the fluid equation $(9.3)_{1,2}$ by $(\boldsymbol{v}_f, q)$, integrating by parts and taking into account the boundary conditions, we get

$$\begin{aligned}\int_{\Omega_f(t)} \rho_f \frac{\partial \boldsymbol{u}_f}{\partial t}_{|\widetilde{\mathcal{A}}} \cdot \boldsymbol{v}_f \,\mathrm{d}\boldsymbol{x} &+ \int_{\Omega_f(t)} \rho_f (\boldsymbol{u}_f - \boldsymbol{w}) \cdot \boldsymbol{\nabla} \boldsymbol{u}_f \cdot \boldsymbol{v}_f \,\mathrm{d}\boldsymbol{x} \\ &+ \int_{\Omega_f(t)} \boldsymbol{\sigma}_f(\boldsymbol{u}_f, P) : \boldsymbol{\nabla} \boldsymbol{v}_f \,\mathrm{d}\boldsymbol{x} - \int_{\Gamma_{f,N}(t)} \boldsymbol{g}_{f,N} \cdot \boldsymbol{v}_f \,\mathrm{d}\gamma \\ &- \int_{\Gamma(t)} \boldsymbol{\sigma}_f(\boldsymbol{u}_f, P) \boldsymbol{n}_f \cdot \boldsymbol{v}_f \,\mathrm{d}\gamma + \int_{\Omega_f(t)} q \operatorname{div} \boldsymbol{u}_f \,\mathrm{d}\boldsymbol{x} = 0. \end{aligned} \tag{9.11}$$

Using a change of variables in the first integral in combination with (9.10) and since ρ_f is assumed to be constant, it follows that

$$\begin{aligned}\int_{\Omega_f(t)} \rho_f \frac{\partial \boldsymbol{u}_f}{\partial t}_{|\widetilde{\mathcal{A}}} \cdot \boldsymbol{v}_f \, \mathrm{d}\boldsymbol{x} &= \int_{\widehat{\Omega_f}} \rho_f \widetilde{J}_{\widetilde{\mathcal{A}}} \frac{\partial \widehat{\boldsymbol{u}_f}}{\partial t} \cdot \widehat{\boldsymbol{v}_f} \, \mathrm{d}\hat{\boldsymbol{x}} \\ &= \frac{\mathrm{d}}{\mathrm{d}t} \int_{\widehat{\Omega_f}} \widetilde{J}_{\widetilde{\mathcal{A}}} \rho_f \widehat{\boldsymbol{u}_f} \cdot \widehat{\boldsymbol{v}_f} \, \mathrm{d}\hat{\boldsymbol{x}} - \int_{\widehat{\Omega_f}} \widetilde{J}_{\widetilde{\mathcal{A}}} \rho_f \widehat{\operatorname{div} \boldsymbol{w} \boldsymbol{u}_f} \cdot \widehat{\boldsymbol{v}_f} \, \mathrm{d}\hat{\boldsymbol{x}} \\ &= \frac{\mathrm{d}}{\mathrm{d}t} \int_{\Omega_f(t)} \rho_f \boldsymbol{u}_f \cdot \boldsymbol{v}_f \, \mathrm{d}\boldsymbol{x} - \int_{\Omega_f(t)} \rho_f \operatorname{div} \boldsymbol{w} \boldsymbol{u}_f \cdot \boldsymbol{v}_f \, \mathrm{d}\boldsymbol{x}.\end{aligned}$$

In addition, using the properties of the Piola transformation (see Proposition 3.2 in Chapter 3) we have

$$\int_{\Gamma(t)} \boldsymbol{\sigma}_f(\boldsymbol{u}_f, P)\boldsymbol{n}_f \cdot \boldsymbol{v}_f \, \mathrm{d}\gamma = \int_{\widehat{\Gamma}} \widetilde{J}_{\widetilde{\mathcal{A}}} \widehat{\boldsymbol{\sigma}(\boldsymbol{u}_f, P)} \widetilde{\boldsymbol{F}}_{\widetilde{\mathcal{A}}}^{-T} \widehat{\boldsymbol{n}}_f \cdot \hat{\boldsymbol{v}}_f \, \mathrm{d}\hat{\gamma}.$$

Finally, by inserting these two equalities in (9.11), we can see that $(\boldsymbol{u}_f, P)$ satisfies

$$\begin{aligned}&\frac{\mathrm{d}}{\mathrm{d}t} \int_{\Omega_f(t)} \rho_f \boldsymbol{u}_f \cdot \boldsymbol{v}_f \, \mathrm{d}\boldsymbol{x} + \int_{\Omega_f(t)} \rho_f (\boldsymbol{u}_f - \boldsymbol{w}) \cdot \boldsymbol{\nabla} \boldsymbol{u}_f \cdot \boldsymbol{v}_f \, \mathrm{d}\boldsymbol{x} \\ &- \int_{\Omega_f(t)} \rho_f (\operatorname{div} \boldsymbol{w}) \boldsymbol{u}_f \cdot \boldsymbol{v}_f \, \mathrm{d}\boldsymbol{x} + \int_{\Omega_f(t)} \boldsymbol{\sigma}_f(\boldsymbol{u}_f, P) : \boldsymbol{\nabla} \boldsymbol{v}_f \, \mathrm{d}\boldsymbol{x} - \int_{\Gamma_{f,N}} \boldsymbol{g}_{f,N} \cdot \boldsymbol{v}_f \, \mathrm{d}\gamma \\ &\qquad - \int_{\widehat{\Gamma}} \widetilde{J}_{\widetilde{\mathcal{A}}} \widehat{\boldsymbol{\sigma}(\boldsymbol{u}_f, P)} \widetilde{\boldsymbol{F}}_{\widetilde{\mathcal{A}}}^{-T} \widehat{\boldsymbol{n}}_f \cdot \hat{\boldsymbol{v}}_f \, \mathrm{d}\hat{\gamma} + \int_{\Omega_f(t)} q \operatorname{div} \boldsymbol{u}_f \, \mathrm{d}\boldsymbol{x} = 0. \qquad (9.12)\end{aligned}$$

On the other hand, multiplying the solid equation $(9.4)_1$ by a smooth function $\hat{\boldsymbol{v}}_s : \widehat{\Omega_s} \longrightarrow \mathbb{R}^3$ vanishing on $\widehat{\Gamma}_{s,D}$, integrating by parts and taking into account the boundary conditions of (9.4), we get

$$\int_{\widehat{\Omega_s}} \hat{\rho}_{s,0} \frac{\partial^2 \widehat{\boldsymbol{\eta}}_s}{\partial t^2} \cdot \hat{\boldsymbol{v}}_s \, \mathrm{d}\hat{\boldsymbol{x}} + \int_{\widehat{\Omega_s}} \widehat{\boldsymbol{F}}_s \widehat{\boldsymbol{\Sigma}} : \boldsymbol{\nabla}_{\hat{\boldsymbol{x}}} \hat{\boldsymbol{v}}_s \, \mathrm{d}\hat{\boldsymbol{x}} - \int_{\widehat{\Gamma}} \widehat{\boldsymbol{F}}_s \widehat{\boldsymbol{\Sigma}} \widehat{\boldsymbol{n}}_s \cdot \hat{\boldsymbol{v}}_s \, \mathrm{d}\hat{\gamma} = 0. \qquad (9.13)$$

After summation of (9.12)–(9.13), taking into account the coupling condition $(9.5)_3$ and assuming that $\hat{\boldsymbol{v}}_f = \hat{\boldsymbol{v}}_s$ on $\widehat{\Gamma}$, we have

$$\begin{aligned}&\frac{\mathrm{d}}{\mathrm{d}t} \int_{\Omega_f(t)} \rho_f \boldsymbol{u}_f \cdot \boldsymbol{v}_f \, \mathrm{d}\boldsymbol{x} + \int_{\Omega_f(t)} \rho_f (\boldsymbol{u}_f - \boldsymbol{w}) \cdot \boldsymbol{\nabla} \boldsymbol{u}_f \cdot \boldsymbol{v}_f \, \mathrm{d}\boldsymbol{x} \\ &- \int_{\Omega_f(t)} \rho_f \operatorname{div} \boldsymbol{w} \, \boldsymbol{u}_f \cdot \boldsymbol{v}_f \, \mathrm{d}\boldsymbol{x} + \int_{\Omega_f(t)} \boldsymbol{\sigma}_f(\boldsymbol{u}_f, P) : \boldsymbol{\nabla} \boldsymbol{v}_f \, \mathrm{d}\boldsymbol{x} - \int_{\Gamma_{f,N}} \boldsymbol{g}_{f,N} \cdot \boldsymbol{v}_f \, \mathrm{d}\gamma \\ &\quad + \int_{\Omega_f(t)} q \operatorname{div} \boldsymbol{u}_f \, \mathrm{d}\boldsymbol{x} + \int_{\widehat{\Omega_s}} \hat{\rho}_{s,0} \frac{\partial^2 \widehat{\boldsymbol{\eta}}_s}{\partial t^2} \cdot \hat{\boldsymbol{v}}_s \, \mathrm{d}\hat{\boldsymbol{x}} + \int_{\widehat{\Omega_s}} \widehat{\boldsymbol{F}}_s \widehat{\boldsymbol{\Sigma}} : \boldsymbol{\nabla}_{\hat{\boldsymbol{x}}} \hat{\boldsymbol{v}}_s \, \mathrm{d}\hat{\boldsymbol{x}} = 0, \\ &\qquad (9.14)\end{aligned}$$

for all $(\hat{\boldsymbol{v}}_f, \widehat{q}) \in [H^1(\widehat{\Omega_f})]^3 \times L^2(\widehat{\Omega_f})$ and $\hat{\boldsymbol{v}}_s \in [H^1_{\widehat{\Gamma}_{s,D}}(\widehat{\Omega_s})]^3$ with $\hat{\boldsymbol{v}}_f = \hat{\boldsymbol{v}}_s$ on $\widehat{\Gamma}$, where L^2 denotes the space of square integrable functions and H^1 the standard Sobolev space of L^2 functions which have first derivatives in L^2.

In what follows, we will make explicit the dependence of $\Omega_f(t)$ and $\Gamma(t)$ on $\widetilde{\boldsymbol{\eta}}_f$ by introducing the notations

$$\Omega_f(\widetilde{\boldsymbol{\eta}}_f) = \Omega_f(t) = (I + \widetilde{\boldsymbol{\eta}}_f)(\widehat{\Omega_f}), \quad \Gamma(\widetilde{\boldsymbol{\eta}}_f) = \Gamma(t).$$

Therefore, after summation of (9.14)–(9.62) we obtain the following global weak formulation of problem (9.3)–(9.5): Find $\widehat{\boldsymbol{u}}_f : \widehat{\Omega_f} \times \mathbb{R}^+ \to \mathbb{R}^3$, $\widehat{P} : \widehat{\Omega_f} \times \mathbb{R}^+ \to \mathbb{R}$, $\widetilde{\boldsymbol{\eta}}_f : \widehat{\Omega_f} \times \mathbb{R}^+ \to \mathbb{R}^3$ and $\widehat{\boldsymbol{\eta}}_s : \widehat{\Omega_s} \times \mathbb{R}^+ \to \mathbb{R}^3$ such that

$$\begin{aligned}
&\widetilde{\boldsymbol{\eta}}_f = \mathrm{Ext}(\widehat{\boldsymbol{\eta}}_{s|\widehat{\Gamma}}), \quad \widehat{\boldsymbol{w}} = \frac{\partial \widetilde{\boldsymbol{\eta}}_f}{\partial t}, && \text{in } \widehat{\Omega_f}, \\
&\boldsymbol{u}_f = \boldsymbol{w}, && \text{on } \Gamma(\widetilde{\boldsymbol{\eta}}_f), \\
&\widehat{\boldsymbol{\eta}}_s = \boldsymbol{0}, && \text{on } \Gamma_{s,D},
\end{aligned} \tag{9.15}$$

and

$$\begin{aligned}
&\frac{\mathrm{d}}{\mathrm{d}t} \int_{\Omega_f(\widetilde{\boldsymbol{\eta}}_f)} \rho_f \boldsymbol{u}_f \cdot \boldsymbol{v}_f \,\mathrm{d}\boldsymbol{x} + \int_{\Omega_f(\widetilde{\boldsymbol{\eta}}_f)} \rho_f (\boldsymbol{u}_f - \boldsymbol{w}) \cdot \boldsymbol{\nabla} \boldsymbol{u}_f \cdot \boldsymbol{v}_f \,\mathrm{d}\boldsymbol{x} \\
&\quad - \int_{\Omega_f(\widetilde{\boldsymbol{\eta}}_f)} \rho_f (\operatorname{div} \boldsymbol{w}) \boldsymbol{u}_f \cdot \boldsymbol{v}_f \,\mathrm{d}\boldsymbol{x} + \int_{\Omega_f(\widetilde{\boldsymbol{\eta}}_f)} \boldsymbol{\sigma}_f(\boldsymbol{u}_f, P) : \boldsymbol{\nabla} \boldsymbol{v}_f \,\mathrm{d}\boldsymbol{x} \\
&\quad - \int_{\Gamma_{f,N}} \boldsymbol{g}_{f,N} \cdot \boldsymbol{v}_f \,\mathrm{d}\gamma + \int_{\Omega_f(\widetilde{\boldsymbol{\eta}}_f)} q \operatorname{div} \boldsymbol{u}_f \,\mathrm{d}\boldsymbol{x} \\
&\quad + \int_{\widehat{\Omega_s}} \hat{\rho}_{s,0} \frac{\partial^2 \widehat{\boldsymbol{\eta}}_s}{\partial t^2} \cdot \hat{\boldsymbol{v}}_s \,\mathrm{d}\hat{\boldsymbol{x}} + \int_{\widehat{\Omega_s}} \widehat{\boldsymbol{F}}_s \widehat{\boldsymbol{\Sigma}} : \boldsymbol{\nabla}_{\hat{\boldsymbol{x}}} \hat{\boldsymbol{v}}_s \,\mathrm{d}\hat{\boldsymbol{x}} = 0,
\end{aligned} \tag{9.16}$$

with $\boldsymbol{u}_f = \widehat{\boldsymbol{u}}_f \circ \widetilde{\mathcal{A}}_t^{-1}$, $P = \widehat{P} \circ \widetilde{\mathcal{A}}_t^{-1}$, and for all $(\hat{\boldsymbol{v}}_f, \widehat{q}) \in [H^1(\widehat{\Omega_f})]^3 \times L^2(\widehat{\Omega_f})$, $\hat{\boldsymbol{v}}_s \in [H^1_{\widehat{\Gamma}_{s,D}}(\widehat{\Omega_s})]^3$ with $\hat{\boldsymbol{v}}_f = \hat{\boldsymbol{v}}_s$ on $\widehat{\Gamma}$.

9.2 Strong *versus* weak coupling

The purpose of this section, mainly based on [70], is to address stability issues of both strongly and loosely coupled methods applied to a "toy model" which can be regarded as a simplified version of (9.3)–(9.5). This model represents the interaction between a potential fluid and a linear elastic thin tube. It cannot describe complex situations, like fluid-structure interaction in arteries, since, for example, it does not include nonlinearities and dissipation phenomena. Nevertheless, it retains important physical features of more complex models: in particular, it reproduces propagation phenomena and takes into account the added-mass effect of the fluid on the structure, which is known to induce numerical difficulties [272]. This model problem is simple enough to perform mathematical and numerical studies but, at the same time, complex enough to mimic more realistic situations, at least in the case of incompressible fluids. As will be shown in Sections 9.2.4 and 9.2.5, starting from this simple FSI model, we are able to derive stability and convergence conditions that are in excellent agreement with the numerical observations collected in much more complex situations. Moreover, this simplified FSI model is also helpful in devising new and more efficient coupled algorithms, as will been shown in Section 9.4.

9.2.1 Motivations

In order to motivate the subsequent discussions, we recall some empirical observations made on a basic FSI test case proposed in previous studies (see [155,188,351]). The goal of this test case is to simulate, in a very idealised framework, the mechanical interaction between blood and arterial wall. The geometry at rest is a cylinder. The fluid is described by the incompressible Navier-Stokes equations in Arbitrary Lagrangian Eulerian formulation (9.3). The structure is described either by a 1D generalised string model (see Section 3.4.4) when the fluid is 2D or by a nonlinear shell model when the fluid is 3D (see [75, 189]). An overpressure is applied at the inlet of the fluid for a short duration of time. Due to the fluid-structure coupling, the overpressure propagates along the cylinder. All the details regarding this test case can be found in the above-cited references.

We first tried explicit coupled methods. It was observed that these algorithms exhibit numerical instabilities:

(R1) for a given geometry, as soon as the density of the structure is lower than a certain threshold;
(R2) for a given structure density, as soon as the length of the domain is greater than a certain threshold.

We then tried "strongly" coupled methods, i.e., we ensured at each time step an exact balance of energy by sub-iterating several times between the fluid and the structure. When the sub-iterations consisted of a relaxed fixed-point method, it was observed that an increasing amount of relaxation is needed when:

(R3) the density of the structure decreases;
(R4) the length of the domain increases.

All the details concerning these observations (values of parameters, algorithms, experiments, etc.) can be found in [351, Chapter 4].

The fact that the numerical stability depends on the structure density has a clear physical interpretation. This is not the same for the dependence on the geometry, which is quite unexpected: since the main physical phenomenon is a wave propagation with a *finite* velocity, it is surprising that the length of the domain modifies the stability of the algorithm (independently of the space and time steps).

Since it is difficult to explain these observations on the original fully non-linear equations (9.3)–(9.5), we propose in the next section a simplified model which exhibits an analogous behaviour and which is simple enough to be analysed in detail.

9.2.2 A simplified model

We consider a rectangular domain $\Omega_f \subset \mathbb{R}^2$ whose boundary is split into different subsets Γ_F^1, Γ_F^2, Γ_F^3 and Γ, the last one corresponding to the fluid-structure interface (see Fig. 9.1). In this simplified model, the domain Ω_s occupied by the structure is such that $\overline{\Omega_s} = \Gamma$. We set $\Gamma_f = \Gamma_f^1 \cup \Gamma_f^2$. Finally, we denote by $\boldsymbol{n}_f$ the unit outward normal vector on $\partial\Omega_f$.

In the domain Ω_s, we use the generalised string model derived in Section 3.4.4: find the displacement $\eta = \eta(x,t)$ such that

$$\begin{cases} \rho_s h_s \dfrac{\partial^2 \eta}{\partial t^2} + a\eta - b\dfrac{\partial^2 \eta}{\partial x^2} = f & \text{in } \Omega_s, \\ \eta = 0 & \text{on } (0,T) \times \partial\Omega_s \end{cases} \tag{9.17}$$

where h_s is the thickness of the structure, $a = Eh_s/R^2(1-\xi^2)$, E is the Young modulus, ξ the Poisson coefficient, $b = \kappa_T G h_s$, G is the shear stress modulus, κ_T the Timoshenko shear correction factor and f the external forcing term coming from the fluid (whose expression will be made precise below). Equation (9.17) must be supplied with initial conditions

$$\eta(x,0) = \eta_0(x), \qquad \frac{\partial \eta}{\partial t}(x,0) = \dot{\eta}_0(x) \quad \text{in } \Omega_s, \tag{9.18}$$

and boundary conditions $\eta(0,t) = \eta(L,t) = 0, \forall t \in (0,T)$.

For the fluid, we use a linear incompressible inviscid model. Moreover, the deformation η of the structure is assumed to be very small, so that the fluid domain Ω_f can be considered fixed. Thus, the fluid problem reads: find the

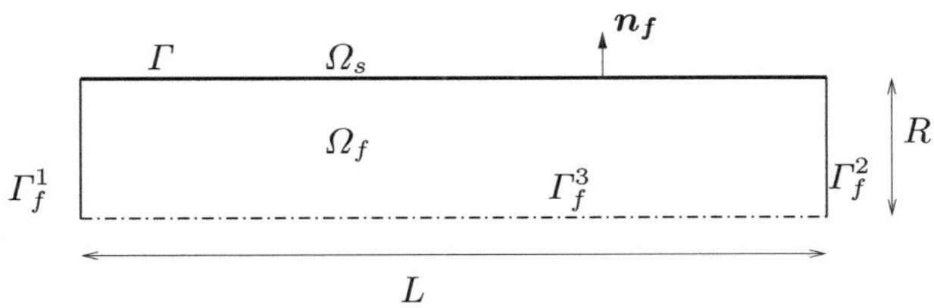

Fig. 9.1. Schematic representation of the computational domain

fluid velocity $\boldsymbol{u}_f = \boldsymbol{u}_f(x,y,t)$ and the pressure $P = P(x,y,t)$ such that

$$\begin{cases} \rho_f \dfrac{\partial \boldsymbol{u}_f}{\partial t} + \boldsymbol{\nabla} P = 0 & \text{in } \Omega_f, \\ \operatorname{div} \boldsymbol{u}_f = 0 & \text{in } \Omega_f, \\ P = \overline{P} & \text{on } \Gamma_f^1 \cup \Gamma_f^2, \\ \boldsymbol{u}_f \cdot \boldsymbol{n}_f = 0 & \text{on } \Gamma_f^3, \\ \boldsymbol{u}_f \cdot \boldsymbol{n}_f = w & \text{on } \Gamma, \end{cases} \tag{9.19}$$

where $\overline{P}$ and w are given functions (we refer to Fig. 9.1 for the notations). System (9.19) may be conveniently reformulated as follows:

$$\begin{cases} -\Delta P = 0 & \text{in } \Omega_f, \\ P = \overline{P} & \text{on } \Gamma_f^1 \cup \Gamma_f^2, \\ \dfrac{\partial P}{\partial \boldsymbol{n}_f} = 0 & \text{on } \Gamma_f^3, \\ \dfrac{\partial P}{\partial \boldsymbol{n}_f} = -\rho_f \dfrac{\partial w}{\partial t} & \text{on } \Gamma. \end{cases} \tag{9.20}$$

The fluid and structure systems are coupled by the following transmission conditions

$$\begin{cases} \boldsymbol{u}_f \cdot \boldsymbol{n}_f = w = \dfrac{\partial \eta}{\partial t} & \text{on } \Gamma, \\ f = P & \text{on } \Gamma. \end{cases} \tag{9.21}$$

Using $(9.21)_1$, condition $(9.20)_4$ can be written as

$$\frac{\partial P}{\partial \boldsymbol{n}_f} = -\rho_f \frac{\partial^2 \eta}{\partial t^2} \quad \text{on } \Gamma. \tag{9.22}$$

9.2.3 The added-mass operator

We introduce the functional spaces

$$\begin{aligned} V &= H_0^1(\Omega_s), \\ Q &= \{q \in H^1(\Omega_f), q|_{\Gamma_f^1 \cup \Gamma_f^2} = 0\}. \end{aligned}$$

We denote by $(\cdot,\cdot)$ the $L^2(\Omega_f)$ or $L^2(\Omega_s)$ inner products and we define the bi-linear forms:

$$\begin{aligned} a_f(p,q) &= \int_{\Omega_f} \nabla p \cdot \nabla q \, dx\, dy, & \forall p, q \in H^1(\Omega_f), \\ a_s(\eta,\xi) &= \int_{\Omega_s} a\, \eta\, \xi \, dx + \int_{\Omega_s} b \frac{\partial \eta}{\partial x} \frac{\partial \xi}{\partial x} \, dx, & \forall \eta, \xi \in H^1(\Omega_s). \end{aligned}$$

Throughout this section, the Hilbert space V will be endowed with the scalar product defined by $a_s(\cdot,\cdot)$. We make the following regularity assumptions on the boundary data for the fluid

$$\overline{P} \in C^0(0,\infty; H^{1/2}(\Gamma_f)), \tag{9.23}$$

and on the initial data for the structure

$$\eta_0 \in V, \dot{\eta}_0 \in V. \tag{9.24}$$

In the sequel, the notation q_Γ will indicate the restriction of an arbitrary function $q : \Omega_f \to \mathbb{R}$ to the interface Γ.

A variational formulation of the fluid-structure problem introduced in the previous section is:

Find $(P(t), \eta(t)) \in H^1(\Omega_f) \times V$ such that (9.18) is satisfied, $P(t)|_{\Gamma_f^1 \cup \Gamma_f^2} = \overline{P}(t), \ \ \forall t \in (0,\infty)$ and for all $(q,\xi) \in Q \times V$:

$$\begin{cases} a_f(P,q) = -\rho_f \displaystyle\int_\Gamma \frac{\partial^2 \eta}{\partial t^2} q, \\ \left(\rho_s h_s \dfrac{\partial^2 \eta}{\partial t^2}, \xi\right) + a_s(\eta,\xi) = (P|_\Gamma, \xi). \end{cases} \tag{9.25}$$

In order to write problem (9.25) in a more compact form, further notations are needed. We introduce the following operators: for $\eta, \xi \in V$, we define

$$\langle \mathcal{L}\eta, \xi \rangle = a_s(\eta,\xi), \tag{9.26}$$

and for $\ell \in L^2(\Omega_s)$, we denote by $T\ell$ the element of V such that

$$\langle \mathcal{L}(T\ell), \xi \rangle = (\ell, \xi). \tag{9.27}$$

Using the above definitions, the structure problem reads:
find η such that

$$\rho_s h_s \frac{\partial^2 \eta}{\partial t^2} + \mathcal{L}\eta = P_\Gamma. \tag{9.28}$$

Next, for any $w \in H^{-1/2}(\Gamma)$, we denote by $\mathcal{R}w$ the element of Q solution of the following problem

$$\begin{cases} -\Delta \mathcal{R}w = 0 \quad \text{in } \Omega_f, \\ \mathcal{R}w = 0 \quad \text{on } \Gamma_f^1 \cup \Gamma_f^2, \\ \dfrac{\partial \mathcal{R}w}{\partial \boldsymbol{n}_f} = 0 \quad \text{on } \Gamma_f^3, \\ \dfrac{\partial \mathcal{R}w}{\partial \boldsymbol{n}_f} = w \quad \text{on } \Gamma. \end{cases} \tag{9.29}$$

We define the *added-mass operator* $\mathcal{M}_{\mathcal{A}} : H^{-1/2}(\Gamma) \to H^{1/2}(\Gamma)$ by

$$\mathcal{M}_{\mathcal{A}} w = \mathcal{R} w|_{\Gamma}. \tag{9.30}$$

Note that, for $w, v \in L^2(\Gamma)$,

$$\langle \mathcal{M}_{\mathcal{A}} w, v \rangle = a_f(\mathcal{R} w, \mathcal{R} v).$$

The operator T is compact, self-adjoint and positive on V. The operator $\mathcal{M}_{\mathcal{A}}$ is compact, self-adjoint and positive on $L^2(\Gamma)$ (see [51,220]).

Let us now introduce an arbitrary continuous extension operator E_F: $H^{1/2}(\Gamma_f) \to H^1(\Omega_f)$. By definition, there exists a positive constant C such that, for all $q \in H^{1/2}(\Gamma_f)$, $E_F q|_{\Gamma_f} = q$ and $\|E_F q\|_{H^1(\Omega_f)} \leq C \|q\|_{H^{1/2}(\Gamma_f)}$.

We define $p^*(t) \in H^1(\Omega_f)$ as the solution to

$$\begin{cases} -\Delta p^* = \Delta E_F \overline{P} & \text{in } \Omega_f, \\ p^* = 0 & \text{on } \Gamma_f^1 \cup \Gamma_f^2, \\ \dfrac{\partial p^*}{\partial \boldsymbol{n}_f} = -\dfrac{\partial E_F \overline{P}}{\partial \boldsymbol{n}_f} & \text{on } \Gamma_f^3, \\ \dfrac{\partial p^*}{\partial \boldsymbol{n}_f} = -\dfrac{\partial E_F \overline{P}}{\partial \boldsymbol{n}_f} & \text{on } \Gamma. \end{cases} \tag{9.31}$$

Using equations (9.29) and (9.31), the solution to (9.20) is given by

$$P = p^* + E_F \overline{P} - \rho_f \mathcal{R} \frac{\partial^2 \eta}{\partial t^2}. \tag{9.32}$$

Then, defining

$$P_{ext} = p^*|_{\Gamma} + E_F \overline{P}|_{\Gamma}, \tag{9.33}$$

and using (9.30), we have

$$P_{\Gamma} = P_{ext} - \rho_f \mathcal{M}_{\mathcal{A}} \frac{\partial^2 \eta}{\partial t^2}. \tag{9.34}$$

Let $\boldsymbol{I}$ denote the identity operator. Inserting (9.34) into (9.28), we see that (9.25) can be written in the following form:
Find η such that

$$(\rho_s h_s Id + \rho_f \mathcal{M}_{\mathcal{A}}) \frac{\partial^2 \eta}{\partial t^2} + \mathcal{L} \eta = P_{ext}, \tag{9.35}$$

the pressure in the fluid being given by (9.32).

Equation (9.35) is very close to the structure equation (9.28) except for the extra operator $\rho_f \mathcal{M}_{\mathcal{A}}$ in front of the second-order time derivative. This operator encompasses the effect that the fluid has on the structure and acts as an extra mass, whence the name of "added-mass" operator (see e.g., [271,341]).

In view of carrying out the stability analysis of the numerical schemes, it is convenient to consider the maximum eigenvalue of $\mathcal{M}_{\mathcal{A}}$ denoted by $\mu_{\max}$. Note that the inverse of $\mu_{\max}$ is the smallest eigenvalue of the standard Steklov-Poincaré operator [408]. Note also that $\mu_{\max}$ is a purely geometric quantity. When dealing with an arbitrary geometry, a closed expression for $\mu_{\max}$ cannot be found. In the case of the simple geometry of Fig. 9.1, $\mu_{\max}$ can be computed analytically (see [70]):

$$\mu_{\max} = \frac{L}{\pi \tanh\left(\dfrac{\pi R}{L}\right)}. \tag{9.36}$$

This expression will be useful in the sequel to understand qualitatively the behaviour of coupling schemes, in particular to comment on observations (R2) and (R4) above.

9.2.4 Weak coupling for the simplified model

In this section, we present the stability analysis, proposed in [70], for an explicit coupling scheme for the temporal discretisation of the FSI problem presented above. For the sake of simplicity we assume that the coefficient b in (9.17) is equal to zero. The differential structural operator defined in (9.26) therefore reduces to $\mathcal{L}\eta = a\eta$. The results obtained in the following sections can be generalised to the case $b \neq 0$ and to other time discretisation schemes (see [164]).

By explicit coupling schemes we mean time discretisation algorithms of the coupled FSI problem (9.17), (9.18), (9.19), (9.21) that allow the fluid and the structure equations to be solved only once (or just a few times) within each time step, without enforcing exactly the coupling conditions.

Our goal is to show that such kinds of algorithms can be *unconditionally unstable* in certain cases, depending on the relative mass density of the structure and the fluid and on some geometric properties of the domain.

As a prototype of an explicit algorithm, we consider the one obtained by employing a Leap-Frog scheme for the structure and an Implicit Euler scheme for the fluid. Denoting by δt the time step, at every time-level we obtain the following systems:

$$\left\{\begin{aligned} \rho_f \frac{\boldsymbol{u}_f^n - \boldsymbol{u}_f{}^{n-1}}{\delta t} + \boldsymbol{\nabla} P^n &= 0 && \text{in } \Omega_f, \\ \operatorname{div} \boldsymbol{u}_f^n &= 0 && \text{in } \Omega_f, \\ P^n &= \overline{P}(t^n) && \text{on } \Gamma_f^1 \cup \Gamma_f^2, \\ \boldsymbol{u}_f^n \cdot \boldsymbol{n}_f &= 0 && \text{on } \Gamma_f^3, \end{aligned}\right. \tag{9.37}$$

and

$$\boldsymbol{u}_f^n \cdot \boldsymbol{n}_f = \frac{\eta^n - \eta^{n-1}}{\delta t} \qquad \text{on } \Gamma, \tag{9.38}$$

$$\rho_s h_s \frac{\eta^{n+1} - 2\eta^n + \eta^{n-1}}{\delta t^2} + a\eta^n = P^n \qquad \text{in } \Omega_s. \tag{9.39}$$

Observe that, given the wall displacement η^n at time t^n, the fluid equation (9.37) with boundary condition (9.38) allows the fluid velocity $\boldsymbol{u}_f^n$ and the pressure P^n to be computed. With the latter, we can now solve the structure equation (9.39) and get the new wall displacement η^{n+1} at time t^{n+1}. Hence, this coupling algorithm is explicit.

We now analyse its stability. We proceed as in Section 9.2.3 and we reduce the coupled problem to a single structure equation with an added-mass term. We have:

$$\begin{cases} \Delta P^n = 0 & \text{in } \Omega \\ \dfrac{\partial P^n}{\partial \boldsymbol{n}_f} = -\rho_f \dfrac{(\boldsymbol{u}_f^n - \boldsymbol{u}_f{}^{n-1}) \cdot \boldsymbol{n}_f}{\delta t} = -\rho_f \dfrac{\eta^n - 2\eta^{n-1} + \eta^{n-2}}{\delta t^2} & \text{on } \Gamma \\ \dfrac{\partial P^n}{\partial \boldsymbol{n}_f} = 0 & \text{on } \Gamma_f^3 \\ P^n = \overline{P}(t^n) & \text{on } \Gamma_f. \end{cases}$$

Hence, with the notation introduced in (9.33), we have

$$P^n\big|_\Gamma = P_{ext}^n - \rho_f \mathcal{M}_{\mathcal{A}} \frac{\eta^n - 2\eta^{n-1} - \eta^{n-2}}{\delta t^2},$$

and

$$\rho_s h_s \frac{\eta^{n+1} - 2\eta^n + \eta^{n-1}}{\delta t^2} + \rho_f \mathcal{M}_{\mathcal{A}} \frac{\eta^n - 2\eta^{n-1} + \eta^{n-2}}{\delta t^2} + a\eta^n = P_{ext}^n, \tag{9.40}$$

on Ω_s. The following result holds (see [70]).

Proposition 9.2. *Let $\mu_{\max}$ be the largest eigenvalue of the operator $\mathcal{M}_{\mathcal{A}}$. Then, the scheme (9.40), and hence the explicit coupling scheme (9.37)–(9.39), is unconditionally unstable if* $\dfrac{\rho_s h_s}{\rho_f \mu_{\max}} < 1$.

Observe that the "instability condition" in Proposition 9.2 confirms empirical observations (R1) and (R2) of Section 9.2.1. Indeed, this condition is more and more restrictive as ρ_s/ρ_f decreases and as $\mu_{\max}$ increases, the connection of the latter with the geometry being shown in (9.36). More precisely, the more Ω_f becomes a slender geometry (that is, when, for a fixed radius R, L increases or when, for a fixed length L, R decreases), the larger $\mu_{\max}$ becomes.

9.2.5 Strong coupling for the simplified model

Proposition 9.2 suggests that explicit coupling schemes might not work for fluid-structure interaction problems in certain conditions. An obvious remedy consists in switching to implicit couplings. As a prototype of implicit coupling algorithms we choose here the one obtained by combining the Implicit Euler scheme for the fluid with the first-order backward difference scheme for the structure. The time-discrete problem reads:

$$\begin{cases} \rho_f \dfrac{\boldsymbol{u}_f^{n+1} - \boldsymbol{u}_f{}^n}{\delta t} + \boldsymbol{\nabla} P^{n+1} = 0 & \text{in } \Omega_f, \\ \operatorname{div} \boldsymbol{u}_f^{n+1} = 0 & \text{in } \Omega_f, \\ P^{n+1} = \overline{P}(t^{n+1}) & \text{on } \Gamma_f^1 \cup \Gamma_f^2, \\ \boldsymbol{u}_f^{n+1} \cdot \boldsymbol{n}_f = 0 & \text{on } \Gamma_f^3, \end{cases} \tag{9.41}$$

and

$$\boldsymbol{u}_f^{n+1} \cdot \boldsymbol{n}_f = \frac{\eta^{n+1} - \eta^n}{\delta t} \qquad \text{on } \Gamma, \tag{9.42}$$

$$\rho_s h_s \frac{\eta^{n+1} - 2\eta^n + \eta^{n-1}}{\delta t^2} + a\eta^{n+1} = P^{n+1} \qquad \text{on } \Omega_s. \tag{9.43}$$

This problem corresponds to the following discrete added-mass problem for the structure

$$(\rho_s h_s \boldsymbol{I} + \rho_f \mathcal{M}_A) \frac{\eta^{n+1} - 2\eta^n + \eta^{n-1}}{\delta t^2} + a\eta^{n+1} = P_{ext}^{n+1} \qquad \text{in } \Omega_s. \tag{9.44}$$

It is straightforward to show that problem (9.44), and hence the coupled problem (9.41)–(9.43), is stable for any choice of the time step δt.

In this simple example, at each time step, the coupled problem (9.41)–(9.43) turns into a linear system in the unknowns $(\boldsymbol{u}_f^{n+1}, P^{n+1}, \eta^{n+1})$ (after spatial discretisation) and can be assembled and solved quite easily. Yet, since we are interested in partitioned schemes, we propose to solve the simplified problem (9.41)–(9.43) in the following way:

Given an initial guess η_0^{n+1}, *solve for each* $k = 1, 2, \ldots$

1. Fluid step: find $(\boldsymbol{u}_{f_k}, p_k)$ s.t.

$$\begin{cases} \rho_f \dfrac{\boldsymbol{u}_{f_k} - \boldsymbol{u}_f{}^n}{\delta t} + \boldsymbol{\nabla} P_k = 0 & \text{in } \Omega_f, \\ \operatorname{div} \boldsymbol{u}_{f_k} = 0 & \text{in } \Omega_f, \\ P_k = \overline{P}(t^{n+1}) & \text{on } \Gamma_f^1 \cup \Gamma_f^2, \\ \boldsymbol{u}_{f_k} \cdot \boldsymbol{n}_f = 0 & \text{on } \Gamma_f^3, \\ \boldsymbol{u}_{f_k} \cdot \boldsymbol{n}_f = \dfrac{\eta_{k-1} - \eta^n}{\delta t} & \text{on } \Gamma. \end{cases}$$

2. Structure step: find $\tilde{\eta}_k$ s.t.

$$\rho_s h_s \frac{\tilde{\eta}_k - 2\eta^n + \eta^{n-1}}{\delta t^2} + a\tilde{\eta}_k = P_k \qquad \text{in } \Omega_s.$$

3. Relaxation step:

$$\eta_k = \omega \tilde{\eta}_k + (1-\omega)\eta_{k-1}.$$

4. Convergence test:
   - if $||\eta_k - \eta_{k-1}|| < tol$ then set $\eta^{n+1} = \eta_k$, $\boldsymbol{u}_f^{n+1} = \boldsymbol{u}_{f\,k}$ and $P^{n+1} = P_k$;
   - else set $k = k+1$ and go to step 1.

We can eliminate the unknowns $\boldsymbol{u}_{f\,k}$ and P_k, using the same technique as was employed before. We obtain in this case:

$$P_{\Gamma,k} = -\rho_f \mathcal{M}_A \left(\frac{\eta_{k-1} - 2\eta^n + \eta^{n-1}}{\delta t^2} \right) + P_{ext}^{n+1}.$$

Keeping in mind that $\tilde{\eta}_k = \frac{\eta_k}{\omega} - \frac{1-\omega}{\omega}\eta_{k-1}$, the previous algorithm corresponds to the following iterative method to solve the added-mass problem (9.44):

$$\begin{aligned}\frac{\rho_s h_s}{\delta t^2}\left(\frac{\eta_k}{\omega} - 2\eta^n + \eta^{n-1}\right) + a\frac{\eta_k}{\omega} &= \frac{1-\omega}{\omega}\left(\frac{\rho_s h_s}{\delta t^2} + a\right)\eta_{k-1} \\ &- \rho_f \mathcal{M}_A \left(\frac{\eta_{k-1} - 2\eta^n + \eta^{n-1}}{\delta t^2} \right) + P_{ext}^{n+1}, \qquad k = 1, 2, \dots\end{aligned}$$

or, equivalently, the fixed-point iteration

$$\frac{1}{\omega}\left(\frac{\rho_s h_s}{\delta t^2} + a\right)\eta_k = \left[\frac{1-\omega}{\omega}\left(\frac{\rho_s h_s}{\delta t^2} + a\right) - \frac{\rho_f \mathcal{M}_A}{\delta t^2}\right]\eta_{k-1} + g(\eta^n, \eta^{n+1}, P_{ext}^{n+1}). \tag{9.45}$$

Concerning the convergence of the fixed point iteration (9.45), the following result can be proved (see [70]). Notice that it confirms the empirical observations (R3) and (R4) of Section 9.2.1.

Proposition 9.3. *The implicit partitioned method converges to the solution to (9.41)–(9.43) if and only if*

$$0 < \omega < \frac{2(\rho_s h_s + a\delta t^2)}{\rho_s h_s + \rho_f \mu_{\max} + a\delta t^2}. \tag{9.46}$$

Remark 9.2.1 *It is possible to investigate a possible alternative to the standard Dirichlet-to-Neumann iterations on the above toy model: if, in contrast to what has been done above, a load is applied to the fluid and a displacement* *to the structure, it can be shown that the relaxation parameter ω tends to zero with the space discretisation parameter. Therefore, such an algorithm seems not to be of practical use. We refer to [70] for the details.*

9.2.6 Conclusions

The above considerations show that it is difficult to achieve stability with weakly (or explicit) coupled schemes, at least in some physical situations (Proposition 9.2). In the context of blood flows, this fact has been confirmed by several numerical experiments using realistic models and various time schemes. Moreover, the computational cost of naive strongly coupled schemes – typically fixed point methods – can be prohibitive (Proposition 9.3). The following section presents various attempts to efficiently and implicitly couple the fluid and the structure.

Nevertheless, we must keep in mind that these conclusions have been obtained on a *simplified* problem. The results only show that a strong coupling is necessary, in some situations, as far as the added-mass part is concerned. A further analysis, considering different time discretisation schemes, has been reported in [164]. In particular, it is advocated that no sequentially staggered scheme can be constructed that is unconditionally stable irrespective of the fluid-solid density ratio.

Finally, let us stress that a more complex fluid model involves many other features, like viscosity and nonlinear advection, that could be coupled explicitly with the structure without significantly compromising stability. This will be investigated in Section 9.4.

9.3 Implicit coupling

In the previous section, it has been shown that explicit coupling schemes may lead to numerical instabilities. We now focus on an implicit coupling scheme for the general coupled problem (9.15)–(9.16). As we shall see, this scheme can be proved to be unconditionally stable (under mild conditions). We also address the numerical solution of the resulting nonlinear system using different iterative procedures.

9.3.1 An implicit coupling scheme

Let $\delta t > 0$ be a given time step. We aim at approximating the solution $\big(\widehat{\boldsymbol{u}}_f, \widehat{P}, \widetilde{\boldsymbol{\eta}}_f, \widehat{\boldsymbol{\eta}}_s\big)$ of (9.16) at time $t^n = n\delta t$, for $n \in \mathbb{N}$. In what follows, the quadruplet $\big(\widehat{\boldsymbol{u}}_f^n, \widehat{P}^n, \widetilde{\boldsymbol{\eta}}_f^n, \widehat{\boldsymbol{\eta}}_s^n\big)$ will stand for an approximation of the solution of (9.16) at time t^n.

We use an implicit Euler scheme for the ALE Navier-Stokes equations and a mid-point rule for the structural equation. Thus, the semi-discretised coupled problem writes: given $\left(\widehat{\boldsymbol{u}}_f^n, \widehat{P}^n, \widetilde{\boldsymbol{\eta}}_f^n, \widehat{\boldsymbol{\eta}}_s^n\right)$, find $\left(\widehat{\boldsymbol{u}}_f^{n+1}, \widehat{P}^{n+1}, \widetilde{\boldsymbol{\eta}}_f^{n+1}, \widehat{\boldsymbol{\eta}}_s^{n+1}\right)$

such that

$$\begin{cases} \widetilde{\boldsymbol{\eta}}_f^{n+1} = \operatorname{Ext}(\widehat{\boldsymbol{\eta}}^{n+1}_{s|\widehat{\Gamma}}), \quad \widehat{\boldsymbol{w}}(\widetilde{\boldsymbol{\eta}}_f^{n+1}) = \dfrac{1}{\delta t}\left(\widetilde{\boldsymbol{\eta}}_f^{n+1} - \widetilde{\boldsymbol{\eta}}_f^{n}\right), & \text{in} \quad \widehat{\Omega_f}, \\ \boldsymbol{u}_f^{n+1} = \boldsymbol{w}(\widetilde{\boldsymbol{\eta}}_f^{n+1}), \quad \text{on} \quad \Gamma(\widetilde{\boldsymbol{\eta}}_f^{n+1}), \\ \widehat{\boldsymbol{\eta}}_s^{n+1} = \boldsymbol{0}, \quad \text{on} \quad \Gamma_{s,D}, \end{cases} \tag{9.47}$$

and

$$\begin{aligned} a_f\left(\widetilde{\boldsymbol{\eta}}_f^{n+1}; (\boldsymbol{u}_f^{n+1}, P^{n+1}), (\boldsymbol{v}_f, q)\right) + a_s\left(\widehat{\boldsymbol{\eta}}_s^{n+1}, \hat{\boldsymbol{v}}_s\right) = \langle F_f, (\boldsymbol{v}_f, q)\rangle \\ + \langle F_s, \hat{\boldsymbol{v}}_s\rangle, \end{aligned} \tag{9.48}$$

for all $(\hat{\boldsymbol{v}}_f, \widehat{q}, \hat{\boldsymbol{v}}_s) \in [H^1(\widehat{\Omega_f})]^3 \times L^2(\widehat{\Omega_f}) \times [H^1_{\Gamma_{s,D}}(\widehat{\Omega_s})]^3$ such that $\hat{\boldsymbol{v}}_f = \hat{\boldsymbol{v}}_s$ on $\widehat{\Gamma}$, where the fluid terms are defined by

$$\begin{aligned} a_f\left(\widetilde{\boldsymbol{\eta}}_f^{n+1}; (\boldsymbol{u}_f^{n+1}, P^{n+1}), (\boldsymbol{v}_f, q)\right) &= \frac{1}{\delta t}\int_{\Omega_f(\widetilde{\boldsymbol{\eta}}_f^{n+1})} \rho_f \boldsymbol{u}_f^{n+1} \cdot \boldsymbol{v}_f \,\mathrm{d}\boldsymbol{x} \\ &+ \int_{\Omega_f(\widetilde{\boldsymbol{\eta}}_f^{n+1})} \rho_f \left(\boldsymbol{u}_f^{n+1} - \boldsymbol{w}(\widetilde{\boldsymbol{\eta}}_f^{n+1})\right) \cdot \boldsymbol{\nabla}\boldsymbol{u}_f^{n+1} \cdot \boldsymbol{v}_f \,\mathrm{d}\boldsymbol{x} \\ &- \int_{\Omega_f(\widetilde{\boldsymbol{\eta}}_f^{n+1})} \rho_f \left(\operatorname{div} \boldsymbol{w}(\widetilde{\boldsymbol{\eta}}_f^{n+1})\right) \boldsymbol{u}_f^{n+1} \cdot \boldsymbol{v}_f \,\mathrm{d}\boldsymbol{x} \\ &+ \int_{\Omega_f(\widetilde{\boldsymbol{\eta}}_f^{n+1})} \boldsymbol{\sigma}_f(\boldsymbol{u}_f^{n+1}, P^{n+1}) : \boldsymbol{\nabla}\boldsymbol{v}_f \,\mathrm{d}\boldsymbol{x} + \int_{\Omega_f(\widetilde{\boldsymbol{\eta}}_f^{n+1})} q \operatorname{div} \boldsymbol{u}_f^{n+1} \,\mathrm{d}\boldsymbol{x}, \end{aligned} \tag{9.49}$$

and

$$\langle F_f, (\boldsymbol{v}_f, q)\rangle = \int_{\Omega_f(\widetilde{\boldsymbol{\eta}}_f^{n})} \rho_f \boldsymbol{u}_f^{n} \cdot \boldsymbol{v}_f \,\mathrm{d}\boldsymbol{x} + \int_{\Gamma_{f,N}} \boldsymbol{g}_{f,N}(t_{n+1}) \cdot \boldsymbol{v}_f \,\mathrm{d}\boldsymbol{\gamma},$$

and the structure terms are defined by

$$\begin{aligned} a_s(\widehat{\boldsymbol{\eta}}_s^{n+1}, \hat{\boldsymbol{v}}_s) =& \frac{2}{\delta t^2}\int_{\widehat{\Omega_s}} \hat{\rho}_{s,0} \widehat{\boldsymbol{\eta}}_s^{n+1} \cdot \hat{\boldsymbol{v}}_s \,\mathrm{d}\hat{\boldsymbol{x}} \\ &+ \frac{1}{2}\int_{\widehat{\Omega_s}} \widehat{\boldsymbol{F}}_s(\widehat{\boldsymbol{\eta}}_s^{n+1}) \widehat{\boldsymbol{\Sigma}}(\widehat{\boldsymbol{\eta}}_s^{n+1}) : \boldsymbol{\nabla}_{\widehat{\boldsymbol{x}}} \hat{\boldsymbol{v}}_s \,\mathrm{d}\hat{\boldsymbol{x}}, \end{aligned} \tag{9.50}$$

and

$$\begin{aligned} \langle F_s, \hat{\boldsymbol{v}}_s\rangle =& \frac{2}{\delta t^2}\int_{\widehat{\Omega_s}} \hat{\rho}_{s,0} \left(\widehat{\boldsymbol{\eta}}_s^{n} + \delta t \hat{\boldsymbol{u}}_s^{n}\right) \cdot \hat{\boldsymbol{v}}_s \,\mathrm{d}\hat{\boldsymbol{x}} \\ &+ \frac{1}{2}\int_{\widehat{\Omega_s}} \widehat{\boldsymbol{F}}_s(\widehat{\boldsymbol{\eta}}_s^{n}) \widehat{\boldsymbol{\Sigma}}(\widehat{\boldsymbol{\eta}}_s^{n}) : \boldsymbol{\nabla}_{\widehat{\boldsymbol{x}}} \hat{\boldsymbol{v}}_s \,\mathrm{d}\hat{\boldsymbol{x}}. \end{aligned} \tag{9.51}$$

The structure velocity is defined by:

$$\frac{1}{2}\left(\hat{\boldsymbol{u}}_s^{n+1} + \hat{\boldsymbol{u}}_s^{n}\right) = \frac{1}{\delta t}\left(\widehat{\boldsymbol{\eta}}_s^{n+1} - \widehat{\boldsymbol{\eta}}_s^{n}\right).$$

This implicit coupling scheme leads to a highly nonlinear system. As a matter of fact, in addition to the common nonlinearities of the fluid and solid equations, implicit coupling induces geometrical nonlinearities within the fluid equations, due to the dependence of $\Omega_f(\widetilde{\boldsymbol{\eta}}_f^{n+1})$ on $\widetilde{\boldsymbol{\eta}}_f^{n+1}$. The numerical approximation of problem (9.47)–(9.48) using iterative methods is addressed in §9.3.3.

The rest of this paragraph is devoted to the stability analysis of the implicit coupling scheme (9.47)–(9.48). The next result (see [272,344]) states its unconditional stability.

Proposition 9.4. *Let us assume that*

1. *The coupled fluid-structure system is isolated, i.e.,*
   - $\boldsymbol{u}_f^{n+1} = \boldsymbol{0}$ *on* $\partial\Omega_f(\widetilde{\boldsymbol{\eta}}_f^{n+1})\backslash\Gamma(\widetilde{\boldsymbol{\eta}}_f^{n+1})$;
   - $\widehat{\boldsymbol{F}}_s(\widehat{\boldsymbol{\eta}}_s^{n+1})\widehat{\boldsymbol{\Sigma}}(\widehat{\boldsymbol{\eta}}_s^{n+1})\widehat{\boldsymbol{n}}_s = \boldsymbol{0}$ *on* $\partial\widehat{\Omega}_s\backslash\widehat{\Gamma}$.
2. *The structure is hyperelastic with a quadratic energy density* $\widetilde{W}(\widehat{\boldsymbol{F}}_s)$:

$$\widehat{\boldsymbol{F}}_s\widehat{\boldsymbol{\Sigma}} = \frac{\partial \widetilde{W}(\widehat{\boldsymbol{F}}_s)}{\partial \widehat{\boldsymbol{F}}}. \tag{9.52}$$

3. *Given a smooth function* $\widehat{v} : \widehat{\Omega}_f \longrightarrow \mathbb{R}$, *we have*

$$\frac{1}{\delta t}\left[\int_{\Omega_f(\widetilde{\boldsymbol{\eta}}_f^{n+1})} v \,\mathrm{d}\boldsymbol{x} - \int_{\Omega_f(\widetilde{\boldsymbol{\eta}}_f^{n})} v \,\mathrm{d}\boldsymbol{x}\right] = \int_{\Omega_f(\widetilde{\boldsymbol{\eta}}_f^{n+1})} v \operatorname{div} \boldsymbol{w}(\widetilde{\boldsymbol{\eta}}_f^{n+1}) \,\mathrm{d}\boldsymbol{x}, \tag{9.53}$$

with $v(\cdot, t^n) = \widehat{v} \circ \widetilde{\mathcal{A}}_n^{-1}$ *for all* $n \geq 0$.

Then, the following energy inequality holds

$$\begin{aligned}
&\frac{1}{\delta t}\left[\int_{\Omega_f(\widetilde{\boldsymbol{\eta}}_f^{n+1})} \frac{\rho_f}{2}|\boldsymbol{u}_f^{n+1}|^2 \,\mathrm{d}\boldsymbol{x} - \int_{\Omega_f(\widetilde{\boldsymbol{\eta}}_f^{n})} \frac{\rho_f}{2}|\boldsymbol{u}_f^{n}|^2 \,\mathrm{d}\boldsymbol{x}\right] \\
&+ \frac{1}{\delta t}\left[\int_{\widehat{\Omega}_s} \frac{\hat{\rho}_{s,0}}{2}|\hat{\boldsymbol{u}}_s^{n+1}|^2 \,\mathrm{d}\hat{\boldsymbol{x}} - \int_{\widehat{\Omega}_s} \frac{\hat{\rho}_{s,0}}{2}|\hat{\boldsymbol{u}}_s^{n}|^2 \,\mathrm{d}\hat{\boldsymbol{x}}\right] \\
&+ \frac{1}{\delta t}\left[\int_{\widehat{\Omega}_s} \tilde{W}(\widehat{\boldsymbol{F}}_s^{n+1}) \,\mathrm{d}\hat{\boldsymbol{x}} - \int_{\widehat{\Omega}_s} \tilde{W}(\widehat{\boldsymbol{F}}_s^{n}) \,\mathrm{d}\hat{\boldsymbol{x}}\right] \\
&+ \int_{\Omega_f(\widetilde{\boldsymbol{\eta}}_f^{n+1})} 2\mu|\boldsymbol{D}(\boldsymbol{u}_f^{n+1})|^2 \leq 0.
\end{aligned} \tag{9.54}$$

Therefore, the implicit coupling scheme is unconditionally stable in the energy norm.

Before giving the proof of this result, some remarks are in order:

1. The energy balance (9.54) constitutes the discrete counterpart of (9.6).
2. The relation (9.53) is known in the literature as the *Geometric Conservation Law* (GCL), see [209, 351]. This constraint on the fluid domain displacement $\widetilde{\boldsymbol{\eta}}_f$ ensures that the continuous ALE transport formula (3.28) holds at the discrete level at each time interval. A deep discussion on (9.53) and its numerical relevance is beyond the scope of this chapter; we refer the interested reader to [209, 351] and the references therein.

Proof. We set

$$\hat{\boldsymbol{v}}_f = \widehat{\boldsymbol{u}}_f^{n+1}, \; \hat{\boldsymbol{v}}_s = \frac{1}{2}\left(\hat{\boldsymbol{u}}_s^{n+1} + \hat{\boldsymbol{u}}_s^n\right) = \frac{1}{\delta t}\left(\widehat{\boldsymbol{\eta}}_s^{n+1} - \widehat{\boldsymbol{\eta}}_s^n\right), \; \widehat{q} = \widehat{P}^{n+1}. \tag{9.55}$$

Thanks to the coupling conditions $(9.47)_{1,2}$, $\hat{\boldsymbol{v}}_f$ and $\hat{\boldsymbol{v}}_s$ are admissible test functions for (9.48), i.e.,

$$\hat{\boldsymbol{v}}_f = \hat{\boldsymbol{v}}_s, \quad \text{on} \quad \widehat{\Gamma}.$$

It is worth noticing that this choice is licit only because the fluid and the structure problems are implicitly coupled (see Remark 9.3.1). This allows us to insert the expressions of (9.55) in (9.48) and proceed term by term.

For the mass term in the fluid we have

$$\begin{aligned}
&\frac{1}{\delta t}\left[\int_{\Omega_f(\widetilde{\boldsymbol{\eta}}_f^{n+1})} \rho_f \left|\boldsymbol{u}_f^{n+1}\right|^2 \mathrm{d}\boldsymbol{x} - \int_{\Omega_f(\widetilde{\boldsymbol{\eta}}_f^{n})} \rho_f \boldsymbol{u}_f^n \cdot \boldsymbol{u}_f^{n+1}\, \mathrm{d}\boldsymbol{x}\right]\\
&\geq \frac{1}{\delta t}\left[\int_{\Omega_f(\widetilde{\boldsymbol{\eta}}_f^{n+1})} \frac{\rho_f}{2} \left|\boldsymbol{u}_f^{n+1}\right|^2 \mathrm{d}\boldsymbol{x} - \int_{\Omega_f(\widetilde{\boldsymbol{\eta}}_f^{n})} \frac{\rho_f}{2} \left|\boldsymbol{u}_f^{n}\right|^2 \mathrm{d}\boldsymbol{x}\right]\\
&\quad + \frac{1}{\delta t}\left[\int_{\Omega_f(\widetilde{\boldsymbol{\eta}}_f^{n+1})} \frac{\rho_f}{2} \left|\boldsymbol{u}_f^{n+1}\right|^2 - \int_{\Omega_f(\widetilde{\boldsymbol{\eta}}_f^{n})} \frac{\rho_f}{2} \left|\boldsymbol{u}_f^{n+1}\right|^2 \mathrm{d}\boldsymbol{x}\right].
\end{aligned}$$

By applying (9.53) with $\widehat{v} = \widehat{\boldsymbol{u}_f^{n+1}}$ to the last term, we finally get

$$\begin{aligned}
&\frac{1}{\delta t}\left[\int_{\Omega_f(\widetilde{\boldsymbol{\eta}}_f^{n+1})} \rho_f \left|\boldsymbol{u}_f^{n+1}\right|^2 \mathrm{d}\boldsymbol{x} - \int_{\Omega_f(\widetilde{\boldsymbol{\eta}}_f^{n})} \rho_f \boldsymbol{u}_f^n \cdot \boldsymbol{u}_f^{n+1}\, \mathrm{d}\boldsymbol{x}\right]\\
&\geq \frac{1}{\delta t}\left[\int_{\Omega_f(\widetilde{\boldsymbol{\eta}}_f^{n+1})} \frac{\rho_f}{2} \left|\boldsymbol{u}_f^{n+1}\right|^2 \mathrm{d}\boldsymbol{x} - \int_{\Omega_f(\widetilde{\boldsymbol{\eta}}_f^{n})} \frac{\rho_f}{2} \left|\boldsymbol{u}_f^{n}\right|^2 \mathrm{d}\boldsymbol{x}\right]\\
&\quad + \int_{\Omega_f(\widetilde{\boldsymbol{\eta}}_f^{n})} \frac{\rho_f}{2} \operatorname{div} \boldsymbol{w}(\widetilde{\boldsymbol{\eta}}_f^{n+1}) \left|\boldsymbol{u}_f^{n+1}\right|^2 \mathrm{d}\boldsymbol{x}.
\end{aligned} \tag{9.56}$$

For the convective term, integrating by parts and using the coupling condition $(9.47)_2$, we have

$$\begin{aligned}
&\int_{\Omega_f(\widetilde{\boldsymbol{\eta}}_f^{n+1})} \frac{\rho_f}{2}\left(\boldsymbol{u}_f^{n+1} - \boldsymbol{w}(\widetilde{\boldsymbol{\eta}}_f^{n+1})\right)\cdot \boldsymbol{\nabla}|\boldsymbol{u}_f^{n+1}|^2 \,\mathrm{d}\boldsymbol{x} \\
&\quad - \int_{\Omega_f(\widetilde{\boldsymbol{\eta}}_f^{n+1})} \rho_f \left(\operatorname{div} \boldsymbol{w}(\widetilde{\boldsymbol{\eta}}_f^{n+1})\right)|\boldsymbol{u}_f^{n+1}|^2 \,\mathrm{d}\boldsymbol{x} \\
&= \int_{\partial\Omega_f(\widetilde{\boldsymbol{\eta}}_f^{n+1})} \frac{\rho_f}{2}\left(\boldsymbol{u}_f^{n+1} - \boldsymbol{w}(\widetilde{\boldsymbol{\eta}}_f^{n+1})\right)\cdot \boldsymbol{n}_f|\boldsymbol{u}_f^{n+1}|^2 \,\mathrm{d}\gamma \\
&\quad - \int_{\Omega_f(\widetilde{\boldsymbol{\eta}}_f^{n+1})} \frac{\rho_f}{2} \left(\operatorname{div} \boldsymbol{w}(\widetilde{\boldsymbol{\eta}}_f^{n+1})\right)|\boldsymbol{u}_f^{n+1}|^2 \,\mathrm{d}\boldsymbol{x} \\
&= - \int_{\Omega_f(\widetilde{\boldsymbol{\eta}}_f^{n+1})} \frac{\rho_f}{2} \left(\operatorname{div} \boldsymbol{w}(\widetilde{\boldsymbol{\eta}}_f^{n+1})\right)|\boldsymbol{u}_f^{n+1}|^2 \,\mathrm{d}\boldsymbol{x}.
\end{aligned} \tag{9.57}$$

On the other hand, using the expression of the fluid Cauchy stress tensor (3.38) and the symmetry of $\boldsymbol{D}(\boldsymbol{u}_f^{n+1})$, we have

$$\begin{aligned}
&\int_{\Omega_f(\widetilde{\boldsymbol{\eta}}_f^{n+1})} \boldsymbol{\sigma}_f(\boldsymbol{u}_f^{n+1}, P^{n+1}) : \boldsymbol{\nabla}\boldsymbol{u}_f^{n+1}\,\mathrm{d}\boldsymbol{x} + \int_{\Omega_f(\widetilde{\boldsymbol{\eta}}_f^{n+1})} P^{n+1} \operatorname{div} \boldsymbol{u}_f^{n+1}\,\mathrm{d}\boldsymbol{x} \\
&= \int_{\Omega_f(\widetilde{\boldsymbol{\eta}}_f^{n+1})} 2\nu \left|\boldsymbol{D}(\boldsymbol{u}_f^{n+1})\right|^2 \mathrm{d}\boldsymbol{x}.
\end{aligned} \tag{9.58}$$

The mass term of the structure gives directly

$$\frac{1}{\delta t}\int_{\widehat{\Omega}_s} \frac{\hat{\rho}_{s,0}}{2}\left(\hat{\boldsymbol{u}}_s^{n+1} - \hat{\boldsymbol{u}}_s^{n}\right)\cdot\left(\hat{\boldsymbol{u}}_s^{n+1} + \hat{\boldsymbol{u}}_s^{n}\right)\mathrm{d}\hat{\boldsymbol{x}} = \frac{1}{\delta t}\int_{\widehat{\Omega}_s} \frac{\hat{\rho}_{s,0}}{2}\left(|\hat{\boldsymbol{u}}_s^{n+1}|^2 - |\hat{\boldsymbol{u}}_s^{n}|^2\right)\mathrm{d}\hat{\boldsymbol{x}}. \tag{9.59}$$

On the other hand, we have

$$\begin{aligned}
&\frac{1}{\delta t}\int_{\widehat{\Omega}_s} \widehat{\boldsymbol{F}}_s(\widehat{\boldsymbol{\eta}}_s^{n})\widehat{\boldsymbol{\Sigma}}(\widehat{\boldsymbol{\eta}}_s^{n}) : \boldsymbol{\nabla}_{\hat{\boldsymbol{x}}}\left(\widehat{\boldsymbol{\eta}}_s^{n+1} - \widehat{\boldsymbol{\eta}}_s^{n}\right)\mathrm{d}\hat{\boldsymbol{x}} \\
&= \frac{1}{\delta t}\int_{\widehat{\Omega}_s} \widehat{\boldsymbol{F}}_s(\widehat{\boldsymbol{\eta}}_s^{n})\widehat{\boldsymbol{\Sigma}}(\widehat{\boldsymbol{\eta}}_s^{n}) : \left(\widehat{\boldsymbol{F}}_s(\widehat{\boldsymbol{\eta}}_s^{n+1}) - \widehat{\boldsymbol{F}}_s(\widehat{\boldsymbol{\eta}}_s^{n})\right)\mathrm{d}\hat{\boldsymbol{x}} \\
&= \frac{1}{\delta t}\int_{\widehat{\Omega}_s} \frac{\partial \widetilde{W}(\widehat{\boldsymbol{F}}_s(\widehat{\boldsymbol{\eta}}_s^{n}))}{\partial \widehat{\boldsymbol{F}}} : \left(\widehat{\boldsymbol{F}}_s(\widehat{\boldsymbol{\eta}}_s^{n+1}) - \widehat{\boldsymbol{F}}_s(\widehat{\boldsymbol{\eta}}_s^{n})\right)\mathrm{d}\hat{\boldsymbol{x}}.
\end{aligned}$$

Therefore, since the density $\tilde{W}$ is assumed to be quadratic, we finally obtain

$$
\begin{aligned}
&\frac{1}{2}\int_{\widehat{\Omega}_s} \widehat{\boldsymbol{F}}_s(\widehat{\boldsymbol{\eta}}_s^n)\widehat{\boldsymbol{\Sigma}}(\widehat{\boldsymbol{\eta}}_s^n) : \boldsymbol{\nabla}_{\widehat{\boldsymbol{x}}}\hat{\boldsymbol{v}}_s \,\mathrm{d}\hat{\boldsymbol{x}} + \frac{1}{2}\int_{\widehat{\Omega}_s} \widehat{\boldsymbol{F}}_s(\widehat{\boldsymbol{\eta}}_s^{n+1})\widehat{\boldsymbol{\Sigma}}(\widehat{\boldsymbol{\eta}}_s^{n+1}) : \boldsymbol{\nabla}_{\widehat{\boldsymbol{x}}}\hat{\boldsymbol{v}}_s \,\mathrm{d}\hat{\boldsymbol{x}} \\
&= \frac{1}{\delta t}\int_{\widehat{\Omega}_s} \frac{1}{2}\left(\frac{\partial \tilde{W}(\widehat{\boldsymbol{F}}_s(\widehat{\boldsymbol{\eta}}_s^{n+1}))}{\partial \widehat{\boldsymbol{F}}} + \frac{\partial \tilde{W}(\widehat{\boldsymbol{F}}_s(\widehat{\boldsymbol{\eta}}_s^{n}))}{\partial \widehat{\boldsymbol{F}}}\right) : \left(\widehat{\boldsymbol{F}}_s(\widehat{\boldsymbol{\eta}}_s^{n+1}) - \widehat{\boldsymbol{F}}_s(\widehat{\boldsymbol{\eta}}_s^{n})\right) \mathrm{d}\hat{\boldsymbol{x}} \\
&= \frac{1}{\delta t}\int_{\widehat{\Omega}_s} \left(\tilde{W}(\widehat{\boldsymbol{F}}_s(\widehat{\boldsymbol{\eta}}_s^{n+1})) - \tilde{W}(\widehat{\boldsymbol{F}}_s(\widehat{\boldsymbol{\eta}}_s^{n}))\right) \mathrm{d}\hat{\boldsymbol{x}}.
\end{aligned}
\tag{9.60}
$$

Finally, the energy balance (9.54) is obtained after summation of (9.56)–(9.60), which completes the proof.

Remark 9.3.1 *The key ingredient in the above proof lies in the admissibility of the test functions (9.55). For an explicit coupling scheme, a correction term needs to be introduced to cope with the fact that the fluid and structure velocities do not match:*

$$
\hat{\boldsymbol{v}}_f = \widehat{\boldsymbol{u}}_f^{n+1} - \mathcal{L}_f\left(\widehat{\boldsymbol{u}}_f^{n+1} - \frac{1}{\delta t}\left(\widehat{\boldsymbol{\eta}}_s^{n+1} - \widehat{\boldsymbol{\eta}}_s^{n}\right)\right),
$$

where $\mathcal{L}_f$ denotes a fluid lifting operator. This term leads to an artificial power at the interface (see [146]).

9.3.2 Abstract formulations

Problem (9.48) can be rewritten in a more compact form in terms of the fluid, solid and interface state operators. With this aim, we first reformulate the coupling conditions $(9.47)_{1,2}$ in weak form. The geometry coupling condition $(9.47)_1$ is rewritten in terms of the interface displacement $\gamma^{n+1} \in [H^{\frac{1}{2}}(\widehat{\Gamma})]^3$ as

$$
\int_{\widehat{\Omega}_f} \left(\widetilde{\boldsymbol{\eta}}_f^{n+1} - \mathrm{Ext}(\gamma^{n+1})\right) \cdot \widehat{\boldsymbol{\tau}} \,\mathrm{d}\hat{\boldsymbol{x}} + \int_{\widehat{\Gamma}} (\widehat{\boldsymbol{\eta}}_s^{n+1} - \gamma^{n+1}) \cdot \widehat{\boldsymbol{\zeta}} \,\mathrm{d}\hat{\gamma} = 0, \tag{9.61}
$$

for all $\widehat{\boldsymbol{\tau}} \in [L^2(\widehat{\Omega}_f)]^3$ and $\widehat{\boldsymbol{\zeta}} \in [L^2(\widehat{\Gamma})]^3$. Finally, the continuity of the velocities at the interface $(9.47)_2$ is reformulated on the reference configuration as

$$
\int_{\widehat{\Gamma}} \left(\widehat{\boldsymbol{u}}_f^{n+1} - \hat{\boldsymbol{w}}(\widetilde{\boldsymbol{\eta}}_f^{n+1})\right) \cdot \widehat{\boldsymbol{\xi}} \,\mathrm{d}\hat{\gamma} = 0, \tag{9.62}
$$

for all $\widehat{\boldsymbol{\xi}} \in [L^2(\widehat{\Gamma})]^3$.

Thus, the semi-discretised coupled problem (9.47)–(9.48) writes:

given $(\widehat{\boldsymbol{u}}_f^n, \widehat{P}^n, \widetilde{\boldsymbol{\eta}}_f^n, \widehat{\boldsymbol{\eta}}_s^n, \gamma^n)$, find $(\widehat{\boldsymbol{u}}_f^{n+1}, \widehat{P}^{n+1}, \boldsymbol{\eta}_f^{n+1}, \widehat{\boldsymbol{\eta}}_s^{n+1}, \gamma^{n+1})$ such that

$$
\begin{aligned}
& a_f\left(\widetilde{\boldsymbol{\eta}}_f^{n+1}; (\boldsymbol{u}_f^{n+1}, P^{n+1}), (\boldsymbol{v}_f, q)\right) + a_s\left(\widehat{\boldsymbol{\eta}}_s^{n+1}, \hat{\boldsymbol{v}}_s\right) \\
& + \int_{\widehat{\Omega_f}} \left(\widetilde{\boldsymbol{\eta}}_f^{n+1} - \operatorname{Ext}\left(\gamma^{n+1}\right)\right) \cdot \widehat{\boldsymbol{\tau}}\, \mathrm{d}\hat{\boldsymbol{x}} + \int_{\widehat{\Gamma}} (\widehat{\boldsymbol{\eta}}_s^{n+1} - \gamma^{n+1}) \cdot \widehat{\boldsymbol{\zeta}}\, \mathrm{d}\hat{\gamma} \\
& + \int_{\widehat{\Gamma}} \left(\widehat{\boldsymbol{u}_f^{n+1}} - \widehat{\boldsymbol{w}}\left(\widetilde{\boldsymbol{\eta}}_f^{n+1}\right)\right) \cdot \widehat{\boldsymbol{\xi}}\, \mathrm{d}\hat{\gamma} = \langle F_f, (\boldsymbol{v}_f, q)\rangle + \langle F_s, \hat{\boldsymbol{v}}_s\rangle,
\end{aligned}
\tag{9.63}
$$

for all $(\hat{\boldsymbol{v}}_f, \widehat{q}, \widehat{\boldsymbol{\xi}}, \widehat{\boldsymbol{\tau}}, \widehat{\boldsymbol{\zeta}}, \hat{\boldsymbol{v}}_s) \in [H^1(\widehat{\Omega_f})]^3 \times L^2(\widehat{\Omega_f}) \times [L^2(\widehat{\Gamma})]^3 \times [L^2(\widehat{\Omega_f})]^3 \times [L^2(\widehat{\Gamma})]^3 \times [H^1_{\Gamma_{s,D}}(\widehat{\Omega_s})]^3$ such that $\hat{\boldsymbol{v}}_f = \hat{\boldsymbol{v}}_s$ on $\widehat{\Gamma}$.

Based on the discrete weak formulation (9.63) we introduce the fluid operator

$$
\begin{aligned}
\mathcal{F} : [H^1(\widehat{\Omega_f})]^3 \times L^2(\widehat{\Omega_f}) \times [H^1(\widehat{\Omega_f})]^3 \times [H^{\frac{1}{2}}(\widehat{\Gamma})]^3 \\
\longrightarrow \left([H^1_{\widehat{\Gamma}}(\widehat{\Omega_f})]^3 \times L^2(\widehat{\Omega_f}) \times [L^2(\widehat{\Gamma})]^3 \times [L^2(\widehat{\Omega_f})]^3\right)',
\end{aligned}
$$

defined by

$$
\begin{aligned}
\left\langle \mathcal{F}\left(\widehat{\boldsymbol{u}_f}, \widehat{p}, \widetilde{\boldsymbol{\eta}}_f, \gamma\right), (\widehat{\boldsymbol{v}_f}, \widehat{q}, \widehat{\boldsymbol{\xi}}, \widehat{\boldsymbol{\tau}})\right\rangle = a_f\left(\widetilde{\boldsymbol{\eta}}_f; (\boldsymbol{u}_f, P), (\boldsymbol{v}_f, q)\right) \\
+ \int_{\widehat{\Gamma}} \left(\widehat{\boldsymbol{u}_f} - \widehat{\boldsymbol{w}}\left(\widetilde{\boldsymbol{\eta}}_f\right)\right) \cdot \widehat{\boldsymbol{\xi}}\, \mathrm{d}\hat{\gamma} + \int_{\widehat{\Omega_f}} \left(\widetilde{\boldsymbol{\eta}}_f - \operatorname{Ext}(\gamma)\right) \cdot \widehat{\boldsymbol{\tau}}\, \mathrm{d}\hat{\boldsymbol{x}} - \langle F_f, (\boldsymbol{v}_f, q)\rangle
\end{aligned}
\tag{9.64}
$$

for all $(\hat{\boldsymbol{v}}_f, \widehat{q}, \widehat{\boldsymbol{\xi}}, \widehat{\boldsymbol{\tau}}) \in [H^1(\widehat{\Omega_f})]^3 \times L^2(\widehat{\Omega_f}) \times [L^2(\widehat{\Gamma})]^3 \times [L^2(\widehat{\Omega_f})]^3$. By taking $(\hat{\boldsymbol{v}}_s, \widehat{\boldsymbol{\zeta}}) = \mathbf{0}$ in (9.63), and using the definition (9.64), it follows that the fluid state $\left(\boldsymbol{u}_{f,h}^{n+1}, \widehat{p}^{n+1}, \widetilde{\boldsymbol{\eta}}_f^{n+1}\right)$ satisfies the following Dirichlet (fluid) sub-problem:

$$
\mathcal{F}\left(\widehat{\boldsymbol{u}_f^{n+1}}, \widehat{p}^{n+1}, \widetilde{\boldsymbol{\eta}}_f^{n+1}, \gamma^{n+1}\right) = 0. \tag{9.65}
$$

Similarly, from (9.63), we define the solid operator

$$
\mathcal{S} : [H^1(\widehat{\Omega_s})]^3 \times [H^{\frac{1}{2}}(\widehat{\Gamma})]^3 \longrightarrow \left([H^1_{\Gamma_D \cup \widehat{\Gamma}}(\widehat{\Omega_s})]^3 \times [L^2(\widehat{\Gamma})]^3\right)',
$$

through

$$
\left\langle \mathcal{S}(\widehat{\boldsymbol{\eta}}_s, \gamma), (\hat{\boldsymbol{v}}_s, \widehat{\boldsymbol{\zeta}})\right\rangle = a_s\left(\widehat{\boldsymbol{\eta}}_s^{n+1}, \hat{\boldsymbol{v}}_s\right) - \langle F_s, \hat{\boldsymbol{v}}_s\rangle + \int_{\widehat{\Gamma}} (\widehat{\boldsymbol{\eta}}_s - \gamma) \cdot \widehat{\boldsymbol{\zeta}}\, \mathrm{d}\hat{\gamma}, \tag{9.66}
$$

for all $(\hat{\boldsymbol{v}}_s, \widehat{\boldsymbol{\zeta}}) \in [H^1_{\Gamma_D}(\widehat{\Omega_s})]^3 \times [L^2(\widehat{\Gamma})]^3$. Now, by taking $(\hat{\boldsymbol{v}}_f, \widehat{q}, \widehat{\boldsymbol{\xi}}, \widehat{\boldsymbol{\tau}}) = \mathbf{0}$ in (9.63), and using the definition (9.66), it follows that the solid displacement $\widehat{\boldsymbol{\eta}}_s^{n+1}$ satisfies the following Dirichlet (solid) sub-problem:

$$
\mathcal{S}\left(\widehat{\boldsymbol{\eta}}_s^{n+1}, \gamma^{n+1}\right) = 0. \tag{9.67}
$$

Finally, let $\mathcal{L}_f : [H^{\frac{1}{2}}(\widehat{\Gamma})]^3 \to [H^1_{\Gamma_{\text{in}-\text{out}}}(\widehat{\Omega_f})]^3$ and $\mathcal{L}_s : [H^{\frac{1}{2}}(\widehat{\Gamma})]^3 \to [H^1_{\partial\widehat{\Omega_s}\setminus\widehat{\Gamma}}(\widehat{\Omega_s})]^3$ be two given continuous linear lift operators. The interface operator

$$\mathcal{I} : [H^1(\widehat{\Omega_f})]^3 \times L^2(\widehat{\Omega_f}) \times [H^1(\widehat{\Omega_f})]^3 \times [H^1(\widehat{\Omega_s})]^3 \longrightarrow [H^{-\frac{1}{2}}(\widehat{\Gamma})]^3,$$

is then defined by

$$\begin{aligned}\left\langle \mathcal{I}\left(\widehat{\boldsymbol{u}_f}, \widehat{p}, \widetilde{\boldsymbol{\eta}}_f, \widehat{\boldsymbol{\eta}}_s\right), \boldsymbol{\mu}\right\rangle &= \left\langle \mathcal{F}(\widehat{\boldsymbol{u}_f}, \widehat{p}, \widetilde{\boldsymbol{\eta}}_f, \gamma), (\mathcal{L}_f\boldsymbol{\mu}, 0, \mathbf{0}, \mathbf{0})\right\rangle \\ &\quad + \left\langle \mathcal{S}(\widehat{\boldsymbol{\eta}}_s, \gamma), (\mathcal{L}_s\boldsymbol{\mu}, \mathbf{0})\right\rangle,\end{aligned} \tag{9.68}$$

for all $\boldsymbol{\mu} \in [H^{\frac{1}{2}}(\widehat{\Gamma})]^3$.

Remark 9.3.2 *The interface operator* (9.68) *does not depend on γ since, due to the choice of the test functions, the terms involving γ vanish in the right-hand side of* (9.68).

For each $\boldsymbol{\mu} \in [H^{\frac{1}{2}}(\widehat{\Gamma})]^3$, taking $\hat{\boldsymbol{v}}_f = \mathcal{L}_f\boldsymbol{\mu}$, $\hat{\boldsymbol{v}}_s = \mathcal{L}_s\boldsymbol{\mu}$ and $(\widehat{q}, \widehat{\boldsymbol{\xi}}, \widehat{\boldsymbol{\tau}}, \widehat{\boldsymbol{\zeta}}) = \mathbf{0}$ in (9.63), it can be seen that the fluid structure state $(\widehat{\boldsymbol{u}}_f^{n+1}, \widehat{P}^{n+1}, \boldsymbol{\eta}_f^{n+1}, \widehat{\boldsymbol{\eta}}_s^{n+1})$ satisfies

$$\mathcal{I}\left(\widehat{\boldsymbol{u}_f^{n+1}}, \widehat{p}^{n+1}, \widetilde{\boldsymbol{\eta}}_f^{n+1}, \widehat{\boldsymbol{\eta}}_s^{n+1}\right) = 0, \tag{9.69}$$

which is a variational form of (9.2).

According to (9.65)–(9.69), and by noticing that the test-functions space:

$$\left\{(\hat{\boldsymbol{v}}_f, \hat{\boldsymbol{v}}_s) \in [H^1(\widehat{\Omega_f})]^3 \times [H^1_{\Gamma_D}(\widehat{\Omega_s})]^3,\ \hat{\boldsymbol{v}}_f = \hat{\boldsymbol{v}}_s \text{ on } \widehat{\Gamma}\right\},$$

can be decomposed as the direct sum

$$\left([H^1_{\widehat{\Gamma}}(\widehat{\Omega_f})]^3 \times [H^1_{\Gamma_D\cup\widehat{\Gamma}}(\widehat{\Omega_s})]^3\right) \oplus \left\{(\mathcal{L}_f\boldsymbol{\mu}, \mathcal{L}_s\boldsymbol{\mu}),\ \boldsymbol{\mu} \in [H^{\frac{1}{2}}(\widehat{\Gamma})]^3\right\},$$

it follows that problem (9.48) is equivalent to

$$\left\{\begin{aligned} \mathcal{F}\left(\widehat{\boldsymbol{u}_f^{n+1}}, \widehat{p}^{n+1}, \widetilde{\boldsymbol{\eta}}_f^{n+1}, \gamma^{n+1}\right) &= 0, \\ \mathcal{S}\left(\widehat{\boldsymbol{\eta}}_s^{n+1}, \gamma^{n+1}\right) &= 0, \\ \mathcal{I}\left(\widehat{\boldsymbol{u}_f^{n+1}}, \widehat{p}^{n+1}, \widetilde{\boldsymbol{\eta}}_f^{n+1}, \widehat{\boldsymbol{\eta}}_s^{n+1}\right) &= 0. \end{aligned}\right. \tag{9.70}$$

Steklov-Poincaré operators

In order to describe partitioned methods for the numerical solution of (9.70), we now introduce the nonlinear fluid and solid Steklov-Poincaré operators, also called *Dirichlet-to-Neumann maps*.

The nonlinear fluid Steklov-Poincaré operator

$$S_f : [H^{\frac{1}{2}}(\widehat{\Gamma})]^3 \longrightarrow [H^{-\frac{1}{2}}(\widehat{\Gamma})]^3,$$

is defined by

$$\langle S_f(\gamma), \boldsymbol{\mu}\rangle = \left\langle \mathcal{I}\big(\widehat{\boldsymbol{u}}_f(\gamma), \widehat{P}(\gamma), \widetilde{\boldsymbol{\eta}}_f(\gamma), \mathbf{0}\big), \boldsymbol{\mu}\right\rangle,$$

for all $\boldsymbol{\gamma}, \boldsymbol{\mu} \in [H^{\frac{1}{2}}(\hat{\Sigma})]^3$, where $(\widehat{\boldsymbol{u}}_f(\gamma), \widehat{P}(\gamma), \widetilde{\boldsymbol{\eta}}_f(\gamma))$ is the solution of the Dirichlet fluid problem:

$$\mathcal{F}\left(\widehat{\boldsymbol{u}}_f(\gamma), \widehat{P}(\gamma), \widetilde{\boldsymbol{\eta}}_f(\gamma), \boldsymbol{\gamma}\right) = 0. \tag{9.71}$$

In an analogous way, we introduce the nonlinear solid Steklov-Poincaré operator

$$S_s : [H^{\frac{1}{2}}(\hat{\Sigma})]^3 \longrightarrow [H^{-\frac{1}{2}}(\hat{\Sigma})]^3,$$

given by

$$\langle S_s(\gamma), \boldsymbol{\mu}\rangle = \langle \mathcal{I}\big(\mathbf{0}, 0, \mathbf{0}, \widehat{\boldsymbol{\eta}}_s(\gamma)\big), \boldsymbol{\mu}\rangle,$$

for all $\boldsymbol{\gamma}, \boldsymbol{\mu} \in [H^{\frac{1}{2}}(\hat{\Sigma})]^3$ and where $\widehat{\boldsymbol{\eta}}_s(\gamma)$ is the solution of the Dirichlet solid problem:

$$\mathcal{S}\left(\widehat{\boldsymbol{\eta}}_s(\gamma), \boldsymbol{\gamma}\right) = 0. \tag{9.72}$$

From the above definitions, it follows that problem (9.48) (or (9.70)) is equivalent to

$$S_f(\gamma^{n+1}) + S_s(\gamma^{n+1}) = 0. \tag{9.73}$$

The composition of (9.73) with the inverse operators S_s^{-1} gives rise to the Dirichlet-to-Neumann formulation, namely

$$S_s^{-1}\big(-S_f(\gamma^{n+1})\big) - \gamma^{n+1} = 0. \tag{9.74}$$

We could also consider the Neumann-to-Dirichlet formulation

$$S_f^{-1}\big(-S_s(\gamma^{n+1})\big) - \gamma^{n+1} = 0,$$

by composing (9.73) with S_f^{-1}. Nevertheless it is rarely used in practice and it is known to lead to poor algorithms in some cases, as pointed out in Remark 9.2.1.

9.3.3 Solution methods

In this section, we review some existing algorithms for the numerical solution of the nonlinear system arising in the time discretisation of the fluid-structure problem with an implicit coupling scheme. These methods are typically based on the application of a particular nonlinear iterative method to the formulations (9.70), (9.73) or (9.74).

In what follows, we only consider one time step of (9.63) so we omit the upper index $n+1$ in the unknowns. Moreover, we introduce the following compact notations for the fluid and solid state variables:

$$\boldsymbol{x} = (\widehat{\boldsymbol{u}}_f, \widehat{P}, \widetilde{\boldsymbol{\eta}}_f), \quad \boldsymbol{y} = \widehat{\boldsymbol{\eta}}_s.$$

Monolithic formulation

A common approach in the numerical solution of nonlinear systems arising in implicit coupling consists of applying a Newton-based algorithm to the global formulation (9.70). This yields the following procedure:

1. Initialise: $\boldsymbol{x}_0$, $\boldsymbol{y}_0$, γ_0.
2. For $k \geq 0$ until convergence
   a) Evaluate residual:

$$\boldsymbol{\mathcal{R}}_k = \begin{bmatrix} \mathcal{F}(\boldsymbol{x}_k, \gamma_k) \\ \mathcal{S}(\boldsymbol{y}_k, \gamma_k) \\ \mathcal{I}(\boldsymbol{x}_k, \boldsymbol{y}_k) \end{bmatrix}.$$

   b) Solve tangent problem:

$$\boldsymbol{\mathcal{J}}_k \begin{bmatrix} \delta\boldsymbol{x} \\ \delta\boldsymbol{y} \\ \delta\gamma \end{bmatrix} = -\boldsymbol{\mathcal{R}}_k. \tag{9.75}$$

   c) Update rule:

$$\begin{bmatrix} \boldsymbol{x}_{k+1} \\ \boldsymbol{y}_{k+1} \\ \gamma_{k+1} \end{bmatrix} = \begin{bmatrix} \boldsymbol{x}_k \\ \boldsymbol{y}_k \\ \gamma_k \end{bmatrix} + \begin{bmatrix} \delta\boldsymbol{x} \\ \delta\boldsymbol{y} \\ \delta\gamma \end{bmatrix}.$$

Here, $\boldsymbol{\mathcal{J}}_k$ stands for the Jacobian, or an approximation of the Jacobian, of the coupled nonlinear operator $(\mathcal{F}, \mathcal{S}, \mathcal{I})$.

The *exact* Newton method involves repeated solutions of problem (9.75) with an exact Jacobian $\boldsymbol{\mathcal{J}}_k$, having the following block structure:

$$\boldsymbol{\mathcal{J}}_k = \begin{bmatrix} \mathrm{D}_{\boldsymbol{x}}\mathcal{F}(\boldsymbol{x}_k, \gamma) & \boldsymbol{0} & \mathrm{D}_\gamma\mathcal{F}(\boldsymbol{x}_k, \gamma) \\ \boldsymbol{0} & \mathrm{D}_{\boldsymbol{y}}\mathcal{S}(\boldsymbol{y}_k, \gamma) & \mathrm{D}_\gamma\mathcal{S}(\boldsymbol{y}_k, \gamma) \\ \mathrm{D}_{\boldsymbol{x}}\mathcal{I}(\boldsymbol{x}_k, \boldsymbol{y}_k) & \mathrm{D}_{\boldsymbol{y}}\mathcal{I}(\boldsymbol{x}_k, \boldsymbol{y}_k) & \boldsymbol{0} \end{bmatrix}. \tag{9.76}$$

The main difficulty in the evaluation of $\boldsymbol{\mathcal{J}}_k$ is the evaluation of the following cross-derivative in (9.76):

$$\mathrm{D}_{\widetilde{\boldsymbol{\eta}}_f}\mathcal{F}(\widehat{\boldsymbol{u}}_f, \widehat{P}, \widetilde{\boldsymbol{\eta}}_f, \gamma)\delta\widetilde{\boldsymbol{\eta}}_f, \tag{9.77}$$

which corresponds to the directional derivative of the fluid equations with respect to fluid-domain perturbations. The evaluation of (9.77) requires shape derivative calculus within the fluid [148,149,473]. For the sake of completeness, we give the expression of (9.77) in the next equation and refer to [148–150] for the details:

$$
\begin{aligned}
&\left\langle \mathrm{D}_{\widetilde{\boldsymbol{\eta}}_f} \mathcal{F}(\widehat{\boldsymbol{u}}_f, \widehat{P}, \widetilde{\boldsymbol{\eta}}_f, \gamma)\delta\widetilde{\boldsymbol{\eta}}_f, \left(\widehat{\boldsymbol{v}_f}, \widehat{q}, \widehat{\boldsymbol{\xi}}, \widehat{\boldsymbol{\tau}}\right)\right\rangle \\
&= \frac{1}{\delta t}\int_{\Omega_f(\widetilde{\boldsymbol{\eta}}_f)} (\operatorname{div}\delta\boldsymbol{\eta}_f)\rho_f \boldsymbol{u}_f \cdot \boldsymbol{v}_f \,\mathrm{d}\boldsymbol{x} \\
&\quad + \int_{\Omega_f(\widetilde{\boldsymbol{\eta}}_f)} \mathbf{div}\left\{\rho_f \boldsymbol{u}_f \otimes \left(\boldsymbol{u}_f - \boldsymbol{w}(\widetilde{\boldsymbol{\eta}}_f)\right)\left[\boldsymbol{I}\operatorname{div}\delta\boldsymbol{\eta}_f - (\boldsymbol{\nabla}\delta\boldsymbol{\eta}_f)^t\right]\right\}\cdot \boldsymbol{v}_f \,\mathrm{d}\boldsymbol{x} \\
&\quad + \int_{\Omega_f(\widetilde{\boldsymbol{\eta}}_f)} \boldsymbol{\sigma}_f(\boldsymbol{u}_f, P)\left[\boldsymbol{I}\operatorname{div}\delta\boldsymbol{\eta}_f - (\boldsymbol{\nabla}\delta\boldsymbol{\eta}_f)^t\right] : \boldsymbol{\nabla}\boldsymbol{v}_f \,\mathrm{d}\boldsymbol{x} \\
&\quad - \int_{\Omega_f(\widetilde{\boldsymbol{\eta}}_f)} \mu\left[\boldsymbol{\nabla}\boldsymbol{u}_f \boldsymbol{\nabla}\delta\boldsymbol{\eta}_f + (\boldsymbol{\nabla}\delta\boldsymbol{\eta}_f)^t(\boldsymbol{\nabla}\boldsymbol{u}_f)^t\right] : \boldsymbol{\nabla}\boldsymbol{v}_f \,\mathrm{d}\boldsymbol{x} \\
&\quad - \int_{\Omega_f(\widetilde{\boldsymbol{\eta}}_f)} q \operatorname{div}\left\{\boldsymbol{u}_f\left[\boldsymbol{I}\operatorname{div}\delta\boldsymbol{\eta}_f - (\boldsymbol{\nabla}\delta\boldsymbol{\eta}_f)^t\right]\right\}\mathrm{d}\boldsymbol{x} - \frac{1}{\delta t}\int_{\widehat{\Gamma}} \delta\widetilde{\boldsymbol{\eta}}_f \cdot \widehat{\boldsymbol{\xi}}\,\mathrm{d}\widehat{\gamma} \\
&\quad + \int_{\widehat{\Omega_f}} \delta\widetilde{\boldsymbol{\eta}}_f \cdot \widehat{\boldsymbol{\tau}}\,\mathrm{d}\widehat{\boldsymbol{x}},
\end{aligned}
\tag{9.78}
$$

for all $(\hat{\boldsymbol{v}}_f, \widehat{q}, \widehat{\boldsymbol{\xi}}, \widehat{\boldsymbol{\tau}}) \in [H^1(\widehat{\Omega_f})]^3 \times L^2(\widehat{\Omega_f}) \times [L^2(\widehat{\Gamma})]^3 \times [L^2(\widehat{\Omega_f})]^3$.

In contrast, *inexact* Newton methods deal with approximations of (9.76), for instance, using finite difference approximations of (9.77) (see [217, 496]), by neglecting the corresponding sub-block in (9.76) (see [30, 217, 496, 557]).

Newton algorithms based on the numerical solution of (9.75) in a *monolithic* fashion, i.e., using global direct or iterative methods, have been reported in [30, 122, 217, 496, 557]. It is worth noticing that such a monolithic approach makes the use of separate solvers for the fluid and structure sub-problems difficult. Alternatively, system (9.75) can be solved in a *partitioned* manner through a block-Gauss elimination of $\delta\boldsymbol{x}_f$, which leads to the so-called block-Newton methods [148, 149], or, more generally, using domain decomposition methods [145].

Dirichlet-to-Neumann formulation

Formulation (9.74) reduces problem (9.70) to the determination of a fixed point of the *Dirichlet-to-Neumann* operator $\gamma \mapsto S_s^{-1}\big(-S_f(\gamma)\big)$. This motivates the use of fixed-point based iterations [272, 336, 337, 351]:

1. initialise γ_0;
2. for $k \geq 0$ until convergence

$$
\gamma_{k+1} = \omega_k S_s^{-1}\big(-S_f(\gamma_k)\big) + (1-\omega_k)\gamma_k. \tag{9.79}
$$

Here, ω^k stands for a given relaxation parameter which is chosen in order to enhance convergence of the method [117, 272, 336, 337].

Remark 9.3.3 *After space discretisation of problem* (9.47)–(9.48), *a common expression for the relaxation parameter ω_k is the one given by a multidimensional Aitken's formula [117, 337]:*

$$\omega_k = \frac{(\gamma_k - \gamma_{k-1}) \cdot \left(S_s^{-1}\big(-S_f(\gamma_k)\big) - \gamma_k - S_s^{-1}\big(-S_f(\gamma_{k-1})\big) - \gamma_{k-1}\right)}{\|S_s^{-1}\big(-S_f(\gamma_k)\big) - \gamma_k - S_s^{-1}\big(-S_f(\gamma_{k-1})\big) - \gamma_{k-1}\|},$$

with $\cdot$ and $\|\cdot\|$ standing for the Euclidean scalar product and norm.

Even though relaxation techniques may improve their efficiency, fixed-point based iterations are very expensive and might fail to converge in real applications. Alternatively, one can use Newton-based methods [150, 188] for a fast convergence towards the solution of (9.74). This gives the algorithm:

1. Initialise γ_0;
2. For $k \geq 0$ until convergence
   a) Evaluate residual:
   $$\mathcal{R}_k = S_s^{-1}\big(-S_f(\gamma_k)\big) - \gamma_k.$$
   b) Solve tangent problem:
   $$\big(\mathcal{J}(\gamma_k) - \boldsymbol{I}\big)\,\delta\gamma = -\mathcal{R}_k. \tag{9.80}$$
   c) Update rule:
   $$\gamma_{k+1} = \gamma_k + \delta\gamma.$$

where $\mathcal{J}(\gamma)$ stands for the Jacobian, or approximated Jacobian, of the composed operator

$$\gamma \mapsto S_s^{-1}\big(-S_f(\gamma)\big). \tag{9.81}$$

In practice, the linear problem (9.80) can be solved using an operator-free iterative method (e.g., GMRES [439, 440]), which only requires repeated evaluations of $\mathcal{J}(\gamma)$ against given interface displacements $\boldsymbol{\lambda}$. As in the previous paragraph, exact Jacobian evaluations of (9.81) require shape derivative calculus within the fluid. Indeed, by the chain rule we have

$$\mathcal{J}(\gamma)\boldsymbol{\lambda} = -\left(S_s^{-1}\right)'\big(-S_f(\gamma)\big)S_f'(\gamma)\boldsymbol{\lambda},$$

whose expression can be obtained by implicit derivation of (9.71) and (9.72). More precisely, the evaluation of $S_f'(\gamma)\boldsymbol{\lambda}$ makes necessary expression (9.78); we refer to [150] for the details. One of the simplest ways of approximating $S_f'(\gamma)\boldsymbol{\lambda}$ consists in using finite differences, for instance,

$$S_f'(\gamma)\boldsymbol{\lambda} \approx \frac{1}{\epsilon}\Big(S_f(\gamma + \epsilon\lambda) - S_f(\gamma)\Big),$$

for a small enough given parameter $\epsilon > 0$. However, as noticed in [188, Remark 5.1], such a strategy may lead to inefficient inexact Newton iterations. Alternatively, one can derive approximations based on simplified models. For instance, as reported in [188], we can provide very efficient approximations of $S_f'(\gamma)\boldsymbol{\lambda}$

in terms of the added-mass operator associated to the simplified fluid problem (9.20)–(9.22), by solving

$$\begin{cases} -\Delta \delta P = 0, & \text{in} \quad \Omega_f(\widetilde{\boldsymbol{\eta}}_f), \\ \quad P = 0, & \text{on} \quad \Gamma_{f,N}, \\ \dfrac{\partial \delta P}{\partial \boldsymbol{n}_f} = -\frac{\rho_f}{\delta t^2} \boldsymbol{\lambda} \cdot \boldsymbol{n}_f, & \text{on} \quad \Gamma(\widetilde{\boldsymbol{\eta}}_f). \end{cases} \tag{9.82}$$

Finally, let us stress the fact that all the methods discussed in this paragraph are naturally partitioned.

Steklov-Poincaré formulation

The Dirichlet-Neumann formulations share a common feature: their implementation is purely sequential. The Steklov-Poincaré formulation (9.73) may allow parallel algorithms to be set up to solve the interface equation.

Following the presentation of [118], the nonlinear problem (9.73) can be solved through nonlinear Richardson iterations:

$$P_k(\gamma_{k+1} - \gamma_k) = \omega_k(-S_f(\gamma_k) - S_s(\gamma_k)), \tag{9.83}$$

for an appropriate choice of the preconditioner P_k, namely

$$P_k^{-1} = \alpha_k \left[S_f'(\gamma_k)\right]^{-1} + (1 - \alpha_k) \left[S_s'(\gamma_k)\right]^{-1}, \tag{9.84}$$

where $\boldsymbol{\lambda} \mapsto S_f'(\beta) \cdot \boldsymbol{\lambda}$ is the differential of S_f at β, and $\left[S_f'(\beta)\right]^{-1}$ its inverse. This choice generalises the standard preconditioners of linear domain decomposition methods (for which $S' = S$). If α_k is $0, 1$ or 0.5 we retrieve respectively Dirichlet-Neumann, Neumann-Dirichlet or Neumann-Neumann preconditioners [408]. On the other hand, since equation (9.73) is nonlinear, one can apply a Newton method,

$$\left(S_f'(\gamma_k) + S_s'(\gamma_k)\right)(\gamma_{k+1} - \gamma_k) = -S_f(\gamma_k) - S_s(\gamma_k), \tag{9.85}$$

which corresponds to the nonlinear Richardson iteration (9.83) preconditioned with $P_k = S_f'(\gamma_k) + S_s'(\gamma_k)$. This linear equation can be solved, for example, by a GMRES algorithm, with or without preconditioning. For instance, in [118] the authors propose to use the preconditioners (9.84).

The Newton method applied to the Dirichlet-Neumann formulation is not equivalent to the Newton method applied to the Steklov formulation, since the roles played by the fluid and by the structure are not symmetric in the first approach whereas they are in the second. After linearisation, one cannot compose (9.80) with S_s to retrieve (9.85). Finally, let us emphasise that (9.83)–(9.84) is not equivalent to (9.85) since in general $(A + B)^{-1} \neq A^{-1} + B^{-1}$.

The advantage of (9.73) compared to formulation (9.74) is that the fluid and the structure sub-problems can be solved simultaneously and independently for the residual computation (right-hand sides of (9.83)) and the application of the preconditioner (S_f' and S_s') as soon as $\alpha \notin \{0, 1\}$.

9.4 Semi-implicit coupling

The method that we introduce in this paragraph is *not* strongly coupled, in the sense that (9.1) and (9.2) are not exactly enforced, but it exhibits very good stability properties. It basically relies upon two ideas. The first one is to couple implicitly the pressure stress to ensure stability. This is suggested in Section 9.2 where it is shown that explicit coupling of the added mass term yields instabilities. The remaining terms of the fluid equations – dissipation, convection and geometrical nonlinearities – are *explicitly* coupled to the structure (of course, these terms may be implicit within the fluid solver). This drastically reduces the cost of the coupling without affecting the stability too much. The second idea relies upon the fact that this kind of implicit-explicit splitting can be conveniently performed using a Chorin-Temam projection scheme (see [89, 495] for the original papers and [207] for a review) in the fluid: at each time step the projection sub-step (carried out in a known fluid domain) is strongly coupled with the structure, so accounting for the added-mass effect in an implicit way, while the expensive ALE-advection-viscous sub-step is explicitly, i.e., weakly, coupled. The main advantages of the resulting algorithm are its simplicity of implementation and its efficiency compared to the methods presented in the previous section. Obviously, the main drawbacks are: first, it assumes the fluid to be solved with a projection scheme and, second, the energy is not perfectly balanced, at least from a theoretical viewpoint. In spite of that, theoretical and numerical evidence shows that, for a wide range of physical and discrete parameters, the scheme is numerically stable.

We denote by δt the time step, and for the sake of clarity we present the time semi-discrete version of the algorithm. Assuming that Ω_f^n, $\boldsymbol{u}_f^n$, P^n, $\widehat{\boldsymbol{\eta}}_s^n$ are known at time t^n, we propose to compute Ω_f^{n+1}, $\boldsymbol{u}_f^{n+1}$, P^{n+1}, $\widehat{\boldsymbol{\eta}}^{n+1}$ according to the following procedure:

- **Step 1:** Definition of the new domain:

$$\widetilde{\boldsymbol{\eta}}_f^{n+1} = \mathrm{Ext}(\widehat{\boldsymbol{\eta}}^n_{s|\widehat{\Gamma}}), \quad \widehat{\boldsymbol{w}}(\widetilde{\boldsymbol{\eta}}_f^{n+1}) = \frac{1}{\delta t}\left(\widetilde{\boldsymbol{\eta}}_f^{n+1} - \widetilde{\boldsymbol{\eta}}_f^{n}\right). \tag{9.86}$$

- **Step 2:** ALE-advection-diffusion step (explicit coupling):

$$\begin{cases} \rho_f \left.\dfrac{\widetilde{\boldsymbol{u}_f^{n+1}} - \boldsymbol{u}_f{}^n}{\delta t}\right|_{\hat{x}} + \rho_f(\widetilde{\boldsymbol{u}_f}^n - \boldsymbol{w}^{n+1}) \cdot \boldsymbol{\nabla}\widetilde{\boldsymbol{u}_f^{n+1}} \\ \qquad\qquad -2\mu\,\mathbf{div}(\boldsymbol{D}(\widetilde{\boldsymbol{u}_f^{n+1}})) = \boldsymbol{0}, \quad \text{in} \quad \Omega_f^{n+1}, \\ \qquad\qquad \widetilde{\boldsymbol{u}_f^{n+1}} = \boldsymbol{w}^{n+1}, \quad \text{on} \quad \Gamma^{n+1}. \end{cases} \tag{9.87}$$

- **Step 3:** Projection step (implicit coupling):
  - **Step 3.1:**

$$\begin{cases} \rho_f \dfrac{\boldsymbol{u}_f^{n+1} - \widetilde{\boldsymbol{u}_f^{n+1}}}{\delta t} + \boldsymbol{\nabla} P^{n+1} = \boldsymbol{0}, & \text{in} \quad \Omega_f^{n+1}, \\ \operatorname{div} \boldsymbol{u}_f^{n+1} = 0, & \text{in} \quad \Omega_f^{n+1}, \\ \boldsymbol{u}_f^{n+1} \cdot \boldsymbol{n}_f = \dfrac{\widehat{\boldsymbol{\eta}}_s^{n+1} - \widehat{\boldsymbol{\eta}}_s^{n}}{\delta t} \cdot \boldsymbol{n}_f, & \text{on} \quad \Gamma^{n+1}. \end{cases} \tag{9.88}$$

  - **Step 3.2:**

$$\begin{cases} \hat{\rho}_{s,0} \dfrac{\hat{\boldsymbol{u}}_s^{n+1} - \hat{\boldsymbol{u}}_s^{n}}{\delta t} - \mathbf{div}_{\hat{\boldsymbol{x}}} \left(\dfrac{\widehat{\boldsymbol{\Pi}}^{n} + \widehat{\boldsymbol{\Pi}}^{n+1}}{2} \right) = \boldsymbol{0}, & \text{in} \quad \widehat{\Omega}_s, \\ \dfrac{\widehat{\boldsymbol{\eta}}_s^{n+1} - \widehat{\boldsymbol{\eta}}_s^{n}}{\delta t} = \dfrac{\hat{\boldsymbol{u}}_s^{n+1} + \hat{\boldsymbol{u}}_s^{n}}{2}, & \text{in} \quad \widehat{\Omega}_s, \\ \widehat{\boldsymbol{\Pi}}^{n+1} \cdot \widehat{\boldsymbol{n}}_s = \hat{J}_f^{n+1} (\boldsymbol{\sigma}_f \, (\widetilde{\boldsymbol{u}_f^{n+1}}, P^{n+1}) \circ \widetilde{\mathcal{A}}^{n+1}) (\widehat{\boldsymbol{F}}_f^{n+1})^{-T} \cdot \widehat{\boldsymbol{n}}_s, & \text{on} \quad \widehat{\Gamma}. \end{cases} \tag{9.89}$$

Note that steps 1 and 2 are performed only *once* per time step. In a partitioned procedure, step 3 is solved by sub-iterating between steps 3.1 and 3.2 (using fixed-point or Newton iterations, for instance) since $\widehat{\boldsymbol{\eta}}_s^{n+1}$ is required in 3.1 while P^{n+1} is required in 3.2. The two sub-problems of steps 3 are therefore solved several times but in contrast to a fully coupled procedure, the part of the fluid solved during the inner iterations reduces to a simple Darcy-like problem. In a standard strongly coupled approach (as shown in Section 9.3) the domain velocity in step 1 is defined from the (unknown) solution of the structure problem by

$$\boldsymbol{w}^{n+1}_{|\widehat{\Gamma}} = \frac{\widehat{\boldsymbol{\eta}}_s^{n+1} - \widehat{\boldsymbol{\eta}}_s^{n}}{\delta t}_{|\widehat{\Gamma}}.$$

The sub-iterations therefore include step 1 and step 2 which dramatically increases the overall computational cost. The key point here is to show that steps 1 and 2 can indeed be treated "outside" the inner loop of sub-iterations, without compromising the stability too much.

Remark 9.4.1 *The idea presented here can be generalised to other fractional step schemes. See for example [22, 400] for an extension to algebraic factorisation methods.*

In a simplified case, when the fluid and the structure are linear, and with a Leap-Frog scheme for the structure, the following stability result can be proved [146].

Proposition 9.5. *Let h and H be the space discretisation steps in the fluid and the solid respectively. Assume that the solid-to-fluid interface matching operator $\pi_h : V_H^s(\Gamma) \longrightarrow V_h^f(\Gamma)$ is L^2-stable. Then, there exists a constant*

$C > 0$, independent of the physical and discretisation parameters, such that under the condition

$$\rho_s \geq C\left(\rho_f \frac{h}{H^\alpha} + 2\frac{\mu\delta t}{hH^\alpha}\right), \quad \textit{with} \quad \alpha = \begin{cases} 0, & \textit{if } \overline{\Omega_s} = \Gamma, \\ 1, & \textit{if } \overline{\Omega_s} \neq \Gamma, \end{cases} \tag{9.90}$$

the following discrete energy estimate holds:

$$\begin{aligned} &\frac{1}{\delta t}\left[\frac{\rho_f}{2}\|\boldsymbol{u}_{f,h}^{n+1}\|_{0,\Omega_f}^2 - \frac{\rho_f}{2}\|\boldsymbol{u}_{f,h}^{n}\|_{0,\Omega_f}^2\right] \\ &+\frac{1}{\delta t}\left[\frac{\rho_s}{2}\left\|\frac{\widehat{\boldsymbol{\eta}_{s,H}^{n+1}} - \widehat{\boldsymbol{\eta}_{s,H}^{n}}}{\delta t}\right\|_{0,\Omega_s}^2 - \frac{\rho^s}{2}\left\|\frac{\widehat{\boldsymbol{\eta}_{s,H}^{n}} - \widehat{\boldsymbol{\eta}_{s,H}^{n-1}}}{\delta t}\right\|_{0,\Omega_f}^2\right] \\ &+\frac{1}{2\delta t}\left[a_s(\widehat{\boldsymbol{\eta}_{s,H}^{n+1}}, \widehat{\boldsymbol{\eta}_{s,H}^{n+1}}) - a_s(\widehat{\boldsymbol{\eta}_{s,H}^{n}}, \widehat{\boldsymbol{\eta}_{s,H}^{n}})\right] + \mu\|\boldsymbol{D}(\boldsymbol{u}_{f,h}^{n+1})\|_{0,\Omega_f}^2 \leq 0. \end{aligned} \tag{9.91}$$

Therefore, the semi-implicit coupling scheme is stable, in the energy-norm, under condition (9.90).

We end this section with a few remarks:

- It is worth noticing that, with this scheme, decreasing δt enhances stability. This property is the main advantage of the semi-implicit algorithm compared to the explicit scheme studied in Section 9.2.4. Indeed, in that case, we have shown in Proposition 9.2 that the coupling may be unstable irrespective of δt.
- The assumption on the L^2-stability of the interface matching operator is satisfied by the standard finite element interpolation operator, for example, whenever the fluid interface triangulation is a sub-triangulation of the solid interface triangulation (see [146]). This includes, in particular, the case of interface matching meshes. By construction, a mortar-based matching operator also fulfils that assumption (see [37]).
- The sufficient condition (9.90) can be satisfied by reducing the ratios $\frac{h}{H^\alpha}$ and $\frac{\delta t}{hH^\alpha}$. The latter might be thought of as a CFL-like condition.
- In the case $\overline{\Omega^s} = \Gamma$, i.e., $\alpha = 0$, condition (9.90) becomes independent of the solid mesh size H. In particular, we can set $H = h$, and stabilise the scheme by simply reducing h (and δt).
- In the case $\overline{\Omega^s} \neq \Gamma$, i.e., $\alpha = 1$, the stability of the scheme can be ensured provided that the fluid mesh size h is small enough compared to the structure mesh size H. Numerical simulations performed in $2D$ and $3D$, with $h = H$, showed however that this condition seems to be unnecessary when dealing with a reasonable range of physical parameters.

9.5 Space discretisation of the coupling conditions

A thorough analysis of the space discretisation of the fluid and structure equations is beyond the scope of this chapter. Nevertheless, we wish to briefly

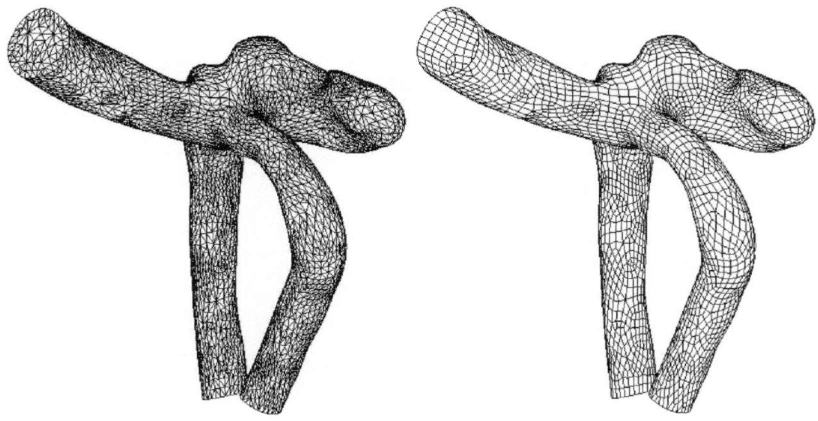

Fig. 9.2. A simple case of nonconformity: tetrahedra for the fluid (left) and quadrilaterals for the structure, but matching nodes (from [189])

address the space discretisation of the transmission conditions (9.1) and (9.2). We assume that the fluid and the structure problems are in a variational form and are discretised by the finite element method.

The simplest situation occurs when the nodes of the fluid and structure meshes match at the interface. The kinematic condition (9.1) can then be imposed straightforwardly, pointwise. Nevertheless, even in this simple case, it may not be obvious to devise a procedure to accurately compute the load for condition (9.2). For example, the aneurysm meshes presented in Fig. 9.2 have been built using tetrahedra for the fluid (convenient for automatic mesh generators) and quadrilaterals for the structure (shell elements). With a special algorithm (see [189]), the meshes can be built in such a way that the nodes lying on the surface wall are matching. Each solid quadrilateral then contains two triangles, which lie on the boundary of fluid tetrahedra. In this configuration, although the nodes are the same on the fluid and structure interfaces, the shape functions are different and the issue of well-balanced load computation is therefore not trivial. Of course, we can also consider completely nonmatching grids, the element size being generally smaller in the fluid than in the structure. Another case of nonconformity can also occur when the structure is immersed in the fluid: in this case, when very large displacements occur, the ALE formulation presented above yields frequent re-meshing. To circumvent this problem, it may be convenient to use completely independent meshes for the fluid and the structure. This of course results in nonconforming meshes.

In all these cases, once the velocity has been imposed – typically on the fluid – the question is how to compute the load on the structure without introducing any spurious energy due to the discretisation. Roughly speaking, the answer is: the operator giving the load has to be the *dual* of the operator defining the velocity. The purpose of the rest of this section is to expound this statement through a few examples.

9.5.1 A general formulation with Lagrange multipliers

In order to reformulate in a slightly different way the fluid-structure problem, we introduce the following notations: For $\widehat{\boldsymbol{v}_f} \in [H^1(\widehat{\Omega_f})]^3$ and $\mu \in [H^{-\frac{1}{2}}(\widehat{\Gamma})]^3$ we define:

$$b_f(\hat{\boldsymbol{v}}_f, \mu) = \langle \mu, \hat{\boldsymbol{v}}_f \rangle_\Gamma,$$

and for $\hat{\boldsymbol{v}}_s \in [H^1(\widehat{\Omega_s})]^3$,

$$b_s(\hat{\boldsymbol{v}}_s, \mu) = \langle \mu, \hat{\boldsymbol{v}}_s \rangle_\Gamma,$$

where $\langle \cdot, \cdot \rangle_\Gamma$ denotes the duality pairing between $[H^{-\frac{1}{2}}(\widehat{\Gamma})]^3$ and $[H^{\frac{1}{2}}(\widehat{\Gamma})]^3$.

The fluid-structure problem reads: find $(\widehat{\boldsymbol{u}}_f, \widehat{P}, \widehat{\boldsymbol{\eta}}_s) \in [H^1(\widehat{\Omega_f})]^3 \times L^2(\widehat{\Omega_f}) \times [H^1(\widehat{\Omega_s})]^3$, $\lambda \in [H^{-\frac{1}{2}}(\widehat{\Gamma})]^3$ such that for all $(\hat{\boldsymbol{v}}_f, \widehat{q}, \hat{\boldsymbol{v}}_s) \in [H^1(\widehat{\Omega_f})]^3 \times L^2(\widehat{\Omega_f}) \times [H^1(\widehat{\Omega_s})]^3$, $\mu \in [H^{-\frac{1}{2}}(\widehat{\Gamma})]^3$

$$\begin{cases} a_f\left(\widehat{\boldsymbol{\eta}}_s; (\widehat{\boldsymbol{u}}_f, \widehat{P}), (\hat{\boldsymbol{v}}_f, \widehat{q})\right) + b_f(\hat{\boldsymbol{v}}_f, \lambda) = \langle F_f, \hat{\boldsymbol{v}}_f \rangle, \\ b_f(\widehat{\boldsymbol{u}}_f, \mu) - b_s(\hat{\boldsymbol{u}}_s, \mu) = 0, \\ a_s(\widehat{\boldsymbol{\eta}}_s, \hat{\boldsymbol{v}}_s) - b_s(\hat{\boldsymbol{v}}_s, \lambda) = \langle F_s, \hat{\boldsymbol{v}}_s \rangle. \end{cases} \tag{9.92}$$

In this formalism, equation $(9.92)_2$ represents the kinematic condition (9.1) while $-b_f(\hat{\boldsymbol{v}}_f, \lambda)$ and $b_s(\hat{\boldsymbol{v}}_s, \lambda)$ are the variational forms of the load acting on the fluid and the structure respectively. Note that (9.2) is implicitly handled since $\lambda = -\boldsymbol{\sigma}_f \cdot \boldsymbol{n}_f$ and $\lambda = \boldsymbol{\sigma}_s \cdot \boldsymbol{n}_s$.

9.5.2 Three configurations of interest

To simplify our notations, we propose to rewrite formally system (9.92) as follows: find $(u_f, u_s, \lambda) \in X_f \times X_s \times X_\Gamma$ such that, for all $(v_f, v_s, \mu) \in X_f \times X_s \times X_\Gamma$,

$$\begin{cases} a_f(u_f, v_f) + b_f(v_f, \lambda) = \langle F_f, v_f \rangle, \\ b_f(u_f, \mu) - b_s(u_s, \mu) = 0, \\ a_s(u_s, v_s) - b_s(v_s, \lambda) = \langle F_s, v_s \rangle. \end{cases} \tag{9.93}$$

Compared to (9.92), the system is now linear, and all the fluid (resp. structure) unknowns are "lumped" in the scalar unknown u_f (resp. u_s). It is easy to extend the ideas presented here to the original fluid-structure problem.

We consider finite element meshes on the fluid and the structure domains and finite element spaces $X_{f,h}$, $X_{s,h}$ and $X_{\Gamma,h}$ approximating X_f, X_s and X_Γ respectively. The fluid (resp. structure) mesh has n_f (resp. n_s) nodes, whose n_f^Γ (resp. n_s^Γ) are located on the fluid-structure interface and n_f^I (resp. n_s^I) are not. The nodes on the fluid-structure interface are numbered from $n_f^I + 1$ to n_f (resp. $n_s^I + 1$ to n_s). We thus have $n_f^\Gamma = n_f - n_f^I$ (resp. $n_s^\Gamma = n_s - n_s^I$). We introduce finite element basis $(v_i^f)_{i=1,\dots,n_f}$, $(v_i^s)_{i=1,\dots,n_s}$ and $(\mu_i)_{i=1,\dots,n_\Gamma}$

of the spaces $X_{f,h}$, $X_{s,h}$ and $X_{\Gamma,h}$ respectively. Then (9.93) can be readily put into the following matrix form:

$$\begin{bmatrix} \mathrm{A_f} & 0 & \mathrm{B_f^T} \\ \mathrm{B_f} & -\mathrm{B_s} & 0 \\ 0 & \mathrm{A_s} & -\mathrm{B_s^T} \end{bmatrix} \begin{bmatrix} \mathrm{U_f} \\ \mathrm{U_s} \\ \Lambda \end{bmatrix} = \begin{bmatrix} \mathrm{F_f} \\ 0 \\ \mathrm{F_s} \end{bmatrix}. \tag{9.94}$$

Note that such a formulation is, by construction, associated to a global energy equality: multiplying $(9.94)_1$ by $\mathrm{U_f}$, $(9.94)_2$ by Λ, $(9.94)_3$ by $\mathrm{U_s}$, and adding, we obtain:

$$(\mathrm{A_f U_f}, \mathrm{U_f}) + (\mathrm{A_s U_s}, \mathrm{U_s}) = (\mathrm{F_f}, \mathrm{U_f}) + (\mathrm{F_s}, \mathrm{U_s}). \tag{9.95}$$

We see that the coupling terms cancel, as in the continuous case (see Section 9.1). In other words, using this formulation, no spurious power appears on the fluid-structure interface due to the space discretisation.

The matrix $\mathrm{B_f}$ has n_Γ rows and n_f columns, but most of the columns are zero. Its block structure is typically the following:

$$\mathrm{B_f} = \left[\begin{array}{c|c} 0 \ldots\ldots 0 & \\ & \mathrm{K_f} \\ 0 \ldots\ldots 0 & \end{array}\right],$$

where $\mathrm{K_f}$ is the $n_\Gamma \times n_f^\Gamma$ matrix whose entries are $b_f(v_j^f, \mu_i)$, $j = n_f^I + 1, \ldots, n_f^\Gamma$ and $i = 1, \ldots, n_\Gamma$. The matrices $\mathrm{B_s}$ and $\mathrm{K_s}$ are defined *mutatis mutandis.*

We propose to address three configurations of interest. We do not claim that formulation (9.94) with Lagrange multipliers is the most convenient in all cases. As we shall see, we can solve the first two configurations without using Lagrange multipliers explicitly. Nevertheless this formulation offers a unified framework and a useful guideline to compute the load at the interface.

Conformal meshes

We first consider the simple case of matching meshes represented in Fig. 9.3. The Lagrange multipliers space can be, for example, defined by:

$$X_{\Gamma,h} = \left\{ \mu_h \text{ measure on } \Gamma,\ \mu_h = \sum_{i=n_f^I+1}^{n_f} \mu_i \delta(\boldsymbol{x}_i), \mu_i \in \mathbb{R} \right\}, \tag{9.96}$$

where $(\boldsymbol{x}_i)_{i=n_f^I+1\ldots n_f}$ denote the fluid nodes on the fluid-structure interface Γ and $\delta(\boldsymbol{x}_i)$ is the Dirac measure on $\boldsymbol{x}_i$ defined by:

$$\langle \delta(\boldsymbol{x}_i), v_h \rangle = v_h(\boldsymbol{x}_i).$$

Note that $X_{\Gamma,h}$ is not a subspace of X_Γ and that this choice requires continuous basis functions. We have $n_\Gamma = n_f^\Gamma = n_s^\Gamma$ and the matrices $\mathrm{K_f}$ and $\mathrm{K_s}$ are the identity:

$$\mathrm{K_f} = \mathrm{K_s} = \mathrm{I}_{n_\Gamma \times n_\Gamma}.$$

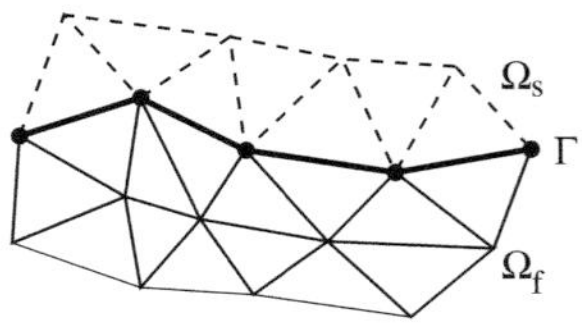

Fig. 9.3. Example of conformal meshes

The second equation of (9.93) is thus simply equivalent to:

$$\mathrm{U}_\mathrm{f}^\Gamma = \mathrm{U}_\mathrm{s}^\Gamma. \tag{9.97}$$

Note that in this case, the Lagrange multiplier space could have been defined equivalently on the structure nodes.

Conformal interface, non-conformal meshes

We now consider the case of non-conformal meshes represented in Fig. 9.4. First suppose that the Lagrange multipliers space is defined as in (9.96). We have

$$[\mathrm{K}_\mathrm{f}]_{ij} = \langle \delta(\boldsymbol{x}_i), v_j^f \rangle = v_j^f(\boldsymbol{x}_i) = \delta_{ij},$$

where $\delta_{ij} = 0$ if $i \neq j$ and 1 otherwise,

$$[\mathrm{K}_\mathrm{s}]_{ij} = \langle \delta(\boldsymbol{x}_i), v_j^s \rangle = v_j^s(\boldsymbol{x}_i).$$

The matrix K_s is the structure-to-fluid interpolation matrix. The kinematic condition thus reads:

$$\mathrm{U}_\mathrm{f}^\Gamma = \mathrm{K}_\mathrm{s}\mathrm{U}_\mathrm{s}^\Gamma. \tag{9.98}$$

Other choices of Lagrange multipliers would lead to different matrices. For example, following [142] and using a mortar approach (see [38]), we could choose

$$X_{\Gamma,h} = \left\{ \mu_h \in L^2(\Gamma),\ \text{trace of the fluid shape functions } v_h^f \right\}.$$

In this case

$$[\mathrm{K}_\mathrm{f}]_{ij} = \langle \mu_i, v_j^f \rangle = \int_\Gamma v_i^f v_j^f,$$

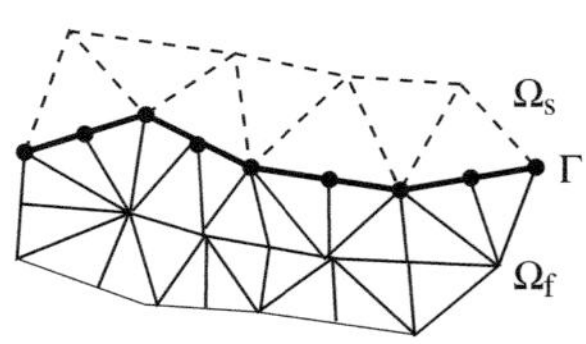

Fig. 9.4. Example of non-conformal meshes

and

$$[\mathrm{K_s}]_{ij} = \langle \mu_i, v_j^s \rangle = \int_\Gamma v_i^s v_j^f .$$

With this choice, the matrix $\mathrm{K_f}$ is a surface mass matrix. It is therefore non-singular. Thus, the kinematic condition reads:

$$\mathrm{U_f^\Gamma} = \mathrm{K_f}^{-1}\mathrm{K_s}\mathrm{U_s^\Gamma}. \tag{9.99}$$

The three previous cases, (9.97), (9.98) and (9.99), can be put in the same form:

$$\mathrm{U_f^\Gamma} = \mathrm{C}\mathrm{U_s^\Gamma} \tag{9.100}$$

where the matrix C is either I, $\mathrm{K_s}$ or $\mathrm{K_f}^{-1}\mathrm{K_s}$, depending on the case and the choice of the Lagrange multipliers space. When using partitioned algorithms, system (9.94) is never solved directly. Nevertheless, we would like to show that this formulation provides a hint to compute the load exerted on the structure when the kinematic condition is imposed on the fluid with relation (9.100).

Let us decompose the matrix $\mathrm{A_f}$, and vectors $\mathrm{U_f}$ and $\mathrm{U_s}$ into blocks corresponding to the internal and fluid-structure nodes:

$$\mathrm{A_f} = \begin{bmatrix} \mathrm{A_f^{II}} & \mathrm{A_f^{I\Gamma}} \\ \mathrm{A_f^{\Gamma I}} & \mathrm{A_f^{\Gamma\Gamma}} \end{bmatrix}, \quad \mathrm{U_f} = \begin{bmatrix} \mathrm{U_f^I} \\ \mathrm{U_f^\Gamma} \end{bmatrix}, \quad \mathrm{U_s} = \begin{bmatrix} \mathrm{U_s^I} \\ \mathrm{U_s^\Gamma} \end{bmatrix}.$$

Consequently, assuming that $\mathrm{U_s^\Gamma}$ is given, we see from (9.94) that $\mathrm{U_f^I}$ is obtained by solving

$$\mathrm{A_f^{II}}\mathrm{U_f^I} = \mathrm{F_f} - \mathrm{A_f^{I\Gamma}}\mathrm{C}\mathrm{U_s^\Gamma}.$$

We introduce the *algebraic residual* $\mathrm{R_f}$ of the fluid problem defined by

$$\mathrm{R_f} = \mathrm{F_f^\Gamma} - \mathrm{A_f^{\Gamma I}}\mathrm{U_f^I} - \mathrm{A_f^{\Gamma\Gamma}}\mathrm{U_f^\Gamma}. \tag{9.101}$$

In the three considered cases, (9.97), (9.98) and (9.99), the Lagrange multiplier is given by:

$$\Lambda = \mathrm{K_f^{-T}}\mathrm{R_f}.$$

In the algebraic system (9.94), formally representing the fluid-structure problem, we see that the algebraic counterpart of the load exerted on the structure is given by:

$$\mathrm{F_{fsi}} = \mathrm{K_s^T}\Lambda.$$

Therefore, as soon as the kinematic continuity is imposed with a relation like (9.100), the load on the structure is given by the dual relation:

$$\boxed{\mathrm{F_{fsi}} = \mathrm{C^T}\mathrm{R_f}} \tag{9.102}$$

where $\mathrm{R_f}$ is the fluid residual defined in (9.101). This corresponds to the *conservative approach* proposed in [142], which, as shown in (9.95), ensures a well-balanced energy transfer at the discrete level.

Let us consider the question raised at the beginning of this section concerning the case of the aneurysm presented in Fig. 9.2. Recall that, with a procedure proposed in [189], we can build a tetrahedral mesh in the fluid and a quadrilateral mesh in the structure with matching nodes. Therefore, the matrix C in (9.100) is the identity. Consequently, relation (9.102) shows that the load on the structure is *exactly* the residual of the fluid problem. Note that this convenient result was not obvious at the beginning since each quadrilateral on the structure corresponds to *two* triangles on the fluid boundary.

Immersed structure

We now address the case of an immersed thin structure, like a valve (see Fig. 9.5). Considering again our simplified system (9.94), we can choose for example the following Lagrange multipliers space:

$$X_{\Gamma,h} = \left\{ \mu_h \text{ measure on } \Gamma,\ \mu_h = \sum_{i=1}^{n_s} \mu_i \delta(\boldsymbol{x}_i), \mu_i \in \mathbb{R} \right\},$$

where $\boldsymbol{x}_i$ denotes the structure nodes lying on the fluid-structure interface (which coincide with the whole structure for a thin solid). We have:

$$[\mathrm{K_f}]_{ij} = \langle \delta(\boldsymbol{x}_i), v_j^f \rangle = v_j^f(\boldsymbol{x}_i),$$

and

$$[\mathrm{K_s}]_{ij} = \langle \delta(\boldsymbol{x}_i), v_j^s \rangle = v_{s,j}(\boldsymbol{x}_i) = \delta_{ij}.$$

The matrix $\mathrm{K_f}$ is the fluid-to-structure interpolation matrix. We have

$$\mathrm{K_f} \mathrm{U_f}^{\Gamma} = \mathrm{U_s}^{\Gamma}. \tag{9.103}$$

Note that the matrix $\mathrm{K_f}$ is rectangular. Thus, in contrast to the previous cases – which can all be put in the form (9.100) – the fluid velocity on the fluid-structure interface cannot be eliminated. Thus, when decoupling the fluid and the structure in a partitioned scheme, the fluid problem has now to be solved as a "genuine" saddle-point problem: given the structure velocity $\mathrm{U_s}$, we have to solve

$$\begin{bmatrix} \mathrm{A_f} & \mathrm{B_f^T} \\ \mathrm{B_f} & 0 \end{bmatrix} \begin{bmatrix} \mathrm{U_f} \\ \Lambda \end{bmatrix} = \begin{bmatrix} \mathrm{F_f} \\ \mathrm{B_s U_s} \end{bmatrix}. \tag{9.104}$$

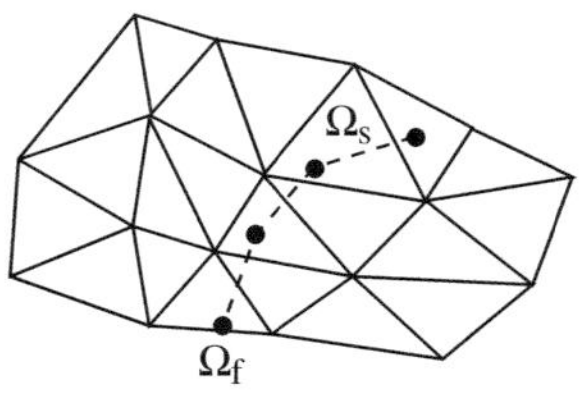

Fig. 9.5. Example of an immersed structure

As before, other Lagrange multipliers spaces can be considered, for example the trace of the structure basis function or more general L^2 functions. Of course, this space has to be carefully chosen in order to have $Ker B_f^T \neq \{0\}$. Once the fluid problem is solved, the load on the structure can be computed following the same guidelines as before.

The use of a Lagrange multipliers for immersed structure is the basis of the so-called Fictitious Domain method, initially used in fluid-structure interaction for rigid solids (see for example [196–198]). It has also been applied for flexible structures, either using Lagrange multipliers located on the structure surface (see [19, 126, 298]) or Lagrange multipliers located on the structure volume for thick solids [553]. It is also possible to simulate valves with the ALE formalism presented in the previous sections ([246, 272]). Another well-known approach is provided by the Immersed Boundary method (see for example [385]).

9.6 Numerical results and discussion

We end this chapter by comparing algorithms presented in the previous sections to solve the benchmark proposed in [155]. The fluid domain is a straight cylinder of radius 0.5 cm and length 5 cm. The wall displacement is described using a nonlinear shell model (based on MITC4 shell elements [75]). The physical parameters are: $\mu = 0.03\,poise$, $\rho_f = 1\,\text{g/cm}^3$, $\rho_s = 1.2\,\text{g/cm}^3$, $E = 3 \times 10^6\,\text{dynes/cm}^2$, $\nu = 0.3$. The thickness of the vessel wall is 0.1 cm. The fluid is initially at rest and a pressure of $1.332 \times 10^4\,\text{dynes/cm}^2$ (10 mmHg) is imposed on the inlet boundary for 0.005 s. The fluid and structure meshes have 3649 and 656 nodes respectively. A pressure wave propagation is observed [150, 155, 188].

We report in Table 9.1 the elapsed CPU time (dimensionless) for each of the approaches used for the simulations. We can notice that the semi-implicit coupling is about 5 times faster than the best implicit coupling (solved through Newton-based iterations). The increase in speed reported in Table 9.1 intensifies greatly when performing physiologic fluid-structure simulations, involving several cardiac beats and realistic boundary conditions based on lumped parameter models (see Chapter 10).

Table 9.1. CPU time: straight cylinder, 50 time steps of length $\delta t = 0.0002$ s.

Coupling	*Algorithm (dimensionless)*	*CPU total*	*Reference in the text*
	FP-Aitken	24.86	(9.79) and Remark 9.3.3
Implicit	inexact-Newton	6.05	(9.80) approx. Jacobian
	Newton	4.77	(9.80) exact Jacobian (9.82)
Semi-Implicit	Newton	1	Section 9.4

In general, the computational cost reduction observed in Table 9.1, with the semi-implicit coupling, is due to: (i) the use of a fractional-step method in the fluid; (ii) the explicit treatment of the ALE-advection-viscous sub-step and (iii) the use of Newton iterations for solving the projection sub-step (9.88)–(9.89). Compared to the implicit case, these iterations are cheap, as they do not require the computation of shape (domain) derivatives (see [150]).

9.7 Conclusions

We have presented various numerical methods to solve fluid-structure interaction problems involving an incompressible fluid. The nonlinear character of the coupled problem is one of the main difficulties that have to be faced when solving this type of problem. Thus, we have presented algorithms to efficiently address this issue. On the other hand, we have also shown that many troubles encountered in practice can be understood in the framework of a simplified *linear* model. This fact has been used to propose a very efficient coupling algorithm in which part of the fluid and the structure solvers are explicitly coupled without compromising the stability. All the proposed approaches have been formulated in the language of domain decomposition techniques.

The design of efficient numerical algorithms for fluid-structure problems in haemodynamics is still a challenging problem. We cite, for instance, recent works [21, 22, 145] that aim at reducing the computational cost of implicit coupling schemes. We refer also to [55, 56], which provide a robust method to stabilise the *explicit* coupling. Alternative approaches consisting in simplifying the structure problem have also been proposed [151, 352].

There are important issues that have not been addressed in the present chapter. Among them, we can mention the definition of appropriate boundary conditions (see e.g., [151, 155, 526]) and the management of contact between valves (see e.g., [16, 126, 521]). The effect of the surrounding tissues, the definition of more realistic constitutive laws and the integration of clinical measurements and of the information provided by medical images are some of the challenges that still have to be addressed.

10

Reduced models of the cardiovascular system

Joaquim Peiró, Alessandro Veneziani

Due to the large number of vessels involved and the multitude of different length scales required to accurately represent the flow in the various regions of the cardiovascular system, simulations of the flow of blood in the system based on full 3D models (see Chapters 2 and 3) are beyond the capability of current computers and they will be for years to come. Moreover, the huge amount of data that would be generated by such simulations is costly to process and of difficult clinical interpretation.

However, it is possible to devise simplified models exploiting specific features of blood flow, such as the basically cylindrical morphology of the vessels. Even though these models are highly simplified with respect to the local dynamics, they can provide reliable numerical results at a low computational cost. Interpretation is much straightforward, thus making them ideal as an everyday tool for use in clinical practice.

Moreover, these models are well-suited for describing systemic dynamics such as *feedback mechanisms* that play an important role in the correct working of the vascular system. These dynamics typically involve mechanical and biochemical phenomena that can be hardly described in terms of complete 3D models.

In this chapter, we address simplified models and in particular we consider:

1. one-dimensional (1D) models in which the space dependence is reduced only to the axial coordinate;
2. lumped parameter (or 0D) models, where the space dependence is discretised, by splitting the cardiovascular system into a set of compartments. The associated mathematical model is typically based on differential algebraic equations (DAE), often represented in terms of hydraulic or electric networks.

It is worth mentioning that studies on one-dimensional models of blood flow were first presented by Leonhard Euler in his seminal article entitled *Pro principa motu sanguinis per arterias determinando* [139]. In spite of the simplifying assumptions behind these models, they are very useful and

Formaggia L, Quarteroni A, Veneziani A (Eds.): Cardiovascular Mathematics. Modeling and simulation of the circulatory system

many of their analytical and numerical aspects still deserve further investigation[1].

10.1 One-dimensional (1D) models

There are several ways of deriving a 1D model of an incompressible fluid flowing in a compliant pipe. One could start from the incompressible Navier-Stokes equations and perform an asymptotic analysis by assuming that the radius of the vessel, R_0, is small compared to its length l, i.e. $\frac{R_0}{L} \ll 1$, that will permit us to simplify the governing equations by discarding the higher order terms in $\frac{R_0}{L}$, as proposed in [25]. Alternatively, the 1D model could be derived by assuming cylindrical symmetry and integrating the Navier-Stokes equations on a generic section as described in [364].

Here we will follow the approach advocated and described in [238,239] and derive the governing equations from conservation principles. This approach is more general and it does not require any simplifying assumptions concerning the geometry of the vessel section.

10.1.1 Derivation of the governing equations

We consider a simple compliant tube, illustrated in Fig. 10.1, as a model of the artery. We assume that the axis of the vessel is rectilinear and coincides with the x axis. The starting point for the derivation of the one-dimensional governing equations is Reynolds' transport theorem for an arbitrary control volume V_t with boundary ∂V_t and outer normal $\boldsymbol{n}$. A formal derivation of this formula can be found in Chapter 2 of this book and in [401]. It states that, for a continuous function $f = f(t, \boldsymbol{x})$, we have

$$\frac{d}{dt} \int_{V_t} f \, dV = \int_{V_t} \frac{\partial f}{\partial t} \, dV + \int_{\partial V_t} f \, \boldsymbol{u}_b \cdot \boldsymbol{n} \, d\sigma, \tag{10.1}$$

where $\boldsymbol{x}$ stands for (x, y, z) and $\boldsymbol{u}_b$ is the velocity of the boundary of volume V_t. This is composed of the arterial wall $\partial V_{t,w}$ and the two end sections S_1 and S_2, that are assumed normal to the axis. On S_1 and S_2 the normal component of $\boldsymbol{u}_b$ is 0, while on $\partial V_{t,w}$ velocity $\boldsymbol{u}_b$ does coincide with the velocity $\boldsymbol{u}_w$ of the arterial wall, so that

$$\int_{\partial V_t} f \, \boldsymbol{u}_b \cdot \boldsymbol{n} \, d\sigma = \int_{\partial V_{t,w}} f \, \boldsymbol{u}_w \cdot \boldsymbol{n} \, d\sigma. \tag{10.2}$$

[1] "Thus in explaining the motion of the blood, we come up against the same insuperable difficulties which clearly prevent us from more accurately investigating all the works of the Creator; wherein we ought constantly to admire and to venerate much more the highest wisdom conjoined with omnipotence since truly not even the greatest human ingenuity avails to understand and explain the true structure of the slightest micro-organism", L. Euler [139].

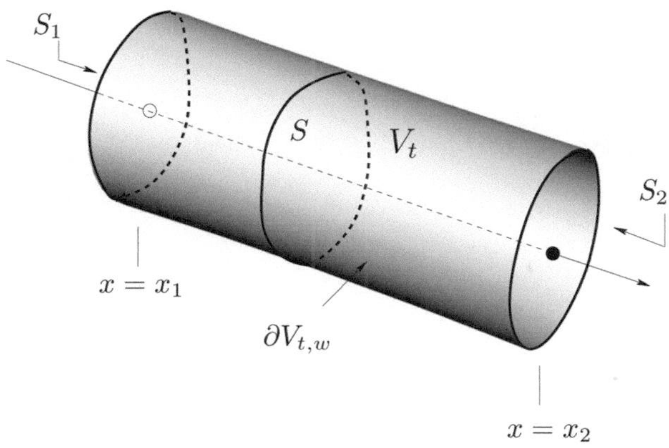

Fig. 10.1. Notation used to describe a simple compliant tube

Here $\boldsymbol{u}_w$ is taken to be different of the fluid velocity $\boldsymbol{u} = (u_1, u_2, u_3)$ to allow for the presence of a permeable lumen. The relative velocity between the arterial wall and the fluid at the lumen is given by

$$\boldsymbol{w} = \boldsymbol{u}_w - \boldsymbol{u}.$$

To obtain the one-dimensional form of the conservation laws, we consider area-averaged values of the relevant variables. The area-averaged value of f is denoted by $\bar{f}$ and given by

$$\bar{f} = \frac{1}{A} \int_S f \, d\sigma, \tag{10.3}$$

where $A = A(x,t) = \int_S d\sigma$ is the area of the cross section S. Using this notation, we write a volume integral as

$$\int_{V_t} f \, dV = \int_{x_1}^{x_2} \left[\int_S f \, d\sigma \right] dx = \int_{x_1}^{x_2} A\bar{f} \, dx, \tag{10.4}$$

where x_1 and x_2 ($x_2 > x_1$) are the $x-$coordinates of the cross sections S_1 and S_2.

Given that x_1 and x_2 are independent of time, the left-hand side term of equation (10.1) can be written as

$$\frac{d}{dt} \int_{V_t} f \, dV = \int_{x_1}^{x_2} \frac{\partial}{\partial t} \left(A\bar{f} \right) dx. \tag{10.5}$$

The presence of a permeable wall makes the evaluation of the second term of the right-hand side of equation (10.1) more involved. After (10.2), this term is calculated as

$$\int_{\partial V_{t,w}} f \boldsymbol{u}_w \cdot \boldsymbol{n} \, d\sigma = \int_{\partial V_{t,w}} f \boldsymbol{w} \cdot \boldsymbol{n} \, d\sigma + \int_{\partial V_{t,w}} f \boldsymbol{u} \cdot \boldsymbol{n} \, d\sigma.$$

Observe that

$$\int_{\partial V_{t,w}} f\boldsymbol{u}\cdot\boldsymbol{n}\,d\sigma = \int_{\partial V_t} f\boldsymbol{u}\cdot\boldsymbol{n}\,d\sigma - \int_{S_1} f\boldsymbol{u}\cdot\boldsymbol{n}\,d\sigma - \int_{S_2} f\boldsymbol{u}\cdot\boldsymbol{n}\,d\sigma =$$
$$\int_{\partial V_t} f\boldsymbol{u}\cdot\boldsymbol{n}\,d\sigma + \int_{S_1} f u_1\,d\sigma - \int_{S_2} f u_1\,d\sigma,$$

where u_1 is the x-component of the velocity $\boldsymbol{u}$. Thanks to the Gauss' theorem, we have

$$\int_{\partial V_{t,w}} f\boldsymbol{u}\cdot\boldsymbol{n}\,d\sigma = \int_{V_t} \nabla\cdot(f\boldsymbol{u})\;dV + \int_{S_1} f u_1\,d\sigma - \int_{S_2} f u_1\,d\sigma,$$

so that using area-averaged quantities, we finally obtain

$$\int_{\partial V_{t,w}} f\boldsymbol{u}_w\cdot\boldsymbol{n}d\sigma = \int_{\partial V_{t,w}} f\boldsymbol{w}\cdot\boldsymbol{n}\,d\sigma - \int_{x_1}^{x_2}\frac{\partial}{\partial x}\left[A\left(\overline{fu_1}\right)\right]dx +$$
$$\int_{V_t} \nabla\cdot(f\boldsymbol{u})\,dV, \tag{10.6}$$

Finally, including the expressions (10.5) and (10.6) into equation (10.1) leads to

$$\int_{x_1}^{x_2}\frac{\partial}{\partial t}\left(A\bar{f}\right)dx = \int_{x_1}^{x_2}\left(\int_S \frac{\partial f}{\partial t}\,d\sigma\right)dx + \int_{x_1}^{x_2}\left(\int_{\partial S} f\boldsymbol{w}\cdot\boldsymbol{n}\,d\gamma\right)dx -$$
$$\int_{x_1}^{x_2}\frac{\partial}{\partial x}\left[A\left(\overline{fu_1}\right)\right]dx + \int_{x_1}^{x_2}\left(\int_S \nabla\cdot(f\boldsymbol{u})\,d\sigma\right)dx,$$

and, given that this is true for any values of the coordinates of the end sections x_1 and x_2, the final form of the one-dimensional transport theorem for a generic variable f is

$$\frac{\partial}{\partial t}\left(A\bar{f}\right) + \frac{\partial}{\partial x}\left[A\left(\overline{fu_1}\right)\right] = \int_S\left[\frac{\partial f}{\partial t} + \nabla\cdot(f\boldsymbol{u})\right]d\sigma + \int_{\partial S} f\boldsymbol{w}\cdot\boldsymbol{n}\,d\gamma. \tag{10.7}$$

This formula is general and applicable to both compressible and incompressible fluids. Now we will proceed to derive the governing equations by invoking the principles of conservation of mass and balance of momentum.

Conservation of mass

The equation representing the conservation of mass in the flexible tube is obtained by taking $f = 1$ in equation (10.7). If we further assume that the fluid is incompressible, i.e. $\nabla\cdot\boldsymbol{u} = 0$, we get

$$\frac{\partial A}{\partial t} + \frac{\partial}{\partial x}\left(A\bar{u}_1\right) = \int_{\partial S} \boldsymbol{w}\cdot\boldsymbol{n}\,d\gamma, \tag{10.8}$$

where the term in the right-hand side could be interpreted as a volumetric outflow per unit length and unit time.

Balance of momentum

Here we take $f = u_1$ in the area-averaged Reynolds' transport expression (10.7), and assume again that the fluid is incompressible, to obtain

$$\frac{\partial}{\partial t}(A\bar{u}_1) + \frac{\partial}{\partial x}\left(A\overline{u_1^2}\right) = \int_S \left[\frac{\partial u_1}{\partial t} + \boldsymbol{u} \cdot \nabla u_1\right] d\sigma + \int_{\partial S} u_1 \boldsymbol{w} \cdot \boldsymbol{n}\, d\gamma\ , \quad (10.9)$$

which we now write as

$$\frac{\partial}{\partial t}(A\bar{u}_1) + \frac{\partial}{\partial x}\left(A\overline{u_1^2}\right) = \int_S \frac{Du_1}{Dt}\, d\sigma + \int_{\partial S} u_1 \boldsymbol{w} \cdot \boldsymbol{n}\, d\gamma\ , \quad (10.10)$$

where $\frac{D}{Dt} = \frac{\partial}{\partial t} + \boldsymbol{u} \cdot \nabla$ denotes the material derivative (see Chapter 3). To calculate the first term on the right-hand side of equation (10.10) we use the balance of momentum derived in Chapter 3 for the control volume V_t in the form

$$\int_{V_t} \frac{D}{Dt}(\rho \boldsymbol{u})\, dV = \int_{V_t} \rho \boldsymbol{f}^b\, dV + \int_{\partial V_t} \boldsymbol{T}\boldsymbol{n}\, d\sigma, \quad (10.11)$$

where $\boldsymbol{f}^b$ represents the body force per unit volume and $\boldsymbol{T}$ is the Cauchy stress tensor. Assuming that the density ρ is constant and using the divergence theorem, the balance of momentum equation (10.11) is written as

$$\int_{V_t} \frac{D\boldsymbol{u}}{Dt}\, dV = \int_{V_t} \boldsymbol{f}^b\, dV + \frac{1}{\rho}\int_{V_t} \nabla \cdot \boldsymbol{T}\, dV. \quad (10.12)$$

Now, invoking the constitutive equation for the fluid, we could write the stress tensor $\boldsymbol{T}$ as

$$\boldsymbol{T} = -p\boldsymbol{I} + \boldsymbol{D}, \quad (10.13)$$

where p denotes the pressure, $\boldsymbol{I}$ is the identity tensor, and $\boldsymbol{D}$ represents the tensor of deviatoric stresses due to the viscosity of the fluid. Setting $\nabla \cdot \boldsymbol{D} = \boldsymbol{d}$ we also write

$$\nabla \cdot \boldsymbol{T} = -\nabla p + \nabla \cdot \boldsymbol{D} = -\nabla p + \boldsymbol{d},$$

and, therefore, equation (10.12) as

$$\int_{x_1}^{x_2} \left(\int_S \frac{D\boldsymbol{u}}{Dt}\, d\sigma\right) dx = \int_{x_1}^{x_2} \left(\int_S \left[\boldsymbol{f}^b + \frac{1}{\rho}(-\nabla p + \boldsymbol{d})\right] d\sigma\right) dx. \quad (10.14)$$

Since x_1 and x_2 can be arbitrarily chosen, the integrands in the left and right-hand sides of equation (10.14) must be equal, therefore we could write the x-component of this equation as

$$\int_S \frac{Du_1}{Dt}\, d\sigma = \int_S \left[f_1^b + \frac{1}{\rho}\left(-\frac{\partial p}{\partial x} + d_1\right)\right] d\sigma, \quad (10.15)$$

where d_1 is the x-component of $\boldsymbol{d}$. Substituting this expression in equation (10.10) gives

$$\frac{\partial}{\partial t}(A\bar{u}_1) + \frac{\partial}{\partial x}\left(A\overline{u_1^2}\right) = \int_S \left[f_1^b + \frac{1}{\rho}(-\frac{\partial p}{\partial x} + d_1)\right] d\sigma + \int_{\partial S} u_1 \boldsymbol{w}\cdot\boldsymbol{n}\, d\sigma, \tag{10.16}$$

which can be expressed using area-averaged values as

$$\frac{\partial}{\partial t}(A\bar{u}_1) + \frac{\partial}{\partial x}\left(A\overline{u_1^2}\right) = \frac{A}{\rho}\left(\rho\bar{f}_1^b - \frac{\partial\bar{p}}{\partial x} + \bar{d}_1)\right) + \int_{\partial S} u_1 \boldsymbol{w}\cdot\boldsymbol{n}\, d\sigma. \tag{10.17}$$

The term $\overline{u_1^2}$ in this equation is handled by defining a momentum-flux correction coefficient α (sometimes called the Coriolis coefficient), which is a function of the velocity profile, as

$$\overline{u_1^2} = \frac{1}{A}\int_S u_1^2\, d\sigma = \alpha\bar{u}_1^2. \tag{10.18}$$

For a flat profile we have $\alpha = 1$ and for a parabolic flow $\alpha = 4/3$.

The term representing the viscous forces $\bar{d}_1$ is taken to be a linear function of the area-averaged velocity $\bar{u}_1$ of the form

$$\frac{A}{\rho}\bar{d}_1 = -K_R\bar{u}_1, \tag{10.19}$$

where K_R is a strictly positive quantity which represents the viscous resistance of the flow per unit length of tube. It is worth observing that for a proper definition of the coefficient, (10.19) is fulfilled by the Poiseuille flow (see Chapter. 5). The final form of the balance of momentum equation is

$$\frac{\partial}{\partial t}(A\bar{u}_1) + \frac{\partial}{\partial x}\left(\alpha\bar{u}_1^2\right) = A\bar{f}_1^b - \frac{A}{\rho}\left(\frac{\partial\bar{p}}{\partial x}\right) - K_R\bar{u}_1 + \int_{\partial S} u_1 \boldsymbol{w}\cdot\boldsymbol{n}\, d\sigma. \tag{10.20}$$

The unknowns in the system given by (10.8) and (10.20) are p, A and $\bar{u}_1$. Their number exceeds the number of equations and a common way to close the system is to explicitly provide a relationship between the pressure of the vessel p and the vessel area A. This relation will be derived from the models introduced in Chapter 3, in particular the algebraic relation (3.94).

Simplified models of wall mechanics

By assuming *static equilibrium* in the radial direction of a cylindrical tube, from one-dimensional models of wall mechanics described in Section 3.4.4 one can derive an algebraic relationship of the form

$$p = P_{ext} + \beta\left(\sqrt{A} - \sqrt{A_0}\right), \tag{10.21}$$

where

$$\beta = \frac{\sqrt{\pi} h_0 E}{(1-\nu^2)A_0}. \tag{10.22}$$

Here h_0 and $A_0 = A_0(x)$ denote the vessel thickness and sectional area, respectively, at the equilibrium state $(p, Q) = (P_{ext}, 0)$, $E = E(x)$ is the Young modulus, P_{ext} is the external pressure, assumed constant, and ν is the Poisson ratio. This ratio is typically taken to be $\nu = 1/2$ since biological tissue is practically incompressible. More generally, we may have

$$p = P_{ext} + \Phi(A; A_0, \beta), \tag{10.23}$$

being Φ a suitable function of the vessel section A and of the reference area A_0 as well as some mechanical parameter β. The main properties of Φ are

$$\frac{\partial \Phi}{\partial A} > 0, \quad \Phi(A_0; A_0, \beta) = 0,$$

for all allowable values of A, A_0 and β.

The algebraic relation (10.23), and in particular (10.21), assumes that the wall is instantaneously in equilibrium with the pressure forces acting on it.

Wall inertia and viscoelasticity can be included, yielding a differential pressure law. For instance, moving from (3.91) we may write

$$p - P_{ext} = \gamma_0 \frac{\partial^2 \eta}{\partial t^2} + \gamma_1 \frac{\partial \eta}{\partial t} + \Phi(A; A_0, \boldsymbol{\beta}), \tag{10.24}$$

where $\gamma_0 = \rho_w h_0$, $\gamma_1 = \frac{\gamma}{r_0^2}$ and the last term is the elastic response, modelled through equation (10.21). Here γ is the same viscoelasticity coefficient of (3.93) and η is the wall position. In the following, we indicate by $\dot{A}$ and $\ddot{A}$ the first and second time derivative of A. By assuming a circular profile $A = \pi\eta^2$, thus

$$\frac{\partial \eta}{\partial t} = \frac{1}{2\sqrt{\pi A}}\dot{A}, \qquad \frac{\partial^2 \eta}{\partial t^2} = \pi^{-\frac{1}{2}}\left(\frac{1}{2\sqrt{A}}\ddot{A} - \frac{1}{4\sqrt{A^3}}\dot{A}^2\right). \tag{10.25}$$

Using these relations into (10.24) we obtain an equation that links the pressure also to the time derivatives of A, which we write in all generality as

$$p - P_{ext} = \tilde{\Phi}_E(A, \dot{A}, \ddot{A}; A_0) + \Phi(A; A_0, \boldsymbol{\beta}),$$

where $\tilde{\Phi}_E$ is a non-linear function which derives from the treatment of the terms containing the time derivative of η. Since it may be assumed that the contribution to the pressure is in fact dominated by the term Φ, we will simplify this relationship by linearizing $\tilde{\Phi}_E$ around the state $A = A_0$, $\dot{A} = \ddot{A} = 0$. By so doing, after some simple algebraic manipulations, one finds

$$p - P_{ext} = \frac{\gamma_0}{2\sqrt{\pi A_0}}\ddot{A} + \frac{\gamma_1}{2\sqrt{\pi A_0}}\dot{A} + \Phi(A; A_0, \boldsymbol{\beta}). \tag{10.26}$$

Replacing this expression for the pressure in the momentum equation requires to compute the term

$$\frac{A}{\rho}\frac{\partial p}{\partial x} = \frac{\gamma_0 A}{2\rho\sqrt{\pi A_0}}\frac{\partial^3 A}{\partial x \partial t^2} + \frac{\gamma_1 A}{2\rho\sqrt{\pi A_0}}\frac{\partial^2 A}{\partial x \partial t} + \frac{A}{\rho}\frac{\partial \Phi}{\partial x}.$$

Wall inertia introduces a *dispersive* term into the momentum equation, while the viscoelasticity has a *diffusive* effect. This has implications on the numerical solution.

In the following we will consider only relation (10.21) to discuss the properties of the resulting scheme and its numerical formulation. Most of the discussion, however, can be extended to any model based on a pressure-area relation of the form (10.23).

10.1.2 Different formulations of the governing equations

In what follows, we will assume that the lumen is impermeable ($\boldsymbol{w} \cdot \boldsymbol{n} = 0$), that body forces are neglegible ($\bar{f}_1^b = 0$), and we will also simplify the notation by denoting the area-averaged axial velocity by u instead of $\bar{u}_1$ and using p instead of $\bar{p}$. Defining the mass flux across a section as $Q = Au = \int_S u_1 d\sigma$, the equations (10.8) and (10.20) now read

$$\begin{aligned} &\frac{\partial A}{\partial t} + \frac{\partial Q}{\partial x} = 0, \\ &\frac{\partial Q}{\partial t} + \frac{\partial}{\partial x}\left(\alpha \frac{Q^2}{A}\right) + \frac{A}{\rho}\left(\frac{\partial p}{\partial x}\right) + K_R \frac{Q}{A} = 0. \end{aligned} \tag{10.27}$$

The couple (A, Q) will be referred to as *conserved variable* since they stem naturally from the application of conservation principles.

The system of equations (10.27) can be expressed alternatively in terms of the variables (A, u). By simple manipulations one gets

$$\begin{aligned} &\frac{\partial A}{\partial t} + \frac{\partial Au}{\partial x} = 0, \\ &\frac{\partial u}{\partial t} + (2\alpha - 1)u\frac{\partial u}{\partial x} + (\alpha - 1)u^2\frac{\partial A}{\partial x} + \frac{1}{\rho}\frac{\partial p}{\partial x} + K_R \frac{u}{A} = 0. \end{aligned} \tag{10.28}$$

Both systems (10.27) and (10.28) may be written in *conservation form*. Let us assume for instance that the wall mechanics is described by the algebraic pressure-wall relationship (10.21).

For the system (A, Q) we have

$$\frac{\partial \mathbf{Q}}{\partial t} + \frac{\partial \mathbf{G}}{\partial x}(\mathbf{Q}) = \mathbf{B}(\mathbf{Q}), \tag{10.29}$$

with

$$\mathbf{Q} = \begin{bmatrix} A \\ Q \end{bmatrix}, \; \mathbf{G} = \begin{bmatrix} Q \\ \alpha \frac{Q^2}{A} + \int_{A_0}^{A} \frac{a}{\varphi} \frac{\partial \rho}{\partial a} da \end{bmatrix} \quad \text{and}$$

$$\mathbf{B} = \begin{bmatrix} 0 \\ -K_R \frac{Q}{A} + \frac{A}{\varphi} \left(\frac{\partial \rho}{\partial A_0} \frac{\partial A_0}{\partial x} + \frac{\partial \rho}{\partial \beta} \frac{\partial \beta}{\partial x} \right) \end{bmatrix}. \tag{10.30}$$

For the (A, u) system, if for the sake of simplicity we assume $\alpha = 1$, we have

$$\frac{\partial \boldsymbol{U}}{\partial t} + \frac{\partial \boldsymbol{F}}{\partial x}(\boldsymbol{U}) = \boldsymbol{S}(\boldsymbol{U}), \tag{10.31}$$

with

$$\boldsymbol{U} = \begin{bmatrix} A \\ u \end{bmatrix}, \quad \boldsymbol{F} = \begin{bmatrix} Au \\ p_t \end{bmatrix} \quad \text{and} \quad \boldsymbol{S} = \begin{bmatrix} 0 \\ -K_R \frac{u}{A} \end{bmatrix}. \tag{10.32}$$

Here

$$p_t = \frac{u^2}{2} + \frac{p}{\rho}, \tag{10.33}$$

denotes the *total pressure* (scaled by the constant density).

In the case $\alpha = 1$ the two weak forms are equivalent for smooth solutions, in particular when A and Q are C^1 continuous functions with respect to both arguments and A is strictly positive. Nevertheless, the assumption $\alpha = 1$ is quite realistic in the problems at hand since the velocity profile is in fact almost flat (see Chapter 1 and [350]) and the solutions within each of the approaches presented in this chapter will be sufficiently smooth to favour the use of the (A, u) system which has a simpler structure.

The (A, u) and the (A, Q) systems given respectively by equations (10.28) and (10.27), together with the algebraic pressure-area relationship (10.21), will be starting points of the numerical schemes discussed in Section 10.1.8.

Remark 10.1.1 *Even though the values of the coefficients α, K_R and β are fixed a priori once we make assumptions on the velocity profile and on the wall mechanics, it is also possible to interpret them as parameters of the model that can be obtained by fitting the results of the 1D model to available in vivo or 3D computational data as proposed in [314].*

10.1.3 1D models for blood solutes

The relevance of the dynamics of blood solutes and its coupling with haemodynamics have been extensively addressed in Chapter 7. Since the dynamics of these solutes is relevant for regulatory mechanisms that involve large parts of the cardiovascular system and are fundamental for its proper working (see Section 10.2.4), it is worth to devise simple models also for biochemical dynamics (see [108]). As done in Section 7.1 of Chapter 7, we assume that the solute concentration $c(\mathbf{x}, t)$ satisfies a (linear) advection-diffusion equation in the form

$$\frac{\partial c}{\partial t} - \mu_s \triangle c + \mathbf{u} \cdot \nabla c = 0,$$

in the domain Ω_t ($\mathbf{u}$ is the blood velocity), together with a suitable initial condition $c(\mathbf{x}, 0) = c_0(\mathbf{x})$. We assume that a Robin condition $\nu \nabla c \cdot \mathbf{n} = \chi(c_{ext} - c)$ is given on the vascular wall. Here coefficient χ denotes the *permeability*. For the sake of simplicity, we will assume that $c_{ext} = 0$.

By using area-averaged quantities, in a way similar to the one adopted for the Navier-Stokes equations, and setting $\Gamma = A\bar{c}$, it is possible to obtain the following 1D solute equation

$$\frac{\partial \Gamma}{\partial t} + \frac{\partial}{\partial x}\left(\omega \frac{\Gamma Q}{A}\right) + K_c \frac{\Gamma}{A} = 0, \quad x_1 < x < x_2, \tag{10.34}$$

to be completed with suitable boundary conditions. Coefficient ω depends on the axial velocity and concentration profiles (similar to the Coriolis coefficient) and K_c is a coefficient depending on the viscosity μ_s and the permeability χ. Equation (10.34) can be therefore coupled to (10.27) for a complete model of the blood and solutes dynamics. For an extensive analysis see [108].

10.1.4 Characteristic variables

Considering the pressure-area relationship (10.21) and assuming that $\beta = \beta(x)$ and $A_0 = A_0(x)$ we recall that applying the chain rule we obtain

$$\frac{\partial p}{\partial x} = \frac{\partial p}{\partial A}\frac{\partial A}{\partial x} + \frac{\partial p}{\partial \beta}\frac{\partial \beta}{\partial x} + \frac{\partial p}{\partial A_0}\frac{\partial A_0}{\partial x},$$

where

$$\frac{\partial p}{\partial A} = \frac{\beta}{2\sqrt{A}}.$$

System (10.28) can therefore be written inquasi-linear form as

$$\frac{\partial \boldsymbol{U}}{\partial t} + \boldsymbol{H}\frac{\partial \boldsymbol{U}}{\partial x} = \mathbf{f}(\mathbf{U}), \tag{10.35}$$

or, more explicitely

$$\begin{bmatrix} A \\ u \end{bmatrix}_t + \begin{bmatrix} u & A \\ c^2/A & u \end{bmatrix} \begin{bmatrix} A \\ u \end{bmatrix}_x = \begin{bmatrix} 0 \\ f \end{bmatrix},$$

where

$$c^2 = \frac{A}{\rho}\frac{\partial p}{\partial A} = \frac{\beta\sqrt{A}}{2\rho} \quad \text{and} \quad f = \frac{1}{\rho}\left[K_R u - \frac{\partial p}{\partial \beta}\frac{\partial \beta}{\partial x} + \frac{\partial p}{\partial A_0}\frac{\partial A_0}{\partial x}\right].$$

Under the assumption that $A > 0$, which is indeed a necessary condition to have a physically relevant solution, the matrix $\mathbf{H}$ has two real eigenvalues $\lambda_{1,2} = u \pm c$ and the corresponding left eigenmatrix $\mathbf{L}$ is

$$\mathbf{L} = \begin{bmatrix} \mathbf{l}_1^T \\ \mathbf{l}_2^T \end{bmatrix} = \begin{bmatrix} \frac{c}{A} & 1 \\ -\frac{c}{A} & 1 \end{bmatrix}, \tag{10.36}$$

where $\mathbf{l}_i$ indicates the i-th left eigenvector such that $\mathbf{l}_i^T \mathbf{H} = \lambda_i \mathbf{l}_i^T$. We will also indicate by $\mathbf{R} = \begin{bmatrix} \mathbf{r}_1 \, \mathbf{r}_2 \end{bmatrix} = \mathbf{L}^{-1}$ the corresponding right eigenmatrix. For the typical values of velocity, vessel area and elastic parameter β encountered in arteries under physiological conditions, we have that $\lambda_1 > 0$ and $\lambda_2 < 0$. Therefore our system is *strictly hyperbolic* and *subcritical* (see [277] for these definitions).

The characteristic variables can be determined by integrating the differential system $\partial_{\mathbf{U}} \mathbf{W} = \mathbf{L}$. It may be shown that this is possible for our problem and that the two characteristic variables are

$$W_1 = u + 4c = u + 4A^{1/4}\sqrt{\frac{\beta}{2\rho}}, \tag{10.37}$$

$$W_2 = u - 4c = u - 4A^{1/4}\sqrt{\frac{\beta}{2\rho}}. \tag{10.38}$$

Since $\beta > 0$, we may write, as previously reported in [160], the variables (A, u) in terms of (W_1, W_2) as

$$A = \left[\frac{(W_1 - W_2)}{4}\right]^4 \left(\frac{\rho}{2\beta}\right)^2 \qquad u = \frac{(W_1 + W_2)}{2}. \tag{10.39}$$

In the case where $f = 0$ equations (10.35) can be transformed in a decoupled system of equations for the characteristic variables, which componentwise reads

$$\begin{aligned} \frac{\partial W_1}{\partial t} + \lambda_1 \frac{\partial W_1}{\partial x} &= 0, \\ \frac{\partial W_2}{\partial t} + \lambda_2 \frac{\partial W_2}{\partial x} &= 0. \end{aligned} \tag{10.40}$$

We recall that the expression of the characteristic variables, as well as that of the λ_i are independent from the choice of the governing variables of our problem. This is not the case for $\mathbf{L}$ and $\mathbf{R}$.

Remark 10.1.2 Smoothness of the solution. *We recall some of the main results regarding the hyperbolic system at hand. It has been shown in [7, 524] that, using a pressure-area relationship of the form*

$$p - P_{ext} = G_0 \left[\left(\frac{A}{A_0}\right)^{\frac{\delta}{2}} - 1\right],$$

where $\delta > 1$ *and* G_0 *is a constant elasticity parameter, and under some reasonable conditions on the smoothness of boundary and initial data, the solution of system (10.27) remains smooth. Two critical assumptions to reach this conclusion are the pulsatility of the inflow data and a bound on the length of the tube; both are verified for physiological flow in the human arterial tree. In the same work it is shown that, if the solution is smooth and the initial and boundary data are such that* $A > 0$, A *remains strictly positive for all times. In [155] an energy inequality was derived which bounds a measure of the energy of the hyperbolic system in terms of the initial and boundary data. Furthermore, in the same work it has been found that the quantity*

$$s = \frac{1}{2}\rho A u^2 + \int_{A_0}^{A} (p - P_{ext}) dA,$$

is an entropy function for the system with associated flux equal to $\boldsymbol{F}_s = \boldsymbol{Q}\, p_t$.

10.1.5 Boundary conditions

The characteristic analysis and the fact that for physiological conditions the flow is subcritical (i.e. $\lambda_1 > 0$ and $\lambda_2 < 0$) leads us to the conclusion that only one boundary condition has to be imposed at each end of the tube. Different type of boundary conditions may be envisaged. For the sake of simplicity let us focus on the boundary $x = x_1$, the arguments being easily extended to the other boundary point. Here, the sign of the eigenvalues tell us that W_1 is associated to the characteristics entering the domain, while W_2 to the one exiting. Let here $\mathbf{U} = \mathbf{U}(t)$ indicate the vector of primitive variables at the boundary point $x = x_1$, either in the form (A, Q) or (A, u), depending on the choice of the adopted differential model. A boundary condition may take the general form

$$\varphi(\mathbf{U}(t)) = g(t), \quad \text{for } t > 0, \tag{10.41}$$

being φ a C^1 function defined for all allowed values of $\mathbf{U}$ and g a given function of time. Not all the choices are possible, indeed we require that the boundary be not characteristic, a condition that in our case is satisfied if for all admissible $\mathbf{U}$

$$\mathbf{r}_1^T(\mathbf{U}) \frac{\partial \varphi(\mathbf{U})}{\partial \mathbf{U}} \neq 0, \tag{10.42}$$

where $\mathbf{r}_1$ is the right eigenvector associated to λ_1.

In practice we are interested in specific types of boundary conditions, some of which are detailed in the following paragraphs.

Non-reflecting boundary conditions

Non-reflecting boundary conditions are those that allow the simple wave associated with the characteristics exiting the domain to leave without spurious reflections. Typically those conditions are expressed in terms of the characteristic variables. Again, let us focus on one of the two boundary points, here we choose $x = x_2$, and on problem (10.31), the modifications for system (10.29) and for the other vessel end being immediate.

Following [502] and [216] non-reflecting boundary conditions at $x = x_2$ are provided as

$$\mathbf{l}_2^T \left[\frac{\partial \mathbf{U}}{\partial t} - \mathbf{S}(\mathbf{U}) \right]_{x=x_2} = 0,$$

which indeed is equivalent to state that at $x = x_2$

$$\frac{dW_2(t)}{dt} = \mathbf{l}_2^T \mathbf{S}(W_2(\mathbf{U}(t))), \quad \text{for } t > 0.$$

Here we have set $W_2(t) = W_2(x_2, t)$, $\mathbf{U}(t) = \mathbf{U}(x_2, t)$ and we have recalled that the characteristic variable may in our case be expressed in function of the primitive variables of our differential problem. Being basically a condition on the incoming characteristics, relation (10.42) is satisfied. Numerically, this ordinary differental equation will be discretised in time, for instance the computation of W_2 in $x = x_2$ and at time $t^{n+1} = t^n + \Delta t$ may be carried out as

$$W_2^{n+1} = W_2^n + \Delta t \mathbf{l}_2^T \mathbf{S}^n,$$

where $\mathbf{l}_2$ and $\mathbf{S}$ are computed from the solution at time t^n.

For the notable case $\mathbf{S}(\mathbf{U}) = \mathbf{0}$, or $\mathbf{B}(\mathbf{Q}) = \mathbf{0}$ if we use (10.29), we have $W_2 = \text{const}$, that is a constant incoming characteristic variable.

In our case a condition of this type may be convenient at the distal section (typically $x = x_2$) whenever one can neglect possible contributions of waves coming from the distal circulation, while at the proximal section ($x = x_1$) we would like to prescribe some given values of pressure or flux data coming either from measurement or other models. When the peripheral circulation is taken into account, we need specific models for the terminal vessels that will be discussed later.

Proximal conditions

It is immediate to verify that the prescription of either a flux Q (or velocity u) or area A at $x = x_1$ is allowable. For instance, we may impose

$$A(x_1, t) = g(t), \quad t > 0,$$

where $g(t)$ is a known function obtained, for instance, from the knowledge of the pressure time variation at $x = x_1$. This type of condition is clearly of reflective type and the simple wave associated to the outgoing characteristic (W_2 in this case) may be partly reflected back into the computational domain. Yet, in the case where the measurements are accurate enough, this reflection is indeed a physical one.

It is also possible to have available values of both pressure (and thus area) and flux variations at the proximal section. For instance, measurements of pressure pulse together with flux data could be obtained from Doppler ultrasound. Clearly the hyperbolic system does not allow to impose both conditions at the same time. However, one may construct a set of allowable boundary conditions through the exact or approximate solution of a Riemann problem [199] at the boundary using the computed values and the known values at the inlet. We will go back to this technique when we discuss the numerical treatment of the boundary data. Alternatively, one may set the incoming characteristics variables as

$$W_1(x_1, t) = W_1(\tilde{p}(t), \tilde{u}(t)),$$

where $\tilde{p}(t)$ and $\tilde{u}(t)$ are the given (measured) values of pressure and velocity, while $W_1(p, u)$ denotes the analytic expression of W_1 as function of these two variables. In both cases we are not enforcing pressure and velocity exactly (it is not compatible with the hyperbolic character of the differential problem).

Distal boundary of terminal vessels: coupling with a model of peripheral circulation

The human arterial system is a network of large arteries branching out into many smaller arteries, arterioles and capillaries. We are usually interested in the results in the larger arteries in the network. Blood vessels further down the arterial tree are very small and numerous. They have, all together, an important role in determining the haemodynamics in the large arteries since they offer flow resistance and pressure wave is partially reflected at each bifurcation. An accurate description of all these vessels and districts although virtually possible is unfeasible for the huge amount of data required not to mention the computational costs. For these reasons, the downstream circulation is usually described in terms of lumped parameter models. In Section 10.2 we will introduce extensively these kind of models and their derivation. So, in general terms, an appropriate way for accounting outflow conditions is to resort to *multiscale models*, namely coupling 1D and lumped parameter models. Chapter 11 will be devoted to this topic. Here we limit ourselves to some considerations when the role of the lumped parameter models is only limited to provide a boundary condition for the 1D model, without further details on the peripheral circulation.

Denoting by $\pi_T(\omega)$ and $\chi_T(\omega)$ the Fourier transform of $P_T(t) = P(x_{\text{out}}, t)$ and $Q_T(t) = Q(x_{\text{out}}, t)$ respectively (see Chapter 2) at the end of the 1D network, the behaviour of the downstream network can be represented by the *terminal impedance* (see Fig. 10.14, left) as

$$\zeta_T(\omega) = \frac{\pi(\omega)}{\chi(\omega)}, \tag{10.43}$$

that in general is a complex-valued function. An extensive discussion about the role of the impedance function in describing the vascular tree haemodynamics can be found in Chapter 13 of [350]. Here the impedance is the *transfer function* describing in a simplified way the downstream blood dynamics that actually influences the hemodynamics in the proximal district represented by our 1D model. The counterpart of (10.43) in the time domain is obtained by computing the inverse Fourier transform of the terminal impedance, $Z_T = \mathcal{F}^{-1}(\zeta_T)$ and by applying the convolution theorem

$$p_T(t) = \int_{t-H}^{t} Z_T(t-\tau)Q_T(\tau)d\tau, \tag{10.44}$$

where H denotes the heart beat duration. Relation (10.44), possibly approximated with suitable numerical quadratures, provides the boundary condition to be used for the 1D network model in correspondence of terminal vessels.

Since possible examples of impedance functions used in the literature stem from the representation of the terminal districts by lumped parameter models, often represented in terms of electrical circuits, we postpone their description to the next section (see Section 10.2.3).

Relation (10.44) is not strictly of the form (10.41) and its admissibility for a general Z_T should be investigated. However, it has proved very effective in the several test cases carried out so far.

10.1.6 Numerical compatibility relations at the boundary

When calculating the numerical solution of our system we need to compute at the boundary points the values of both variables Q and A (or u and A), yet the boundary condition provides only a single relation. We need to complete this piece of information with an additional relation that can only come from the differential equation. A possibility is to project the equation along the outgoing characteristics, giving rise to the so-called compatibility relations [408]. Again, for the sake of simplicity let us consider first the point $x = x_1$ and the differential equation written in the quasi-linear form (10.35). The compatibility relation in this case reads

$$\mathbf{l}_2^T \left[\frac{\partial \boldsymbol{U}}{\partial t} + \boldsymbol{H} \frac{\partial \boldsymbol{U}}{\partial x} - \mathbf{f}(\mathbf{U}) \right] = 0, \quad \text{at } x = x_1, \quad t > 0.$$

By simple manipulations it may be recognised that this expression may be written as

$$\frac{dW_2(x(t),t)}{dt} - \mathbf{l}_2^T \mathbf{f}(\mathbf{U}) = 0, \quad \text{at } x = x_1, \quad t > 0, \tag{10.45}$$

where $\frac{dW_2(x(t),t)}{dt}$ is the total derivative of W_2 along the characteristic curve of equation $\frac{dx(t)}{dt} = \lambda_2$.

In a numerical setting relation (10.45) may be approximated by following the characteristic line backwards. Using a first-order scheme we may set at $t = t^{n+1} = t^n + \Delta t$ that

$$W_2(x_1, t^{n+1}) = W_2(x_1 - \lambda_2 \Delta t, t^n) + \Delta t \mathbf{l}_2^T \mathbf{f}(\mathbf{U}), \tag{10.46}$$

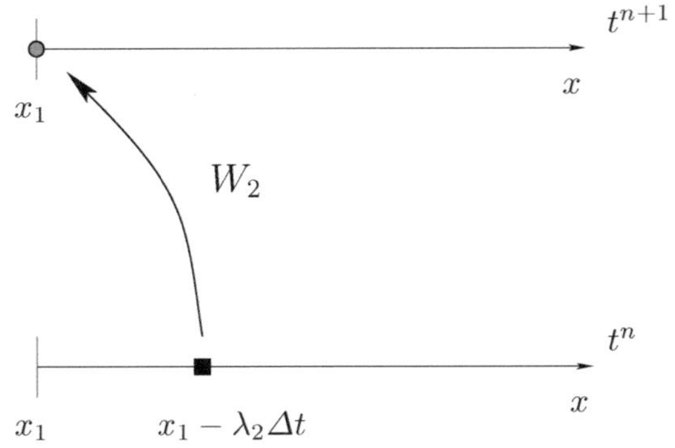

Fig. 10.2. Extrapolation of the characteristic W_2 in x_1

where λ_2 and $\mathbf{U}$ are computed at $x = x_1$ and $t = t^n$. More accurate schemes may be devised following the ideas applied in [48] in the context of Navier-Stokes equations. Relation (10.46) is called *extrapolation of the characteristic variable*, and coupled with the boundary condition provides a full set of (non-linear) equations for the numerical computation of the boundary data. An analogous relation may be found at $x = x_2$ for W_1.

We may note that if $\mathbf{f} = \mathbf{0}$, which is the case if we neglect the friction term, and the dependence of B and A_0 on x, then (10.46) reduces to $W_2(x_1, t^{n+1}) = W_2(x_1 - \lambda_2 \Delta t, t^n)$.

10.1.7 Extensions of the basic model

In the previous sections we have introduced some assumptions on the geometry of the vessel and on the smoothness of the coefficients characterizing the wall dynamics. These hypotheses are acceptable for small segments of the vascular tree, however more general models should be introduced to deal with segments with discontinuous properties, bifurcations and curved vessels. These will be discussed in the following sections.

Discontinuous material properties

In some cases, material properties of the wall are not smooth. In particular, coefficient β introduced in (10.21) features discontinuities for instance in stented arteries (Fig. 10.3) or in by-pass grafts. The Young's modulus E can exhibit jumps due to the differences between the vascular tissue and the prosthesis (see e.g. [269]). It is also possible for the area of the vessel to change abruptly due to certain pathologies, e.g. an aneurysm.

Since the derivative of the elastic coefficient β appears in the balance of momentum equation, the presence of discontinuities in β requires careful treatment in our models. There are basically two approaches for handling material discontinuities.

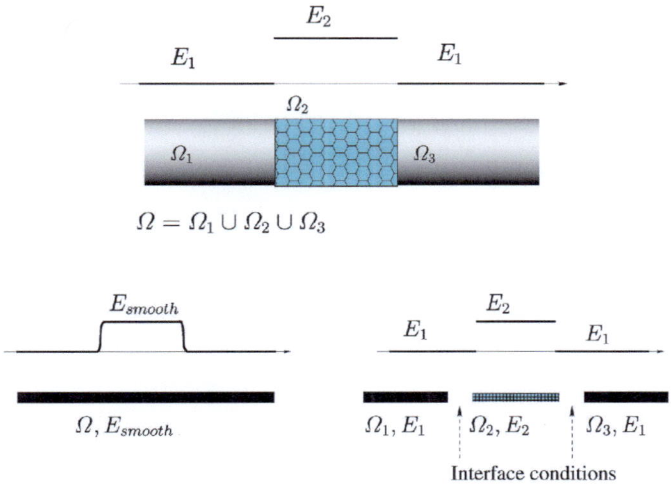

Fig. 10.3. Discontinuity of Young's modulus in the case of a stented artery. Bottom left: regularisation approach; bottom right: domain splitting

1. *Data regularisation*: the discontinuous data are suitably replaced by smooth functions that can be differentiated and the models presented above can be used straightforwardly.
2. *Domain splitting*: the vessel with discontinuous properties is split into a set of smooth segments and the coupling between each pair of segments is accomplished through suitable *matching or interface conditions.* A reasonable choice is to assume continuity of fluxes and thus impose the continuity of mass flux and total pressure across the interface, i.e.

$$Q = u_l A_l = u_r A_r, \tag{10.47}$$

$$P_r = \rho \frac{u_l^2}{2} + \beta_l(\sqrt{A_l} - \sqrt{A_{l_0}}) = \rho \frac{u_r^2}{2} + \beta_r(\sqrt{A_r} - \sqrt{A_{r_0}}). \tag{10.48}$$

These interface conditions will preserve the conservation properties of the (A, u) system.

In practice, the problem can be solved iteratively, by solving the sequence of problems on each segment. In this case, the interface conditions (possibly reformulated in terms of characteristic variables) become boundary conditions on each segment, following a classical domain decomposition approach (see e.g. [408]).

Treatment of bifurcations

The 1D model of the compliant tube can be extended to handle the arterial tree by adopting a domain splitting technique similar to the one used for the discontinuous case. Again we require suitable interface conditions at the bifurcations or branching points of the tree (see Fig. 10.4).

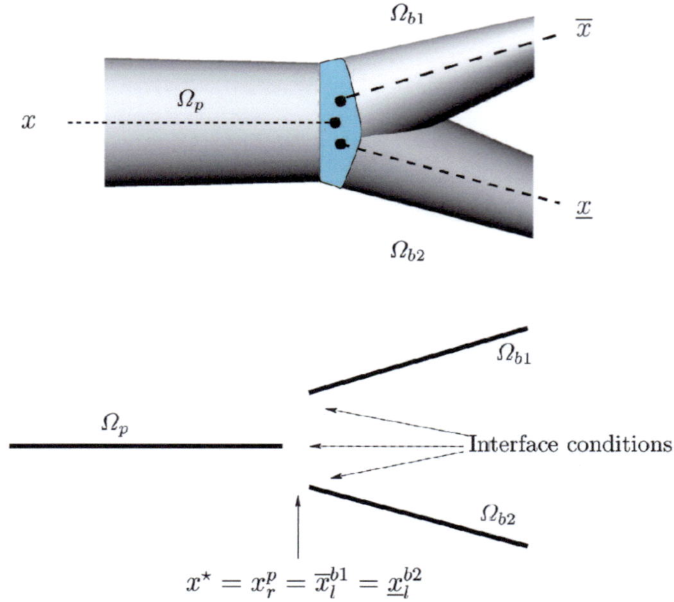

Fig. 10.4. Arterial tree bifurcation: notation

In the bifurcations the problem is only *locally* one-dimensional, in the sense that each branch is associated with its own axis (denoted by x, $\overline{x}$ and $\underline{x}$ in Fig. 10.4). The use of domain splitting techniques allows us to cast the global problem into a set of 1D problems (10.27) or (10.28). If we denote by $x^\star$ the branching point such that it is the right-end point x_r^p of the parent vessel Ω_p, and the left-end point $\overline{x}_l^{b1}$ and $\underline{x}_l^{b2}$ of the branches Ω_{b1} and Ω_{b2}, for a given function f defined over each segment we denote

$$f_l = f\big|_{\Omega_p}(x_r^p), \quad f_{b1} = f\big|_{\Omega_{b1}}(\overline{x}_l^{b1}), \quad f_{b2} = f\big|_{\Omega_{b2}}(\underline{x}_l^{b2}).$$

At the bifurcation we have six unknowns: (A_l, u_l) in the parent vessel, (A_{b1}, u_{b1}) and (A_{b2}, u_{b2}) in the branches Ω_{b1} and Ω_{b2} respectively.

The first three equations required to solve the problem may be obtained by extrapolating the outgoing characteristics like in (10.46) (or alternatively by solving (10.45)), giving

$$W_1 = u_l + 4A_l^{1/4}\sqrt{\frac{\beta_l}{2\rho}} = W_1^*, \tag{10.49}$$

$$W_{21} = u_{b1} - 4A_{b1}^{1/4}\sqrt{\frac{\beta_{b1}}{2\rho}}, \tag{10.50}$$

$$W_{22} = u_{b2} - 4A_{b2}^{1/4}\sqrt{\frac{\beta_{b2}}{2\rho}} = W_{22}^*, \tag{10.51}$$

where the starred quantities are the extrapolated values. The other three equations required to close the problem are obtained from the continuity of mass flux and total pressure across the boundary of the elements at the bifurcation, i.e.

$$Q = u_p A_p = u_{b1} A_{b1} + u_{b2} A_{b2}, \tag{10.52}$$

$$P_r = \rho \frac{u_p^2}{2} + \beta_p(\sqrt{A_p} - \sqrt{A_{po}}) = \rho \frac{u_{b1}^2}{2} + \beta_{b1}(\sqrt{A_{b1}} - \sqrt{A_{b1_0}}), \tag{10.53}$$

$$P_r = \rho \frac{u_p^2}{2} + \beta_p(\sqrt{A_p} - \sqrt{A_{po}}) = \rho \frac{u_{b2}^2}{2} + \beta_{b2}(\sqrt{A_{b2}} - \sqrt{A_{b2_0}}). \tag{10.54}$$

The six equations given by (10.49-10.54) define a non-linear system of algebraic equations which allow to determine the values of (A_l, u_l), (A_{r1}, u_{r1}) and (A_{r2}, u_{r2}) at the bifurcation. These values are then used to evaluate the flux at the elemental interfaces in the numerical discretisation.

We have assumed that the coefficient β could be different in the three vessels, as it is to be expected from the different values of their respective areas at rest A_0.

Remark 10.1.3 *Continuity of the total pressure in (10.53,10.54) can be modified for including pressure losses due to the bifurcation. These typically depend on the bifurcation angle. For more details see [157, 469].*

Accounting for curvature in 1D models (Directors' theory)

One of the most relevant assumptions in devising the basic 1D model is that the axis of the vessel is rectilinear. Actually, if we remove this hypothesis, it is still possible to define a main flow direction in the domain, namely the curvilinear abscissa along the axis, and however the effect of the blood dynamics in the other directions on the main one is no longer negligible (see [373]). Nevertheless, there are some vessels which are significantly curved (aorta, femoral arteries, etc.). For these vessels, the basic 1D model (10.28) or (10.27) can be considered only as a rough description. A possible model relies on introducing a subdivision into subsegments sufficiently short to be considered straight and connected one to the other with a suitable angle $\theta \neq 0$ (see Fig. 10.5). A suitable pressure loss as a function of the angle needs to be introduced in the interface conditions between segments. The other interface conditions will be given by the flow conservation (see (10.47) and Remark 10.1.3).

We would like to briefly address in the following an alternative definition of 1D models that are able to account for the effects of the transversal dynamics on the axial one, still at a reasonable computational cost. The task is not easy, since we want to devise a sort of 1D models for the cheap description of a genuinely 3D dynamics.

Simplified models for curved pipes can be obtained for small curvatures of the vessels with a perturbation analysis of the rectilinear model (see [113]).

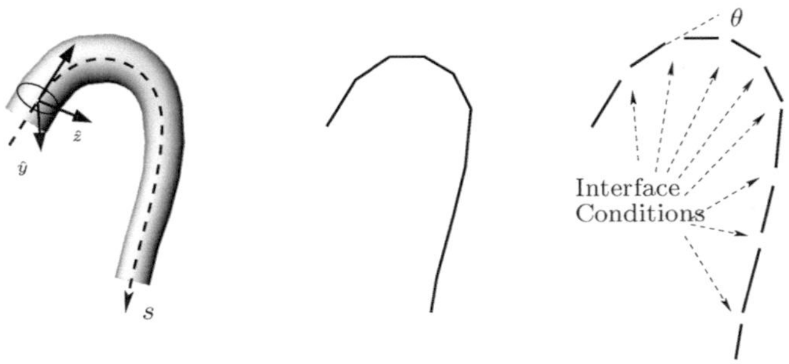

Fig. 10.5. Splitting of a curved domain into a sequence of rectilinear segments

Let us consider the non-dimensional parameter

$$De = 2\sqrt{2}\sqrt{\frac{r_w}{r_c}}\text{Re}, \tag{10.55}$$

where r_w is the vessel radius, r_c is the curvature radius of the vessel axis ($r_c \to \infty$ in the straight case), Re is the *Reynolds number* and *De* the *Dean number* (they have been defined in Chapter 5). Simplified models can be readily obtained for small values of the Dean number. For large values of *De* these models need to be suitably corrected, and the analysis becomes by far more difficult: a complete description of this approach can be found in [373], Chapter 4.

A different approach relies on the *theory of Cosserat* curves considered by Green and Naghdi in [204, 205] (see also [269]). If we consider the reference frame $(s, \hat{y}, \hat{z})$ of Fig. 10.5 left, the basic idea of the Green and Naghdi approach is to represent the velocity field $\mathbf{u}(s, \hat{y}, \hat{z}, t)$ with respect to a set of *shape functions* that depend only on the coordinates in the normal section $\hat{y}, \hat{z}$ and are given by

$$\mathbf{u}(s, \hat{y}, \hat{z}, t) = \sum_{n=0}^{N} \omega_n(s,t)\boldsymbol{\varphi}(\hat{y}, \hat{z}), \tag{10.56}$$

where ω_n are the coefficients of the velocity profile. This can be considered as a generalisation of the straight vessel case, where we set for the axial velocity, $u_z(x, y, z, t) = \varphi(\hat{y}, \hat{z})\overline{u}(x, t)$ being $\overline{u}(x, t)$ the average velocity and $\varphi(\hat{y}, \hat{z})$ a given velocity profile. Once a basis function set is selected the unknowns are the coefficients ω_n, that can be computed by solving a suitable set of equations derived by mass and momentum conservation principles.

In principle, the accuracy of these models can be tuned by choosing a suitably large N, i.e. having a rich enough basis functions set. However, even for small values of N, mathematical difficulties of the obtained model imply high numerical costs (see [269]).

A curved pipe model

Let us consider a curved pipe of circular section and indicate by s the arch length coordinate of the axis, which we assume to be a planar curve. If we integrate any function $f(s,\hat{y},\hat{z},t)$ over the volume of the pipe $V(\varepsilon)$ between normal sections at a distance ε one to the other and let $\varepsilon \to 0$, we get (see [269])

$$\lim_{\varepsilon\to 0}\frac{1}{\varepsilon}\int_{\overline{s}-\varepsilon/2}^{\overline{s}+\varepsilon/2}\int_{\mathcal{S}}\sqrt{g}f(\overline{s},\hat{y},\hat{z},t)d\sigma ds=\int_{\mathcal{S}}\sqrt{g}f(\overline{s},\hat{y},\hat{z},t)d\sigma,$$

where $\mathcal{S}=\mathcal{S}(\overline{s},t)$ is the section normal to the vessel axis and $\sqrt{g}$ is the metric tensor invariant, accounting for the integration over a curved axis. In particular, for a rectilinear pipe $g=1$, while for a curved vessel in the plane (s,y) with a constant curvature radius R_C, $\sqrt{g}=(\hat{y}+R_C)/\hat{y}$.

Associated to this integral over the section $\mathcal{S}$, we introduce the following operators acting on a generic regular enough function $f(\overline{s},\hat{y},\hat{z},t)$

$$P_{00}(f)=\int_{\mathcal{S}}\sqrt{g}fd\hat{y}d\hat{y},$$

$$P_{10}(f)=\int_{\mathcal{S}}\sqrt{g}f\hat{y}d\hat{y}d\hat{z},P_{01}(f)=\int_{\mathcal{S}}\sqrt{g}f\hat{z}d\hat{y}d\hat{z}. \tag{10.57}$$

Consider now the 3D Navier-Stokes equations written with respect to the reference frame $(s,\hat{y},\hat{z})$ with the velocity field represented by (10.56). In particular, we assume for the axial velocity

$$u_s=\left(1-\frac{\hat{y}^2+\hat{z}^2}{R^2}\right)(a(s,t)+b(s,t)\hat{y}+c(s,t)\hat{z}),$$

which is a generalisation of the classical parabolic profile (first term), while for the transversal velocity components, we simply postulate a linear dependence: $u_{\hat{y}}=\dot{\eta}\hat{y}/R$, $u_{\hat{z}}=\dot{\eta}\hat{z}/R$, where $\dot{\eta}$ is the wall velocity. The unknowns of the problem are therefore the coefficients $a(s,t)$, $b(s,t)$ and $c(s,t)$ and the vessel radius $R(s,t)$. A more convenient set of unknowns is

$$A=\pi R^2,\quad Q=\frac{\pi}{2}R^2a,\quad H=\frac{\pi}{12}R^4b,\quad G=\frac{\pi}{12}R^4c.$$

For the determination of these unknowns we need four equations that can be obtained by applying memberwise the average operator P_{00} to the continuity equation and the operators P_{00}, P_{10} and P_{01} to the axial momentum equations.

The resulting 1D model for curved vessels reads

$$\begin{cases} \dfrac{\partial A}{\partial t} + \dfrac{\partial Q}{\partial s} = 0, \\[2ex] \dfrac{\partial Q}{\partial t} + \dfrac{4}{3}\dfrac{\partial}{\partial s}\left(\dfrac{Q^2}{A}\right) + 6\pi\dfrac{\partial}{\partial s}\left(\dfrac{H^2}{A^2}\right) + \\[2ex] \qquad\qquad 6\pi\dfrac{\partial}{\partial s}\left(\dfrac{G^2}{A^2}\right) + \dfrac{\beta\sqrt{A}}{2\rho A_0}\dfrac{\partial A}{\partial s} + 8\pi\nu\dfrac{Q}{A} = 0, \\[2ex] \dfrac{\partial H}{\partial t} + \dfrac{H}{2A}\dfrac{\partial Q}{\partial s} + 2\dfrac{\partial}{\partial s}\left(\dfrac{HQ}{A}\right) + 24\pi\nu\dfrac{H}{A} = 0, \\[2ex] \dfrac{\partial G}{\partial t} + \dfrac{G}{2A}\dfrac{\partial Q}{\partial s} + 2\dfrac{\partial}{\partial s}\left(\dfrac{GQ}{A}\right) + 24\pi\nu\dfrac{G}{A} = 0. \end{cases} \tag{10.58}$$

More complex model can devised for instance by assuming a different profile for the transversal velocity components (see [269]).

10.1.8 The numerical solution of the 1D models

The wave propagation speeds in the large arteries are typically an order of magnitude higher than the average flow speeds. As mentioned previously, the characteristic system is inherently subcritical and does not produce shock under physiological conditions. Therefore the numerical challenge is to propagate waves for many periods without suffering from excessive errors in amplitude (*dissipation*) and in phase (*dispersion*) (see e.g. [277]). If the solution remains smooth then high-order methods are particularly attractive due to the fast convergence of the dispersion and dissipation errors with the order of the scheme [457].

Here, we limit ourselves to present two possible discretisations of the problems. The first one is based on a *Taylor-Galerkin approach* and is essentially a generalisation of the classical *Lax-Wendroff* scheme for systems of conservation laws (see [277]).

The second one is based on more recent techniques for the discretisation of the space variable, in which continuity of the solution at the discretisation nodes is no longer postulated. This *discontinuous Galerkin approach* is well suited for high order approximations.

Taylor-Galerkin method

In this section we describe the numerical discretisation of the (Q, A) system described by equation (10.27) recast in the conservation form (10.31) given by

$$\frac{\partial \boldsymbol{Q}}{\partial t} + \frac{\partial \boldsymbol{G}}{\partial x}(\boldsymbol{Q}) = \boldsymbol{B}(\boldsymbol{Q}).$$

The expressions for $\boldsymbol{Q}$, $\boldsymbol{G}$ and $\boldsymbol{B}$ are given in (10.30).

We proceed to discretise equation (10.31) by adopting a second-order Taylor-Galerkin scheme. To this aim, we write the Taylor expansion truncated up to the second order terms at time t^n such that $\Delta t = t^{n+1} - t^n$, yielding

$$\boldsymbol{Q}^{n+1} = \boldsymbol{Q}^n + \Delta t \left.\frac{\partial \boldsymbol{Q}}{\partial t}\right|^n + \frac{\Delta t^2}{2} \left.\frac{\partial^2 \boldsymbol{Q}}{\partial t^2}\right|^n . \tag{10.59}$$

The time derivatives will be replaced by space derivatives, by exploiting the equations (10.31). In particular, we will use the abridged notation

$$\boldsymbol{G}_{\boldsymbol{Q}} = \frac{\partial \boldsymbol{G}}{\partial \boldsymbol{Q}}, \quad \boldsymbol{B}_{\boldsymbol{Q}} = \frac{\partial \boldsymbol{B}}{\partial \boldsymbol{Q}},$$

and we obtain

$$\frac{\partial \boldsymbol{Q}}{\partial t} = \boldsymbol{B} - \frac{\partial \boldsymbol{G}}{\partial x}, \tag{10.60}$$

$$\frac{\partial^2 \boldsymbol{Q}}{\partial t^2} = \boldsymbol{B}_{\boldsymbol{Q}} \frac{\partial \boldsymbol{Q}}{\partial t} - \frac{\partial^2 \boldsymbol{G}}{\partial t \partial x} = \boldsymbol{B}_{\boldsymbol{Q}} \frac{\partial \boldsymbol{Q}}{\partial t} - \frac{\partial}{\partial x}\left(\boldsymbol{G}_{\boldsymbol{Q}} \frac{\partial \boldsymbol{Q}}{\partial t}\right) =$$

$$\boldsymbol{B}_{\boldsymbol{Q}}\left(\boldsymbol{B} - \frac{\partial \boldsymbol{G}}{\partial x}\right) - \frac{\partial (\boldsymbol{G}_{\boldsymbol{Q}} \boldsymbol{B})}{\partial x} + \frac{\partial}{\partial x}\left(\boldsymbol{G}_{\boldsymbol{Q}} \frac{\partial \boldsymbol{G}}{\partial x}\right). \tag{10.61}$$

Remark 10.1.4 *The presence of a non-constant source term and the explicit dependence of the momentum flux* $\boldsymbol{G}$ *on the variable* x *through* $\beta(x)$ *makes the derivation of the scheme slightly more complex than the standard Lax-Wendroff formulation. In particular we stress that, in contrast to the normal derivation, we have not further developed the* x *derivative of the fluxes, since for our problem*

$$\frac{\partial \boldsymbol{G}}{\partial x} \neq \boldsymbol{G}_{\boldsymbol{Q}} \frac{\partial \boldsymbol{Q}}{\partial x},$$

because of the dependence of $\boldsymbol{G}$ *on* x *through* β*.*

From (10.59), (10.60) and (10.61) we obtain the following time-marching scheme

$$\boldsymbol{Q}^{n+1} = \boldsymbol{Q}^n - \Delta t \frac{\partial}{\partial x}\left[\boldsymbol{G}^n + \frac{\Delta t}{2} \boldsymbol{G}^n_{\boldsymbol{Q}} \boldsymbol{B}^n\right] - \frac{\Delta t^2}{2}\left[\boldsymbol{B}^n_{\boldsymbol{Q}} \frac{\partial \boldsymbol{G}^n}{\partial x}\right.$$

$$\left. - \frac{\partial}{\partial x}\left(\boldsymbol{G}^n_{\boldsymbol{Q}} \frac{\partial \boldsymbol{G}^n}{\partial x}\right)\right] + \Delta t\left(\boldsymbol{B}^n + \frac{\Delta t}{2} \boldsymbol{B}^n_{\boldsymbol{Q}} \boldsymbol{B}^n\right). \tag{10.62}$$

Space discretisation is carried out by using linear finite elements. To that purpose, let us subdivide the domain Ω into N_{el} finite elements Ω_e, of size h_e. We indicate by $\mathbf{V}_h$ the space of continuous vector functions defined on Ω, linear on each element, and with $\mathbf{V}^0_h$ the set formed by functions of $\mathbf{V}_h$ which are zero at $x = x_1$ and $x = x_2$. Furthermore, we omit the subscript Ω in the $\mathbf{L}^2(\Omega)$ vector product.

Using the notation

$$\begin{aligned} \boldsymbol{G}_{LW} &= \boldsymbol{G} + (\Delta t/2)\boldsymbol{G}_{\boldsymbol{Q}}\boldsymbol{B}, \\ \boldsymbol{B}_{LW} &= \boldsymbol{B} + (\Delta t/2)\boldsymbol{B}_{\boldsymbol{Q}}\boldsymbol{B}, \end{aligned}$$

and indicating with

$$(\mathbf{u}, \mathbf{v})_{\Omega} = \int_{\Omega} \mathbf{u}\ \mathbf{v}\ dx,$$

the standard $\mathbf{L}^2(\Omega)$ inner product, the finite element solution of (10.62) requires, for $n \geq 0$, to find $\boldsymbol{Q}_h^{n+1}$ in $\mathbf{V}_h$ which satisfies for all ψ_h in $\mathbf{V}_h^0$ that

$$(\boldsymbol{Q}_h^{n+1}, \psi_h) = (\boldsymbol{Q}_h^n, \psi_h) + \Delta t(\boldsymbol{G}_{LW}^n, \frac{\partial \psi_h}{\partial x}) - \frac{\Delta t^2}{2}(\boldsymbol{B}_{\boldsymbol{Q}}^n \frac{\partial \boldsymbol{G}^n}{\partial x}, \psi_h) - \frac{\Delta t^2}{2}(\boldsymbol{G}_{\boldsymbol{Q}}^n \frac{\partial \boldsymbol{G}^n}{\partial x}, \frac{\partial \psi_h}{\partial x}) + \Delta t(\boldsymbol{B}_{LW}^n, \psi_h). \tag{10.63}$$

The numerical initial condition $\boldsymbol{U}_h^0$ will be taken as the finite element interpolant of the given initial data $\boldsymbol{U}_0$. A possible technique for computing the boundary values $\boldsymbol{U}_h^{n+1}$ is described later on.

In (10.63) we need to numerically integrate the terms containing the fluxes and sources. For the terms involving $\boldsymbol{G}^n$ and $\boldsymbol{G}_{\boldsymbol{Q}}^n$ we have projected each component on the finite element function space V_h via interpolation. The same applies for the other vector products which involve only $\boldsymbol{G}^n$ and $\boldsymbol{G}_{\boldsymbol{Q}}^n$.

The term $d\beta/dx$ in $\boldsymbol{B}^n$ and $\boldsymbol{B}_{\boldsymbol{Q}}^n$ must be approximated in a piecewise constant manner to ensure that our numerical scheme represents constant solutions of the differential problem exactly. Therefore, on each element (x_e^l, x_e^u) we have approximated $d\beta/dx$ by $[\beta(x_i^u) - \beta(x_i^l)]/h_e$. For the remaining terms we have applied the same technique adopted for the fluxes. This gives rise to a piecewise linear discontinuous representation for the source terms.

Discontinuous Galerkin method

The discontinuous Galerkin method is an attractive formulation for high-order discretisation of hyperbolic conservation laws. Following the work of Cockburn and Shu [96] and Lomtev, Quillen and Karniadakis [296] we proceed as follows.

Considering the one-dimensional hyperbolic system (10.28) in conservative form we have

$$\frac{\partial \boldsymbol{U}}{\partial t} + \frac{\partial \boldsymbol{F}}{\partial x} = \boldsymbol{S}(\boldsymbol{U}), \tag{10.64}$$

where

$$\boldsymbol{U} = \begin{bmatrix} U_1 \\ U_2 \end{bmatrix} = \begin{bmatrix} A \\ u \end{bmatrix}, \quad \boldsymbol{F} = \begin{bmatrix} F_1 \\ F_2 \end{bmatrix} = \begin{bmatrix} uA \\ \frac{u^2}{2} + \frac{p}{\rho} \end{bmatrix}, \quad \boldsymbol{S} = \begin{bmatrix} S_1 \\ S_2 \end{bmatrix} = \begin{bmatrix} 0 \\ -K_R \frac{u}{A} \end{bmatrix}.$$

To solve this system in a domain $\Omega = (x_1, x_2)$ discretised into a mesh of N_{el} elemental non-overlapping regions $\Omega_e = (x_e^l, x_e^u)$, such that $x_e^u = x_{e+1}^l$ for $e = 1, \ldots, N_{el}$, and

$$\bigcup_{e=1}^{N_{el}} \overline{\Omega}_e = \overline{\Omega},$$

we start by constructing the weak form of (10.64), i.e.

$$\left(\frac{\partial \boldsymbol{U}}{\partial t}, \boldsymbol{\psi}\right)_\Omega + \left(\frac{\partial \boldsymbol{F}}{\partial x}, \boldsymbol{\psi}\right)_\Omega = (\boldsymbol{S}, \boldsymbol{\psi})_\Omega, \tag{10.65}$$

where $\boldsymbol{\psi}$ represents an arbitrary function in Ω. Decomposing the integral into elemental regions we obtain

$$\sum_{e=1}^{N_{el}} \left[\left(\frac{\partial \boldsymbol{U}}{\partial t}, \boldsymbol{\psi}\right)_{\Omega_e} + \left(\frac{\partial \boldsymbol{F}}{\partial x}, \boldsymbol{\psi}\right)_{\Omega_e} - (\boldsymbol{S}, \boldsymbol{\psi})_{\Omega_e}\right] = 0. \tag{10.66}$$

Integrating the second term by parts leads to

$$\sum_{e=1}^{N_{el}} \left[\left(\frac{\partial \boldsymbol{U}}{\partial t}, \boldsymbol{\psi}\right)_{\Omega_e} - \left(\boldsymbol{F}, \frac{d\boldsymbol{\psi}}{dx}\right)_{\Omega_e} + [\boldsymbol{\psi} \cdot \boldsymbol{F}]_{x_e^l}^{x_e^u} - (\boldsymbol{S}, \boldsymbol{\psi})_{\Omega_e}\right] = 0. \tag{10.67}$$

To get the discrete form of our problem we choose $\boldsymbol{U}$ to be in the finite space of $\mathbf{L}^2(\Omega)$ functions which are polynomial of degree q on each element. We indicate an element of such space using the subscript h. We also note that $\boldsymbol{U}_h$ may be discontinuous across inter-element boundaries. However to attain a global solution in the domain Ω we need to allow information to propagate between the elemental regions. Information is propagated between elements by upwinding the boundary flux, $\boldsymbol{F}$, in the third term of equation (10.67).

More precisely, thanks to the relations (10.39) linking primitive and characteristic variables we may always write the flux $\mathbf{F}$ as function of the characteristic variables, that is $\mathbf{F} = \mathbf{F}(W_1, W_2)$. At the right interface of element Ω_e we set the upwinded flux as $\boldsymbol{F}^u = \mathbf{F}(W_1^-, W_2^+)$, being $W_1^+ = W^1|_{\Omega_e}(x_e^l)$ and $W_2^- = W^2|_{\Omega_{e+1}}(x_{e+1}^r)$, being Ω_{e+1} the adjacent element on the right of Ω_e. On the left interface the relation is analogous with the role of W_1 and W_2 exchanged. In this way we always construct the flux by using the information carried by the two characteristics impinging on the interface. This upwinding process can be conveniently used in the numerical scheme also to impose the boundary conditions, as we will see in the next section. Clearly we are assuming that the flow is subcritical, i.e. $\lambda_1 > 0$ and $\lambda_2 < 0$.

The discrete weak formulation can now be written as

$$\begin{aligned}\textstyle\sum_{e=1}^{N_{el}} \Big\{ \left(\frac{\partial \boldsymbol{U}_h}{\partial t}, \boldsymbol{\psi}_h\right)_{\Omega_e} - \left(\boldsymbol{F}(\boldsymbol{U}_h), \frac{d\boldsymbol{\psi}_h}{dx}\right)_{\Omega_e} + \\ [\boldsymbol{\psi}_h \cdot \boldsymbol{F}^u]_{x_e^l}^{x_e^u} - (\boldsymbol{S}(\boldsymbol{U}_h), \boldsymbol{\psi}_h)_{\Omega_e} \Big\} = 0.\end{aligned} \tag{10.68}$$

Following the traditional Galerkin approach, we choose the test function $\boldsymbol{\psi}_h$ within each element to be in the same discrete space as the numerical solution $\boldsymbol{U}_h$. At this point if we defined our polynomial basis and choose an appropriate quadrature rule we would now have a semi-discrete scheme. However, from an implementation point of view, the calculation of the second term in equation (10.68) can be inconvenient and consequently we choose to integrate this term by parts once more to obtain

$$\sum_{e=1}^{N_{el}} \left\{ \left(\frac{\partial \boldsymbol{U}_h}{\partial t}, \boldsymbol{\psi}_h\right)_{\Omega_e} + \left(\frac{\partial \boldsymbol{F}(\boldsymbol{U}_h)}{\partial x}, \boldsymbol{\psi}_h\right)_{\Omega_e} + [\boldsymbol{\psi}_h \cdot \{\boldsymbol{F}^u - \boldsymbol{F}(\boldsymbol{U}_h)\}]_{x_e^l}^{x_e^u} - \right.$$
$$\left. (\boldsymbol{S}(\boldsymbol{U}_h), \boldsymbol{\psi}_h)_{\Omega_e} \right\} = 0. \tag{10.69}$$

We note that the information between elements is transmitted by the third boundary term as the difference between the upwinded and the local fluxes, $[\boldsymbol{\psi}_h \cdot [\boldsymbol{F}^u - \boldsymbol{F}(\boldsymbol{U}_h)]]_{x_e^l}^{x_e^u}$. This method can be considered as a penalty method with an automatic procedure for determining the penalty parameter.

Finally we select our expansion bases to be polynomials of order q and expand our solution on each element e in terms of Legendre polynomials $L_p(\xi)$, i.e.

$$\boldsymbol{U}_h\big|_{\Omega_e}(x_e(\xi), t) = \sum_{p=0}^{q} L_p(\xi)\hat{\boldsymbol{U}}_e^p(t).$$

where, following standard finite element techniques, we consider ξ in the reference element $\Omega_{\text{ref}} = \{\xi : -1 \le \xi \le 1\}$ and introduce the elemental affine mapping

$$x_e(\xi) = x_e^l \frac{(1-\xi)}{2} + x_e^u \frac{(1+\xi)}{2}$$

whose Jacobian J_e is

$$J_e = \frac{dx_e}{d\xi} = \frac{x_e^u - x_e^l}{2}.$$

We note that the choice of discontinuous discrete solution and test functions allows us to decouple the problem on each element, the only link coming through the upwinded boundary fluxes. Legendre polynomials are particularly convenient because the basis is orthogonal with respect to the $\mathbf{L}^2(\Omega_e)$ inner product and equation (10.69) turns out to be equivalent to solving componentwise, for all elements e, for $i = 1, 2$ and $p = 1, \ldots, P$, the equation

$$J_e \frac{\partial \hat{U}_{i,e}^p}{\partial t} = -J_e \left(\frac{\partial F_i}{\partial x}, L_p\right)_{\Omega_e} - [L_p\,(F_i^u - F_i(\boldsymbol{U}_h))]_{x_e^l}^{x_e^u} + J_e\,(S_i, L_p)_{\Omega_e}. \tag{10.70}$$

To complete the discretisation we require a time integration scheme. Possible choices are the standard Runge-Kutta or the Adams-Bashforth schemes (see e.g. [403]).

The numerical treatment of boundary data

The numerical schemes (10.70) and (10.63) need to be complemented with boundary data $\boldsymbol{Q}$ or $\boldsymbol{U}$ at the boundaries of the domain Ω. The way the boundary data is treated in practice by the two schemes is different.

Taylor-Galerkin method

Let assume that the boundary condition at $x = x_1$ is given by the general form (10.41). A possible way to provide the boundary data on the first node at time $t]t^{n+1}$, here indicated by $\mathbf{Q}_0^{n+1}$ is to solve the system

$$\begin{aligned} \varphi(\mathbf{Q}_0^{n+1}) &= g(t^{n+1}), \\ W_2(\mathbf{Q}_0^{n+1})) &= W_2^* = W_2(x_1 - \lambda_2 \Delta t, t^n) + \Delta t \mathbf{l}_2^T \mathbf{f}, \end{aligned} \qquad (10.71)$$

where λ_2 and $\mathbf{f}$ are computed, for instance, in $x = x_1$ and at $t = t^n$ and $W_2(\mathbf{Q})$ indicates the expression linking the characteristic and primitive variables that can be derived from (10.38).

It is a system of nonlinear equation which may be solved by a few Newton iterations, starning from the values at the previous time step. In practice, we have notices that for our problems three Newton iterations are sufficient.

Similar considerations can be applied to the right boundary x_2.

Discontinuous Galerkin method: Flux upwinding

The procedure illustrated in the previous paragraph may in principle be applied also to the discontinuous Galerkin scheme. However in the latter the technique of flux upwinding at the interface between elements may be of hand also to implement the boundary conditions. Let consider the boundary $x = x_1$ and assume to have at disposal the boundary condition in terms of the entering characteristic, variable, i.e $W_1 = w_1(t)$. Then when computing the upwinded flux for the left interface of the first element we will set $\boldsymbol{F}^u = \mathbf{F}(w(t^n), W_2^+)$. If both primitive variables are provided at the boundary (for instance form experiments) $w_1(t^n)$ could be readily computed from their value. It means that we will not impose the values exactly (it would be impossible because we can impose only a single scalar equation) but their value mediated through the entering characteristic variable. If instead we wish to impose the value of a single primitive variable, for instance the flux, the situation is more complicated.

10.2 Zero-dimensional (0D) or lumped models

As for the 1D models, lumped parameters models can be derived by general conservation principles or directly by averaging 3D and 1D models. In the former case, the key concept is the *compartment*, that is a part of the system at hand that it is worth to be considered as a homogeneous unit. This definition is kept vague since the number and kind of compartments considered depend on the type of analysis at hand. A few compartments, describing the heart, arterial and venous systems and the capillary bed are sufficient for a very general description of the behaviour of the cardiovascular system. More detailed analysis may give rise to models with up to fifty separate compartments accounted for. Following this approach the continuous space dependence is lost, and the emphasis is on the behaviour of the unit with respect to the rest of the system. Input/output relations are formulated via transfer functions based either on physical or empirical relations.

Since we have already considered one-dimensional models of a blood vessel, we will here derive the corresponding lumped model by an averaging procedure. This approach is closer to the physics of the problem, and is useful to understand the role of the parameters of the model and their quantification. We will start from lumped parameter models of a simple vascular compartment formed by a single artery, and then, by application of appropriate matching conditions derived from conservation principles we will be able to build more general models.

Let us consider the single artery Ω, illustrated in Fig. 10.1, of length $l = |x_2 - x_1|$. We define *the (volumetric) mean flow rate over the whole artery* as the quantity

$$\hat{Q} = \frac{\rho}{l}\int_{\Omega} u_1 dv = \frac{\rho}{l}\int_{x_1}^{x_2}\left(\int\limits_{\mathcal{S}(x)} u_x d\sigma\right)dx = \frac{\rho}{l}\int_{x_1}^{x_2} Q(x)dx. \tag{10.72}$$

Similarly, we define the *mean pressure and area* over the artery as

$$\hat{p} = \frac{1}{l}\int\limits_{x_1}^{x_2} P dx, \quad \hat{A} = \frac{1}{l}\int\limits_{x_1}^{x_2} A dx. \tag{10.73}$$

Starting from equations (10.27) for this domain, we integrate the continuity equation along the axial direction ($x_1 \leq x \leq x_2$) to obtain

$$l\frac{d\hat{A}}{dt} + Q_2 - Q_1 = 0, \tag{10.74}$$

where we have set

$$Q_1(t) = Q(t, x_1), \quad Q_2(t) = Q(t, x_2). \tag{10.75}$$

Observe that now $\hat{A}$ depends only on time, so we have an ordinary time derivative.

In considering the momentum equation, we add the following simplifying assumptions:

1. *the contribution of the convective term* $\partial_x(\alpha Q^2/A)$ *may be neglected*; and
2. *the variation of* A *(and* β*) with respect to* x *is small compared to that of* P *and* Q.

The first assumption is particularly suited to represent the peripheral circulation, where blood flow is in general quite slow. The second assumption is reasonable when the axial average is carried out over short segments. It basically amounts to replace A in the momentum equation with a constant value for the area that in general is assumed to be the area at rest A_0. With these assumptions, averaging over x of $(10.27)_2$ yields

$$\frac{\rho l}{A_0}\frac{d\hat{Q}}{dt} + \frac{\rho K_R l}{A_0^2}\hat{Q} + P_2 - P_1 = 0, \tag{10.76}$$

where

$$P_1(t) = P(t, x_1), \quad P_2(t) = P(t, x_2). \tag{10.77}$$

As for 1D models we have now the problem of closing system (10.74, 10.76), by adding a wall mechanics law. In particular, if we assume the simple law (10.21) to hold, we have

$$\int_{x_1}^{x_2} \frac{\partial p}{\partial t} dx = \int_{x_1}^{x_2} \frac{\beta}{2\sqrt{A}} \frac{\partial A}{\partial t} dx.$$

Now, if we exploit the second assumption above, we obtain $l\dfrac{d\hat{p}}{dt} = \dfrac{l\beta}{2\sqrt{A_0}}\dfrac{d\hat{A}}{dt}$, which we write, for convenience, as

$$\frac{d\hat{A}}{dt} = k_1 \frac{d\hat{p}}{dt}, \tag{10.78}$$

where $k_1 = \dfrac{\sqrt{A_0}}{\beta}$. Substituting (10.78) into (10.74) we obtain

$$k_1 l \frac{d\hat{p}}{dt} + Q_2 - Q_1 = 0, \tag{10.79}$$

that together with (10.76) represents the lumped parameter model for a vessel.

Equations of this type are also found in the analysis of electrical circuits. Indeed, before digital computers, early simulations of flow in the vascular system were based on analog electrical circuits, see for instance [539]. In the electric network analogy, the blood flow rate is assimilated to the current, while blood pressure corresponds to voltage, as summarised in Table 10.1.

Table 10.1. Correspondence table of the analogy between electric and hydraulic networks

Hydraulic	*Electric*
Pressure	*Voltage*
Flow rate	*Current*
Blood viscosity	Resistance R
Blood inertia	Inductance L
Wall compliance	Capacitance C

In order to exploit this electrical analogy, we recast the system (10.76,10.79) as

$$\begin{aligned} C\frac{d\hat{p}}{dt} + Q_2 - Q_1 = 0, \\ L\frac{d\hat{Q}}{dt} + R\hat{Q} + P_2 - P_1 = 0. \end{aligned} \tag{10.80}$$

The coefficients R, L and C are associated to elements of a circuit as depicted in Fig. 10.6, where the corresponding equation is recalled at the bottom. We recall hereafter their physical significance.

Resistance. The coefficient $R = \dfrac{\rho K_R l}{A_0^2}$ in equation (10.80) represents the *resistance* induced to the flow by the blood viscosity. Different expressions for R can be obviously obtained for different velocity profiles or if a non-Newtonian rheology is introduced into the model (see e.g. [426], [539], [162]).

Inertia (inductance). The coefficient $L = \dfrac{\rho l}{A_0}$ in equation (10.76) represents the inertial term in the momentum equation and it will be called the *inductance* of the flow.

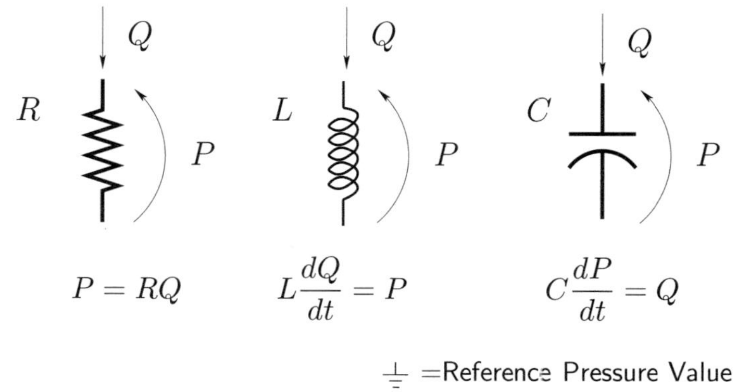

Fig. 10.6. Notation used in the electrical analogy of the circulatory system

Compliance (capacitance). It is characterised by the coefficient $C = k_1 l$ that represents the mass storage term in the mass conservation law, due to the *compliance* of the vessel.

For instance, if we assume Poiseuille flow (i.e. fully developed flow with a constant pressure gradient) and that the vessel is a cylinder of constant circular section we have

$$R = \frac{8\pi\rho\nu l}{\pi^2 r_0^4} = \frac{8\mu l}{\pi r_0^4}; \quad L = \frac{\rho l}{\pi r_0^2}; \quad C = \frac{3\pi r_0^3 l}{2Eh_0}.$$

The system of equations (10.80) involves the mean flow rate and pressure over the vascular segment at hand and the *boundary* values of pressure and flow rate Q_i, P_i, with $i = 1, 2$. Strictly speaking, the term *boundary* is inappropriate, since the continuous space dependence has been lost in the axial average, and they simply represent input/output quantities exchanged by the vessel with the rest of the systems. However, we will retain the term, since it is related to the physical derivation of the equations. In particular, in order to close problem (10.80), we need to introduce some *boundary conditions.* This means that we need to identify the *input data* of the district at hand. For instance, suppose that Q_1 *and* P_2 *are given.* Then, (10.80) represents a system of two equations for four unknowns, $\hat{Q}, \hat{p}, P_1$ and Q_2. The dynamic of the system is represented by $\hat{p}$ and $\hat{Q}$, i.e. by the unknowns that are under time derivative (the *state variables*). We approximate now the unknowns on the upstream and downstream sections with the state variables,

$$\hat{p} \approx P_1, \quad \hat{Q} \approx Q_2,$$

that corresponds to assume that the *output* of the district is given by the *state* variables. With these additional assumptions, which are reasonable for a short pipe, the lumped parameter model becomes:

$$\begin{aligned} C\frac{dP_1}{dt} + Q_2 &= Q_1, \\ L\frac{dQ_2}{dt} + RQ_2 - P_1 &= P_2. \end{aligned} \tag{10.81}$$

where the input data have been put on the right hand side. This system can be illustrated by the electric $\mathcal{L}$-network shown in Fig. 10.7 (left).

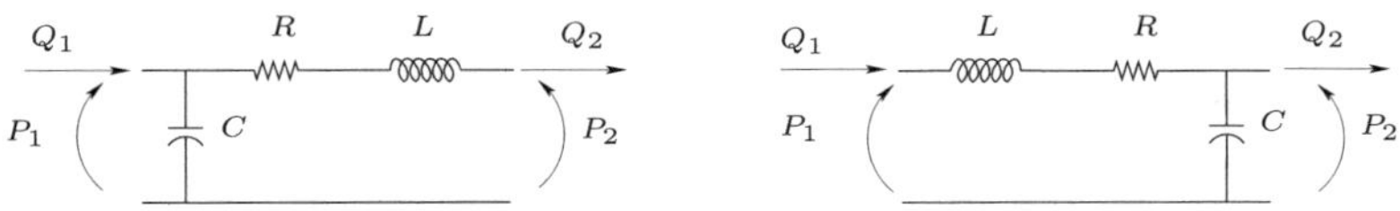

Fig. 10.7. Lumped $\mathcal{L}$-network (top) and $\mathcal{L}$-inverted network (bottom) equivalent to a short pipe

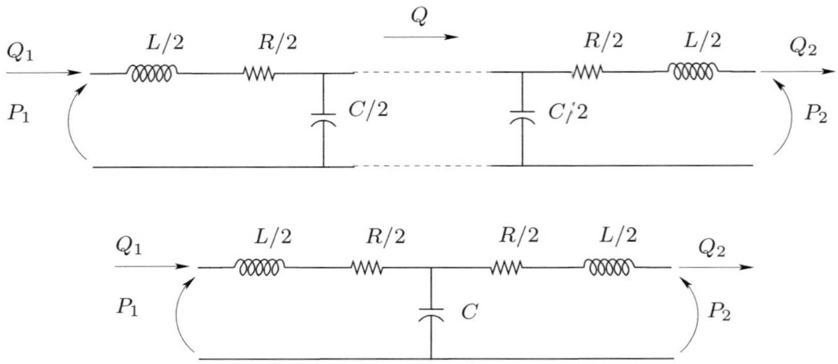

Fig. 10.8. Cascade connection of a $\mathcal{L}$-inverted and a $\mathcal{L}$-network (top), lumped $\mathcal{T}$-network (bottom)

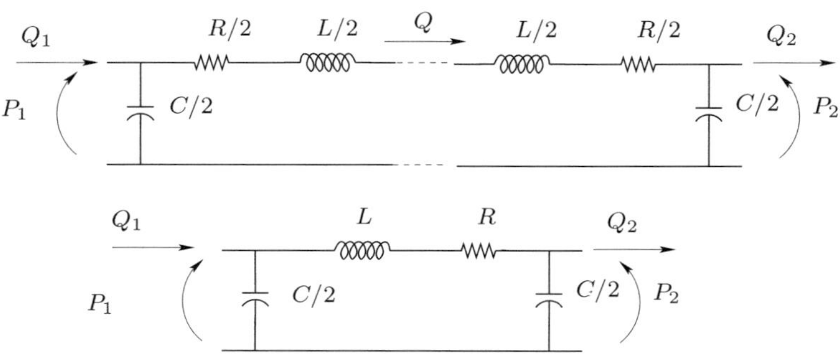

Fig. 10.9. Cascade connection of a $\mathcal{L}$-network and a $\mathcal{L}$-inverted one (top), lumped π-network (bottom)

In a similar way, if the pressure P_1 and the flow rate Q_2 are prescribed, we still approximate the quantities at the upstream and downstream sections by the state variables, i.e. $\hat{p} \approx P_2, \quad \hat{Q} \approx Q_1$, yielding the system represented by an electric analog, called an $\mathcal{L}$-inverted network, depicted in Fig. 10.7(right).

If the mean pressures P_1 and P_2 are prescribed, the system can be modelled by a cascade connection of $\mathcal{L}$ and $\mathcal{L}$-inverted lumped representations, yielding a $\mathcal{T}$-network (Fig. 10.8). Similarly, if both flow rates Q_1 and Q_2 are prescribed, the vessel Ω is described by an electric π-network, obtained as a cascade connection of a $\mathcal{L}$-network and a $\mathcal{L}$-inverted network (Fig. 10.9).

The four different representations of the same vessel arise from four different possible assumptions about the data prescribed at the upstream and downstream sections. In other words, they can be considered as the lumped parameter simplifications of four different "boundary" values problems.

Remark 10.2.1 *Alternative ways can be pursued for devising lumped parameter models. Among the most recent, we mention the one proposed in [359]*

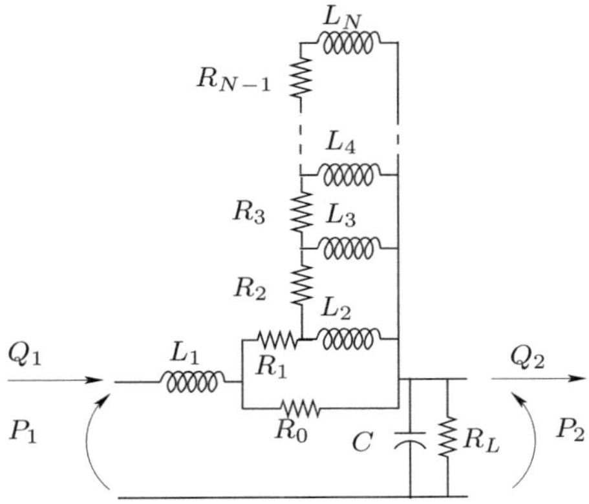

Fig. 10.10. Electric analog network of the Jager, Westerhof and Noordergraf model [244] including the sleeve effect and rheological effects. The larger N is, the more accurate is the model

which is based on suitable approximations of the inverse Laplace transform of the axisymmetric Stokes equations in rigid vessels.

Other lumped parameters models relying on more realistic assumptions have been proposed by different authors. For instance, we mention [244]. In this paper some modifications to the $\mathcal{L}$-inverted network of Fig. 10.7 (right) are proposed that account for the interactions between inertial and viscous phenomena induced by the pulsatility of blood flow (the so-called sleeve effect*) and the non-Newtonian blood rheology (see Chapter 6). In particular, a boundary layer with lower viscosity due to the different concentrations of red cells is accounted for. The set up of the model was based on an explicit computation of the impedance associated to an approximation of the Womersley solution (see Chapter 5). The corresponding electric analog is depicted in Fig. 10.10. More accurate models can be obtained by including more elements, i.e. by taking higher values of N. Resistance R_0 is related to the non-Newton effects, while R_L (where L stands for* leakage*) accounts for secondary vessels that are not accurately described in the model and however are relevant in the mass conservation.*

The picture highlights the remarkably simple modifications to the lumped model required to account for the description of complex phenomena.

10.2.1 Lumped parameters models for the heart

As explained in Chapter 1, Section 1.1.1, the heart is subdivided into the right and the left parts, separated by the septum. The right heart supplies the pulmonary circulation, while the left one pumps the blood into the systemic tree. Each side consists of two chambers, the atrium and the ventricle, separated by the atrioventricular valves (the tricuspid valve in the right side, the mitral valve in the left one). Their role is to receive fluid at low pressure and transfer it to a higher pressure region, acting as a *pump*. A possible representation of heart working is given by left ventricle pressure-volume diagrams (see [227] and Section 1.1).

Each ventricle can be described therefore as a vessel where the most significant feature is the compliance and *the compliance changes with time* (see [227, 256, 443, 509]).

The starting point for a candidate mathematical model is the relation that links internal pressure with the radius of an elastic spherical ball filled with fluid. Here and in the following we take $P_{ext} = 0$. We have

$$\pi R^2 P = 2\pi E h_0 R \frac{R - R_0}{R_0},$$

where R_0 is the reference sphere radius (corresponding to $P = 0$), h_0 is a reference thickness of the ball surface and E denotes the Young's modulus. The contraction of the cardiac muscle may be taken into account by an increase of E (stiffening) and by a shortening of the muscle length (i.e. a reduction of R_0). It is more convenient to express this relation as a function of the volume V, instead of the radius. By recalling that $V = \frac{4}{3}\pi R^3$, a linearisation procedure leads to

$$P = \frac{2E(t)h_0}{3R_0^2}\left(\frac{3}{4\pi}\right)^{1/3} V_0^{-\frac{2}{3}}\left(V - V_0\right),$$

where we have indicated the coefficients that change in time because of the action of the muscle. This simplified model does indeed describe the major characteristic of the ventricle. If we indicate $C(t) = \frac{3R_0^2 V_0^{\frac{2}{3}}}{2E(t)h_0}\left(\frac{4\pi}{3}\right)^{1/3}$ we may re-write the relation in the more compact form

$$V(t) = C(t)P(t) + V_0(t).$$

By differentiating with respect to time we obtain

$$\frac{dV}{dt} = Q = \frac{dC}{dt}P + C\frac{dP}{dt} + M_Q(t), \tag{10.82}$$

where Q represents the (incoming) flow rate and $M_Q = \frac{dV_0}{dt}$ is the action exerted by the contraction of the cardiac muscle.

A lumped representation (electric analog) of each ventricle[2] is given in Fig. 10.11, where R accounts for an additional viscous resistance inside the ventricle. Here, M_Q is represented by a current generator.

The electrical analog of the presence of heart valves has been represented in Fig. 10.11 by *diodes*. Ideally, the behaviour of a diode is described by the

[2] A mechanical representation of the heart working based on the classical Hill's model for the muscle can be found in [262] and [555].

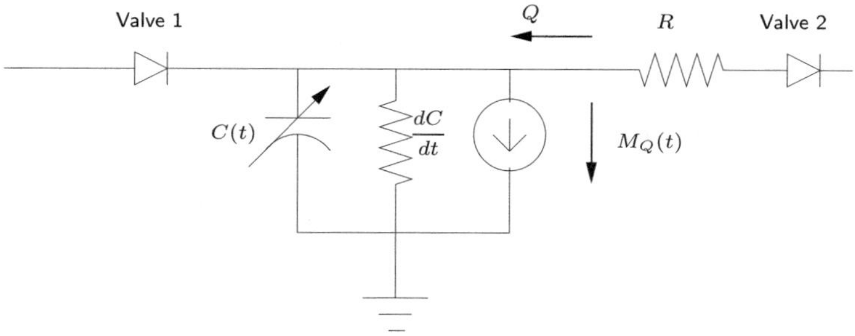

Fig. 10.11. Electric analog of the lumped parameter model of a ventricle

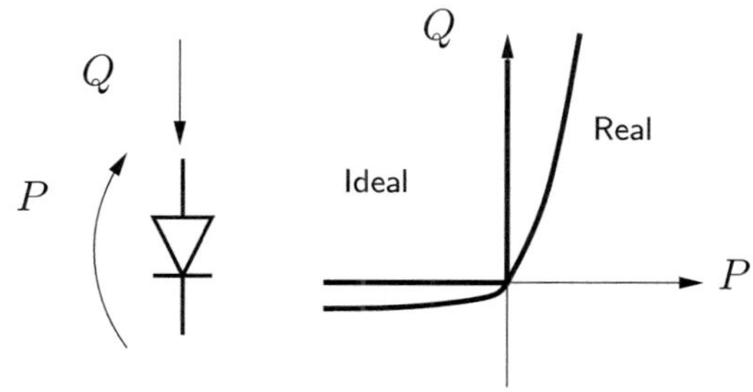

Fig. 10.12. $P-Q$ curve in a diode, representing the electric analog of a heart valve

curve depicted in Fig. 10.12 and given by

$$\begin{aligned} P &= 0 \quad \text{if} \quad Q > 0, \\ Q &= 0 \quad \text{if} \quad P < 0. \end{aligned}$$

This means that the diode representation does not allow flow through the valve if the pressure is higher downstream than upstream. If the upstream pressure is higher, the diode allows the flow without any pressure loss. This is an "ideal" behaviour. Real valves have a different behaviour that can be represented by the curve

$$Q = Q_S \left(e^{\alpha P} - 1\right) \tag{10.83}$$

called *Shockley equation*. In some cases, this equation has been approximated by a piecewise polynomial curve (see e.g. [328]).

The presence of diodes introduces a nonlinear term in the system. However, if we resort to the Shockley model, the nonlinear terms are smooth in terms of mathematical regularity.

10.2.2 Lumped parameters models for the circulatory system

In the previous sections we have introduced lumped parameter description of two basic compartments, a segment of vessel and the heart. A possible model for the vascular network can be derived by "connecting" these compartments

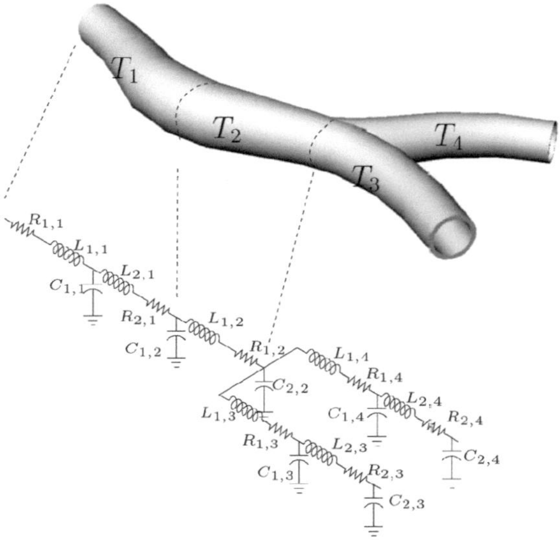

Fig. 10.13. Lumped parameters model for a branched vessel as a cascade of T and π networks

by means of appropriate *matching conditions*, in a way similar to the one pursued for the 1D model of bifurcations in Section 10.1.7. Matching conditions will be actually driven by *continuity of flux* and *balance of momentum* at the interfaces. More precisely, since our lumped parameter models deal with the flow rate Q and the pressure P, matching conditions will essentially state the continuity of these variables at the interfaces. In the electric analog, these relations correspond to the application of the classical *Kirchhoff laws* for the nodes (conservation of current/flow rate) and the nets (conservation of the voltage/pressure). For these reasons, lumped parameter models will also be referred to as *Kirchhoff* (K) models.

A sketch of possible connections of different compartments is given in Fig. 10.13.

More detailed models for the circulation are proposed in [353, 539], where hundreds of elementary compartments are considered.

Mathematical and numerical analysis of lumped parameters models

From the mathematical viewpoint, a general representation of lumped parameters models is a system of differential-algebraic equations (DAE) of the form

$$\begin{aligned} &\frac{d\mathbf{y}}{dt} = \mathbf{b}(\mathbf{y}, \mathbf{z}, t), \quad t \in (0, T], \\ &G(\mathbf{y}, \mathbf{z}) = 0, \end{aligned} \qquad (10.84)$$

together with the *initial condition vector* $\mathbf{y}|_{t=t_0} = \mathbf{y}_0$. Here, $\mathbf{y}$ is the vector of state variables, the vector $\mathbf{z}$ contains the other variables of the network and G represents the algebraic equations derived from the Kirchhoff laws. Differentiating the algebraic equations with respect to time we get

$$\frac{dG(\mathbf{y},\mathbf{z})}{dt} = \mathbf{J}_\mathbf{y}\frac{d\mathbf{y}}{dt} + \mathbf{J}_\mathbf{z}\frac{d\mathbf{z}}{dt} = 0$$

where $\mathbf{J}_\mathbf{y} = \dfrac{\partial G}{\partial \mathbf{y}}$ and $\mathbf{J}_\mathbf{z} = \dfrac{\partial G}{\partial \mathbf{z}}$ are the Jacobian matrices with respect to $\mathbf{y}$ and $\mathbf{z}$. Assuming that $J_\mathbf{z}$ is non singular, the DAE system is said to be *of index 1* (see e.g. [184]). This is the most frequent case in problems concerning lumped parameters models of the vascular system. We can then write

$$\frac{d\mathbf{z}}{dt} = -\mathbf{J}_\mathbf{z}^{-1}\mathbf{J}_\mathbf{y}\frac{d\mathbf{y}}{dt} = -\mathbf{J}_\mathbf{z}^{-1}\mathbf{J}_\mathbf{y}\mathbf{b}(\mathbf{y},\mathbf{z},t). \tag{10.85}$$

Assuming that an initial vector $\mathbf{z}_0$ is available, the first equation of (10.84) and (10.85) can be rewritten as the classical Cauchy problem

$$\begin{aligned} &\frac{d\mathbf{w}}{dt} = \mathbf{a}(\mathbf{w},t), \quad t \in (0,T], \\ &\mathbf{w}(t_0) = \mathbf{w}_0, \end{aligned} \tag{10.86}$$

where $\mathbf{w} = [\mathbf{y},\mathbf{z}]^T$ and $\mathbf{a} = [\mathbf{b}, -\mathbf{J}_\mathbf{z}^{-1}\mathbf{J}_\mathbf{y}\mathbf{b}]^T$. For the analysis of this problem we can refer to classical mathematical results, e.g. [214]. We will recall the following results:

1. if $\mathbf{a}(\mathbf{w},t)$ is continuously differentiable there exists a time interval $[0,T^*]$ in which the solution of the problem exists and is unique;
2. if, moreover, the derivatives $\partial \mathbf{a}_i/\partial w_j$ are bounded in the time interval $[0,T]$, then the solution of the Cauchy problem exists and is unique in $[0,T]$.

Numerical solution of Cauchy problems like (10.86) is an important branch of scientific computing. A general introduction can be found in [268]. Some basic ideas have been given in Section 2.3 in Chapter 2 for the Cauchy problems arising from the space discretisation of unsteady partial differential equations. Beyond the schemes mentioned there, we quote here a class of methods particularly useful for the problems considered here, namely the *Runge-Kutta methods.* Like the Euler and Crank-Nicolson methods, these schemes involve at each time step only the solution of the current and the previous steps, yielding however high accuracy by a splitting of the computation into an appropriate number of stages. These schemes can be explicit or implicit. For instance, the following is an explicit method of order 2 (called *Heun scheme*) given by

$$\begin{aligned} &\mathbf{w}^\star = \mathbf{w}^n + \Delta t\mathbf{a}(\mathbf{w}^n,t^n), \\ &\mathbf{w}^{n+1} = \mathbf{w}^n + \frac{\Delta t}{2}\left(\mathbf{a}(\mathbf{w}^n,t^n) + \mathbf{a}(\mathbf{w}^\star,t^{n+1})\right). \end{aligned}$$

Some Runge-Kutta methods have interesting practical features prone to *time adaptive implementations*. This means that with these methods it is possible to devise competitive a posteriori error estimators that can be used for adapting the time step to the solution dynamics. This feature is particularly useful in vascular problems where a fast transient (*systole*) is followed by a relatively steady phase (*diastole*). Furthermore, implicit Runge-Kutta schemes can be succesfully used in *stiff problems*, i.e. problems where different components of the solution $\mathbf{w}$ have so different dynamics that the fulfillment of stability and accuracy requirements could ask for an intensive computational effort (see e.g. [455]). These kind of problems can arise for instance when the lumped parameter representation of the vascular system couples a precise description of a district of interest with a rough description of the rest of the system. Other stiff problems arise when the dynamics of blood solutes (see the next section) is included in the mathematical model.

When the DAE problem (10.84) is of index higher than one, which is not the usual situation in this kind of problems, both the mathematical and numerical analyses become more involved. We refer the interested readers to [14, 184].

10.2.3 Lumped parameter models for modelling terminal vessels

By using the electrical analogy presented above, we now consider briefly some possible model for the terminal vessels to be used as stand-alone models or for computing boundary conditions to 1D networks (Section 10.1.5).

Pure resistive load: In some cases, the dynamics of blood in peripheral vessels is adequately represented by a simple algebraic law, see Fig. 10.14(right), given by

$$p(t) = RQ(t), \tag{10.87}$$

corresponding to the impedance $Z_T(t-\tau) = R\delta(\tau - t)$, where δ denotes the Dirac delta. This is particularly true for small vessels where the heart pulsatil-

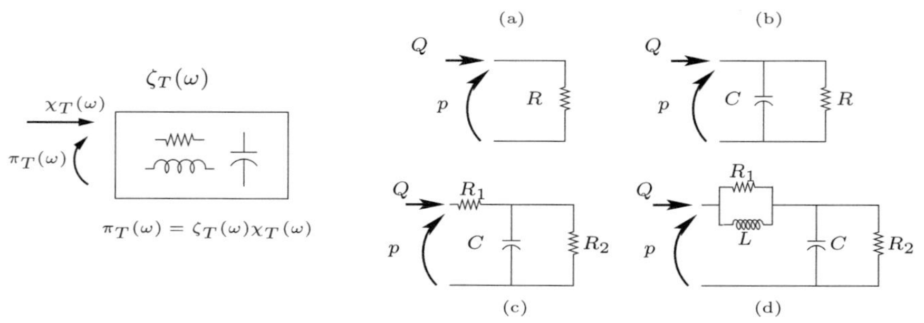

Fig. 10.14. Left: Terminal impedance for the peripheral circulation. Right: Lumped parameters representation (electrical networks) of possible impedances: (a) pure resistive load; (b) original windkessel model; (c) three elements windkessel; (d) four elements windkessel

ity has been almost completely attenuated by the larger vessel compliance and the motion is almost steady. An effective way of including this condition into the 1D model is based on the introduction of a *reflection coefficient.*

The reflection coefficient, R_t, is defined in [290] as the ratio of the magnitude of change of pressure across the reflected wave, δP, to the magnitude of change of pressure in the incident wave, ΔP. By an appropriate linearisation and assuming that the pressure in the venous system is zero, it has been found that this ratio can be expressed as function of the terminal resistance at the vessel outflow and is related to the resistance R by the expression

$$R_t = \frac{\delta P}{\Delta P} = \frac{A_0 R - \rho c_0}{A_0 R + \rho c_0} = \frac{R - \rho c_0 / A_0}{R + \rho c_0 / A_0}.$$

The suffix 0 indicates the at rest state, i.e $Q = 0$ and $A = A_0$.

The value of R_t may vary between a free outflow when $R_t = 0$ and a blockage when $R_t = 1$. The use of this parameter to characterise wave reflections caused by peripheral vessels is described in [535]. An advantage of using R_t instead of R is that it is related to pressure data only.

There is another possible definition for the reflection coefficient which is more suitable for prescribing boundary conditions based on the characteristic variables. More precisely, R_c is defined as

$$R_c = -\frac{W_{inc} - W_{inc,0}}{W_{out} - W_{out,0}},$$

where W_{inc} and W_{out} are the incoming and the outgoing characteristic variables at the boundary point, respectively. The negative sign is necessary to have a positive coefficient under normal conditions. A zero value of R_c indicates a perfectly non-reflecting boundary: the incoming characteristic variable is kept constant and equal to the value at rest, while $R_c = 1$ is again associated to a perfect blockage (indeed, it can be verified that in this case $u = 0$).

If we consider the right boundary $x = x_2$ and use (10.87) we have the following expressions

$$W_{out} = W_1 = \frac{p}{RA} + 4c \quad \text{and } W_{inc} = W_2 = \frac{p}{RA} - 4c.$$

Thus, if the rest value of the pressure is taken equal to 0, we have

$$R_c = -\frac{W_2 - W_{2,0}}{W_1 - W_{1,0}} = \frac{R_0 - p/4A(c - c_0)}{R + p/4A(c - c_0)}.$$

Using equations (10.39) and (10.87) in can be shown that $R_c \simeq R_t$ and indeed we have an equality by linearising c around the rest configuration. At the numerical level, W_1 can be computed for instance by extrapolation along the characteristic curves, refer to equation (10.46), the condition

$$W_2 = W_{2,0} - R_c(W_1 - W_{1,0}), \tag{10.88}$$

thus readily yields a boundary value for W_2.

Windkessel models: A more accurate representation of the terminal load is provided by the models including some possible dynamics related to vessel compliance and blood inertia. The first model was introduced by Otto Frank in 1899 [170]. It included a peripheral resistance and a compliance (see Fig. 10.14(b)) which yields a value of the impedance

$$\zeta_T(\omega) = \frac{R}{1+\sqrt{-1}\omega RC}.$$

This model has been called *Windkessel* in analogy with the device (made of a reservoir and an air chamber) converting the alternate (periodic) water pumping of firemen into a steady flow. In order to better fit the experimental results (see [350, 539]), this basic model has been successively refined by Westerhof and his co-workers with the introduction of a second resistance (see Fig. 10.14(c)). The model has been called a *three-element Windkessel* or also familiarly *Westkessel*, and corresponds to an impedance value of

$$\zeta_T(\omega) = \frac{R_1 + R_2 + \sqrt{-1}\omega R_1 R_2 C}{1+\sqrt{-1}\omega R_2 C}.$$

More recently (see [53, 483]), it has been pointed out that the fitting of experimental data with the three elements Windkessel model requires values that are not clearly related to the physical properties of the arteries. A new improvement of the model has been therefore proposed, leading to a four-element network (Fig. 10.14 right, (d)) that includes an inductor for inertial effects. The impedance of the model is

$$\zeta_T(\omega) = \frac{R_1 R_2 - C R_1 R_2 L\omega^2 + \sqrt{\omega}(R_1+R_2)}{R_1 - C R_2 L\omega^2 + \sqrt{\omega}(L + C R_1 R_2)}.$$

The determination of an appropriate estimate of the parameters of these models is a difficult problem. The interested reader is referred to [53, 350, 483]. An intuitive and systematic approach to estimate the parameters of a three-element model is presented in [5].

The moduli of impedances and angles of the four networks considered in Fig. 10.14 are drawn in Fig. 10.15.

Remark 10.2.2 *For including this kind of conditions in the 1D model, an alternative to equation (10.44) consists in formulating a condition in the time-domain for the Riemann variables (see the previous remark). For instance, by setting $R = R_1 + R_2$, the three-element Windkessel model corresponds to the boundary condition*

$$R_2 C \frac{R_a + R_1}{R_a + R} \frac{dW_2}{dt} + W_2 = R_2 C \frac{R_a - R_1}{R_a + R} \frac{dW_1}{dt} - R_c W_1,$$

that generalises (10.88) (see [158]).

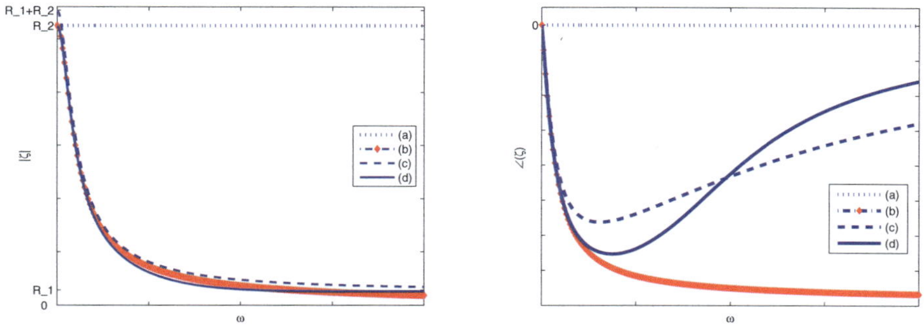

Fig. 10.15. Modulus (left) and angle (right) for the transfer function of the four networks in Fig. 10.14 (right)

Structured tree model: The dynamics spanned by family of Windkessel models is quite crude and in particular the wave propagation in the peripheral circulation is not well represented. A possible way for accounting these effects is the introduction of lumped parameters models with many elements, following the *geometrical multiscale approach* discussed in Chapter 11. A different approach, still resorting to the definition of an appropriate impedance function has been introduced in [358] and it is based on the representation of the terminal vessels as a structured tree (see Fig. 10.16).

By classical arguments in the wave theory (see e.g. [373]), the impedance at the beginning of a vessel with length l can be written as a function of the

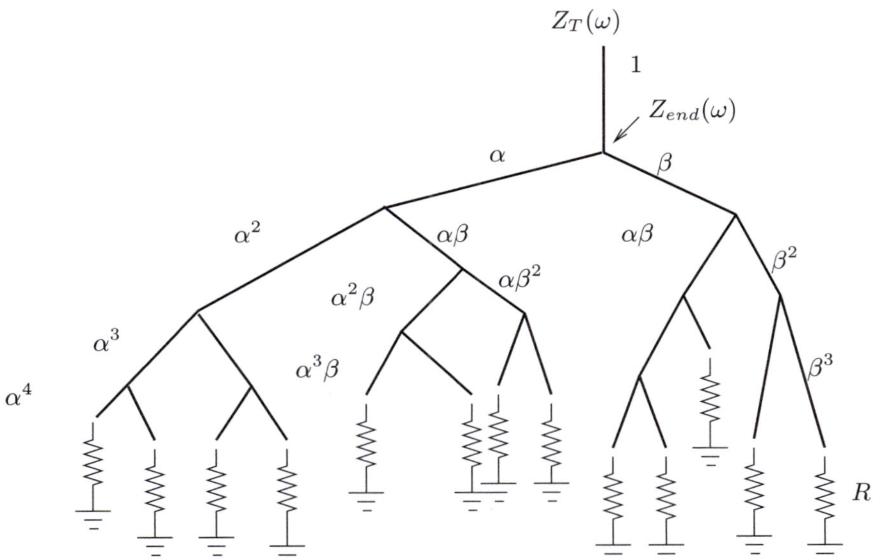

Fig. 10.16. Structured asymmetric tree representation of peripheral circulation

impedance at the end:

$$\zeta_{beg}(\omega) = \frac{g^{-1}\sqrt{-1}\sin(\omega l/c) + \zeta_{end}(\omega)\cos(\omega l/c)}{\cos(\omega l/c) + g\sqrt{-1}\zeta_{end}(\omega)\sin(\omega l/c)}, \tag{10.89}$$

where

$$g = A_0\sqrt{\frac{3\sqrt{A_0}K}{2E\pi h\rho}}, \quad c = \sqrt{\frac{2E\pi hK}{3\sqrt{A_0}\rho}},$$

and K is an appropriate function of the Womersley number. The basic idea of this peripheral model is therefore to apply this formula for the terminal impedance ζ_T that is expressed in this way as a function of the impedance at the end of the first peripheral vessel. The latter will be computed recursively by:

1. giving a model for the bifurcations in terms of impedance of parent and daughters vessels;
2. applying (10.89) for each branch of the vascular tree.

Continuity of pressure and flow rate at the bifurcation yields the condition linking the impedance of the parent vessel to the impedances of the daughter vessels (we assume branching with only two daughters)

$$\zeta_{parent} = \left(\frac{1}{\zeta_{d1}} + \frac{1}{\zeta_{d1}}\right)^{-1}.$$

Each branch of the tree is then scaled on the basis of the following assumptions:

1. at each bifurcation, the daughters branches scale asymmetrically with respect to the parent one with radius factors α, β that can be determined on the basis of optimal branching considerations (see [358]);
2. under a certain threshold on the radius it is possible to assume that the impedance is purely a resistive load, known by experimental data.

Observe that the threshold is applied to the vessel radii and not to the number of branchings, so the number of branches is in general a function of the position of the interface with the 1D model and will be not assumed to be known a priori.

A more detailed code for this impedance modelling can be found in [364]. Results presented in [360] show that this approach for terminal outflow boundary conditions provide reliable results. In particular, it provides a closer physiological behaviour than the Windkessel models, with a correct phase-lag between flow and pressure.

See also [477] for an advanced application of this approach.

10.2.4 Modelling the interaction between cardiovascular system and chemical species

In the previous sections we have assumed that the parameters of the models depend on the morphological features and are *constant in time* (see equation (10.76)). This is a strong simplification since daily experience indicates that these parameters change in different physiological situations. Heavy exercise requires a body's response that involves biochemical reactions, chemicals transport (oxygen in particular) and definitely adjustments in blood flow. The cardiovascular system has feedback mechanisms that regulate its working activity and are essential for life (see e.g. [227]). The dynamics underlying these phenomena is extremely heterogeneous and complex, involving different chemical species, the cardiovascular and the nervous systems from peripheral to central districts (see [364], Chapter 7). There are *long-term* mechanisms that are essentially driven by the renal activity. Presence of water and salt or hormones can be adjusted by the kidneys for controlling arterial pressure. Other mechanisms belong to the *short term regulation effects.* In the latter case, the *central nervous system* (CNS) is the main mediator, involving *baroreceptors, mechanoreceptors* and *chemoreceptors.* The latter are sensitive to chemicals in blood (see Section 10.1.3). When the oxygen concentration drops, chemoreceptors increases cardiac strength and vasoconstriction. Baroreceptors are sensitive to the pressure alterations. They are located in the carotid sinus and the aortic arch. The role of the *baroreflex effect* is to keep the pressure within a physiological range. Mechanoreceptors are located in the atria and in the pulmonary veins and control arterial pressure by acting on the venous volume.

Other tuning dynamics are specifically present in the cardiovascular system. In particular, the *autoregulation* is a mechanism for maintaining an almost constant oxygen supply (in particular in the brain), driven by the smooth muscles in the vascular walls (see [2,227]).

Lumped parameter models are an affordable mathematical and numerical tool for modelling these complex phenomena. Here we address some basic ideas for including feedback mechanisms in the models introduced so far. We essentially need:

1. lumped parameter models for chemical species, and
2. constitutive equations establishing the dependence of the parameters of the cardiovascular model on the concentration of chemicals.

We present these topics by means of an example based on Chapter 1 of reference [108].

Cardiovascular model

We assume the the cardiovascular system is represented by means of a set of four compartments (see Fig. 10.17):

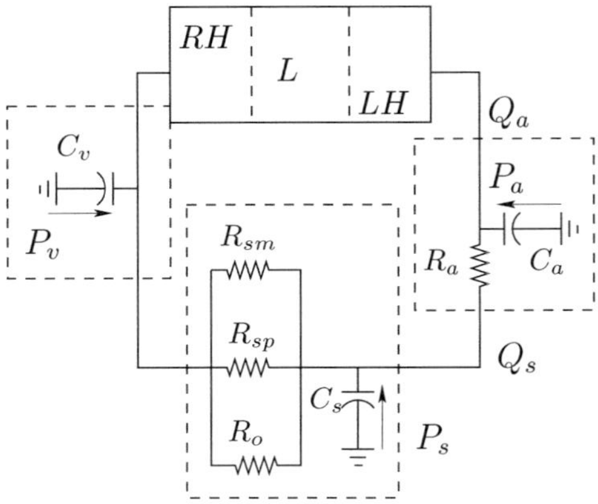

Fig. 10.17. Simplifed compartment model of the circulation

Right heart/lungs/left heart acting as a forcing term for the whole system.

Large arteries represented by a resistance R_a and a compliance C_a.

Systemic arteries that are represented by the compliance C_s and three sub-districts:

1. *skeletal muscle* represented by the resistance R_{sm} and with flow rate Q_{sm};
2. *splanchnic compartment* with resistance R_{sp} and flow rate Q_{sp};
3. *other organs* with resistance R_o and flow rate Q_o.

The total systemic resistance will be given by

$$R_s = \left(R_{sm}^{-1} + R_{sp}^{-1} + R_o^{-1}\right)^{-1}.$$

Venous system that is represented by the compliance C_v as their deformability is the more relevant feature of the veins.

The cardiovascular system will be therefore modelled by a lumped parameter model of the form

$$\begin{aligned}
C_a \frac{dP_a}{dt} &= Q_a - \frac{P_a - P_s}{R_a}, \\
C_s \frac{dP_s}{dt} &= \frac{P_a - P_s}{R_a} - \frac{P_s - P_v}{R_s}, \\
C_v \frac{dP_v}{dt} &= Q_a - C_a \frac{dP_a}{dt} - C_s \frac{dP_s}{dt}, \\
Q_{sm} &= \frac{P_s - P_v}{R_{sm}}, \quad Q_{sp} = \frac{P_s - P_v}{R_{sp}}, \quad Q_o = \frac{P_s - P_v}{R_o}.
\end{aligned} \tag{10.90}$$

Here Q_a is driven by the heart activity that can be simply given by

$$\begin{aligned} Q_a &= \frac{V_{str}}{T}, \\ V_{str} &= V_{ed}(P_v) - V_{u,vent} - \frac{P_a}{E}. \end{aligned} \tag{10.91}$$

Here, T is the *heart period*, V_{str} is the stroke volume of the heart. The latter is assumed to be a function of the end-of-diastole volume V_{ed}, which is in turn a function of the venous pressure P_v, of the (constant) unstressed ventricular volume $V_{u,vent}$ and of the arterial pressure P_a by means of the heart *elastance*+E.

Chemical model

Let us start considering only the dynamics of oxygen. We denote by $[O_2]_i$ the oxygen concentration in compartment i ($i \in (a, v, sm, sp, o)$) and by V_i is the volume of the i compartment. A possible law for the dynamics of oxygen in the systemic compartments ($i = sm, sp, o$) is

$$V_i \frac{d[O_2]_i}{dt} = -r_i([O_2]_i, t) + Q_i(t)\left([O_2]_a - \sigma_i [O_2]_i\right), \tag{10.92}$$

where r_i is the oxygen consumption rate and σ_i is a partition (constant) coefficient, function of the oxygen concentration in the different compartments *at rest.* The first term on the right-hand side is driven by the chemical reactions, while the second one is related to the *transport* associated to the blood flow. In the arterial compartment it is reasonable to assume that the oxygen consumption is negligible, so that $[O_2]_a$ is constant. In the venous compartment, by mass conservation, we collect the residual oxygen coming from the systemic compartments and its concentration is thus given by

$$[O_2]_v = \sum_{i=sm,sp,o} \frac{Q_i}{Q_a} \sigma_i [O_2]_i.$$

A possible generalisation of this equation to the multi-chemical case is the following. We introduce a *vector* of chemical concentration $\mathbf{c}_i$ so that c_{ki} is the concentration of the kth species in compartment i. This model is given by

$$\begin{aligned} V_i \frac{d\mathbf{c}_i}{dt} &= A\boldsymbol{\psi}_i(\mathbf{c}_i, t) + \mathbf{b}_i(\mathbf{c}_a, \mathbf{c}_i, Q_i, t), \quad i = sm, sp, o, \\ \mathbf{c}_v &= \sum_{i=sm,sp,o} \frac{Q_i}{Q_a} S_i \mathbf{c}_i, \\ \mathbf{c}_a &= \mathbf{c}_a(\mathbf{c}_a^0, \mathbf{c}_v), \end{aligned} \tag{10.93}$$

where S_i is a diagonal matrix with entries given by the partition coefficients σ_{ki} and $\mathbf{c}_a^0$ is the arterial vector concentration at rest. Moreover, $\boldsymbol{\psi}_i$ is the vector of consumption rates associated to chemical reactions and A_i is the so-called *stoichiometric matrix* representing the weighed connection of the species involved in the chemical reactions. Term $\mathbf{b}_i$ represents the convection contribution to the chemical dynamics, driven by the blood flow. It is worth pointing out that since chemical reactions can have different time scales associated with each reaction, differential systems like (10.93) can in practice be *stiff*.

Feedback model

The dependence of chemical dynamics on fluid dynamics is clearly defined in the transport term $\mathbf{b}_i$ of equation (10.93). Let us consider now how the chemical dynamics can affect the blood flow (see Fig. 10.18). To this aim, following [516], we introduce some new unknowns:

f_{es} represents the *efferent sympathetic activity*;

f_{ev} is the *efferent vagal activity*;

f_{cs} is the *carotid sinus firing rate*, that is the action generated by pressure alterations at the level of the carotid sinus;

f_{cm} is the *chemoreflex activity*;

$\widetilde{R}_i$ with $i = sm, sp, o$ the state variables determining the systemic resistances and influenced by the vagal activity;

x_i with $i = sm, sp, o$ the state variables determining the systemic resistances and influenced by the chemoreflex activity;

P_n a reference pressure value.

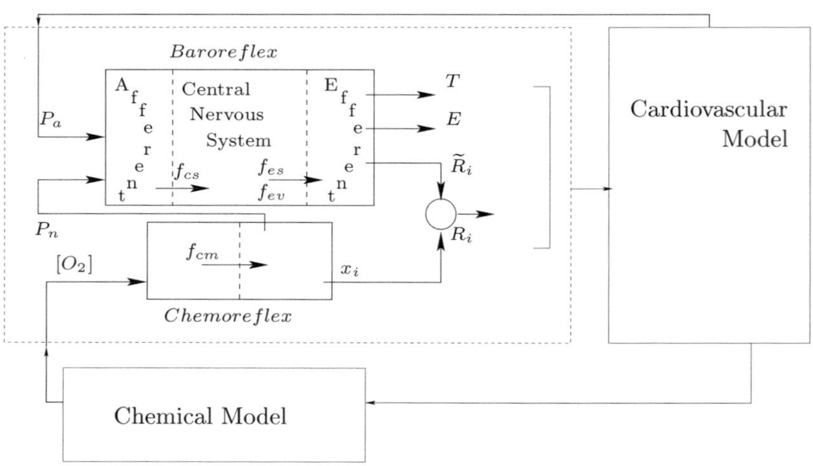

Fig. 10.18. Three compartments representation of the feedback cardiovascular model

We assume that the heart period T and the elastance E are influenced by the efferent vagal and sympathetic activities. In particular, we assume that

$$\begin{aligned}
\frac{dT}{dt} &= \frac{1}{\tau_T}\left(T_0 - T - \sigma_{T,s}(f_{es}) - \sigma_{T,v}(f_{ev})\right), \\
\frac{dE}{dt} &= \frac{1}{\tau_E}\left(E_0 - E - \sigma_{T,s}(f_{es})\right), \\
f_{es} &= f_{es,\infty} + (f_{es,0} - f_{es,\infty})\exp(-k_{es} f_{cs}), \\
f_{ev} &= \frac{f_{ev,0} + f_{ev,\infty}\exp((f_{cs} - f_{cs,0})/k_{ev})}{1 + \exp((f_{cs} - f_{cs,0})/k_{ev}))}, \\
f_{cs} &= \frac{f_{\min} + f_{\max}\exp((P_a - P_n)/k_a)}{1 + \exp((P_a - P_n)/k_a}.
\end{aligned} \tag{10.94}$$

where σ, E_0, T_0, $f_{,\infty}$, $f_{,0}$, $f_{\min}$, $f_{\max}$ and k (with their respective indices) represent appropriate functions and constants. The reference pressure P_n is driven by the chemoreflex activity and its temporal variation is given by

$$\frac{dP_n}{dt} = \frac{1}{\tau_{P_n}}\left(P_{n,0} - P_n - \sigma_{P_n,cm}(f_{cm})\right). \tag{10.95}$$

The systemic resistances are influenced both by the baroreflex and chemoreflex activities. More precisely, for $i = sm, sp, o$ we have

$$\begin{aligned}
\frac{d\widetilde{R}_i}{dt} &= \frac{1}{\tau_{\widetilde{R}_i}}\left(\widetilde{R}_{i,0} - \widetilde{R}_i - \sigma_{\widetilde{R}_i,s}(f_{es})\right), \\
\frac{dx_i}{dt} &= \frac{1}{\tau_{x_i}}\left(x_{i,0} - x_i - \sigma_{x_i,cm}(f_{cm})\right),
\end{aligned} \tag{10.96}$$

where finally we "assemble" the resistances

$$\begin{aligned}
R_{sm} &= \frac{\widetilde{R}_{sm}}{1 + x_{sm}}, \\
R_{sp} &= \widetilde{R}_{sp}(1 + x_{sp}), \\
R_o &= \frac{\widetilde{R}_o}{1 + x_o}.
\end{aligned} \tag{10.97}$$

Finally, the chemoreflex control is driven by the oxygen concentration:

$$f_{cm} = \begin{cases} 0 & \text{if} \quad [O_2]_{sm} > [O_2]^0_{sm}, \\ k_{cm}\left([O_2]_{sm} - [O_2]^0_{sm}\right)^2 & \text{otherwise.} \end{cases} \tag{10.98}$$

Equations (10.90), ... (10.98) represent a possible simplified model of feedback mechanisms in the cardiovascular system More details can be found in [108, 363, 515, 516].

A major concern in the devise of this kind of models is the parameter identification based on experimental data. There are different approaches for pursuing this aim. Basically, the problem is recast into the form of the minimisation of the distance between an experimental data set and the corresponding results predicted by the theory, by acting on the values of the parameters to be estimated. The "optimal values" can be found by means of:

- *line search algorithms* (see e.g. [403]), that are quite cheap and however can found local (i.e. non global) optimal values;
- *genetic algorithms*, that compute the global optimal solution, even if with a larger computational cost. See [109] for more details.

10.3 Conclusions

Although this Chapter is limited to a basic introduction to simplified models of the circulatory system, we should stress that these models represent an important tool for quantitative cardiovascular investigations. The simple representation of a single vessel or a compartment makes these models well suited for an affordable description of complex dynamics among different vessels or compartments. As a matter of fact, in practice these models have been used in *cardiovascular mathematics* before the Navier-Stokes based models, because the latter require so many complex numerical techniques (and computational time) for providing quantitative results. In particular, 1D models are appropriate for describing pressure wave propagation along the vascular tree [316], and at which extent this can be affected by some pathologies, prostheses or aging [3, 4, 158]. Lumped parameter models, on the other hand, are extremely useful for describing complex dynamics among compartments, in particular when the space details are not so relevant, like in the case of estimation of blood flow reserves in some compartment (usually the coronary reserve) or the feedback mechanisms.

The main drawback of these models is the loss of some details that could be relevant at the systemic level, despite of their local nature. For this problem, a possible approach is to couple together local and systemic models, as it is addressed in the next chapter.

11

Multiscale models of the vascular system

Luca Formaggia, Alfio Quarteroni, and Alessandro Veneziani

As we have illustrated in the previous chapters, there are essentially three classes of models for the vascular system: fully three dimensional models, based on the Navier-Stokes (NS) equations, one dimensional models, including the space dependence on the vessel axial coordinate, based on the Euler (E) equations, and the lumped parameter or zero-dimensional models, based on the Kirchhoff laws (K) for hydraulic networks. Navier-Stokes based models can account for many different features of blood flow problems, such as the blood rheology (Chapter 6), the vascular wall dynamics (Chapter 3), the interaction between blood flow and wall deformation (Chapters 8 and 9). These models are perfectly adequate for investigating qualitatively and quantitatively the effects of the geometry on the blood flow (Chapters 5) and the possible relations between local haemodynamics and the development of some pathologies (Chapter 1). On the other hand, the high computational costs (Chapters 2, 3 and 9) restrict their use to cover few contiguous vascular districts only.

Euler-based models provide an optimal tool for the analysis of wave propagation phenomena in the vascular tree. In particular, they are convenient when the local flow details are less relevant than the accounting for propagative phenomena on large parts of the vascular tree and the numerical results are needed in a relatively short time. These models outline the role of the vascular system as a sort of telegraph line with the task of transmitting nutrients as well as biological signals along the body. On the other hand, the space dependence still retained in these models inhibits their use in the whole vascular system. In fact, it would be impossible to follow the geometrical details of the capillary network (not to mention the specific rheological assumptions required by capillary circulation – see Chapter 6).

On the contrary, Kirchhoff-based models can provide a representation of a large part or even the whole circulatory system, since they get rid of the explicit space dependence (see Section 10.2 and [364]). In a simple and however still quantitative way, these models can include the presence of the heart, the venous system, but also account for self-regulating and metabolic dynamics, as we have seen in Section 10.2.4.

Formaggia L, Quarteroni A, Veneziani A (Eds.): Cardiovascular Mathematics. Modeling and simulation of the circulatory system

If NS, E and K models provide such a different tools, reliable numerical methods for real life applications need to overcome the drawbacks and weakness of each individual class of models. This can be done by resorting to the *geometrical multiscale representation* of the circulatory system.

11.1 What do we mean with *geometrical multiscale models*?

Geometrical multiscale[1] approach is a strategy for modelling the circulatory system, including the reciprocal interactions between local and systemic haemodynamics by exploiting the complementary features of the different possible models. Indeed, these features suggest in a natural way to couple detailed local models with coarser models able to describe the dynamics over a large part or the whole system with acceptable computational costs (see Fig. 11.1).

Multiscale modelling can be regarded as a refinement of models, or a sort of "models zoom" in a specific region of interest, moving from a rough description of the whole system (*bottom-up approach*). From a different point of view, it

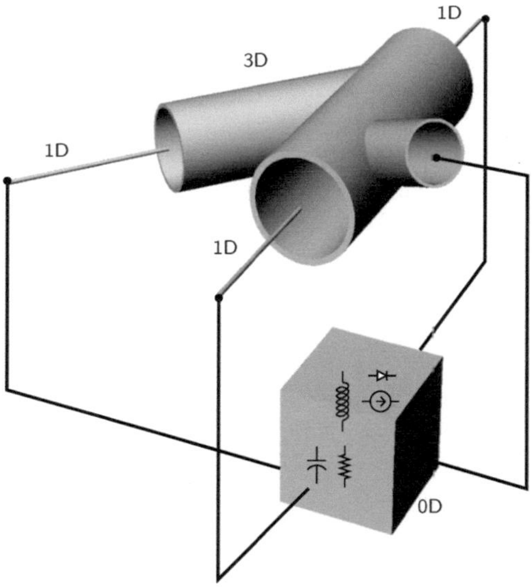

Fig. 11.1. A schematic representation of a geometrical multiscale model

[1] Term "multiscale" is often used with a different meaning in many fields of mathematical and numerical modelling, whenever two or more time and/or spatial scales are present. Typical examples are the modelling of turbulence or multiresolution representations. In order to avoid ambiguities, we have added the term *geometrical* for identifying the multiscale perspective illustrated in this chapter.

can be regarded as a sophisticated and reliable method for computing correct boundary conditions at the artificial boundaries of a district of interest, that is the non-physical boundaries needed to bound the computational domain (*top-down approach*). In the latter perspective, it can be considered also as a specific numerical tool to avoiding, or at least reduce, spurious effects caused by the presence of artificial boundaries (see also Chapter 2). Indeed, the propagative nature of blood flow in large vessels require appropriate techniques to avoid artificial wave reflections at those boundaries. In this perspective the geometrical multiscale approach can be regarded as a new method for solving a class of problems, whose application goes beyond those addressed in this book.

Despite the simplicity of the basic idea, the coupling of NS, E and K models lead to nontrivial problems at both the mathematical and the numerical level. After a quick review of geometrical multiscale models of the cardiovascular system and the coupling conditions based on some intuitive formulations, we will consider in more details the mathematical aspects of this approach, leading to less immediate and however more accurate solutions.

11.2 Setting up of geometrical multiscale models

A main issue of the geometrical multiscale modelling is to devise mathematically and physically sound coupling conditions among the models, and develop efficient techniques for their numerical computation.

11.2.1 Coupling of 3D and 1D models

According to the top-down approach introduced above, let us consider the coupling of 3D and 1D models for haemodynamics (see Fig. 11.2). This technique is of interest for instance when an endograft prosthesis or a stent is deployed in a specific district (abdominal aorta, carotid, etc.) and one is interested to the alterations induced by this operations on the pressure propagation over the vascular tree.

As already mentioned, this is also an effective way to implement physically based absorbing conditions, in particular for a 3D compliant model. As it has been pointed out in Chapter 3 (see also [155]) the solution of the fluid-structure interaction problem in a compliant vessel Ω_{3D} features a propagative behaviour, similar to that of a compressible flow in a rigid pipe. We have seen in the previous chapter that two pulse waves travel along the circulatory system, in opposite directions. The domain Ω_{3D} normally represents just a tiny portion of the whole cardiovascular system, for instance a specific artery. The pulse waves outgoing the artery are partially reflected by the remaining part of the system and give rise to a backward wave (see Chapter 10) which eventually re-enters the artery under consideration. Forward and backward components are related to the structure of vascular tree and their correct mathematical description is crucial to avoid artifacts in the numerical solution

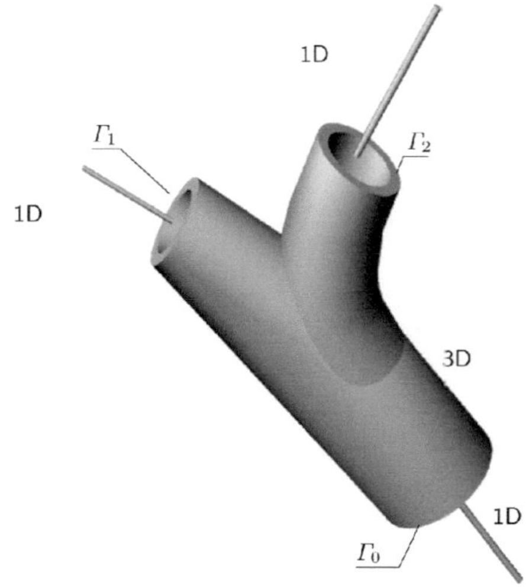

Fig. 11.2. A 3D-1D model

induced by a wrong decomposition of incoming and outgoing waves. Coupling of 3D and 1D models is a possible and reliable approach to achieve this goal and requires the introduction of a proper 1D representation of the vascular tree around Ω_{3D}.

Appropriate matching conditions drive the data exchange between NS and E models at the interface Γ (see Fig. 11.3). Different conditions in fact can be considered. In particular we refer to the following quantities defined on Γ (see [155])

$$
\begin{aligned}
A &= \text{meas}(\Gamma), \quad Q = \int_\Gamma \boldsymbol{u}\cdot\mathbf{n}d\gamma, \\
\overline{\boldsymbol{u}} &= \frac{1}{A}\int_\Gamma \boldsymbol{u}\cdot\mathbf{n}d\gamma = \frac{Q}{A}, \quad \overline{p} = \frac{1}{A}\int_\Gamma p d\gamma.
\end{aligned}
\tag{11.1}
$$

A priori, it is reasonable to prescribe the continuity of the following quantities at the interface:

[A] area: $A_{3D} = A_{1D}$;
[B] mean pressure: $\overline{p}_{3D} = \overline{p}_{1D}$;
[C] flux: $Q_{3D} = Q_{1D}$;
[D] incoming characteristic: $\overline{\boldsymbol{u}}_{3D} + \frac{8}{\rho}\left(\sqrt{\overline{p} - p_{ext} + p^*} - \sqrt{p^*}\right) = W_{1,1D}$;
[E] mean total pressure: $\overline{p}_{3D} + \frac{1}{2}\overline{\boldsymbol{u}}_{3D}^2 = \overline{p}_{1D}\frac{1}{2}\overline{\boldsymbol{u}}_{1D}^2$,

where $W_{1,1D}$ is the incoming characteristic variable[2] introduced in (10.37), p_{ext} is the pressure external to the vessel and p^* depends on the physical

[2] The incoming characteristic variable is W_1 because we are considering an interface which is an outflow (distal) boundary for the 3D model and correspondingly an

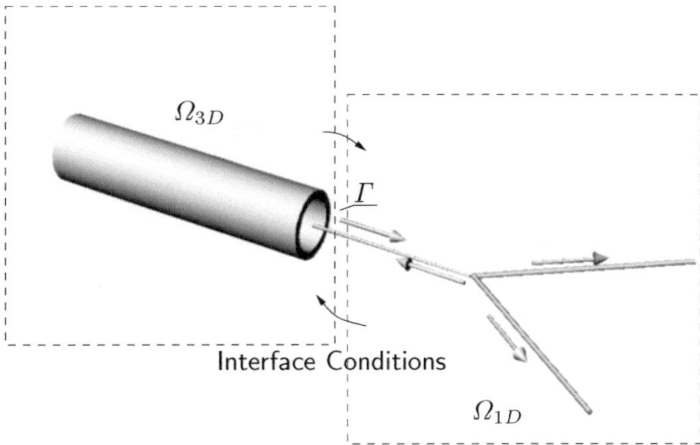

Fig. 11.3. 3D-1D model: detail of the coupling at the outflow of Ω_{3D}

features of vascular walls (see Chapter 3). The conditions above are not all independent. For instance, [A],[B] and [D] imply conditions [C]. Similarly, conditions [A], [C] and [D] imply [B]. Moreover, it is worth observing that, following the derivation of 1D models carried out in Chapter 10, conditions [B], [D] and [E] can be replaced by similar conditions where the mean pressure on the 3D side is replaced by the averaged normal stresses (see Chapter 3 and [155]), yielding:

[B1] $\overline{\sigma_{\mathbf{n}}}_{3D} = \overline{p}_{1D}$;

[D1] $\overline{\boldsymbol{u}}_{3D} + \frac{8}{\rho}\left(\sqrt{\overline{\sigma_{\mathbf{n}}} - p_{ext} + p^*} - \sqrt{p^*}\right) = W_{1,1D}$;

[E1] mean total pressure: $\overline{\sigma_{\mathbf{n}}}_{3D} + \frac{1}{2}\overline{\boldsymbol{u}}^2_{3D} = \overline{p}_{1D}\frac{1}{2}\overline{\boldsymbol{u}}^2_{3D}$.

In practise, we can identify different (alternative) sets of independent interface conditions:

a) [A], [B], [D];
b) [A], [C], [D];
c) [A], [B1], [D1];
d) [A], [C], [D1];
e) [A], [E], [D];
f) [A], [E1], [D].

Different possible choices that are equivalent form the mathematical viewpoint can however lead to different numerical schemes.

inflow (proximal) boundary for the 1D model. Should we swap the sequence of 1D and 3D models, the incoming characteristic variable would be W_2.

Some numerical issues

In numerical solution of multiscale models presented above it is natural to split the scheme into the iterative sequence of dimensionally homogeneous problems, namely 3D and 1D separately. In this way, we can figure out for instance the following algorithm to be carried out at each time step[3]. We focus our attention on interface between the two models. In particular, we refer to interface conditions (b) of the previous list. The conditions on the other boundaries are assumed to be standard (see Chapter 3 and 10).

`Initialisation.` Set $k = 0$ and select an initial guess for the mean velocity $\overline{\boldsymbol{u}}_{3D}^{(0)}$ and pressure $\overline{p}^{(0)}$ at the interface. Typically, this guess is given by the same quantities at the end of the previous time step.

`Loop.`

1. *Solve* the 1D model, using [D] as boundary condition at the interface, by computing $W_1^{(k)}$ as a function of the current guess of the mean velocity and pressure (or normal stress). The other boundaries of the 1D model will be properly managed (see Section 10.1.5). In this step, $A_{1D}^{(k+1)}$ and $Q_{1D}^{(k+1)}$ are computed.
2. *Solve* the 3D fluid-structure interaction model, with [A] as a boundary condition for the structure and [C] for the fluid by using $A_{1D}^{(k+1)}$ and $Q_{1D}^{(k+1)}$. At the end of this step, compute the new guess $W_1^{(k+1)}$. Set $k = k + 1$.

`Test.` The loop ends when:

$$|W_1^{(k)} - W_1^{(k-1)}| \leq \varepsilon, \quad |A^{(k)} - A^{(k-1)}| \leq \varepsilon, \quad |Q^{(k)} - Q^{(k-1)}| \leq \varepsilon \tag{11.2}$$

being ε a given tolerance.

Analogous algorithms can be devised for the other interface conditions.

While the boundary conditions in step (1) of the loop lead to a mathematically well posed problem, step (2) in this form does not, since these averaged data on the boundary are not enough to guarantee uniqueness of solution for the associated 3D problem. A specific treatment of these problems is required. To be more concrete, let us use condition [A] for the structure at step 2. On the 3D compliant model we would need pointwise data for the wall displacement $\boldsymbol{\eta}$. On the other hand, when the area of the interface $\Gamma(t)$ is known from the computation of the 1D model, we have the average condition:

$$\int_{\Gamma(t)} d\gamma = A_{1D}(t). \tag{11.3}$$

We need to "spread" the average data to pointwise conditions on the displacements $\boldsymbol{\eta}$. To this aim we can assume a shape for the displacement depending

[3] We will not put in evidence explicitly the temporal level for the sake of notation.

on a single parameter to be tuned so to force (11.3). For instance, assume that Γ is circular with centre on the axis of coordinates (x_c, y_c, z_c), and belongs to the plane identified by the equation $z = z_c$. In this way the component η_3 along z of $\boldsymbol{\eta}$ is constant and equal to zero and we can set:

$$\eta_1(x,y,z,t) = \Delta R(t) \cos\left(\tan^{-1}\left(\frac{y}{x}\right)\right) = \sqrt{\frac{A_{1D}(t) - A_0}{\pi}} \cos\left(\tan^{-1}\left(\frac{y}{x}\right)\right),$$

$$\eta_2(t) = \Delta R(t) \sin\left(\tan^{-1}\left(\frac{y}{x}\right)\right) = \sqrt{\frac{A_{1D}(t) - A_0}{\pi}} \sin\left(\tan^{-1}\left(\frac{y}{x}\right)\right). \tag{11.4}$$

Here A_0 is the reference area of section Γ, corresponding to a zero displacement, and $\Delta R(t) = R(t) - R_0$ is the difference between the current and the reference radius. With this choice the average condition has been extended to pointwise data by assuming a priori a planar circular shape for the interface Γ. This technique can be extended to more general shapes.

In a similar way we can address condition [C], by assuming, for instance, a velocity profile depending on a single parameter. For instance, let us assume again that Γ has a circular shape in the xy–plane. Then, we can resort to the Poiseuille velocity field (see Chapter 5):

$$u_1 = u_2 = 0, \quad u_3(x,y,t) = \frac{2Q_{1D}(t)}{\pi \rho R^2}\left(1 - \frac{(x-x_c)^2 + (y-y_c)^2}{R^2}\right), \tag{11.5}$$

where Q_{1D} is the flow rate computed by the 1D model. Again, the arbitrary selection of a velocity profile converts the average conditions into pointwise Dirichlet conditions for the fluid problem.

Numerical results (see Fig. 11.4 and 11.5) show that this approach is actually able to reduce spurious back-reflections at the boundaries, in particular when the arbitrary assumptions on the displacement shape or the chosen velocity profile are realistic. However, in general, the arbitrary selection of a shape for the displacement or the velocity profile strongly affects the numerical solution. Hence, the reliability of results obtained in this way is sometimes questionable. More sophisticated mathematical and numerical techniques that are able to expand average data to pointwise conditions are required for ensuring better accuracy. We will address these techniques in Section 11.3.

Another drawback of this multiscale coupling still relies on the limited capability of E models of covering the capillary network, which on the other hand is the main source of the back reflections propagating in the arterial tree and of including the action of the heart. More sophisticated multiscale models are therefore needed.

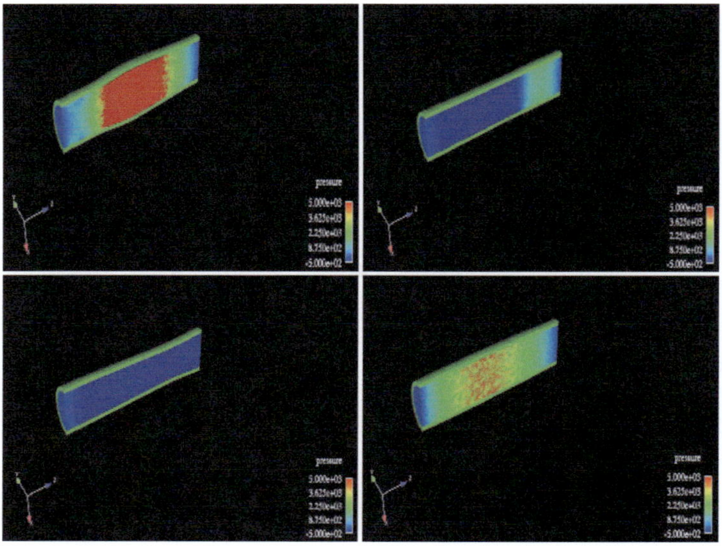

Fig. 11.4. 3D simulation: pressure wave propagation along a compliant vessel. Spurious effects arise at the artificial downstream boundary

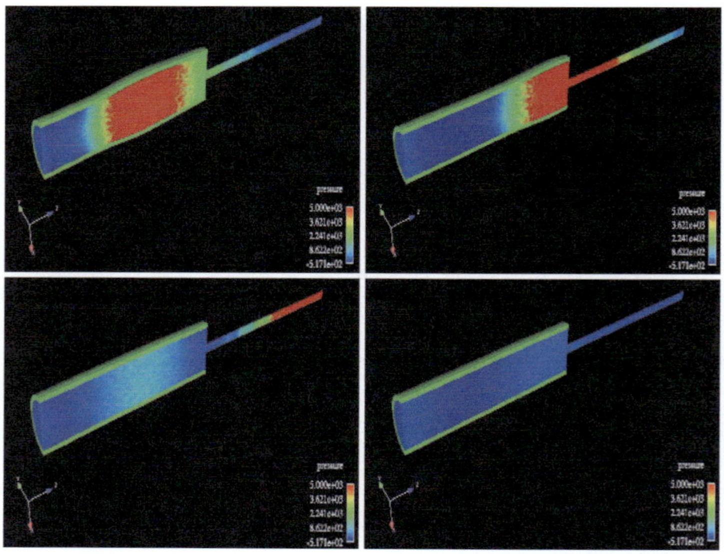

Fig. 11.5. Multiscale 3D-1D simulation: pressure wave propagation along the two submodels. Spurious effects at the artificial boundary are small

11.2.2 Coupling of 1D-0D and 3D-1D-0D models

A possible way to account for the presence of the capillary bed and the action of the heart is to close the 3D-1D network with K models. This requires in particular the coupling of 1D and lumped parameter models, through interface conditions. A simplified version of this coupling has been already addressed in Chapter 10. In that case, lumped parameter models were represented by a simple terminal impedance for prescribing boundary conditions in the frequency domain at the downstream sections of a 1D network. Here, we want to give an insight of models and numerical issues arising from a precise and accurate inclusion of the dynamics in K models. In the multiscale framework they are described in terms of a system of differential-algebraic equations (DAE – see (10.84)) in the time variable.

For the sake of simplicity, we consider the multiscale model represented in Fig. 11.6, where the 1D model represents a simple cylindrical domain. More complex problems, featuring a network of 1D segments or even a coupled 3D-1D model can be considered as well within the same framework.

In the model at hand we have two interfaces, Γ_0 and Γ_1, where it is reasonable to prescribe the continuity of:

[A] area: $A_{1D} = A_{0D}$;
[B] pressure: $P_{1D} = P_{0D}$;
[C] flow rate: $Q_{1D} = Q_{0D}$.

Moreover, we could require the continuity of the Riemann variables:

[D] characteristic variable propagating from the heart to the peripheries:
$$\frac{Q_{0D}}{A_{0D}} + \frac{8}{\rho}\left(\sqrt{P_{0D} - p_{ext} + p^*} - \sqrt{p^*}\right) = W_{1,1D};$$
[E] characteristic variable propagating from the peripheries to the heart:
$$\frac{Q_{0D}}{A_{0D}} - \frac{8}{\rho}\left(\sqrt{P_{0D} - p_{ext} + p^*} - \sqrt{p^*}\right) = W_{2,1D}.$$

Again, these conditions are not all independent. This is the case for instance of [A] and [B], since both the E and K models include a wall law linking together pressure and area. Should these wall laws be the same, the continuity of the area would imply the continuity of the pressure and vice-versa. More in general, only one between [A] and [B] can be explicitly prescribed.

Similarly, only two conditions among [B], [C], [D] and [E] can be selected, for instance:

1. conditions [B], [D] at the upstream interface Γ_0;
2. conditions [C], [E] at the downstream interface Γ_1.

Some numerical issues

A possible approach for solving this multiscale model still resorts to splitting the computation into the sequence of dimensionally homogeneous problems.

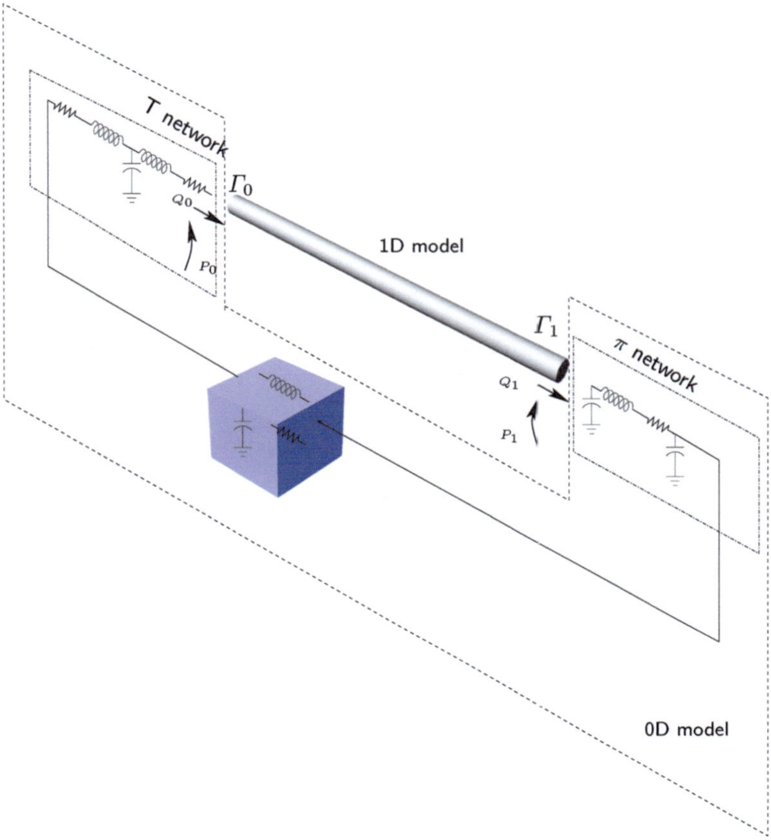

Fig. 11.6. 1D-0D model: the 1D model is given by a simple compliant straight cylinder, the 0D model is composed by the network in the cube and two bridging regions (upstream and downstream). Upstream bridging region is given by a T network, featuring the flow rate Q_0 as state variable. Downstream bridging region has the pressure P_1 as state variable. These interface compartments are compatible with the splitting scheme described in the text

In the case of Fig. 11.6, this means that we solve separately the DAE system arising from the lumped parameter model and the Euler hyperbolic system. Let us consider preliminarily the simple case in which a 1D straight cylinder is split into a 1D-0D model as illustrated in Fig. 11.7. In particular, let us consider the multiscale model at the top of Fig. 11.7, where the 0D model is represented by a $\mathcal{L}$ inverted network (see Chapter 10). The lumped parameter model is therefore described by the following equations:

$$\begin{aligned} C\frac{dP}{dt} &= Q_{up} - Q, \\ L\frac{dQ}{dt} + RQ &= P - P_{dw}. \end{aligned} \qquad (11.6)$$

A possible iterative scheme reads as follows. At each time step:

`Initialisation.` Set $k = 0$ and fix an initial guess for the interface flow rate $Q_{up}^{(0)}$.

`Loop.`

1. *Solve* the 0D model (11.6), by using $Q_{up}^{(k)}$ as forcing term. This yields the estimates of $Q^{(k)}$ and $P^{(k)}$. On the basis of this computation, Riemann variable $W_2^{(k)}$ at the interface entering the 1D model can be computed.
2. *Solve* the 1D model by using incoming Riemann variable $W_2^{(k)}$ as boundary condition. At the end of this step, a new guess for $Q_{up}^{(k+1)}$ is available. Set $k = k + 1$.

`Test.` The loop ends when the solution fulfils an appropriate test, for instance:

$$|P^{(k)} - P^{(k-1)}| \leq \varepsilon, \quad |Q_{up}^{(k)} - Q_{up}^{(k-1)}| \leq \varepsilon.$$

Let us consider now the multiscale model on the bottom of Fig. 11.7. Here 0D model is represented by a $\mathcal{L}$ network, described by system

$$\begin{aligned} L\frac{dQ}{dt} + RQ &= P_{up} - P, \\ C\frac{dP}{dt} &= Q - Q_{dw}. \end{aligned} \tag{11.7}$$

We can still use an iterative approach as follows.

`Initialisation.` Set $k = 0$ and fix an initial guess for interface pressure $P_{up}^{(0)}$.

`Loop.`

1. *Solve* the 0D model (11.7), by using $P_{up}^{(k)}$ as forcing term. This yields the estimates of $Q^{(k)}$ and $P^{(k)}$. On the basis of this computation, Riemann variable $W_2^{(k)}$ at the interface entering the 1D model can be computed.
2. *Solve* 1D model by using incoming Riemann variable $W_2^{(k)}$ as boundary condition. At the end of this step, a new guess for $P_{up}^{(k+1)}$ is available. Set $k = k + 1$.

`Test.` The loop ends when the solution fulfils an appropriate test, for instance:

$$|P_{up}^{(k)} - P_{up}^{(k-1)}| \leq \varepsilon, \quad |Q^{(k)} - Q^{(k-1)}| \leq \varepsilon.$$

Several remarks are in order. First of all the use of characteristic variables has the advantage of prescribing (at least approximately) absorbing boundary conditions, well suited for avoiding numerical reflections at the boundary of the E model (see Chapter 10).

Secondly, interface conditions are by definition localised in a specific position in space. On the other hand, K models have lost an explicit space dependence. Therefore, in managing matching conditions with K models:

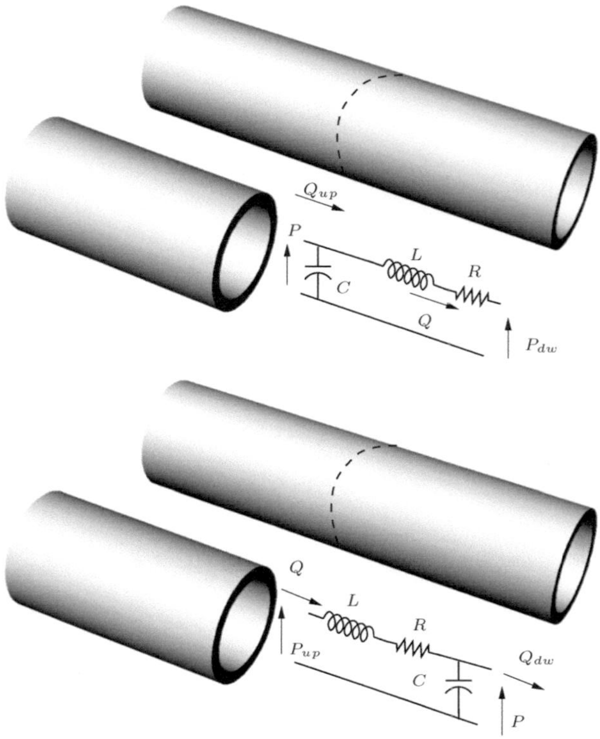

Fig. 11.7. Two simple examples of 1D-0D multiscale models. At the top, the lumped parameter model is given by a $\mathcal{L}$-inverted network. On the bottom, it is given by a $\mathcal{L}$ network. The two network configurations are appropriate for different iterative solvers (see text)

1. interface conditions yield a forcing term in the 0D model;
2. different configurations of the 0D models are associated with different iterative schemes: in the first case the 0D model is forced by the flow rate Q_{up} and provides the pressure P; in the latter case, it is forced by the pressure P_{up} and provides the flow rate Q.

The latter item deserves some further remarks. In lumped parameter problems, interfaces between E and K models are represented by the boundary of the 1D domain and the compartments placed in the neighbourhood of the 1D models[4]. The type of network used in these compartments defines implicitly the state variables and forcing terms for the 0D model. In an iterative scheme, the latter will be provided to the 0D model by the 1D problem, while the former are the variables that will be computed by the 0D and used to build the boundary condition for the 1D model.

[4] In the two oversimplified examples above they in fact corresponds to the entire 0D models.

We call *bridging regions* those compartments of the 0D model that play the role of the interfaces with the other models. The link between the graph of the bridging regions and the numerical scheme will be called *bridging region compatibility* (see [409]). More precisely, we say that a numerical scheme is *bridging region compatible* if it is consistent with the topology of the bridging regions.

For instance, for the multiscale model of Fig. 11.6, where the upstream bridging region is given by a T network and the downstream one is given by a π network, a bridging region compatible scheme reads as follows.

`Initialisation.` Set $k = 0$ and fix an initial guess for the upstream pressure $P_0^{(0)}$ and the downstream flow rate $Q_1^{(0)}$.

`Loop.`

1. *Solve* the 0D model, by using the available upstream pressure and the downstream flow rate as forcing terms. Compute in particular the upstream flow rate $Q_0^{(k)}$ and the downstream pressure $P_1^{(k)}$. After this computation, the incoming characteristic variables, $W_1^{(k)}$ upstream and $W_2^{(k)}$ downstream are available.
2. *Solve* the 1D model by using the incoming characteristic variables as boundary conditions. At the end of this step, new guesses for the upstream pressure $P_0^{(k+1)}$ and the downstream flow rate $Q_1^{(k+1)}$ are available.

`Test.` The loop ends when the solution fulfils an appropriate test, for instance:

$$|P_i^{(k)} - P_i^{(k-1)}| \leq \varepsilon, \quad |Q_i^{(k)} - Q_i^{(k-1)}| \leq \varepsilon, \qquad i = 0, 1.$$

Remark 11.2.1 *Step 1 can be regarded as a stand-alone lumped parameter model, represented by the circuit of Fig. 11.8, where input variables of the 1D model are represented by a current and a voltage generator respectively. In terms of circuit analysis bridging region compatibility in fact implies that no voltage/pressure generator is in parallel with a capacitor and no current/flow rate generator is in series with an inductance. Under these assumptions it is possible to prove that the DAE system associated with this stand-alone network is of index 1 and it can be reduced to a well posed Cauchy problem for a system of ordinary differential equations (see [121, Chap. 12]).*

Aortic valve function

As we have pointed out, an advantage of K models is their capability of representing in relatively simple terms complex systems like the heart or the action of control dynamics. Moving from the observation that "the left ventricle and arterial circulation represent two mechanical units that are joined together to form a coupled biological system" [350, Chap. 13], it makes sense to consider a 1D model for the aorta coupled with the lumped parameter model of the

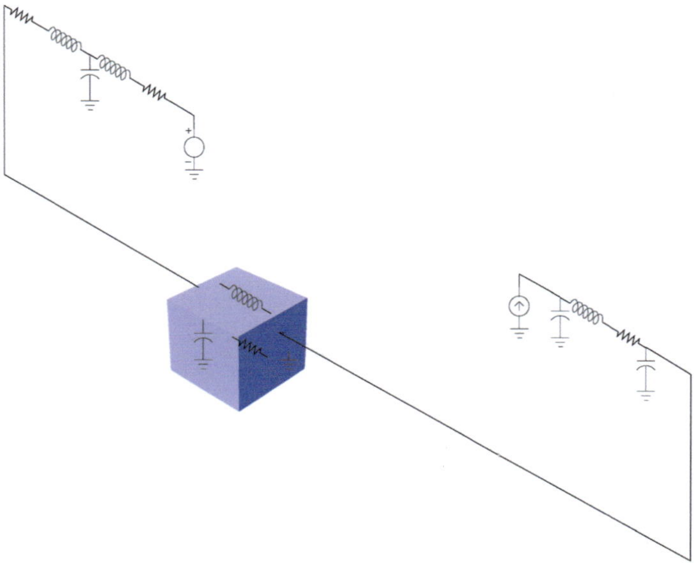

Fig. 11.8. Stand alone 0D model corresponding to step 2 of the splitting iterative algorithm (see text)

heart presented in Section 10.2.1. Since the coupling is mediated by the aortic valve, we assume that there are two possible working states for the system Heart-Aorta.

1. *Closed valve (CV) condition*: when the aortic valve is closed, the two systems are actually decoupled; in particular, for the arterial tree we have a null flow rate condition at the aorta inflow, which in terms of the characteristic variables implies
$$W_1 = -W_2.$$
2. *Open valve (OV) condition*: the ventricular pressure is related to the 1D problem by solving equation (10.82) which we recall here for the sake of clarity:
$$\frac{1}{E_v}\frac{dP_v}{dt} + \frac{d}{dt}\left(\frac{1}{E_v}\right) P_v = -Q_v.$$
During this phase, we assume that ventricular flow rate Q_v and pressure P_v are equal to the arterial ones at the aorta inflow (see Fig. 11.9), corresponding to conditions
$$Q_v = Q_{1D}, \quad P_v = P_{1D}.$$
A numerical implementation of these conditions by using the incoming characteristic variable in the 1D network is addressed in [158].

Transition between OV and CV conditions cannot be prescribed a priori. We assume that the valve opens under the action of a differential pressure

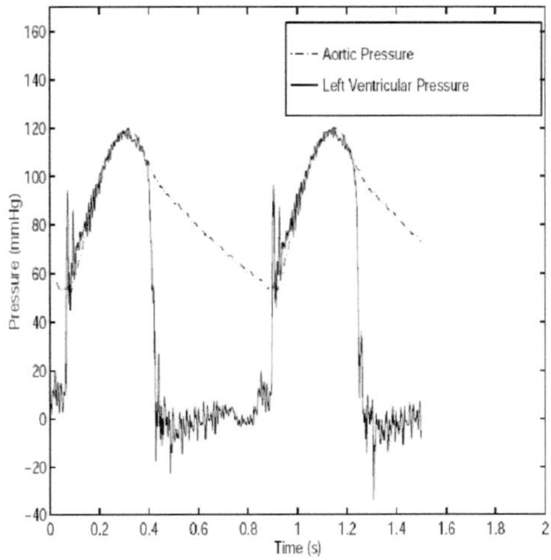

Fig. 11.9. Ventricular and arterial pressures during the heart beat. When the aortic valve is open, the two pressures can be assumed to be the same

and it closes when forced by a flow reversal. This means that when the valve is closed we need to compare at each time step the aortic and ventricular pressure. If $P_v - P_{1D} < 0$ the valve is kept closed (CV conditions), otherwise we switch to the OV conditions until the next closure. To determine the instant of valve closure (end of systole) we check the sign of the flux at the aortic proximal node. At the first time step when Q_v becomes negative we "close" the valve by adopting again CV boundary condition, up to the next heart cycle (see Fig. 11.10).

In [158] this multiscale model has been used for simulating a 1D network of the largest 55 arteries, coupled with the heart. The microcirculation is represented by simple Windkessel models at every 1D terminal section. Figure 11.11 pinpoints the relevance of the multiscale model (right column) in comparison with a standard approach, in which the action of the heart is described as a boundary condition, not sensible to the real functioning of the arterial network. The standard model actually damps wave reflection, in particular in the pathological case in which right femoral artery is supposed to be surgically closed.

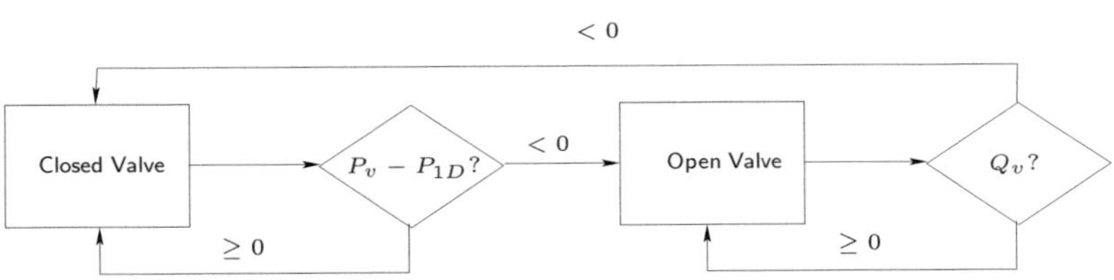

Fig. 11.10. Flow chart representation of the aortic valve modelling

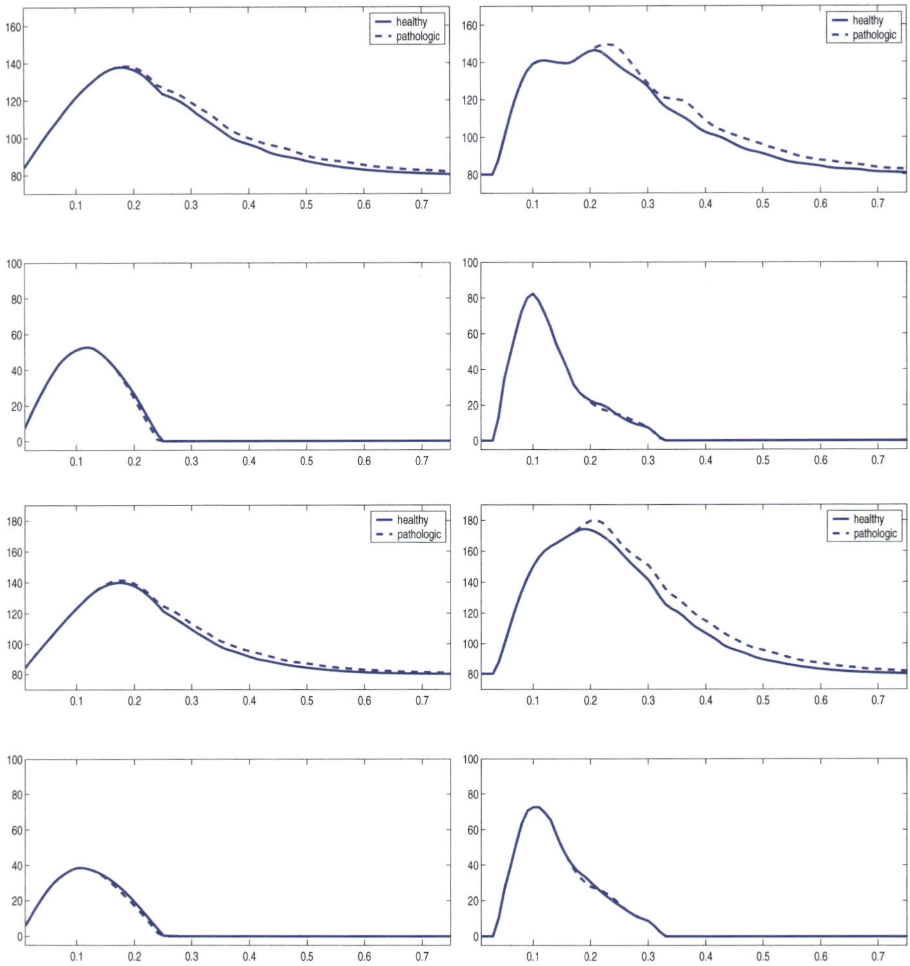

Fig. 11.11. Comparison between the results obtained with standard proximal conditions (left) and the coupling with the ventricular model (right). Values of velocity (first and third rows) and pressure (second and fourth rows) in the mid-point of the aorta are presented. We have simulated circulation in a physiologic (solid) and pathologic (dotted) test case. The pathologic case corresponds to a total occlusion of the right femoral artery. The first two rows refer to an adult patient, the other ones to an elder patient. Pictures taken from [158], reproduced with permission

11.2.3 Coupling of 3D-0D models

In our top-down approach, we have coupled the three kind of models, moving from the finest 3D down to the coarsest 0D. In some applications a sort of *shortcut modelling* can be pursued, coupling together directly 3D and 0D models. This is, for instance, the case when the wave propagation phenomena

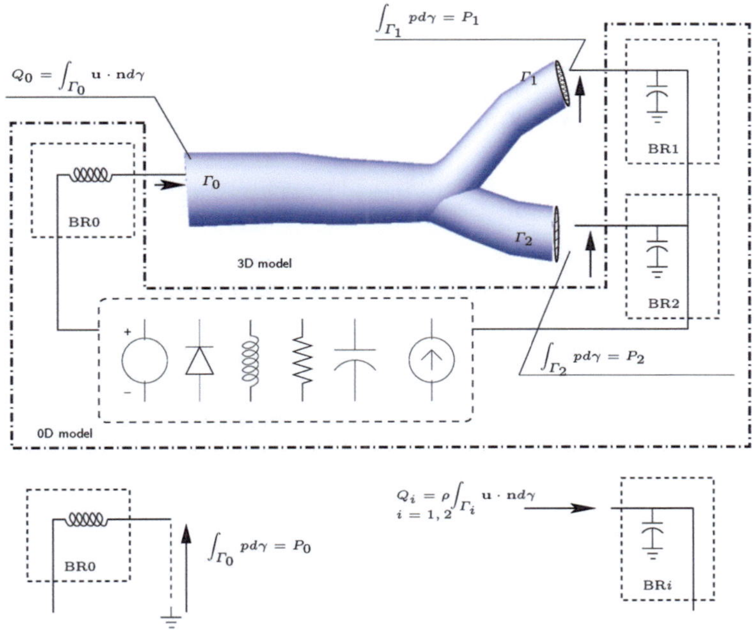

Fig. 11.12. Representation of a 3D rigid-0D geometrical multiscale model with three bridging regions (BR0, BR1, BR2). At the inlet of the 3D domain, the bridging region has the current/flow rate Q_0 as state variable. The latter is computed by the 0D model and provided to the NS model. In the other bridging regions, the voltage/pressures p_i, $i = 1, 2$, are the state variables. The 0D model is forced by the mean pressure at the interface Γ_0 and by the flow rates at Γ_1 and Γ_2

are not of interest, and a 3D simulation needs boundary conditions that could account in a precise way the dynamics of the complete vascular tree. An example of clinical relevance of this situation is given in Chapter 12.

Consider for instance the model obtained by coupling a 3D model of a region of interest and a lumped parameter model like in Fig. 11.12. Again, three model ingredients can be identified:

K model, represented by a system of ordinary differential equations in the form

$$\frac{d\mathbf{y}}{dt} + A\mathbf{y} = \mathbf{f}.$$

NS model, represented by the Navier-Stokes equations with appropriate boundary conditions on the vascular walls Γ_w;

interface conditions represented by continuity conditions.

In particular, at each interface we consider the following conditions:

[A] area: $A_{3D,i} = \text{meas}(\Gamma_i) = A_{0D,i}$;

[B] mean pressure: $\overline{p}_{3D,i} = \dfrac{1}{A_{3D,i}} \displaystyle\int_{\Gamma_i} pd\gamma = P_{0D,i}$;

[C] flow rate: $Q_{3D,i} = \rho \int_{\Gamma_i} \boldsymbol{u} \cdot \mathbf{n}_i d\gamma = Q_{0D,i}$.

As we have already pointed out for the 3D-1D coupling, condition [B] can be replaced by a condition on the normal component of the stress

[B1] $\frac{1}{A_{3D,i}} \int_{\Gamma_i} (p\mathbf{n}_i - (\nabla \mathbf{u} + \nabla \mathbf{u}^T) \cdot \mathbf{n}_i) d\gamma = P_{0D,i}$.

Possible interface conditions are therefore represented by [A], [B] and [C], or else by [A], [B1] and [C]. If the 3D model is assumed to be rigid, the three conditions are not independent and in particular [A] and [B] (or [B1]) cannot be prescribed together. Actually, in the 3D model the area at the interface is constant, while in the 0D model is not. Indeed it is related to the pressure by an algebraic law like (10.21). For this reason, typical interface conditions in the 3D rigid-0D coupling are [B] (or [B1]) and [C].

Some numerical issues

We consider the problem represented in Fig. 11.12 where the 3D model is assumed to be rigid and interface conditions [B1] and [C] are prescribed. We consider the following algorithm for the numerical coupling at each time step.

`Initialisation.` Select an initial guess for the pressure $P_0^{(0)} = P_0$ and the flow rates $Q_1^{(0)} = Q_1$ and $Q_2^{(0)} = Q_2$ at the interfaces. Typical choice is to take these quantities from the previous time step. Set the iteration index $k = 0$.

`Loop.`
1. *Solve* the 0D model by using the forcing terms $P_0^{(k)}$, $Q_1^{(k)}$ and $Q_2^{(k)}$. This step, in particular, computes the state variables of the K model $Q_0^{(k+1)}$, $P_1^{(k+1)}$ and $P_2^{(k+1)}$.
2. *Solve* the 3D model by using the boundary conditions given by $Q_0^{(k+1)}$, $P_1^{(k+1)}$ and $P_2^{(k+1)}$. Compute the average normal stress on Γ_0, $P_0^{(k+1)} = \int_{\Gamma_0} (p^{(k+1)}\mathbf{n}_0 - (\nabla \mathbf{u}^{(k+1)} + \nabla \mathbf{u}^{(k+1),T}) \cdot \mathbf{n}_0) d\gamma$ and the flow rates $Q_i^{(k+1)} = \rho \int_{\Gamma_i} \mathbf{u}^{(k+1)} \cdot \mathbf{n}_i d\gamma$, for $i = 1, 2$.

`Test.` The iteration continues up to the fulfilment of a convergence test, for instance:

$$|P_i^{(k+1)} - P_i^{(k)}| \leq \varepsilon, \qquad |Q_i^{(k+1)} - Q_i^{(k)}| \leq \varepsilon, \quad i = 0, 1, 2.$$

As done previously, several remarks are in order.

1. *Bridging region compatibility.* The compartment that stands at the interfaces with the 3D model (bridging region) has to be devised appropriately. More precisely, it should allow the calculation of the quantities required by the splitting scheme. For instance, in the example presented in Fig. 11.12

the flow rate on Γ_0 and the pressures P_1 and P_2 on Γ_1 and Γ_2, respectively, must be state variables of the lumped parameter model. As we have pointed out, this ensures well posedness of the problem solved at step 1.

2. *3D defective boundary data problems.* The K model (as well as the E model) computes averaged quantities that do not provide enough boundary data to the 3D model in step (2) of the loop. As for the coupling between 3D and 1D models, we could postulate a priori single parameter profile for the velocity or the normal stress and use the average data to set the parameter appropriately. For instance, we could "expand" average data into pointwise data in the following manner:

   Flow rate conditions $\rightarrow$ Poiseuille parabolic profile $\rightarrow$ (Standard) Dirichlet conditions (see (11.5));

   Average pressure conditions $\rightarrow$ Constant normal stress $\rightarrow$ (Standard) Neumann conditions:

$$p\mathbf{n} - \nu \nabla \boldsymbol{u} \cdot \mathbf{n} = P\mathbf{n} \tag{11.8}$$

   where P is constant over the interface.

   At which extent numerical results are affected by this arbitrary profile selection is a crucial question for the reliability of multiscale modelling. We will address this problem in the next sections.

Fig. 11.13 illustrates some numerical results with a multiscale model (2D coupled with a 0D model) with the aim of computing the flow distribution in a by-pass anastomosis for different levels of occlusions in the stenotic vessel (results taken from [402]). This distribution strongly depends on the behaviour of the whole vascular system. Consequently, the multiscale 3D-0D coupling is an appropriate numerical tool for investigating the effectiveness of the by-pass.

Remark 11.2.2 *The same algorithm for the 3D-0D coupling can be extended to the compliant case. If the 3D compliant model adopts an algebraic model for the vascular walls, no further interface conditions are needed. In the case of a differential (in space) structure model, conditions on the displacements should be prescribed. Again, as we have seen in the 3D-1D coupling, a condition on the section area is not enough for the structure problem. A workaround is to expand it into a pointwise Dirichlet condition as we have done in (11.4).*

11.2.4 Improving multiscale models

So far, we have proposed different coupled models, with some basic ideas for their numerical implementation. A mismatch of mathematical characteristics of the submodels we want to couple requires specific strategies to obtain feasible and efficient multiscale simulations. In particular, we have already outlined the role of the characteristic variables as interface conditions in the coupling of E models. They allow to formulate absorbing boundary conditions for the E model, allowing a better description of wave propagation dynamics at the interface. Another crucial issue is the role played by bridging regions in coupling with K models.

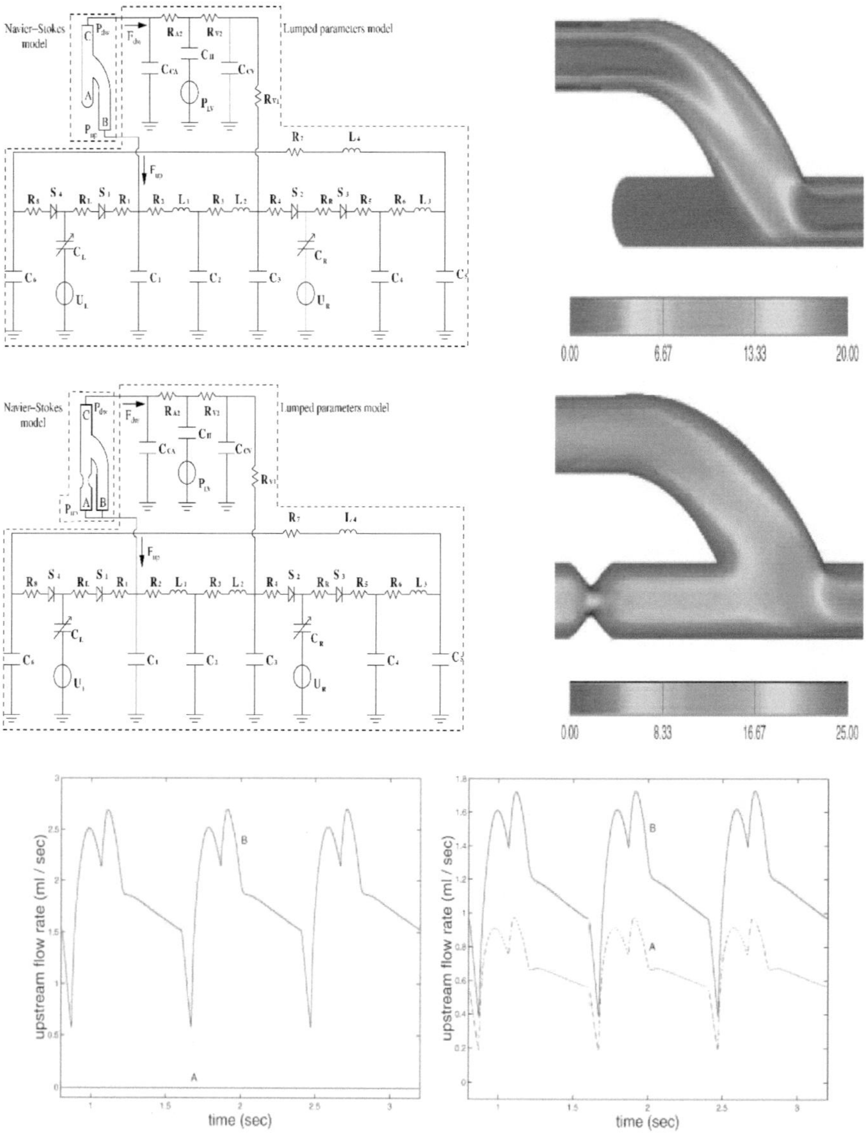

Fig. 11.13. Top: Left, multiscale problem with a completely occluded host artery and a by-pass; Right: results in the fine domain at the end of a heart beat. Centre: as in the Top line, but for a partially occluded case. Bottom: Flow division in the host artery and in the graft for the two cases. On the left, the completely occluded case. On the right, the partially occluded case. Pictures taken from [402]

There are two further issues that deserve a further investigation, for the improvements of multiscale modelling.

Average data expansion: when coupling 3D with 1D or 0D models, we need to convert average data into proper boundary conditions for a differential problem that requires "pointwise data" instead. We have proposed some practical strategies, which however introduce a level of arbitrariness in the final numerical solution. Indeed, numerical results in [342, 527] show how the prescription of an arbitrary velocity profile can sometimes induce incorrect results (and maybe lead a medical researcher to wrong conclusions). We need therefore to understand if there is an optimal approach able to reduce the impact on the final solution of the unavoidable arbitrariness. To be more precise, if we select an arbitrary parabolic profile at the inlet of a cylindrical pipe, as done in (11.5), we could expect that this choice will not affect the numerical results far away from that inlet boundary. This "entry problem" has been studied mathematically and a review of the theory and main results may be found in [181]. In practise, for steady problems and in conditions akin to that in the cardiovascular system, it is commonly accepted that the effects of the profile chosen at the inlet are no more significant after an entry length $L \approx 0.06D$ where D is the diameter of the pipe (see [542]). However, for unsteady problems it has been verified in [423] that an entry length of $40D$ may be not enough to recover the analytical (Womersley) solution from a prescription of an inlet parabolic profile. Different strategies, able to force a given flow rate *without* the prescription of a velocity profile are then necessary to improve the reliability of multiscale results.

Efficiency of coupling iterative schemes: we have presented some basic iterative schemes, resorting to the successive solution of standard subproblems. The effectiveness of this kind of schemes (in terms of number of iterations required for the convergence) can be improved for instance by introducing appropriate relaxation strategies. Convenience of such splitting schemes in comparison with non-splitting or monolithic solvers is another relevant point in devising multiscale models.

We investigate these two items in the next sections. We also discuss mathematical well posedness of multiscale models.

11.3 Defective boundary data problems

Let us consider the 3D Navier-Stokes equations (see Chapter 2):

$$\begin{aligned} &\rho\frac{\partial \boldsymbol{u}}{\partial t} + \rho\boldsymbol{u}\cdot\nabla\boldsymbol{u} - \mu\triangle\boldsymbol{u} + \nabla P = \mathbf{f}, \\ &\operatorname{div}\boldsymbol{u} = 0, \end{aligned} \tag{11.9}$$

that we assume to hold in the 3D domain Ω. The boundary $\partial\Omega$ still consists of the vascular wall Γ_w and the artificial boundaries Γ_i, with $i = 1, 2, \dots, m$. For the time being, we assume that the vessel is rigid, i.e.

$$\boldsymbol{u}|_{\Gamma_w} = \boldsymbol{0}, \tag{11.10}$$

where Γ_w denotes the part of the boundary corresponding to the vascular wall. The initial conditions

$$\boldsymbol{u}(\boldsymbol{x}, 0) = \boldsymbol{u}_0(\boldsymbol{x}) \tag{11.11}$$

are assigned.

We will consider the two kind of averaged data encountered in the previous section, namely conditions on mean velocity or flow rates and on mean pressures.

11.3.1 Flow rate problem

Consider problem given by (11.9), (11.10), (11.11), together with boundary conditions:

$$\rho \int_{\Gamma_i} \boldsymbol{u} \cdot \boldsymbol{n} \, \mathrm{d}\gamma = Q_i, \quad i = 0, 1, \dots, m,$$

where Q_i are given functions of time. In the case of a rigid domain, the incompressibility of the fluid implies the following constraint on the data:

$$\sum_{i=0}^{m} Q_i = 0.$$

To avoid dealing with this constraint we will consider a slightly different problem, namely

$$P\boldsymbol{n} - \nu \frac{\partial \boldsymbol{u}}{\partial \boldsymbol{n}} = \boldsymbol{0}, \text{ on } \Gamma_0, \qquad \rho \int_{\Gamma_i} \boldsymbol{u} \cdot \boldsymbol{n} \, \mathrm{d}\gamma = Q_i, \quad i = 1, \dots, m. \tag{11.12}$$

In the analysis of this problem, we will prove however that there is no loss of generality with these conditions.

In the sequel, for the sake of simplicity, we set $\rho = 1$.

We have already pointed out that conditions (11.12) are not enough to guarantee the existence of a solution. Three scalar conditions should be required for the well posedness of the problem, while (11.12) provides only a scalar value for each Γ_i, for $i = 1, 2, \dots m$. The approach advocated in the previous section was based on a-priori selection of a velocity profile fitting the given flow rate (see for instance [72, 151]).

This approach is in fact pretty simple, since it actually reduces the defective boundary problem to a classical Dirichlet one. Nevertheless there are several limitations. Real geometries (see e.g. Chapter 4) are typically far from being cylindrical circular and rectilinear, which are the assumptions for the Womersley and Poiseuille solutions. Moreover, a-priori selection of a profile may affect the entire numerical solution.

In general, a practical workaround is to expand the computational domain (flow extensions), so that the arbitrary velocity profile is prescribed far away from the zone of interest. The downstream section of the extension is often made circular to apply a parabolic profile. However, this technique affects the computational costs, in particular for unsteady computations where, as we have pointed out, we need a rather long extension to damp out the effects of the arbitrary choice of the velocity profile.

Different approaches that do not require arbitrary prescription of a velocity profile are therefore very helpful.

A variational approach

A strategy proposed in [218] relies on the selection of an appropriate variational formulation for the problem at hand including all the available data. Variational formulation by itself will complete the boundary data set with homogeneous natural conditions. These conditions have been called sometimes *do nothing conditions*, since they are obtained spontaneously as a result of the chosen variational formulation[5]. They are indeed less perturbing (or "invasive") on the (unknown) solution, since they are natural conditions for the chosen variational formulation.

To introduce this approach for the flow rate problem, we need some functional spaces and a specific notation. Set:

$$\widehat{\mathbf{V}}_f \equiv \left\{ \mathbf{v} \in \boldsymbol{V}_f : \int_{\Gamma_j} \mathbf{v} \cdot \boldsymbol{n} = 0, \ \forall j = 1, 2, \dots, m \right\},$$

and let us denote by $\mathbf{b}_i$, $i = 1, \dots, m$ the functions of $\boldsymbol{V}_f$ such that, for all $j = 1, \dots, m$

$$\int_{\Gamma_j} \mathbf{b}_i \cdot \boldsymbol{n} \, d\gamma = \delta_{ij}, \qquad \nabla \cdot \mathbf{b}_i = 0.$$

These functions are commonly called *flux carriers* and act as a lifting of the flow rate data. We set $\boldsymbol{u} = \widehat{\boldsymbol{u}} + \sum_{i=1}^{m} Q_i \mathbf{b}_i$. A possible variational formulation of the flow rate problem is the following: find $\widehat{\boldsymbol{u}} \in L^2(0, T, \widehat{\mathbf{V}}_f) \cap L^\infty(0, T, \mathbf{L}^2(\Omega))$

[5] This denomination is effective but also a little bit misleading, since in any case these conditions "*do something*". This is the reason why we do not adopt this name here.

and $p \in L^2(0,T,Q_f)$ such that for all $\mathbf{v} \in \widehat{\mathbf{V}}_f$ and $q \in Q_f$:

$$\begin{aligned}
&\left(\frac{\partial \widehat{\boldsymbol{u}}}{\partial t}, \mathbf{v}\right) + a(\boldsymbol{u}, \mathbf{v}) + c\left(\widehat{\mathbf{u}}, \widehat{\boldsymbol{u}}, \mathbf{v}\right) + c\left(\widehat{\mathbf{u}}, \sum_{j=1}^{m} Q_j \mathbf{b}_j, \mathbf{v}\right) + \\
&\quad c\left(\sum_{j=1}^{m} Q_j \mathbf{b}_j, \widehat{\boldsymbol{u}}, \mathbf{v}\right) + b(\mathbf{v}, p) = \\
&\qquad (\mathbf{f}, \mathbf{v}) - \sum_{j=1}^{m}\left(\left(\frac{\partial Q_j}{\partial t}\mathbf{b}_j, \mathbf{v}\right) + Q_j\, a(\mathbf{b}_j, \mathbf{v})\right) - c\left(\sum_{j=1}^{m} Q_j \mathbf{b}_j, \sum_{j=1}^{m} Q_j \mathbf{b}_j, \mathbf{v}\right), \\
&b(\widehat{\mathbf{u}}, q) = 0,
\end{aligned} \tag{11.13}$$

with $\widehat{\mathbf{u}}(\boldsymbol{x}, 0) = \boldsymbol{u}_0 - \sum_{j=1}^{m} Q_j(0)\mathbf{b}_j$.

In fact, this formulation forces some conditions implicitly, as stated by the following proposition (for the proof see [218]).

Proposition 11.3.1 *The solution of the flow problems (11.13) fulfills the following boundary conditions on Γ_i, $i = 1, \ldots m$ and for all $t > 0$,*

$$p\boldsymbol{n} - \mu \boldsymbol{\nabla} \boldsymbol{u} \cdot \boldsymbol{n} = C_i \boldsymbol{n}, \quad i = 1, \ldots, m,$$

where $C_i = C_i(t)$ are unknown functions of time.

Remark 11.3.1 *In the case of a problem with flow conditions also on Γ_0, with the constraint on the data $\sum_{i=0}^{m} Q_i = 0$, the previous proposition still holds with $C_0 = C_0(t)$ an arbitrary function of time. The case considered in (11.12) is therefore a special case where we choose $C_0 = 0$. Problem associated to conditions (11.12) is of the same type of the one with all flow boundary conditions and it does not require to force the flow rate compatibility explicitly.*

Concerning the well posedness, we have the following result, proved in [218].

Proposition 11.3.2 *Under suitable assumptions on the smoothness of the domain and the initial data, there exists a time interval in which the flow problem (11.13) is well posed. If $||\boldsymbol{\nabla} \boldsymbol{u}_0||$ and $|Q_i|$ for all i are sufficiently small the solution exists for each $t > 0$.*

This approach has *a practical drawback*. The functional space $\widehat{\mathbf{V}}_f$ is not standard. In view of the numerical approximation, the construction of finite dimensional functional subspaces of $\widehat{\mathbf{V}}_f$, as well as that of the flux carriers is rather problematic.

Different strategies have been proposed that do not suffer from these limitations even if they present other drawbacks.

Augmented formulation

A second approach, proposed in [156], considers the flux conditions as constraints for the solution, to be forced by means of Lagrange multipliers (in a way similar to the treatment of the incompressibility constraint in the mixed formulation of the Navier-Stokes). In practise, we introduce a vector function $\boldsymbol{\lambda}(t)$ and resort to the following problem: find $\mathbf{u} \in L^2(0,T,\boldsymbol{V}_f) \cap L^\infty(0,T,\mathbf{L}^2(\Omega))$, $p \in L^2(0,T,Q_f)$ and $\boldsymbol{\lambda} \in (L^2(0,T))^m$ such that for all $\mathbf{v} \in \boldsymbol{V}_f$, $q \in Q_f$:

$$
\begin{aligned}
&\left(\frac{\partial \boldsymbol{u}}{\partial t}, \mathbf{v}\right) + a(\mathbf{u},\mathbf{v}) + c(\boldsymbol{u},\boldsymbol{u},\mathbf{v}) + b(\mathbf{v},p) + \sum_{i=1}^{m} \lambda_i \int_{\Gamma_i} \mathbf{v}\cdot\boldsymbol{n}\, d\gamma = (\mathbf{f},\mathbf{v}),\\
&b(\boldsymbol{u},q) = 0,\\
&\int_{\Gamma_i} \mathbf{u}\cdot\boldsymbol{n}\, d\gamma = Q_i \qquad i = 1,2,\ldots m,
\end{aligned}
\tag{11.14}
$$

Well posedness of this augmented formulation can be proven by means of classical arguments (see [195]). In particular, moving from the well posedness result of Prop. 11.3.2, it can be shown that an inf-sup condition holds for the augmented problem, leading to the following result (see [526]).

Proposition 11.3.3 *Under the same assumptions of Proposition 11.3.2, the augmented formulation (11.14) is well posed.*

Moreover, the investigation of the boundary conditions forced in the augmented formulation so that the problem has a unique solution highlights the physical significance of the Lagrange multiplier. We have in fact the following Proposition (for the proof see [156]).

Proposition 11.3.4 *The solution of problem (11.14) fulfils the following conditions on the artificial boundaries Γ_i, $i = 1,2,\ldots,m$ and for $t > 0$,*

$$
P\boldsymbol{n} - \mu\boldsymbol{\nabla}\boldsymbol{u}\cdot\boldsymbol{n} = \lambda_i\boldsymbol{n}. \tag{11.15}
$$

In other words, the Lagrange multipliers λ_i do coincide with the functions C_i and play the role of normal stresses on the artificial boundaries.

The augmented formulation is based on standard functional spaces, whose finite dimensional approximations are readily built (and present in most of the commercial packages). However the indefinite saddle point nature of the associated problem needs a specific analysis. Discretisation of (11.14) leads indeed to an algebraic problem that in general is not practical to solve in a monolithic way, i.e. with the simultaneous computation of $\boldsymbol{u}$, P and λ_i.

On the one hand the resulting linear system is in general ill conditioned, on the other hand problem (11.14) is not standard, since it deals with velocity, pressure and the Lagrange multipliers at the same time. Therefore, the use of existing software packages is complex, if not impossible, in this setting.

These remarks suggest to split apart the computation of the fluid dynamics quantities ($\boldsymbol{u}/P$) from that of the λ_i, yielding the so-called *segregated methods.* In this perspective, some numerical methods have been proposed in [156,526, 528] to this aim. We limit ourselves to consider algebraic splittings of the matrix obtained after discretisation/linearisation of the problem at hand at each time step. This system reads $\mathrm{A}\mathbf{y} = \mathbf{c}$, with

$$\mathrm{A} = \begin{bmatrix} \mathrm{C} & \mathrm{D}^T & \mathrm{L}^T \\ \mathrm{D} & \mathbf{0} & \mathbf{0} \\ \mathrm{L} & \mathbf{0} & \mathbf{0} \end{bmatrix}, \qquad \mathbf{c} = \begin{bmatrix} \mathbf{b} \\ \mathbf{0} \\ \mathbf{q} \end{bmatrix}, \tag{11.16}$$

and represents the discrete counterpart of (11.14). Matrix L corresponds to the discretisation of the boundary integrals on Γ_i, D is the discretisation of the divergence operator and C is the result of the discretisation and linearisation of $\left(\frac{\partial \boldsymbol{u}}{\partial t}, \mathbf{v}\right) + a(\mathbf{u}, \mathbf{v}) + c\,(\boldsymbol{u}, \boldsymbol{u}, \mathbf{v})$. Correspondingly, $\mathbf{y} = [\mathbf{U}, \mathbf{P}, \boldsymbol{\Lambda}]^T$, contains the nodal values of the unknowns of velocity, pressure and Lagrange multipliers respectively. Finally $\mathbf{b}$ derives from the discretisation of source terms in the momentum equation, and the entries of vector $\mathbf{q}$ are the prescribed flow rates Q_i. Using the notation

$$\mathcal{C} = \begin{bmatrix} \mathrm{C} & \mathrm{D}^T \\ \mathrm{D} & \mathbf{0} \end{bmatrix}, \qquad \mathcal{L} = [\mathrm{L}, \mathbf{0}].$$

matrix A can be rewritten in the form:

$$\mathrm{A} = \begin{bmatrix} \mathcal{C} & \mathcal{L}^T \\ \mathcal{L} & \mathbf{0} \end{bmatrix}.$$

Correspondingly, we set $\mathbf{x}_1 = [\mathbf{U},\ \mathbf{P}]^T$ and $\mathbf{x}_2 = \boldsymbol{\Lambda}$, $\mathbf{f}_1 = [\mathbf{b}, \mathbf{0}]^T$ and $\mathbf{f}_2 = \mathbf{q}$.

A possible way for splitting velocity/pressure and multipliers computations is based on the following classical block LU factorisation:

$$\begin{bmatrix} \mathcal{C} & \mathcal{L}^T \\ \mathcal{L} & \mathbf{0} \end{bmatrix} = \begin{bmatrix} \mathcal{C} & \mathbf{0} \\ \mathcal{L} & -\mathcal{L}\mathcal{C}^{-1}\mathcal{L}^T \end{bmatrix} \begin{bmatrix} I & \mathcal{C}^{-1}\mathcal{L}^T \\ \mathbf{0} & I \end{bmatrix},$$

which yields the following three-step algorithm

$$\begin{aligned} &1)\ \mathcal{C}\widehat{\mathbf{x}}_1 = \mathbf{f}_1, \\ &2)\ \mathcal{L}\mathcal{C}^{-1}\mathcal{L}^T\mathbf{x}_2 = \mathcal{L}\widehat{\mathbf{x}}_1 - \mathbf{f}_2, \\ &3)\ \mathcal{C}\mathbf{x}_1 = \mathbf{f}_1 - \mathcal{L}^T\mathbf{x}_2. \end{aligned}$$

We can observe that:

a) steps (1) and (3) require to solve a system in $\mathcal{C}$, i.e. a standard Navier-Stokes problem (see [526]);

b) step (2) consists of solving a problem governed by the $m \times m$ matrix $\mathcal{L}\mathcal{C}^{-1}\mathcal{L}^T$, being m the number of artificial sections where the flow rate is assigned. This is typically a small number in haemodynamics problems (≤ 5). Therefore, a small number of GMRES iterations is in general enough to reach convergence. However, the explicit computation of this matrix is not convenient, since $\mathcal{C}$ is large and sparse and its inversion is expensive and memory consuming due to the well known phenomenon of fill-in. However, iterative methods can avoid the explicit calculation of the matrix, since they only need the application of the current matrix to a vector. This can be done in the following way ($\mathbf{v}, \mathbf{r}, \mathbf{z}$ and $\mathbf{w}$ are vectors of proper dimensions)

$$\mathbf{r} = \mathcal{L}\mathcal{C}^{-1}\mathcal{L}^T\mathbf{v} \Rightarrow \begin{cases} \mathbf{z} = \mathcal{L}^T\mathbf{v}, \\ \mathbf{w} = \mathcal{C}^{-1}\mathbf{z} \Rightarrow \mathcal{C}\mathbf{w} = \mathbf{z}, \\ \mathbf{r} = \mathcal{L}\mathbf{w}. \end{cases}$$

The second step on the right hand side requires again to solve a standard Navier-Stokes problem;

c) step (3) can be rewritten in the form:

$$\mathbf{x}_1 = \mathcal{C}^{-1}\mathbf{f}_1 - \mathcal{C}^{-1}\mathcal{L}^T\mathbf{x}_2 = \widehat{\mathbf{x}}_1 - \mathbf{w}$$

where vector $\mathbf{w} = \mathcal{C}^{-1}\mathcal{L}^T\mathbf{x}_2$ is a by-product of the last iteration of step (2), so this step requires a simple vector sum.

This approach can still be computationally expensive, because of the numerous Navier-Stokes solves involved. The cost is particularly high for unsteady problems, since the algorithm must be applied at each time step. For this reason, some specific techniques for computing an approximate solution to $A\mathbf{y} = \mathbf{c}$ have been devised, like the one in [527] that guarantees that the error introduced is confined in a small neighbourhood of the sections where flow rate are prescribed. In Fig. 11.14 we present an example of solution in a realistic geometrical model of a carotid bifurcation. The heuristic approach based on the prescription of an inlet velocity parabolic profile and a constant pressure profile at the outlet of the internal carotid (on the left) yields a different solution of the velocity field computed than that obtained with the Lagrange multiplier approach (centre). The solution computed by the inexact approach [527] (on the right) is very similar to the Lagrange multiplier one, yet it requires about half of the computational time.

Control approach

Finally, we address a different approach that is in some sense "dual" to the Lagrange multiplier strategy. While in the Lagrangian approach the flow rate boundary conditions are regarded as constraints to the Navier-Stokes equations in the new approach the latter play the role of *state equations*. They act

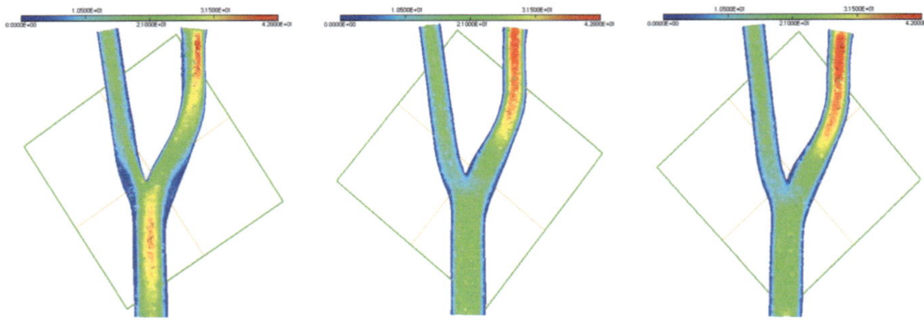

Fig. 11.14. Computations in a 3D carotid bifurcation (the square identifies the cutting plane). Velocity field obtained with the prescription of an inlet parabolic profile (left), the augmented Lagrangian scheme (centre), the inexact approach of [527] (right)

as "constraints" to minimisation of a functional which enforces the desired boundary conditions.

Clearly, for this to work we need to make Navier-Stokes problem function of some parameters, called *control variables*, over which the minimum is sought. The defective boundary problem in this way is formulated as a *control problem* (see e.g. [210]).

For the sake of simplicity, we introduce this approach for the case of the steady Stokes problem. The extension to the unsteady Navier-Stokes problem can be found in [163].

Let us consider the following functional associated with flux conditions (11.12)

$$J_Q : \boldsymbol{V}_f \to \mathbb{R}^+, \quad J_Q(\mathbf{w}) = \frac{1}{2}\sum_{i=1}^{m}\left(\int_{\Gamma_i} \mathbf{w}\cdot \boldsymbol{n} d\gamma - Q_i\right)^2. \tag{11.17}$$

We can formulate the defective boundary problem as follows: minimise $J_Q(\boldsymbol{u}(\mathbf{k}))$ where $\boldsymbol{u}(\mathbf{k})$ is subject to the constraint

$$\begin{aligned}
&-\mu\triangle\boldsymbol{u}(\mathbf{k}) + \nabla P = \mathbf{f}, && \text{in } \Omega\\
&\nabla\cdot\boldsymbol{u}(\mathbf{k}) = 0, && \text{in } \Omega\\
&\boldsymbol{u}(\mathbf{k}) = \mathbf{0}, && \text{on } \Gamma\\
&-P\boldsymbol{n} + \mu\nabla\boldsymbol{u}(\mathbf{k})\cdot\boldsymbol{n} = \mathbf{0}, && \text{on } \Gamma_0\\
&-P\boldsymbol{n} + \mu\nabla\boldsymbol{u}(\mathbf{k})\cdot\boldsymbol{n} = -k_i\boldsymbol{n} && \text{on } \Gamma_i\, i = 1,\ldots,m.
\end{aligned} \tag{11.18}$$

Here, $\mathbf{f} \in \mathbf{L^2(\Omega)}$ is given and the control variables is the vector $\boldsymbol{k}$ whose elements $k_i \in \mathbb{R}$ are the normal components of the stress on the artificial boundaries. In other words, we look for the values of k_i such that the solution of (11.18) minimises J_Q.

To this aim, following e.g. [210], we introduce the constrained functional:

$$\mathcal{L}(\mathbf{w}, s; \boldsymbol{\lambda}_{\mathbf{w}}, \lambda_s; \boldsymbol{\eta}) = J_Q(\mathbf{w}) + \mu(\nabla \mathbf{w}, \nabla \boldsymbol{\lambda}_w) + \\ b(s, \nabla \cdot \boldsymbol{\lambda}_w) + \sum_{i=1}^{m} \int_{\Gamma_i} \eta_i \boldsymbol{\lambda}_w \cdot \boldsymbol{n}\, d\gamma - (\mathbf{f}, \boldsymbol{\lambda}_w) - (\lambda_s, \nabla \cdot \mathbf{w}).$$

Here $\boldsymbol{\lambda}_{\mathbf{w}}$ and λ_s are the so-called *adjoint* variables associated with $\mathbf{w}$ and s respectively. Solution is sought by looking for stationary points of $\mathcal{L}$. This turns to be equivalent to solve the following problem[6], where for the sake of brevity we omit to specify that the differentials are computed in $[\mathbf{u}, \mathbf{p}; \boldsymbol{\lambda}_{\mathbf{u}}, \lambda_{\mathbf{p}}; \mathbf{k}]$, while we put into evidence the dependence on the control variables.

Given $\mathbf{f} \in \mathbf{L^2(\Omega)}$ and $\mathbf{Q} \in \mathbb{R}^{\mathbf{m}}$, find $\boldsymbol{u}(\mathbf{k}) \in \mathbf{V}, \mathbf{p}(\mathbf{k}) \in \mathbf{L^2(\Omega)}$, $\boldsymbol{\lambda}_{\boldsymbol{u}} \in \mathbf{V}, \lambda_p \in L^2(\Omega)$ and $\mathbf{k} \in \mathbb{R}^m$, such that, for all $\mathbf{v} \in \mathbf{V}$, $q \in L^2(\Omega)$ and $\nu \in \mathbb{R}$:

$$(P) \quad \langle d\mathcal{L}_{\boldsymbol{\lambda}_{\mathbf{w}}}, \mathbf{v}\rangle = \mu(\nabla \mathbf{u}, \nabla \mathbf{v}) + b(p, \nabla \cdot \mathbf{v}) + \\ \sum_{i=1}^{m} \int_{\Gamma_i} k_i \mathbf{v} \cdot \mathbf{n}\, d\gamma - (\mathbf{f}, \mathbf{v}) = 0,$$

$$\begin{cases} \langle d\mathcal{L}_{\mathbf{u}}, \mathbf{v}\rangle = \mu(\nabla \mathbf{v}, \nabla \boldsymbol{\lambda}_{\boldsymbol{u}}) + b(\lambda_p, \nabla \cdot \mathbf{v}) - \\ (A) \quad \displaystyle\sum_{i=1}^{m} \Big(\int_{\Gamma_i} \boldsymbol{u} \cdot \mathbf{n}\, d\gamma - Q_i\Big) \int_{\Gamma_i} \mathbf{v} \cdot \mathbf{n}\, d\gamma = 0, \\ \langle d\mathcal{L}_s, q\rangle = b(q, \nabla \cdot \boldsymbol{\lambda}_{\boldsymbol{u}}) = 0, \end{cases}$$

$$(C_j) \quad \langle d\mathcal{L}_{\eta_j}, \nu\rangle = \int_{\Gamma_j} \nu \boldsymbol{\lambda}_{\boldsymbol{u}} \cdot \mathbf{n}\, d\gamma = 0, \quad j = 1, \ldots, m.$$

Here, $\langle d\mathcal{L}_{\mathbf{u}}, \mathbf{v}\rangle$ indicates the Gateaux differential with respect to $\boldsymbol{u}$ applied to $\boldsymbol{v}$.

This system couples a steady Stokes problem (P), its adjoint (A) and m scalar equations (*optimality conditions*, denoted by (C_j)). Observe that the last condition forces the adjoint variable $\boldsymbol{\lambda}_{\boldsymbol{u}}$ to have a null flux on the artificial boundaries. Well posedness of this problem can be proven by resorting to fixed point arguments (see [163]).

The numerical solution of this problem is not a trivial task. A possible approach is to resort to the *steepest descent method* applied to the minimisation of the functional at hand. For more details see [163].

In Fig. 11.15 we report the computation for the same case of Fig. 11.14, solved with the control approach. The differences with the solution computed with the Lagrange multiplier approach, reported in the figure on the right, are below the discretisation errors. The computational cost of this approach

---

[6] Rigorously speaking, the problem is obtained by forcing the Gateaux differentials of $\mathcal{L}$ evaluated along the direction of any test function to vanish in correspondence of the solution $[\mathbf{u}, \mathbf{p}; \boldsymbol{\lambda}_{\mathbf{u}}, \lambda_{\mathbf{p}}; \mathbf{k}]$ (see [210]).

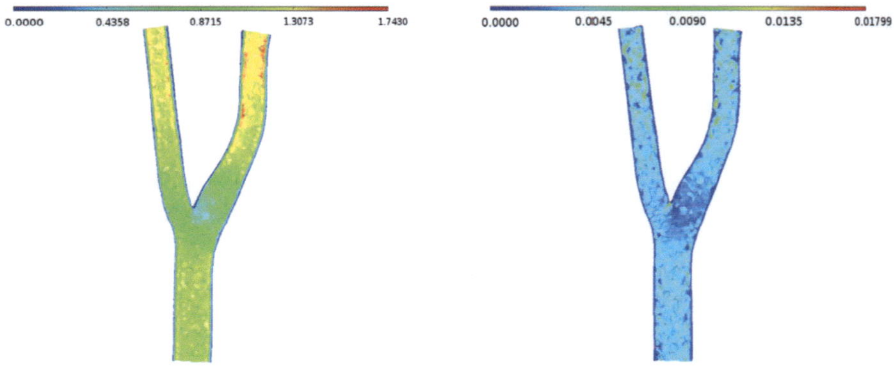

Fig. 11.15. Control approach applied to a flow rate problem in a 3D carotid bifurcation. On the left, the solution obtained by solving the minimisation problem. On the right, plot of the differences with the solution obtained by the Lagrange multiplier approach. The differences are below the discretisation error

can be made comparable with that of the augmented formulation (solved by the splitting scheme) thanks to a proper selection of the iterative solver (see [163]) for the sequence of problems (P), (A) and (C_j). The control approach is however more versatile, as we will illustrate when considering the mean pressure problems.

11.3.2 Mean pressure problem

Let us consider now the following problem: look for $(\boldsymbol{u}, p)$ such that equation (11.9) is satisfied with conditions (11.10) and (11.11) and

$$\int_{\Gamma_i} p d\gamma = P_i, \quad i = 0, 1, \ldots, m, \tag{11.19}$$

where P_i are given functions of time. As for flow rate problem, conditions (11.19) are not enough and some further information need to be prescribed to obtain a well posed problem. Let us illustrate some approaches that aim at completing these conditions in a mathematically sound way.

Again, we will introduce a simple variational approach at first, then we will consider a possible Lagrange multiplier formulation. Both approaches are affected by some important drawbacks that the formulation based on control approach overcomes.

A variational approach

In [218] the following variational formulation of the mean pressure problem is proposed: given $P_i(t)$, $i = 1, 2, \ldots m$, find $(\boldsymbol{u}, P) \in L^2(0, T; \mathbf{H}^1(\Omega)) \times$

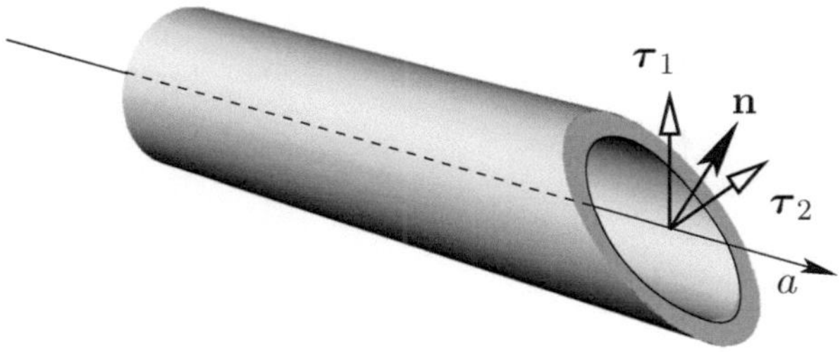

Fig. 11.16. A domain where variational formulation (11.20) for the mean pressure problem is not exact. τ_1 and τ_2 are the directions orthogonal to the axis a and $\mathbf{n}$ is the unit vector orthogonal to the artificial boundary

$L^2(0,T;L^2(\Omega))$ such that for all $\mathbf{v} \in \mathbf{H}^1(\Omega)$ and $q \in L^2(\Omega)$

$$\begin{aligned} &\left(\frac{\partial \boldsymbol{u}}{\partial t}, \mathbf{v}\right) + a(\boldsymbol{u}, \mathbf{v}) + c\,(\boldsymbol{u}, \boldsymbol{u}, \mathbf{v}) + b(\mathbf{v}, p) = (\mathbf{f}, \mathbf{v}) - \sum_{j=1}^{m} P_j \int_{\Gamma_j} \mathbf{v} \cdot \mathbf{n} d\gamma, \\ &b(\mathbf{u}, q) = 0, \end{aligned} \tag{11.20}$$

with $\boldsymbol{u}(\boldsymbol{x}, 0) = \boldsymbol{u}_0(\boldsymbol{x})$.

The boundary conditions added implicitly by this formulation are identified in the following Proposition (see [218]).

Proposition 11.3.5 *Any smooth solution of (11.20) fulfils the following boundary conditions on the artificial boundaries Γ_i, $i = 0, 1, 2, \ldots m$ and for $t > 0$*

$$P\mathbf{n} - \nu \nabla \mathbf{u} \cdot \mathbf{n} = P_i \mathbf{n}. \tag{11.21}$$

In practise, formulation (11.20) forces the mean pressure data by imposing it as a constant normal stress on the artificial boundaries. This is indeed the expected solution in special domains, like a cylindrical rectilinear pipe where Γ_i is normal to the axis. Here, the analytical solution of the mean pressure problem may be computed and satisfies (11.21).

For a generic domain, however, this technique may force a too strong condition, which does not correspond to what is physically expected. This is for instance the case of a rectilinear cylindrical domain with Γ_i oblique to its axis (see Fig. 11.16). Here, we would like the mean pressure problem to reproduce the Poiseulle flow (in steady situations) or the Womersley solution (in a pulsatile flow), which however in this case do not satisfy (11.21). We should therefore consider different approaches.

Augmented formulation

An augmented formulation for pressure drop problems still stems from regarding mean pressure data as constraints for the Navier-Stokes solution, leading to the problem: find $\mathbf{u} \in L^2(0,T,\boldsymbol{V}_f) \cap L^\infty(0,T,\mathbf{L}^2(\Omega))$, $p \in L^2(0,T,Q_f)$ and $\boldsymbol{\lambda} \in (L^2(0,T))^m$ such that for all $\mathbf{v} \in \boldsymbol{V}_f$, $q \in Q_f$:

$$\left(\frac{\partial \boldsymbol{u}}{\partial t}, \mathbf{v}\right) + a(\mathbf{u},\mathbf{v}) + c(\boldsymbol{u},\boldsymbol{u},\mathbf{v}) + b(\mathbf{v},p) + \sum_{i=1}^m \frac{1}{\Gamma_i}\int_{\Gamma_i} P d\gamma = (\mathbf{f},\mathbf{v}),$$
$$b(\boldsymbol{u},q) + \sum_{j=0}^m \lambda_j \int_{\Gamma_j} q d\gamma = 0, \tag{11.22}$$
$$\frac{1}{|\Gamma_i|}\int_{\Gamma_i} P d\gamma = P_i \qquad i = 1,2,\dots m.$$

Unfortunately, this problem is not well posed. Indeed, it is possible to verify (see [155]) that the conditions forced implicitly by this formulation are

$$\boldsymbol{u}(\mathbf{x},t)\cdot\mathbf{n} = \lambda_i(t) \qquad \text{on} \quad \Gamma_i.$$

In general, since λ_i are non zero constants in space, the latter conditions are incompatible with the fact that $\boldsymbol{u} = \mathbf{0}$ on Γ_w. The discontinuity on $\overline{\Gamma}_i \cap \overline{\Gamma}_w$ leads to a value of the velocity on the boundary which cannot represent a trace for $\mathbf{H}^1(\Omega)$, the natural functional space where we seek the velocity solution of our flow problem. Indeed, the augmented formulation is appropriate in the case where only a slip condition (i.e $\boldsymbol{u}\cdot\boldsymbol{n} = 0$) is imposed on Γ_w, a situation which however is not physical for a Navier-Stokes problem.

For this reason, the augmented formulation for mean pressure drop problems is not investigated any further.

Control approach

The approach based on control theory presented for the flow rate problems can be straightforwardly extended to the mean pressure problem. With this aim, we introduce the following functional

$$J_P(s) = \frac{1}{2}\Big(\sum_{i=0}^m \frac{1}{|\Gamma_i|}\int_{\Gamma_i} s\, d\gamma - P_i\Big)^2 \tag{11.23}$$

and, as for the flow rate conditions, we consider a constrained minimisation problem. Again, we assume that Navier-Stokes equations play the role of constraint for the solution minimising (11.23). As control variables we still assume the constant normal stresses $\mathbf{k} = [k_i]$. It is worth remarking that this is not the only possibility, since other choices for the control variables can be pursued, such as flow rates (see [163]).

Still referring to steady Stokes equations for the sake of simplicity, we introduce the following Lagrange functional:

$$\mathcal{L}(\mathbf{w}, s; \boldsymbol{\lambda}_w, \lambda_s; \boldsymbol{\eta}) = J_P(s) + a(\mathbf{w}, \boldsymbol{\lambda}_w) + d(s, \boldsymbol{\lambda}_w)$$
$$+ \sum_{i=0}^m \int_{\Gamma_i} \eta_i \boldsymbol{\lambda}_w \cdot \mathbf{n}\, d\gamma - (\mathbf{f}, \boldsymbol{\lambda}_w) + d(\lambda_s, \mathbf{w}).$$

A stationary point of $\mathcal{L}$ satisfies the following problem: given $\mathbf{f} \in \mathbf{L}^2(\Omega)$ and $P_j \in \mathbb{R}$, $j = 0, \ldots, m$, find $\mathbf{k} \in \mathbb{R}^m$, $\mathbf{u}(\mathbf{k}) \in \mathbf{V}_{div}, p(\mathbf{k}) \in H^1(\Omega), \boldsymbol{\lambda}_u \in \mathbf{V}_{div}$ and $\lambda_p \in H^1(\Omega)$, such that, for all $\mathbf{v} \in \mathbf{V}_{div}$, $q \in H^1(\Omega)$ and $\nu \in \mathbb{R}$,

$$(P)\begin{cases} \langle d\mathcal{L}_{\boldsymbol{\lambda}_u}, \mathbf{v}\rangle = a(\mathbf{u}, \mathbf{v}) + d(p, \mathbf{v}) + \displaystyle\sum_{i=0}^{m} \int_{\Gamma_i} k_i \mathbf{v} \cdot \mathbf{n}\, \mathbf{d}\gamma - (\mathbf{f}, \mathbf{v}) = \mathbf{0}, \\ \langle d\mathcal{L}_{\lambda_p}, q\rangle = d(q, \mathbf{u}) = \mathbf{0}, \end{cases}$$

$$(A)\begin{cases} \langle d\mathcal{L}_{\mathbf{u}}, \mathbf{v}\rangle = a(\mathbf{v}, \boldsymbol{\lambda}_{\mathbf{u}}) + d(\lambda_p, \mathbf{v}) = 0, \\ \langle d\mathcal{L}_p, q\rangle = \displaystyle\sum_{i=0}^{m} \Big(\frac{1}{|\Gamma_i|} \int_{\Gamma_i} p\, d\gamma - P_i\Big) \frac{1}{|\Gamma_i|} \int_{\Gamma_i} q\, d\gamma + d(q, \lambda_{\mathbf{u}}) = \mathbf{0}, \end{cases}$$

$$(C_j) \quad \langle d\mathcal{L}_{k_i}, \nu\rangle = \int_{\Gamma_i} \nu \lambda_{\mathbf{u}} \cdot \mathbf{n}\, \mathbf{d}\gamma = \mathbf{0}, \quad \mathbf{i} = \mathbf{0}, \ldots, \mathbf{m}.$$

One of the most interesting features of this approach is that functional to be minimised can be adjusted for including some possible a priori information on the behaviour of the solution on artificial boundaries. For instance, for a boundary of a pipe non orthogonal to the axis (see Fig. 11.16), where formulation (11.20) fails, the functional to be minimised can be adapted in order to include the physical evidence of the prevalent axial direction of the flow. We resort in this case to the functional

$$\mathcal{L}(\mathbf{w}, s; \boldsymbol{\lambda}_w, \lambda_s; \boldsymbol{\eta}) = J_P(s) + a(\mathbf{w}, \boldsymbol{\lambda}_w) + d(s, \boldsymbol{\lambda}_w)$$
$$+ \sum_{i=0}^{m} \int_{\Gamma_i} \eta_i \boldsymbol{\lambda}_w \cdot \mathbf{n}\, d\gamma - (\mathbf{f}, \boldsymbol{\lambda}_w) + d(\lambda_s, \mathbf{w}) + \mathcal{S}(\mathbf{w}, \boldsymbol{\tau}_1, \ldots, \boldsymbol{\tau}_m) \quad (11.24)$$

where in a problem with d space dimensions

$$\mathcal{S}(\mathbf{w}, \boldsymbol{\tau}_1, \ldots, \boldsymbol{\tau}_m) = \frac{1}{2} \sum_{l=1}^{d-1} \sum_{i=0}^{m} \int_{\Gamma_i} |\mathbf{w} \cdot \boldsymbol{\tau}_l|^2\, d\gamma, \quad (11.25)$$

and τ_l are the orthogonal directions to the pipe axis a, which in this case do not coincide with the tangential directions to the boundary Γ_i. The term $\mathcal{S}$ forces the velocity components orthogonal to a to be small. With a proper choice of control variables, this procedure yields good numerical results.

For instance, suppose to prescribe a mean pressure $\int_{\Gamma} p d\gamma = P = 1\,\mathrm{g}/(\mathrm{s}^2\,\mathrm{cm})$ at the outlet Γ_{out} of the domain T (see Fig. 11.17 top). Boundary Γ_{out} is supposed to be an artificial boundary in a pipe where a Poiseuille flow holds, so that vertical velocity is zero.

By minimising functional (11.23), an undesirable vertical velocity at the outlet occurs (Fig. 11.17, centre) while this is not anymore the case when using the penalised functional (11.24) with (11.25) and the complete stress (normal and tangential) as control variables. Fig. 11.17, bottom, show that the latter strategy is able to strongly reduce the wrong tangential velocities.

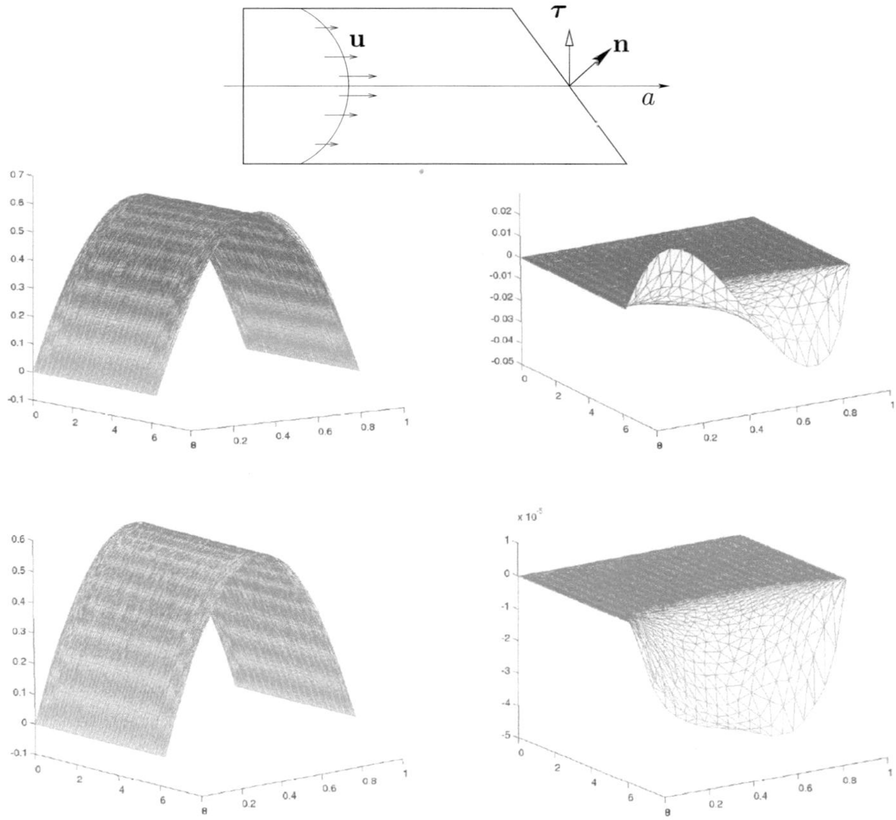

Fig. 11.17. Simulations in a 2D pipe with an oblique boundary: in the centre axial and normal velocity components by solving a mean pressure problem with the minimisation of (11.23). On the bottom the same problem solved by minimising (11.25): the velocity component along $\boldsymbol{\tau}$ is strongly reduced (maximum value in the last figure is 10^{-5})

Remark 11.3.2 *As previously pointed out, different variational formulations lead to different boundary conditions. For instance, if we exploit the vector identity* $\nabla(1/2|\mathbf{u}|^2) = \mathbf{u}\cdot(\nabla\mathbf{u})^T$, *momentum equations can be equivalently reformulated*

$$\frac{\partial \boldsymbol{u}}{\partial t} + \boldsymbol{u}\cdot\nabla\boldsymbol{u} - \boldsymbol{u}\cdot(\nabla\mathbf{u})^T - \nu\triangle\boldsymbol{u} = -\nabla\left(P + \frac{1}{2}|\boldsymbol{u}|^2\right).$$

Variational formulations associated to this form lead to natural conditions where the total pressure $P + \frac{1}{2}|\boldsymbol{u}|^2$ *replaces the pressure* P. *This form of the momentum equations is therefore well suited for defective boundary conditions on the total pressure. Other strong formulations of the momentum equations well suited for other kinds of boundary conditions are considered in [32].*

11.3.3 Defective boundary problems: the compliant case

When describing a compliant domain, different models for the vessel mechanics could be considered, as discussed in Chapter 3. Models which do not involve a differential operator for the space variables, like the algebraic laws considered in Chapter 10 do not need boundary conditions for the wall problem. Models which exhibit second order differential operators in space, on the contrary, require boundary conditions on the artificial boundaries that typically either prescribe the position **d** or the normal stresses (see Chapter 3). In this case, defective problems occur also for the structure problem and a complete analysis is still missing. Here, we limit ourselves to some basic remarks.

Possible approaches are suggested by the strategies presented in the rigid case. For instance, let us assume that a boundary condition is prescribed on the *area* of the i–th artificial section

$$\int_{\Gamma_i(\mathbf{d})} d\gamma = A_i(t). \tag{11.26}$$

This condition can come from coupling a 3D compliant model with a 1D model or can be inferred by measurements. It is clear that (11.26) can be regarded in general as an *average* condition for the vascular wall position. As a matter of fact, assume that the interface Γ_i is planar and the z-axis is aligned along its normal. Then, we may write

$$\boldsymbol{d}(x,y,z,t) = \begin{cases} \sqrt{x^2(t)+y(t)^2} = R_i(\theta,t), \\ z = z_i, \end{cases}$$

where $\theta = \tan^{-1}(y/x)$. In this case, condition (11.26) provides

$$\int_0^{2\pi}\int_0^{R(\theta,t)} \rho d\rho d\theta = A_i(t). \tag{11.27}$$

As done in Section 11.2 (eq. (11.4)), we can pursue a heuristic approach similar to the one for flow rates. The latter was essentially based on the a-priori selection of a velocity profile, so that condition (11.27) can be fulfilled by arbitrarily selecting a profile for $R_i(\theta,t)$. In particular, assumption of a circular shape implies to take R_i independent of θ. In this way, (11.27) reduces to

$$\pi R_i^2(t) = A_i(t) \Rightarrow R_i(t) = \sqrt{\frac{A_i(t)}{\pi}}.$$

More in general, one can set $R_i(t,\theta) = C_i(t)R_0(\theta)$ where $C_i(t)$ is selected in such a way that:

$$C_i^2(t)\int_0^{2\pi} \frac{R_0^2(\theta)}{2} d\theta = A_i(t).$$

In practise, this amounts to assume that boundary area evolves according to a homothety of the reference area described by $R_0(\theta)$ (see [52]).

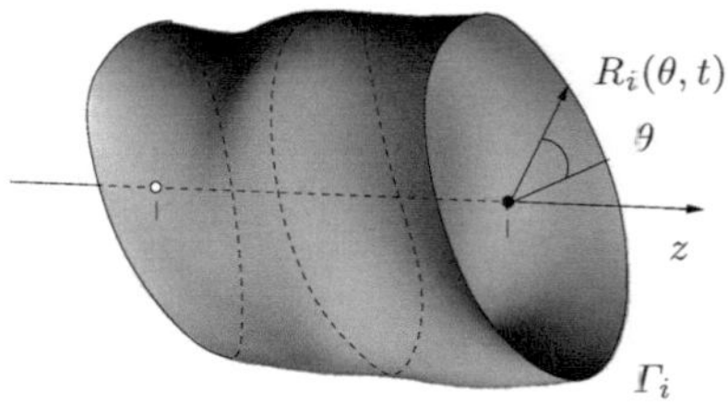

Fig. 11.18. "Artificial" section of a compliant domain

As for the case of flow rate conditions, this strategy upgrades defective data for the displacement to classical Dirichlet conditions and actually requires low computational costs. This is an important feature in particular for fluid-structure interaction problems which are usually computationally very expensive.

However, different mathematically sound approaches can still be pursued. Control approach can be extended to the compliant case, by including conditions on structure in the functional to be minimised. For instance, pressure and area conditions in the form

$$\int_{\Gamma_i} P da = P_i, \qquad \int_{\mathbf{x}\in\Gamma_i(\boldsymbol{d})} d\gamma = A_i \tag{11.28}$$

can be faced by resorting to the minimisation of

$$\mathcal{J}_{p,A} = \frac{1}{2}\left(\int_{\Gamma_i} P da - P_i\right)^2 + \left(\int_{\mathbf{x}\in\Gamma_i(\boldsymbol{d})} d\gamma - A_i\right)^2$$

with the constraint given by fluid-structure equations.

Another possible approach refers to the augmented formulation. In [352] an augmented formulation for a compliant 3D model is considered with flow rate boundary conditions. Since no data were available for the structure, homogeneous natural conditions have been introduced. In Fig. 11.19 we report the

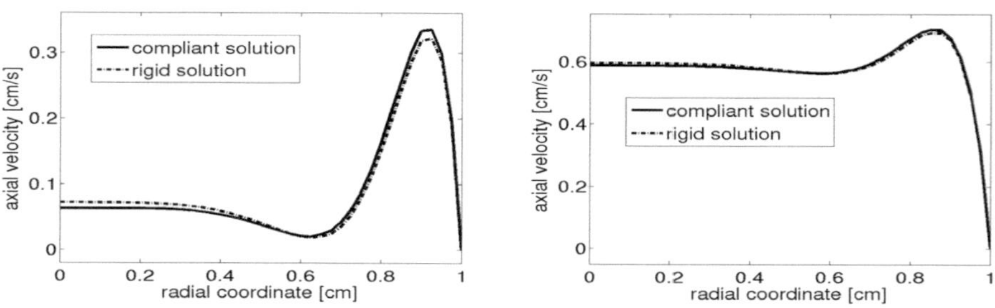

Fig. 11.19. Comparison between the inlet profiles in a rigid and compliant simulation. The results are obtained by prescribing the sinusoidal in time flow rates with a Lagrange multiplier approach [352]

velocity profile computed with this approach at the inlet of a compliant vessel, compared to the solution of the corresponding rigid case. The solution is axial-symmetric, so that only half profile is reported.

11.4 Some well posedness results

In this section we recall some theoretical results on multiscale models. We illustrate in particular some stability properties concerning the coupling of 3D and 1D models. Then we will present a general well posedness analysis of 3D/0D models and its extension to the 1D/0D case.

11.4.1 Coupling of 3D and 1D models

Referring to Fig. 11.20, let us consider a $3D-1D$ coupling, where for the sake of simplicity we assume that the interface between the models is normal to the z axis. The $3D$ model is given by

$$\begin{aligned} &\frac{\partial \boldsymbol{u}}{\partial t} + \left(\frac{1}{2}\nabla|\boldsymbol{u}|^2 + (\nabla \times \boldsymbol{u}) \times \boldsymbol{u}\right) - \nabla \cdot (2\nu \mathbf{D}(\boldsymbol{u})) + \nabla P = \mathbf{f} \quad \mathbf{x} \in \Omega_f, t > 0, \\ &\nabla \cdot \boldsymbol{u} = 0 \qquad \mathbf{x} \in \Omega_f, t > 0, \\ &\rho_w \frac{\partial^2 \eta_r}{\partial t^2} + \sigma \eta_r = \Phi_r - \Phi_{ext} \quad \mathbf{x} \in \Gamma_w, t > 0, \end{aligned} \tag{11.29}$$

where ρ_w is the wall density, η_r is the radial displacement, while we assume that axial and circumferential displacements are null, and $\Phi_r - \Phi_{ext}$ is the difference of stresses in the radial direction induced by the fluid and the external organs. Observe that the structure is modelled by the *independent rings model* (structure is considered as a stack of independent slices or rings), while the convective term of the fluid problem has been rearranged in order to have natural conditions associated with the total pressure (see Remark 11.3.2). System is completed by the initial conditions $\eta_r(\mathbf{x}, 0) = \eta_0$, $\dfrac{\partial \eta_r}{\partial t}(\mathbf{x}, 0) = u_r$ for $\mathbf{x} \in \Gamma_w$

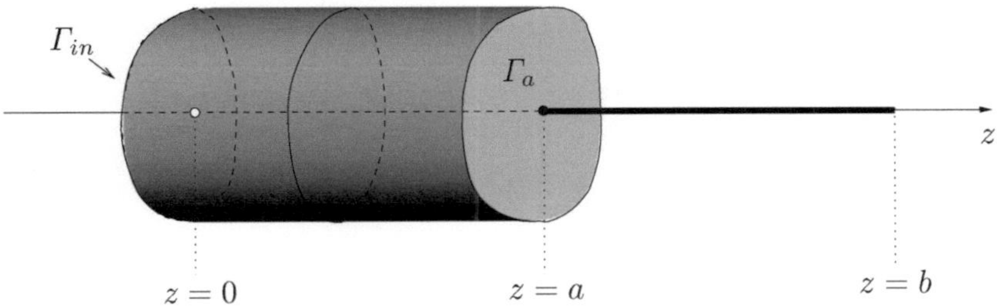

Fig. 11.20. Domain for the coupled 3D/1D problem

and $\boldsymbol{u}(\mathbf{x},0) = \boldsymbol{u}_0$ for $\mathbf{x} \in \Omega$. At the inlet Γ_{in} of the 3D domain we can assume both Dirichlet and Neumann conditions for the Navier-Stokes equations.

For $z \in (a,b)$ we assume the 1D model to satisfy equations (10.27) that we report here for completeness

$$\frac{\partial A}{\partial t} + \frac{\partial Q}{\partial x} = 0,$$

$$\frac{\partial Q}{\partial t} + \frac{\partial}{\partial x}\left(\alpha \frac{Q^2}{A}\right) + \frac{A}{\rho}\left(\frac{\partial p}{\partial x}\right) + K_R \frac{Q}{A} = 0.$$

We assume also that area and pressure are related by the algebraic law (see Section 10.1.1)

$$P - P_{ext} = \psi(A, A_0, \beta) = \beta \frac{\sqrt{A} - \sqrt{A_0}}{A_0}.$$

On $z = b$ we assume absorbing boundary conditions, while in $z = a$ we set

$$\begin{aligned} &\left(\left(P + \frac{1}{2}|\boldsymbol{u}|^2\right)\mathbf{I} - 2\nu \mathbf{D}(\boldsymbol{u})\right) \cdot \boldsymbol{n} = P_{1D} + \frac{1}{2}|\overline{u}_{1D}|^2, \\ &\int\limits_{\Gamma_f} \boldsymbol{u} \cdot \boldsymbol{n} d\gamma = Q_{1D}. \end{aligned} \tag{11.30}$$

To the 3D model we associate the following energy functional

$$\mathcal{E}_{3D} = \frac{1}{2}||\boldsymbol{u}||^2_{L^2(\Omega_f(t))} + \frac{\rho_w}{2}||\frac{\partial \eta_r}{\partial t}||^2_{L^2(\Gamma_{w,0})} + \frac{b}{2}||\eta_r||^2_{L^2(\Gamma_{w,0})}$$

where $\Omega_f(t)$ is the fluid domain at time t while $\Gamma_{w,0}$ is the reference structure domain, which here reduces to the wall boundary of $\Omega_f(0)$. For the 1D model, we select the following energy

$$\mathcal{E}_{1D} = \frac{1}{2}\int_a^b \frac{Q^2}{A} dz + \int_a^b \int_{A_0}^A \psi(\tau, A_0, \beta) d\tau dz.$$

We have then (see [159]) the following Proposition.

Proposition 11.4.1

1. *If homogeneous Dirichlet conditions for the velocity are prescribed on Γ_{in}, the following (*energy decay property*) holds*

$$\mathcal{E}_{3D}(t) + \nu \int_0^t ||\mathbf{D}(\boldsymbol{u})||^2_{L^2} dt + \mathcal{E}_{1D}(t) K_r \int_0^t \int_a^b \frac{Q^2}{A^2} dz dt \leq \mathcal{E}_{3D}(0) + \mathcal{E}_{1D}(0).$$

2. If non homogeneous Neumann conditions for the fluid are prescribed on Γ_{in} with data $\mathbf{g}$*, we have (*energy estimate*)*

$$\mathcal{E}_{3D}(t) + \nu \int_0^t ||\mathbf{D}(\boldsymbol{u})||^2_{L^2} dt + \mathcal{E}_{1D}(t) K_r \int_0^t \int_a^b \frac{Q^2}{A^2} dz dt \leq$$

$$\left(\mathcal{E}_{3D}(0) + \mathcal{E}_{1D}(0) + C \int_0^t ||\mathbf{g}||^2_{L^2(\Gamma_in)} \right) e^{2\nu t}.$$

Remark 11.4.1 *The previous results can be extended to more complex domains with many interfaces between 3D and 1D models. As a matter of fact, they can be applied locally at each interface.*

11.4.2 Coupling of 3D and 0D models

We consider now the multiscale 3D/0D depicted in Fig. 11.18. In particular we make the following basic assumptions.

1. The NS model is given in terms of classical primitive variable formulation of Navier-Stokes equations. We assume that initial data and forcing terms are small enough, for the sake of well-posedness of the problem (see [218]).
2. Nonlinear terms of K model (introduced by the modelling of valves and of the heart action) are described by suitable smooth functions (see Chapter 10).

This coupled problem can be analysed by a fixed point strategy represented in Fig. 11.21. Precisely, we regard the solution as the fixed point of an operator $\mathcal{T}$ given by the sequence of NS and K problems (denoted respectively as $\mathcal{P}_{NS}$ and $\mathcal{P}_K$). Setting $\mathcal{T} = \mathcal{P}_K \cdot \mathcal{P}_{NS}$ the solution to the coupled multiscale problem satisfies

$$\overline{\mathbf{s}} = \mathcal{T}\overline{\mathbf{s}} = \mathcal{P}_K \cdot \mathcal{P}_{NS}\overline{\mathbf{s}}.$$

In this framework, we add two further assumptions.

3. The splitting into subproblems $\mathcal{P}_{NS}$ and $\mathcal{P}_K$ represented in Fig. 11.21 is bridging region compatible. With reference to Fig. 11.18, the role of interface variables in the splitting is given in Table 11.1.
4. Defective boundary problem $\mathcal{P}_{NS}$ is formulated in terms of variational formulations following the variational approach advocated in Section 11.3.

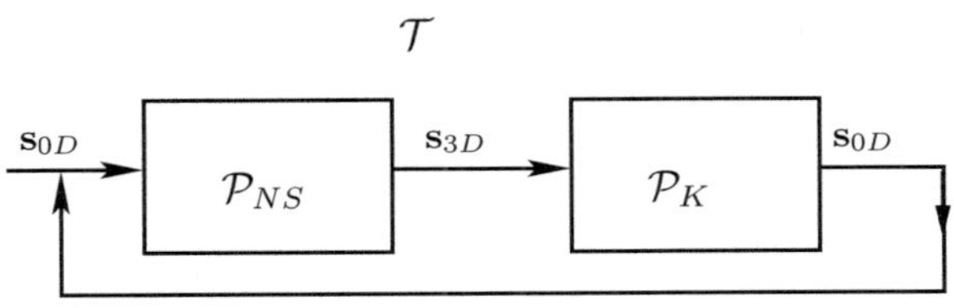

Fig. 11.21. Splitting/fixed point reformulation of multiscale model of Fig. 11.18

Table 11.1. Role of matching data in a bridging region compatible splitting for multiscale model depicted in Fig. 11.12

	Input $\mathcal{P}_{NS}$ = *Output* $\mathcal{P}_K$	*Input* $\mathcal{P}_K$ = *Output* $\mathcal{P}_{NS}$
Γ_0	pressure P_0	flow rate Q_0
Γ_1	flow rate Q_1	pressure P_1
Γ_2	flow rate Q_2	pressure P_2

More precisely, let $\widehat{\mathbf{V}}_f$ denote the space

$$\widehat{\mathbf{V}}_f \equiv \left\{ \mathbf{v} \in \boldsymbol{V}_f : \int_{\Gamma_0} \mathbf{v} \cdot \boldsymbol{n} = 0 \right\},$$

and $\mathbf{b}_0$ a function of $\boldsymbol{V}_f$ such that $\displaystyle\int_{\Gamma_0} \mathbf{b}_0 \cdot \boldsymbol{n}\, d\gamma = 1$. Set $\boldsymbol{u} = \widehat{\boldsymbol{u}} + Q_0 \mathbf{b}_0$. The following variational formulation holds. Find $\widehat{\boldsymbol{u}} \in L^2(0,T,\widehat{\mathbf{V}}_f) \cap L^\infty(0,T,\mathbf{L}^2(\Omega))$ and $p \in L^2(0,T,Q_f)$ such that for all $\mathbf{v} \in \widehat{\mathbf{V}}_f$ and $q \in Q_f$:

$$\begin{aligned}
&\left(\frac{\partial \widehat{\boldsymbol{u}}}{\partial t}, \mathbf{v}\right) + a(\boldsymbol{u}, \mathbf{v}) + c\,(\widehat{\boldsymbol{u}}, \widehat{\boldsymbol{u}}, \mathbf{v}) + c\,(\widehat{\boldsymbol{u}}, Q_0\mathbf{b}_0, \mathbf{v}) + c\,(Q_0\mathbf{b}_0, \widehat{\boldsymbol{u}}, \mathbf{v}) + \\
&b(\mathbf{v}, p) = (\mathbf{f}, \mathbf{v}) - \left(\frac{\partial Q_0}{\partial t}\mathbf{b}_0, \mathbf{v}\right) + Q_0\; a(\mathbf{b}_0, \mathbf{v}) - c\,(Q_0\mathbf{b}_0, Q_0\mathbf{b}_0, \mathbf{v}) - \\
&P_1 \int_{\Gamma_1} \mathbf{v} \cdot \boldsymbol{n}\, d\gamma - P_2 \int_{\Gamma_2} \mathbf{v} \cdot \boldsymbol{n}\, d\gamma, \\
&b(\widehat{\mathbf{u}}, q) = 0,
\end{aligned} \tag{11.31}$$

with $\widehat{\mathbf{u}}(\boldsymbol{x}, 0) = \boldsymbol{u}_0 - Q_0(0)\mathbf{b}_0$.

By collecting classical results of calculus and results proven in [218], [121], we have that:

1. **NS Problem:** If initial and forcing data are small enough, $\mathcal{P}_{NS}$ is well posed.
2. **K Problem:** DAE system of $\mathcal{P}_K$ is of index 1 and can be reformulated as a well posed Cauchy problem.
3. **Multiscale:** There exists $T^\star > 0$ such that $\mathcal{T}$ is *compact* in $(0, T^\star]$. This means that the application of $\mathcal{T}$ to bounded sequences of arguments yields *convergent* sequences in appropriate topologies (for a more precise definition of compactness see e.g. [556]).

The latter step actually proves the existence of a fixed point, thanks to the classical *Schauder's fixed point theorem* (see [409]).

11.4.3 Coupling of 1D and 0D models

Following a similar outline as for the 3D-0D coupling, in [147] the coupling between 1D and 0D models is investigated. It is assumed that the 1D model is represented in terms of characteristic variables $\mathbf{W}$ and that the DAE system of lumped parameters model is reduced to an ordinary differential system, so that the coupled model reads

$$\begin{aligned} &\frac{\partial \mathbf{W}}{\partial t} + \begin{bmatrix} \mu(W_1, W_2) & 0 \\ 0 & \lambda(W_1, W_2) \end{bmatrix} \frac{\partial \mathbf{W}}{\partial x} = 0, \qquad \text{in} \quad \mathbb{R}^+ \times [0, T], \\ &\frac{d\mathbf{y}}{dt} = \mathcal{G}(\mathbf{y}, t) + \mathbf{f} \qquad \text{in} \quad [0, T]. \end{aligned} \tag{11.32}$$

System (11.32) is completed by initial conditions $\mathbf{w}(x, 0) = \mathbf{w}_0(x)$, $\mathbf{y}(x, 0) = \mathbf{y}_0(x)$ and the matching conditions:

$$W_1(a, t) = g(\mathbf{y}, W_2), \mathbf{f} = \mathbf{f}(\mathbf{W}),$$

where $x = a$ is the interface between the two submodels, g is a suitable function relating the characteristic variable W_1 with the entry of the state vector $\mathbf{y}$ associated with the interface condition, for instance the interface pressure, and correspondingly forcing term $\mathbf{f}$ would depend on the interface flow rate $Q = Q(\mathbf{W})$.

Results obtained for the 3D/0D coupling can be strengthened in the case of 1D/0D problems. In fact the analysis can be carried out again by reformulating this problem in a fixed point framework. Let $\mathcal{P}_K$ be the operator corresponding to solve the lumped parameter model for a given flow rate Q at the interfaces and $\mathcal{P}_E$ be the operator corresponding to solve 1D model for given pressure interfaces and to compute the associated interface flow rates. Then the problem at hand can be reformulated as the search of the fixed point for the operator:

$$\mathcal{T} = \mathcal{P}_E \cdot \mathcal{P}_K.$$

Under mild assumptions on the regularity of the initial data and on λ and μ it is possible to prove that:

1. $\mathcal{P}_K$ is well posed for $0 < t \leq T_0$ with $T_0 \leq T$;
2. $\mathcal{P}_E$ is well posed for $0 < t \leq T_1$ with $T_1 \leq T$;
3. $\mathcal{T}$ is a *contraction* in $0 < t \leq \hat{T} \leq \min(T_0, T_1)$, i.e.

$$||\mathcal{T}(Q_1) - \mathcal{T}(Q_2)||_{C^0[0,\hat{T}]} \leq K||u_1 - u_2||_{C^0[0,\hat{T}]}$$

with $K < 1$, being Q_1 and Q_2 two interfaces flow rates properly selected.

The latter inequality is stronger than the compactness proved for the corresponding operator in the 3D/0D. In particular, well known *Banach contraction theorem* (see e.g. [556]) proves in this case that the solution to the coupled problem exists and it is unique.

Recent results on the coupled problem stating the existence of local and global classical solutions under assumptions on the data may be found in [435–437].

11.5 Numerical techniques for the coupling

We here consider possible numerical techniques for the coupled problems. In particular we will distinguish between monolithic solvers where the coupled problem is treated as a whole and substructuring-type solvers. In the latter, the solution is sought by an iterative procedure where each model is computed in sequence. Monolithic solvers avoid the problem of setting up a fast convergent sequence of iterates. Yet, they may be more difficult to implement and sometimes give rise to badly conditioned problems. Substructuring procedures, on the other hand, may allow to use existing software already developed for solving subproblems separately.

11.5.1 Monolithic solvers

Let us start by considering the case of a 3D-0D coupled problem where K models describe terminal vessels, as we have done in Section 10.1.5. More precisely, we assume that the presence of terminal vessels is described in the frequency domain by means of an appropriate impedance function $\zeta_i(\omega)$ for $i = 1, 2, \dots, m$ (see Chapter 10) to be coupled to the 3D problem at the m distal boundaries of the latter. On the proximal boundaries of the NS problem we assume for the sake of simplicity that boundary data (pressure or flow rates) are given, for instance by measurements (see Fig. 11.22, where $m = 2$).

If $\pi_i(\omega)$ and $\chi_i(\omega)$ represent the Fourier transform of the interface pressures $P_i(t)$ and flow rates $Q_i(t)$ respectively, the 0D model would provide a relation in the frequency domain of the type

$$\pi_i(\omega) = \zeta_i(\omega)\chi_i(\omega),$$

which, transformed back to the time domain gives

$$P_i(t) = \frac{1}{T}\int_{t-T}^{t} Z_i(t-\tau)Q_i(\tau)d\tau. \tag{11.33}$$

Here Z_i is the inverse Fourier transform of ζ_i and T is the heart beat period. Conditions (11.33) cannot be regarded as mean pressure boundary conditions,

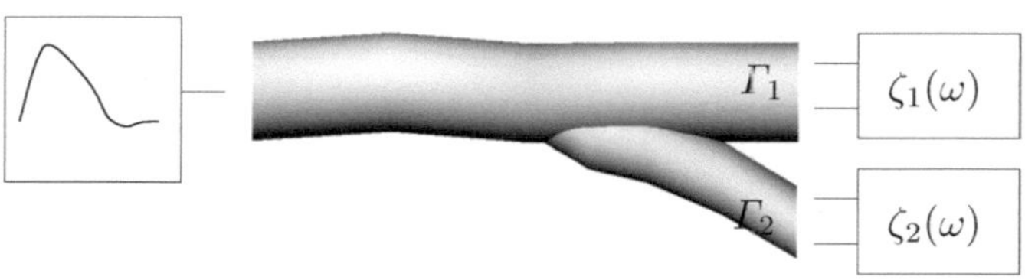

Fig. 11.22. 3D/0D coupling with K models described by impedance functions ζ_1 and ζ_2 in the frequency domain. Here lumped parameters model have the role of describing terminal vessels (see Section 10.1.5)

since the pressure is given as a function of the (unknown) flow rate. However, we can recast (11.33) in the variational formulation of the 3D NS problem in a way similar to the one pursued for the variational formulation of the mean pressure problem (see (11.20)). We set (for $j = 1, \ldots, m$)

$$\int_{\Gamma_j} (P\boldsymbol{n} - \nu \mathbf{D}(\boldsymbol{u}) \cdot \boldsymbol{n}) \cdot \mathbf{v} d\gamma = P_j \int_{\Gamma_j} \boldsymbol{n} \cdot \mathbf{v} d\gamma.$$

In this way, a variational formulation of the 3D/0D coupled problem reads:

$$\left(\frac{\partial \boldsymbol{u}}{\partial t}, \mathbf{v}\right) + a(\boldsymbol{u}, \mathbf{v}) + c\,(\boldsymbol{u}, \boldsymbol{u}, \mathbf{v}) + b(\mathbf{v}, p) + \sum_{j=1}^{m} T_j^{0D} = (\mathbf{f}, \mathbf{v}), \qquad (11.34)$$

$$b(\mathbf{u}, q) = 0,$$

where

$$T_j^{0D} = \frac{1}{T} \int\limits_{t-T}^{t} Z_j(t-\tau) \int_{\Gamma_j} \boldsymbol{u}(\tau) \cdot \mathbf{n} d\tau \int_{\Gamma_j} \mathbf{v} \cdot \mathbf{n} d\gamma. \qquad (11.35)$$

In practise, we obtain special Robin boundary conditions for the Navier-Stokes problem.

Discretisation of this problem can be carried out by means of methods addressed in Chapter 2. For instance, if space discretisation is based on the finite element method and time discretisation on finite differences, then velocity field at time t^n is represented as

$$\boldsymbol{u}_h(\boldsymbol{x}, t^n) = \sum_i \mathbf{U}_i^n \boldsymbol{\varphi}_i(\boldsymbol{x})$$

being $\boldsymbol{\varphi}_k$ the Lagrangian basis functions of the finite element space and $\mathbf{U}_k^n$ the nodal values vector. The term on the right hand side of (11.35) can be discretised in time by resorting to classical quadrature formulae. If the quadrature nodes do coincide with time levels, we have simply

$$\frac{1}{T} \int\limits_{t^{n+1}-T}^{t^{n+1}} Z_j(t^{n+1}-\tau) \int_{\Gamma_j} \boldsymbol{u}(\tau) \cdot \mathbf{n} d\tau \int_{\Gamma_j} \mathbf{v} \cdot \mathbf{n} d\gamma \approx$$

$$\frac{1}{T} \left(\sum_{k=\underline{k}}^{\overline{k}} w_k Z_j(t^{n+1} - t^k) \int_{\Gamma_j} \varphi_j \cdot \mathbf{n} \sum_l \int_{\Gamma_j} \varphi_l \cdot \mathbf{n} \right) \mathbf{U}_j^l,$$

where w_k are the quadrature weights and the quadrature nodes are such that $T - t^{n+1} \leq t^{\underline{k}} \leq t^{\underline{k}+1} \leq \ldots \leq t^{\overline{k}-1} \leq t^{\overline{k}} \leq t^n$.

Remark 11.5.1 *In the oversimplified case of a purely resistive impedance function $Z_j(t) = R_j T \delta(t)$, being δ the Dirac generalised function, and we have*

$$T_j^{0D} = R_j \int_{\Gamma_j} \boldsymbol{u}(t) \cdot \mathbf{n} d\gamma \int_{\Gamma_j} \mathbf{v} \cdot \mathbf{n} d\gamma.$$

This approach has been adopted for instance in [531] where the relevance of an appropriate impedance function is clearly shown by numerical results.

An algebraic formulation

Thus far, we have considered a monolithic formulation of a coupled 3D/0D problem in which however the primal role of K models was to provide boundary conditions which could well represent the general behaviour of the vascular tree external to the 3D model. In particular, blood dynamics in terminal vessels is computed only as far as it influences the 3D solution at the interfaces.

Let us consider now a different approach in which one is interested also to the evolution of the state variables in the lumped parameter model. We assume therefore to describe 0D problems in the time domain as a system of ordinary differential equations.

For the sake of clarity we will consider an example, namely the multiscale problem represented in Fig. 11.23, where the K model is given by a network featuring a capacitance C, three resistances and three inductors. The forcing term in the network is given by a voltage/pressure generator where $P_p(t)$ is a given function. The NS model is given by Navier-Stokes equations and bridging region compatibility requires that flow rate is prescribed at the boundaries of 3D domain. A model for the compliance of the wall can be included as well. For the sake of simplicity however we assume that the pipe is rigid, so that flow rate at inflow must equal that at outflow. Equations associated to the K model are

$$\begin{aligned} L\frac{dQ}{dt} + RQ + P &= P_p - P_1 + P_2, \\ C\frac{dP}{dt} - Q &= 0, \end{aligned} \tag{11.36}$$

where $L = L_1 + L_2 + L_3$ and $R = R_1 + R_2 + R_3$, P is the pressure jump associated with the capacitance C, P_1 and P_2 are computed by the 3D model, and Q is the flow rate in the circuit.

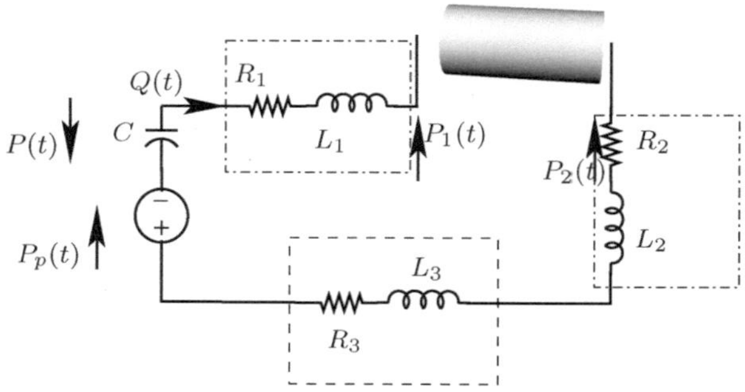

Fig. 11.23. An example of 3D/0D geometrical multiscale model

Assume that both 3D and 0D problems have been properly discretised in time, and the 3D problem also in space, linearised when required. Since the considerations we are going to make are rather general and apply to other couplings like the 3D/1D or the 1D/0D, we indicate with the suffix f the "fine" model (in this case NS) and with c the "coarse" model (here the K model). We also assume that we are using a multistep time advancing scheme for both models, with number of steps p_f+1 and p_c+1, respectively. At each time step we have to solve a linear system in the form

$$\begin{bmatrix} \mathcal{A}_{cc} & \mathcal{A}_{cf} \\ \mathcal{A}_{fc} & \mathcal{A}_{ff} \end{bmatrix} \begin{bmatrix} \mathbf{s}_c^{n+1} \\ \mathbf{s}_f^{n+1} \end{bmatrix} = \begin{bmatrix} \mathbf{b}_c^{n+1} \\ \mathbf{b}_f^{n+1} \end{bmatrix} + \begin{bmatrix} \mathbf{g}_c(\mathbf{s}_c^n, \mathbf{s}_c^{n-1}, \ldots, \mathbf{s}_c^{n-p_c}) \\ \mathbf{g}_f(\mathbf{s}_f^n, \mathbf{s}_f^{n-1}, \ldots, \mathbf{s}_f^{n-p_f}) \end{bmatrix}. \qquad (11.37)$$

Vectors $\mathbf{g}_c$ and $\mathbf{g}_f$ account for the terms due to the time advancing schemes in the two submodels, that depend on the solution $\mathbf{s}$ at the previous time steps. Let us denote by N_u and N_p the number of degrees of freedom for velocity and pressure in the fine (NS) model. Suppose moreover to solve the flow boundary problem by means of a Lagrange multiplier approach, so that $\mathbf{s}_f \in \mathbb{R}^{N_u+N_p+1}$ is here given by $\mathbf{s}_f = [\mathbf{U},\ \mathbf{P},\ \lambda]$, while the vector of the unknowns of the coarse model is formed by the state variables of the network, namely $\mathbf{s}_c = [Q,\ P]$. Finally, suppose to use an implicit Euler time discretisation for both the fine and the coarse models ($p_c = p_f = 0$). From (11.36) we have therefore:

$$\mathcal{A}_{cc} = \begin{bmatrix} \frac{1}{\Delta t}L + R & 1 \\ -1 & C \end{bmatrix}, \quad \mathcal{A}_{ff} = \begin{bmatrix} \frac{1}{\Delta t}\mathrm{M} + \mathrm{K} & D^T & \Lambda \\ \mathrm{D} & \mathbf{0} & \mathbf{0} \\ \Lambda^T & \mathbf{0} & \mathbf{0} \end{bmatrix},$$

where M is the mass matrix, K is the discretisation of the diffusion-convection operator of the momentum equation and D is the discretisation of the divergence operator in the NS problem, while the discretisation of the term related to the Lagrange multiplier has been denoted here by Λ.

Once pressure in 3D model is computed for a given flow rate, mean pressures P_1 and P_2 at the interfaces are usually computed by means of quadrature formulae

$$P_k = |\Gamma_k|^{-1} \int_{\Gamma_k} P d\gamma \approx |\Gamma_k|^{-1} \sum_i w_{i,k} p(x_i, y_i, z_i) \qquad k = 1, 2.$$

It is practically convenient to assume that quadrature nodes x_i, y_i, z_i on Γ_k do coincide with nodes of the space discretisation of the problem[7]. We may

[7] In general quadrature nodes will not correspond to grid nodes and interpolation procedures will be necessary.

finally write (see also (11.14)):

$$\mathcal{A}_{cf} = \begin{bmatrix} \mathbf{0}_{1\times N_u} & a_{cf} & 0 \\ \mathbf{0}_{1\times N_u} & \mathbf{0}_{1\times N_p} & 0 \end{bmatrix}, \quad a_{fc,i} = \begin{cases} 0 & \text{if } (x_i, y_i, z_i) \notin \Gamma_{1,2} \\ w_{i,k} & \text{if } (x_i, y_i, z_i) \in \Gamma_{1,2} \end{cases},$$

$$\mathcal{A}_{fc} = \begin{bmatrix} \mathbf{0}_{N_u\times 1} & \mathbf{0}_{N_u\times 1} \\ \mathbf{0}_{N_p\times 1} & \mathbf{0}_{N_p\times 1} \\ -1 & 0 \end{bmatrix},$$

and

$$\mathbf{b}_c^{n+1} = \begin{bmatrix} P_P(t^{n+1}) \\ 0 \end{bmatrix}, \mathbf{b}_f^{n+1} = \begin{bmatrix} \mathbf{F}^{n+1} \\ 0 \\ 0 \end{bmatrix}, \mathbf{g}_c = \begin{bmatrix} \frac{1}{\Delta t} LQ^n \\ 0 \end{bmatrix}, \mathbf{g}_f = \begin{bmatrix} \frac{1}{\Delta t} M\mathbf{U}^n \\ 0 \\ 0 \end{bmatrix}.$$

A possible solution strategy is to solve the complete system (11.37) as a whole at each time step. As already pointed out, also for simple cases as for the example at hand, this approach can have the drawback of a badly conditioned matrix. An alternative approach is a Schur complement decomposition of the problem. By a formal elimination of the coarse solution $\mathbf{s}_c^{n+1}$, we obtain

$$\left(\mathcal{A}_{ff} - \mathcal{A}_{fc}\mathcal{A}_{cc}^{-1}\mathcal{A}_{cf}\right)\mathbf{s}_f^{n+1} = \mathbf{b}_f^{n+1} + \mathbf{g}_2(\mathbf{s}_f^n) - \mathcal{A}_{fc}\mathcal{A}_{cc}^{-1}\left(\mathbf{b}_c^{n+1} + \mathbf{g}_c(\mathbf{s}_c^n)\right). \tag{11.38}$$

In general, matrix $\mathcal{A}_{cc}^{-1}$ is not available and appropriate techniques of solution are required (see the next section). However, in the simplest coarse models like the one at hand, matrix $\mathcal{A}_{cc}^{-1}$ can be easily computed

$$\mathcal{A}_{cc}^{-1} = \frac{1}{(\Delta t^{-1}L + R) + 1}\begin{bmatrix} C & -1 \\ 1 & \Delta t^{-1}L + R \end{bmatrix}, \tag{11.39}$$

and problem can be solved by (11.38). In fact, by a simple algebraic argument, the Schur complement can be explicitly computed

$$\mathcal{A}_{ff} - \mathcal{A}_{fc}\mathcal{A}_{cc}^{-1}\mathcal{A}_{cf} = \begin{bmatrix} \frac{1}{\Delta t}M + K & D & r \\ D^T & \mathbf{0} & \mathbf{0} \\ r^T & -\frac{\Delta t C}{L + \Delta t(R+1)}a_{cf} & \mathbf{0} \end{bmatrix}. \tag{11.40}$$

System (11.38) can be therefore solved, yielding the fine solution $\mathbf{s}_f^{n+1}$. Coarse solution is then recovered by solving

$$\mathbf{s}_c^{n+1} = \mathcal{A}_{cc}^{-1}\left(\mathbf{b}_c^{n+1} + \mathbf{g}_c(\mathbf{s}_c^n) - \mathcal{A}_{cf}\mathbf{s}_f^{n+1}\right).$$

In this way, the coupled problem is split into a sequence of 3D and 0D problems, each of them being in general smaller and better conditioned than the whole heterogeneous system.

11.5.2 Iterative substructuring approaches

The block Gauss elimination procedure proposed in the previous section is seldom feasible, since in general matrix $\mathcal{A}_{cc}^{-1}$ is neither easy nor convenient to compute explicitly. For this reason, here we address some possible solution schemes resorting to the separate computing of the submodels that do not need the explicit computation of $\mathcal{A}_{cc}^{-1}$.

A first, simple method for solving the problem is the following iterative scheme.

1. Let $\mathbf{s}_{f,0}^{n+1}$ be a time extrapolation of $\mathbf{s}_f^{n+1}$ based on the previous time evaluations of $\mathbf{s}_f$.
2. For $k = 0, 1, 2, \ldots$ solve

$$\begin{cases} \mathcal{A}_{cc}\mathbf{s}_{c,k+1}^{n+1} = \mathbf{b}_c^{n+1} + \mathbf{g}_c(\mathbf{s}_c^n, \ldots, \mathbf{s}_c^{n-p_c}) - \mathcal{A}_{cf}\mathbf{s}_{f,k}^{n+1} \\ \mathcal{A}_{ff}\mathbf{s}_{f,k+1}^{n+1} = \mathbf{b}_f^{n+1} + \mathbf{g}_f(\mathbf{s}_f^n, \ldots, \mathbf{s}_c^{n-f_f}) - \mathcal{A}_{fc}\mathbf{s}_{c,k+1}^{n+1} \end{cases} \tag{11.41}$$

   up to the fulfillment of an appropriate convergence test.

Observe how this splitting approach is essentially based on the same fixed point formulation devised for the proof of well posedness of multiscale problems.

The first issue is the *convergence* of the iterations. This problem can be analysed by regarding this scheme as a *block Gauss-Seidel* scheme for solving system (11.37), or, equivalently, as a Richardson preconditioned scheme (see e.g. [403]). By classical arguments, the convergence of the scheme holds if the spectral radius ρ of matrix

$$\begin{bmatrix} \mathcal{A}_{cc} & \mathbf{0} \\ \mathcal{A}_{fc} & \mathcal{A}_{ff} \end{bmatrix}^{-1} \begin{bmatrix} \mathcal{A}_{cc} & \mathcal{A}_{cf} \\ \mathcal{A}_{fc} & \mathcal{A}_{ff} \end{bmatrix},$$

i.e. the maximum modulus of the matrix eigenvalues, is less than 1.

In practice, it is quite hard to compute ρ, so this convergence analysis is seldom able to give quantitative responses about convergence and it has essentially a theoretical relevance. A practical approach for driving the iterative scheme to the convergence is to introduce a parameter to be properly tuned. In the present case, (11.41) can be modified as follows (for the sake of notation we drop time index $n+1$ from now on)

$$\begin{aligned} \mathcal{A}_{cc}\mathbf{s}_{c,k+1} &= \mathbf{b}_c + \mathbf{g}_c(\mathbf{s}_c^n, \ldots, \mathbf{s}_c^{n-p_c}) - \mathcal{A}_{cf}\mathbf{s}_{f,*}^{n+1}, \\ \mathcal{A}_{ff}\mathbf{s}_{f,k+1} &= \mathbf{b}_f + \mathbf{g}_f(\mathbf{s}_f^n, \ldots, \mathbf{s}_f^{n-p_f}) - \mathcal{A}_{fc}\mathbf{s}_{c,k}^{n+1}, \\ \mathbf{s}_{f,*}^{n+1} &= \theta\mathbf{s}_{f,k+1}^{n+1} + (1-\theta)\mathbf{s}_{f,k}^{n+1}. \end{aligned} \tag{11.42}$$

In the example above, this means that average pressures used as forcing terms for the coarse problem are modulated by the *relaxation parameter* θ. An appropriate choice of θ can yield or improve convergence of the iterative scheme, even if a priori it is not easy to identify its optimal value.

This scheme has been used for 3D/1D coupling illustrated in Fig. 11.24. The 3D model features rigid boundaries and mimics a stented segment of a cylindrical artery. Pressure drop problem is solved for the NS model, being pressure computed as a function of the area computed by E model. The latter receives data on flow rate, that are formulated in terms of the incoming characteristic variables (W_2 at interface Γ_{up} and W_1 at interface Γ_{dw}). Velocity and pressure solutions in 3D model (bottom, centre) are illustrated together with area in upstream (bottom, left) and downstream (bottom, right) of Fig. 11.24. Effects of the stent rigidity on the upstream area can be recognised. Relaxation parameter θ has been tuned in this case by a trial and error approach.

The main drawback of this approach is related to the computational costs. Iterations of these coupling algorithm are nested into the time loop, and this in general implies high computational costs. For this reason, more sophisticated algorithms can be devised to reduce the number of iterations. Possible approaches resort to a dynamical choice of relaxation parameters, or to more effective preconditioners of the coupled problem at hand.

Remark 11.5.2 *Splitting schemes like (11.41) or (11.42) can be regarded as the final result of an approximation process starting from a fully accurate model of blood flow problems. If Ω denotes the cardiovascular system (a) in Fig. 11.25, we can summarise the steps performed as follows.*

1. Domain splitting*: Ω is split into Ω_f and Ω_c subdomains ((b) in Fig. 11.25). Original problem is formulated as a set of subproblems. This is the first step of any* domain decomposition method *(see e.g. [408, 511]). In domain decomposition theory domain splitting can be performed with or without overlap among subdomains. Here we assume that subdomains do not overlap. Appropriate interface conditions describe the link between two subdomain solutions.*
2. Model coarsening*: Fully model in Ω_c is downscaled to a coarse model ((c) in Fig. 11.25). For lumped parameter models this step requires to keep trace of interface conditions that need to be incorporated in K problem by means of a proper selection of bridging regions.*
3. Iterative substructuring schemes*: Solution of the overall problem is pursued by a sequence of subdomain solutions suitably coupled ((d) in Fig. 11.25). In particular, for coarse K models bridging region compatibility guarantees that in the downscaled problem interface conditions are correctly included.*

This picture based on domain decomposition theory can be useful for the set up and analysis of effective ad hoc preconditioners.

Another approach for reducing computational costs is based on the introduction of a fully explicit splitting of subproblems.

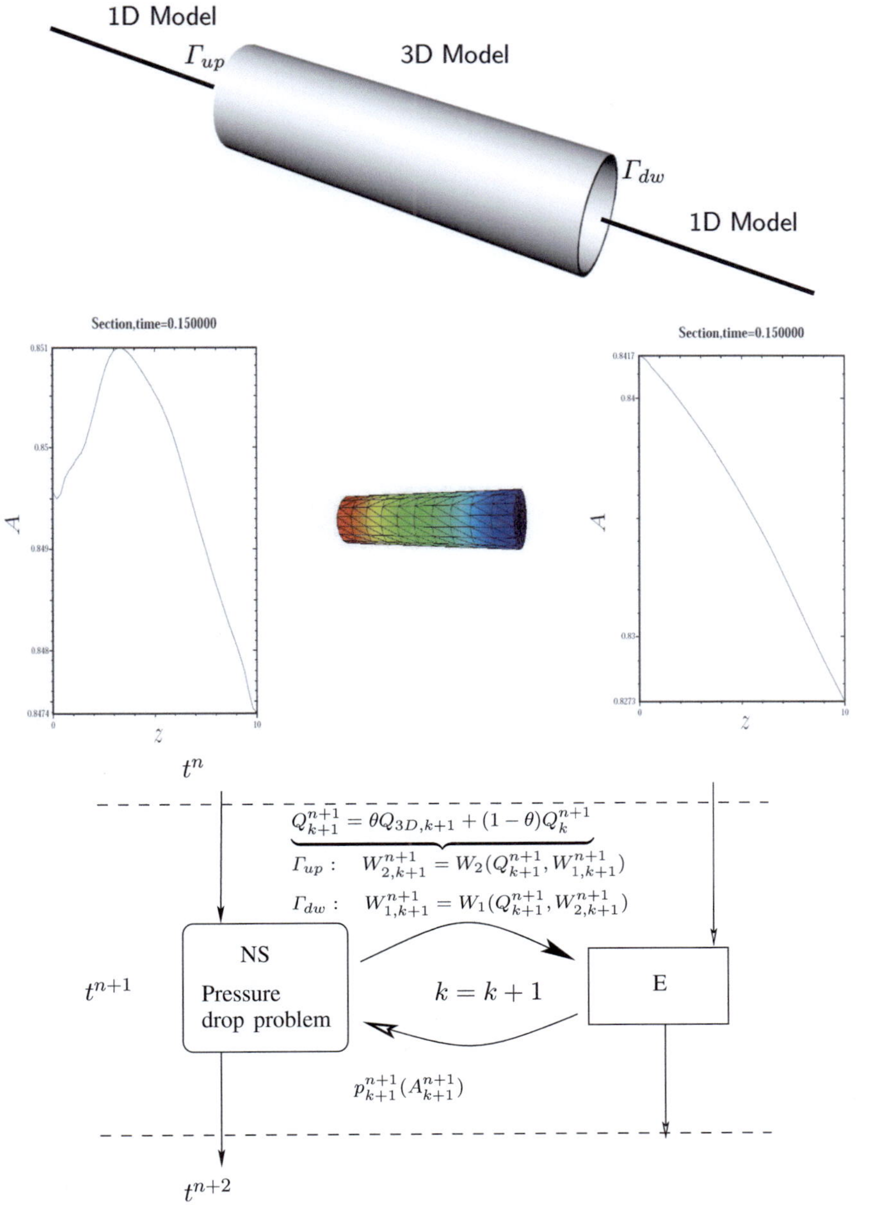

Fig. 11.24. 3D/1D multiscale problem: solution based on an iterative splitting solver with a relaxation parameter θ

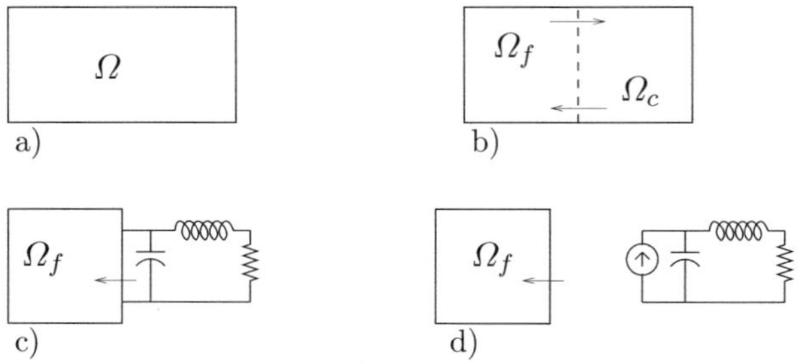

Fig. 11.25. Geometrical multiscale modelling as a domain decomposition method

11.5.3 Decoupled schemes

A simple way for reducing the computational costs essentially relies on the time dependent nature of the problems at hand. At each time step t^{n+1} we compute an extrapolation $\mathbf{s}_f^\star$ of $\mathbf{s}_f^{n+1}$ as a function of the fine solution at the previous time steps and we solve

$$\begin{cases} \mathcal{A}_{cc}\mathbf{s}_c = \mathbf{b}_c + \mathbf{g}_c(\mathbf{s}_c^n, \mathbf{s}_c^{n-1}, \ldots, \mathbf{s}_c^{n-p_c}) - \mathcal{A}_{cf}\mathbf{s}_f^\star \\ \mathcal{A}_{ff}\mathbf{s}_f^{n+1} = \mathbf{b}_f^{n+1} + \mathbf{g}_f(\mathbf{s}_f^n, \mathbf{s}_f^{n-1}, \ldots, \mathbf{s}_f^{n-p_f}) - \mathcal{A}_{fc}\mathbf{s}_c^{n+1}. \end{cases} \tag{11.43}$$

In practise, we perform scheme (11.41) for one time solely. A flow-chart representation of this scheme is given in Fig. 11.26.

The computational advantage is clear, no nested iterations are required. However, both stability and accuracy issues need to be addressed.

1. *Absolute Stability* in time of the scheme is affected by the explicit treatment of the fine solution in the first equation. The region of absolute stability (see Chapter 2) will be reduced even when unconditionally stable time advancing schemes such as implicit Euler are used for the time discretisation.
   A precise quantitative assessment of these stability restrictions is in practise neither easy nor convenient. It is however worth pointing out that in

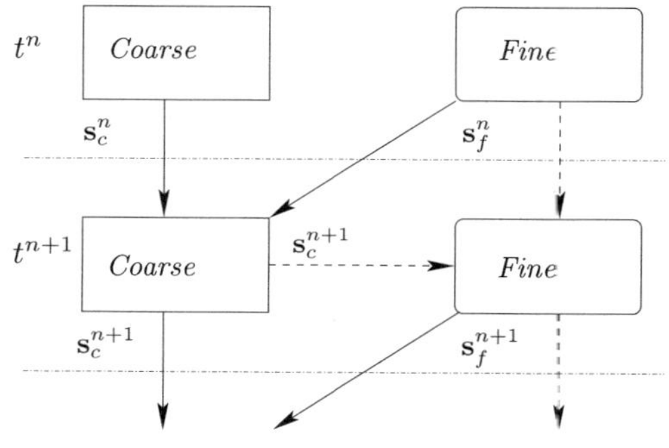

Fig. 11.26. Semi-implicit solver for multiscale problems

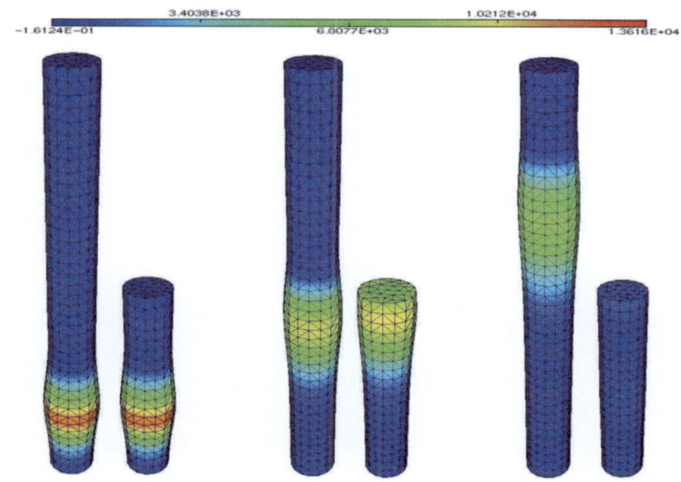

Fig. 11.27. Comparison between the pressure values of the stand-alone and the multiscale solutions at three different times (t=0.005, 0.01 and 0.015), using a 3D linear elastic model for the structure

many situations time advancing schemes used for solving single subproblems are explicit or semi-explicit. This is the case of 3D Navier-Stokes solver with a semi-explicit treatment of the convective term or of Lax-Wendroff schemes for 1D Euler equations (see Chapter 10). Numerical experience suggests that in many situations stability bounds associated with time advancing schemes are not significantly affected by the splitting scheme (11.43). This is the case for instance of results presented in Fig. 11.13.

Another example is provided by the 3D/1D model presented in [159]. In Fig. 11.27 we report a comparison between the pressure computed by a stand-alone 3D compliant model and a multiscale model, solved with a scheme in the form (11.43). Stand-alone model is a 10 cm long tube, the multiscale one is split into two domains (3D and 1D) of 5 cm each. Matching conditions yield the continuity of the total stresses and fluxes. Explicit coupling scheme (11.43) has been successfully used also for the application of multiscale modelling to paediatric surgery, as shown in Section 12.4.

2. *Time Accuracy.* Time accuracy of the scheme (11.43) is not lower than that of the uncoupled scheme (11.41) provided that an appropriate extrapolation $\mathbf{s}_f^\star$ is computed. More precisely, if q_c denotes the accuracy of the time advancing scheme for the coarse problem and q_f the one for the fine problem, an extrapolation of order q_c of $\mathbf{s}_f$ is enough for maintaining an accuracy of order q_c to the solution of the coarse problem. The accuracy of the fine solution will depend both on q_f and q_c. More precisely, on the basis of classical results of numerical analysis (see [268]), it is possible to

prove that accuracy of the fine model is given by:

$$q = \min(q_f, q_c + 1). \tag{11.44}$$

Since it is reasonable that for the fine model one would have a greater accuracy in time than for the coarse model, it follows from (11.44) that, for a desired order of accuracy q for the fine solution, it suffices that the coarse model be solved by a scheme of order $q - 1$.

11.6 Conclusions

Complexity of the vascular system demands for the set up of convenient mathematical and numerical models that go beyond the traditional ones based on Navier-Stokes, Euler or Kirchhoff equations. By themselves, these models have an intrinsic appeal and correctness that make them mathematically and numerically self-consistent. However, when we try to couple them, we face the unusual task of mixing different kind of differential equations, which are not conceived to function in a cooperative model. Many options are possible for yielding a multiscale model, starting from heuristic approaches, that however are often oversimplified and unreliable. From the mathematical and numerical viewpoints, set up of mathematically sound multiscale models raises new challenges both at the theoretical and practical level. The set up of effective and accurate numerical methods for the multiscale modelling and their analysis is not trivial and is actually still an open problem, especially for the simulation of 3D compliant domains. On the other hand, geometrical multiscale approach can play a relevant role in numerical treatment of spurious reflections at the artificial boundaries (see [155]). This approach can be of interest also in other engineering problems, featuring similar geometric multiscale complexity, like the design of intake/out-takes of internal combustion engines, the study of complex hydrological basins for environmental applications, or the design of electrical circuits (see e.g. [6, 116]).

More in general, reliable numerical solution of defective problems is by itself an interesting problem. For instance, in [392] a method for improving the accuracy in blood flow ultrasound measures is proposed, based on the extensive use of numerical simulations with flow rate defective boundary conditions. The focal point of these simulations is the prescription of the flow rate *without* the prescription of a velocity profile that induces a bias in results of ultra sound measurements.

Future perspectives in the mathematics for the vascular system should include *multiscale modelling in time*. Some pathological effects such as plaques formation or aneurysms growth require time scales of weeks, months or even years. Nevertheless, basic mechanisms that could be responsible of these pathologies develop over the time scale of a heart beat (seconds). An adequate multiscale-in-time modelling of these phenomena represents an important challenge for cardiovascular mathematics.

12

Applications and test cases

12.1 Flow in large vessels

J. Alastruey Arimon, Denis Doorly, Sergio Giordana, Joaquim Peiró, and Spencer Sherwin

12.1.1 Flow in an idealised distal anastomosis

Although medical imaging can provide relatively accurate geometric data of *in vivo* bypass grafts, as will be discussed in Section 12.1.2, to obtain an understanding of the general flow features it is instructive to consider an idealisation of a distal bypass graft. In this example we therefore consider the problem shown in Fig. 12.1, which consists of three vessels, all of the same diameter D, where the bypass (connecting) vessel has a centreline length of $3D$ and the host vessel is represented by two co-aligned vessels of lengths $5D$ (distal) and $10D$ (proximal) from the junction.

In this example the upstream (proximal) host vessel is fully occluded. At the inflow to the bypass graft we impose a normal flow rate of the fully

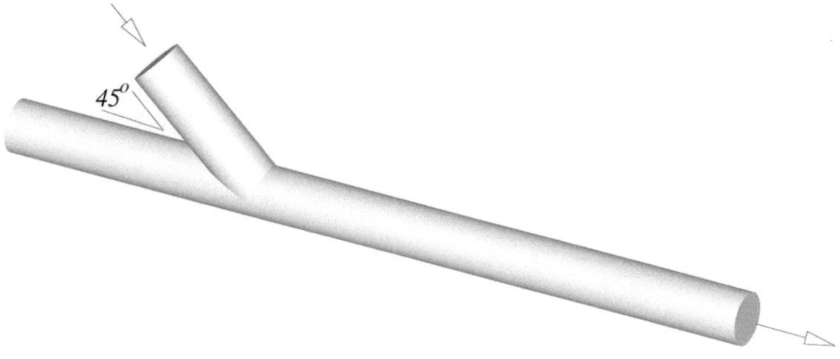

Fig. 12.1. Domain of idealised distal anastomosis

Formaggia L, Quarteroni A, Veneziani A (Eds.): Cardiovascular Mathematics. Modeling and simulation of the circulatory system

developed Hagen-Poiseuille flow, i.e.,

$$u(x,y,z) = u_m\left(1 - \frac{(x-x_0)^2 + (y-y_0)^2 + (z+z_0)^2}{R^2}\right)$$
$$v(x,y,z) = v_m\left(1 - \frac{(x-x_0)^2 + (y-y_0)^2 + (z+z_0)^2}{R^2}\right)$$
$$w(x,y,z) = w_m\left(1 - \frac{(x-x_0)^2 + (y-y_0)^2 + (z+z_0)^2}{R^2}\right)$$

where $(u_m, v_m, w_m) = (\sqrt{2}, -\sqrt{2}, 0)$ and if we take the centreline intersection to be the origin of the coordinate system $(x_0, y_0, z_0) = (3/\sqrt{2}, 3/\sqrt{2}, 0)$ and $R = D/2$. At outflow we impose zero traction conditions by imposing fully developed conditions on the velocity and that pressure within the plane is zero, i.e.,

$$\left.\frac{\partial u}{\partial n}\right|_{\text{outflow}} = 0 \qquad p|_{\text{outflow}} = 0.$$

The requirement for separate conditions on velocity and pressure is a consequence of the velocity correction scheme [208, 252] to discretise the Navier-Stokes equations. Finally we set the Reynolds number, Re_D based on diameter, D, and mean inflow velocity $\bar{u}$ to be $Re_D = \bar{u}D/\nu = 125$.

The flow within this model graft has been extensively discussed in [458] and in Section 5.3.2. In Fig. 12.2(a) we show the Dean vortex structure established in the junction idealised by the λ_2 criterion at a value of $\lambda_2 D^2/\bar{u} = -0.3$ (see 5.2.3). In Fig. 12.2(b) we show the wall shear stress magnitude distribution in the junction normalised with the wall shear stress magnitude at the inflow. The points labelled α, β denote the maximum and minimum (stagnation point) of the wall shear stress magnitude distribution. Finally in Fig. 12.3 we show the axial flow profiles at $x = 1D, 3D$ and $5D$ distal to the centreline intersection in the distal host vessel. In Fig. 12.3 we highlight the distribu-

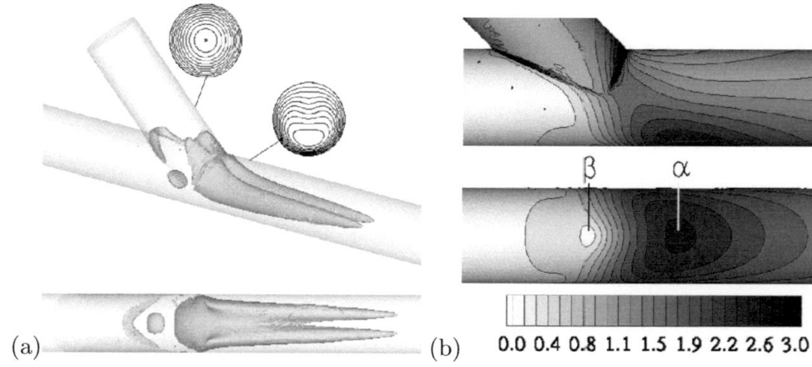

Fig. 12.2. (a) Dean vortex flow structure identified using the λ_2 criterion. (b) Normalised wall shear stress magnitude contours

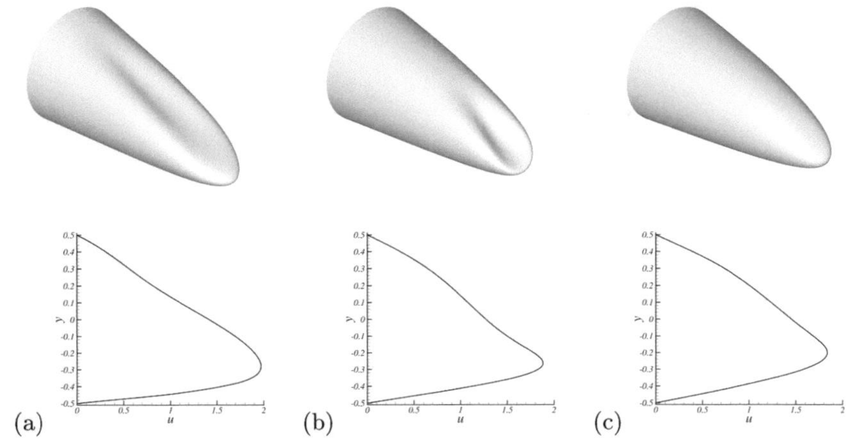

Fig. 12.3. Axial flow profiles in the host vessel located at a distance from the centreline intersection of (a) $1D$, (b) $3D$ and (c) $5D$. The bottom plots show the profile evaluated along the line of symmetry

tion of velocity magnitude as well as the profile evaluated along the plane of symmetry of the flow and geometry.

12.1.2 Flow in an anatomically realistic distal anastomosis

In this section we provide the details of flow within a realistic anastomosis as reported in [193] (see study 3). The domain shown in Fig. 12.4(a) belongs to a graft that runs from the femoral to the popliteal artery. It was located below the knee of the patient, and the graft conduit was an *in situ* long saphenous vein. The geometry was acquired from an MR scan performed one week post-operatively, and, as we can see, the graft meets the host vessel with a reasonably sharp bend. Figure 12.4(a) also illustrates a series of four-sided patches through which a cubic spline fit was enforced. The coordinate of each point in the patches is provided on the web page, and the units are provided in pixels of the original imaging data. In this domain, an inflow was imposed as indicated in Fig. 12.4(a), which corresponds to a fully developed Poiseuille flow which has a radius of 6.476 units. The other two vessels were specified to be outflows with zero pressure conditions, i.e.,

- Inflow: Fully developed Poiseuille flow.

$$u(x,y,z) = u_m \left(1 - \frac{(x-x_0)^2 + (y-y_0)^2 + (z+z_0)^2}{R^2}\right)$$

$$v(x,y,z) = v_m \left(1 - \frac{(x-x_0)^2 + (y-y_0)^2 + (z+z_0)^2}{R^2}\right)$$

$$w(x,y,z) = w_m \left(1 - \frac{(x-x_0)^2 + (y-y_0)^2 + (z+z_0)^2}{R^2}\right)$$

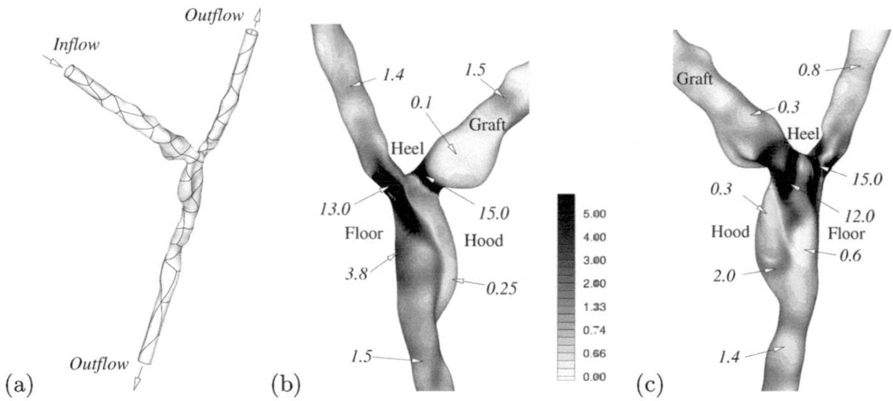

Fig. 12.4. (a) Anatomic bypass geometry, (b,c) relative wall shear stress magnitude relative to inflow wall shear

with constants $R = 6.476$,

$$(x_0, y_0, z_0) = (193.52, 183.87, 369.70)$$

and

$$(u_m, v_m, w_m) = 2\mathbf{n} = (1.3, -0.66, -1.36).$$

This choice of definition for the velocity magnitude ensures that the sectionally average velocity $\bar{u} = 1$.

- Outflow: Zero traction conditions with zero pressure.

$$\frac{\partial u}{\partial n} = \frac{\partial v}{\partial n} = \frac{\partial w}{\partial n} = 0, \qquad p|_{\text{outflow}} = 0.$$

The imposition of zero pressure at both outflows leads to a flow split where 65 % of the flow exits at the distal (downstream) outflow.

The flow was simulated at a Reynolds number, based on the average inflow velocity and inflow diameter of $Re_D = 341$. Figure 12.4(b) shows the normalised wall shear stress magnitude calculated assuming a Newtonian fluid and rigid walls divided by the inflow wall shear stress magnitude. For a point of data comparison in Fig. 12.4(b) we present the wall shear stress magnitude normalised by the wall shear stress at the inflow, i.e., $\mu 4/R$ assuming $\rho = 1$.

12.1.3 Assessment of a 1-D numerical simulation against *in vitro* measurements

The accuracy of the non-linear, one-dimensional (1-D) equations of pulse wave propagation in complaint arteries was tested by comparison against a well defined experimental 1:1 replica of the human arterial tree [316]. The experimental model was a 1:1 replica of the 37 largest systemic arteries in the human,

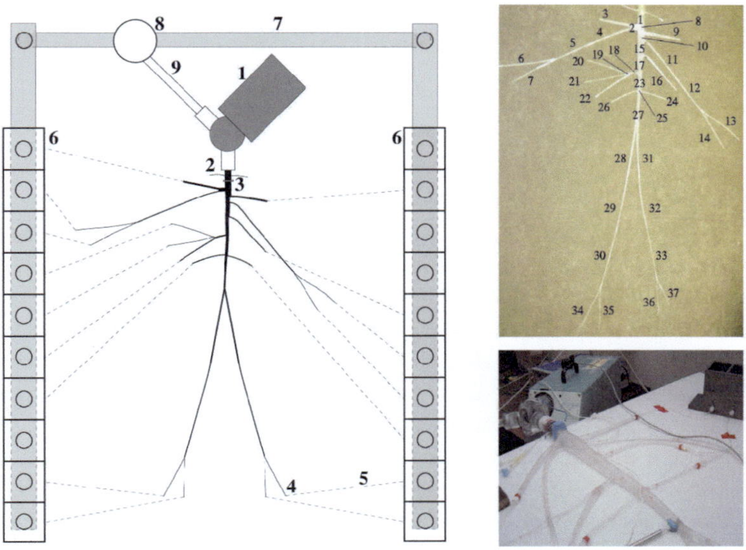

Fig. 12.5. Planview schematic of the hydraulic model (left). 1: Pump (left heart); 2: catheter access; 3: two-leaflet aortic valve; 4: peripheral resistance tube; 5: flexible plastic tubing (veins); 6: venous overflow; 7: venous return conduit; 8: buffering reservoir; 9: pulmonary veins. The 37 arteries simulated (top right). Detail of the pump and the aorta (bottom right). Taken from [316].

including the aorta, carotid arteries and arteries that perfuse the upper and lower limbs and the main abdominal organs (Fig. 12.5).

The *in vitro* arterial network was manufactured using in-house crafted tubular aluminium moulds, which were either linearly tapered or had constant cross-section (for the smallest branches). A two-component silicone material (Fairfield, CT, USA) was hand-painted in six layers on each mould. Curing between subsequent layers was done at 150 °C. The silicone network was manually assembled piece by piece, mounted horizontally and subsequently connected proximally to a Harvard pulsatile pump and distally to a set of terminal resistance tubes connected to overflow reservoirs, creating a closed loop hydraulic system. A 65%–35 % water–glycerol mixture, with a density $\rho = 1050\,\mathrm{kg\,m^{-3}}$ and a viscosity $\mu = 2.5\,\mathrm{mPa\,s}$ at 30 °C, was used to mimic the density and viscosity of blood.

Values of length (l), radius (R) and wall thickness (h) were measured at the inlet, middle point and outlet of each arterial segment (Fig. 12.5, top right) using a ruler, callipers and micrometer. These measurements were taken at the end of the experiment and after having dissected the model. The elastic wall properties were measured by performing a tensile test on 63 silicone sample strips, taken from specimen sheets of various thicknesses and angles with respect to the principal direction of painting the silicone layers. A constant Young modulus $E = 1.2$ MPa was measured within the working interval of pressures. Wave speeds were calculated using

$$c^2 = \frac{2Eh}{3\rho R}. \tag{12.1}$$

Table 12.1 shows these data for each arterial segment.

The *in vitro* inflow boundary condition was imposed by the Harvard pump with the following settings: 70 beats per minute (with a systole-to-diastole ratio of 35/65) and a stroke volume of 70 ml, creating an average pressure of approximately 13.3 kPa at the ascending aorta. Figure 12.6 shows the resulting flow rate measured at the root of the silicone network and enforced as a periodic inflow boundary condition in the numerical model. Each experimental outflow consisted of a single diameter tube (length 250 mm; Ø2 mm) and an overflow reservoir with a constant back pressure $p_{out} = 427$ Pa. The simplicity of this type of outlet allowed for accurate quantification of its parameters, although it induced some non-physiological features in the pressure and flow waveforms because peripheral compliances were not simulated. Numerically, these outflow boundary conditions were modelled using the relation

$$Q_{1\mathrm{D}} = \frac{p_{1\mathrm{D}} - p_{out}}{R_p}, \tag{12.2}$$

where $Q_{1\mathrm{D}}$ and $p_{1\mathrm{D}}$ are the flow rate and pressure at the outlet of the 1-D terminal branch, and R_p is the peripheral resistance to the flow, determined from mean pressure and flow measurements less than 2 cm to the outlet of each terminal branch. The values of R_p are shown in the last column of Table 12.1. Combined, they yield a total peripheral resistance of $2.25 \cdot 10^8$ Pa s m^{-3}. Applying Equation (12.2) with $Q_{1\mathrm{D}}$ and $p_{1\mathrm{D}}$ as the mean flow rate and pressure measured at the inlet of the ascending aorta produced a larger total resistance ($2.37 \cdot 10^8$ Pa s m^{-3}), resulting from the total peripheral resistance plus the effect of viscous dissipation throughout the vessels and junctions of the silicone network. At the bifurcations of the system, conservation of mass and

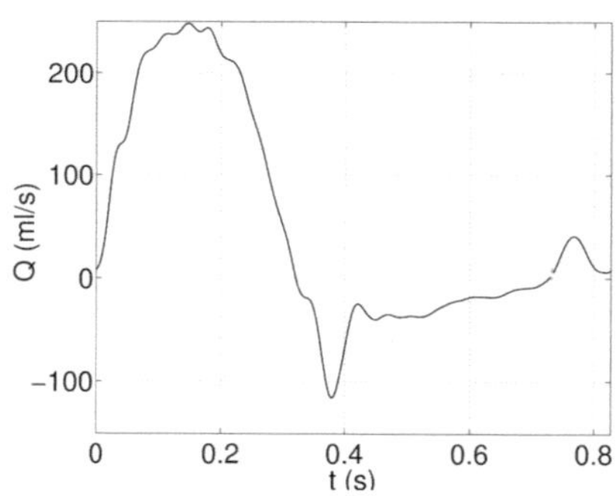

Fig. 12.6. The experimental flow rate measured at the ascending aorta is enforced as the inflow boundary condition of the numerical model. Taken from [316].

Table 12.1. Data of the 37 silicone tubes shown in Fig. 12.5 (top right). l: length; $R_{in} \to R_{out}$: diastolic cross-sectional radii at the inlet and the outlet; h: average wall thickness; $c_{in} \to c_{out}$: wave speed at the inlet and the outlet; R_p: peripheral resistance. Single numbers indicate vessels with a constant cross-section. The interval of confidence of the geometrical measurements is indicated in the heading

Arterial segment	l (mm) ± 2.0 %	$R_{in} \to R_{out}$ (mm) ± 3.5 %	h (mm) ± 2.5 %	$c_{in} \to c_{out}$ (m/s)	R_p (10^9 Pa s m^{-3})
1. Ascending aorta	36	14.40 → 13.00	0.51	5.21 → 5.49	–
2. Innominate	28	11.00 → 7.29	0.35	4.89 → 6.01	–
3. R. carotid	145	5.37 → 3.86	0.28	6.35 → 7.49	2.67
4. R. subclavian I	218	4.36 → 3.34	0.27	6.87 → 7.84	–
5. R. subclavian II	165	3.34 → 2.78	0.16	6.00 → 6.58	–
6. R. radial	235	2.07	0.15	7.43	3.92
7. R. ulnar	177	2.10	0.21	8.81	3.24
8. Aortic arch I	21	13.00 → 12.50	0.50	5.41 → 5.52	–
9. L. carotid	178	5.58 → 3.73	0.31	6.55 → 8.00	3.11
10. Aortic arch II	29	12.50 → 11.80	0.41	4.98 → 5.12	–
11. L. subclavian I	227	4.42 → 3.39	0.22	6.21 → 7.10	–
12. L. subclavian II	175	3.39 → 2.84	0.17	6.26 → 6.84	–
13. L. radial	245	2.07	0.21	8.84	3.74
14. L. ulnar	191	2.07	0.16	7.77	3.77
15. Thoracic aorta I	56	11.80 → 11.00	0.43	5.29 → 5.48	–
16. Intercostals	195	4.12 → 3.22	0.27	7.07 → 7.99	2.59
17. Thoracic aorta II	72	11.00 → 9.26	0.34	4.84 → 5.26	–
18. Coeliac I	38	3.97	0.20	6.20	–
19. Coeliac II	13	4.31	1.25	14.90	–
20. Splenic	191	1.83	0.13	7.24	3.54
21. Gastric	198	1.92	0.11	6.73	4.24
22. Hepatic	186	3.31 → 2.89	0.21	6.95 → 7.44	3.75
23. Abdominal aorta I	62	9.26 → 8.01	0.33	5.19 → 5.59	–
24. L. renal	120	2.59	0.19	7.39	3.46
25. Abdominal aorta II	7	7.90	0.35	5.83	–
26. R. renal	118	2.55	0.16	6.95	3.45
27. Abdominal aorta III	104	7.80 → 5.88	0.30	5.41 → 6.24	–
28. R. iliac-femoral I	205	3.90 → 3.38	0.21	6.47 → 6.94	–
29. R. iliac-femoral II	216	3.38 → 2.31	0.15	5.89 → 7.13	–
30. R. iliac-femoral III	206	2.31 → 2.10	0.20	8.04 → 8.44	–
31. L. iliac-femoral I	201	4.02 → 3.34	0.20	6.19 → 6.79	–
32. L. iliac-femoral II	195	3.34 → 2.26	0.16	6.11 → 7.44	–
33. L. iliac-femoral III	207	2.26 → 2.12	0.13	6.67 → 6.89	–
34. R. anterior tibial	163	1.55	0.15	8.47	5.16
35. R. posterior tibial	151	1.53	0.12	7.73	5.65
36. L. posterior tibial	149	1.58	0.11	7.23	4.59
37. L. anterior tibial	126	1.55	0.10	7.01	3.16

continuity of the total pressure $p + \frac{1}{2}\rho U^2$ were enforced. The initial conditions of the numerical model were $A(x,0) = A_0(x)$ and $U(x,0) = 0$ in all the vessels. The model was run until it converged to a periodic solution, which took about 10 cardiac cycles and of the order of five minutes to run on a standard PC.

Simultaneous pressure and flow measurements were taken at 70 sites along the arterial network. Flow rates were measured using ultrasonic volume flow meters with five different sized probes (Ø24 mm, Ø16 mm, Ø12 mm, Ø8 mm and Ø3 mm). Pressures were measured using micro-tip catheter pressure transducers. Peripheral recording of the pressure and flow was always accompanied by a simultaneous measurement of the pressure and flow just distal to the aortic valve. At least ten successive beats of pressure and the flow were recorded at each measurement location. The signals were first calibrated and subsequently filtered with a 5th-order low-pass (20Hz) Butterworth filter to reduce noise on the signals while maintaining the relevant frequency information. Subsequently, a minimum of 8 beats were selected from the 10–12 recorded beats and ensemble averaged to generate a single beat pressure and flow waveform to be compared with their numerical counterparts.

Figure 12.7 compares experimental and numerical pressure and flow waveforms at three representative locations along the silicone aorta, showing the ability of the 1-D formulation to capture the main features of experimental pulse waves. None of the parameters involved in the simulation was tuned, except for phase matching the onset of the experimental and numerical systolic ejections during data post-processing. Despite the simple terminal boundary conditions used, the experimental model was able to reproduce the main features of *in vivo* pressure and flow waveforms, such as the dicrotic notch, diastolic decay and peaking and steepening of pulse pressure as we move away from the heart [66]. Some backward flow was observed after the closure of the two-leaflet aortic valve, as well as a reduction in the amplitude of the flow with the distance from the heart. These results highlighted the relative independence of aortic pulse waves from the outflow boundary conditions, which was to be expected since the bifurcations of the *in vitro* model were well matched for forward travelling waves.

Typical comparisons between experimental and numerical results in the rest of the vessels of the system are shown in Figs. 12.8–12.10. Each figure compares experimental and numerical results in representative vessels of each generation of bifurcations, going from vessels branching off the experimental aorta (Fig. 12.8) to vessels of the third generation of bifurcations (Fig. 12.10). The 1-D formulation was also able to predict the essential characteristics of the *in vitro* pressure and flow waveforms in more peripheral vessels. Due to the simple resistance boundary conditions used in the experiment, the measured pulse waves became less physiological in the more distal vessels, containing many non-physiological oscillations, in both pressure and the flow, whose frequency was surprisingly well captured by the 1-D model.

Relative errors in pressure and the flow were within 4 % and 19 %, respectively, at all 70 locations studied. The larger relative error in the flow was

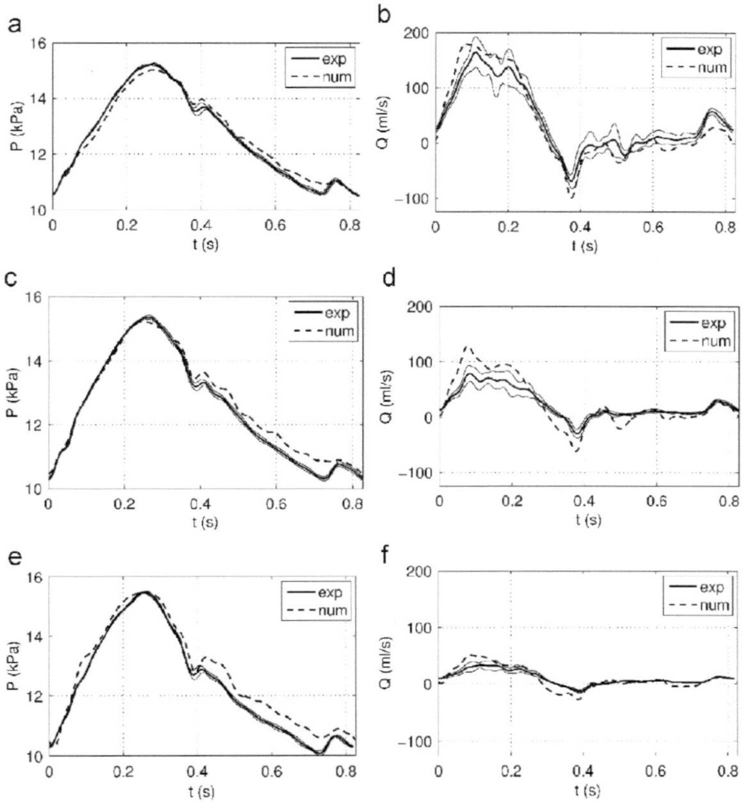

Fig. 12.7. Experimental and theoretical pressure (left) and flow (right) waveforms. (top) Aortic arch II (segment 10 in Table 1), (middle) thoracic aorta II (segment 17) and (bottom) abdominal aorta III (segment 27). The figures also show the standard deviation (thin solid lines) of the ensemble average of each experimental measurement. Taken from [316]

primarily attributed to flow measurement uncertainty. Accurate flow measurements rely upon close contact between the tube and the flow transducer, and since only five different sizes of transducers were available, some mismatches were inevitable at the 70 different measurement sites. In general, relative errors were smaller at locations close to the inflow boundary condition, where the numerical flow matched its experimental counterpart. Discrepancies between experimental and numerical measurements arose from the uncertainties in the experimental measurements and the assumptions and simplifications of the 1-D formulation. The study in [316] showed that these discrepancies could not be a consequence of having neglected energy losses at junctions. In addition, the higher amplitude of the numerical peripheral oscillations could only be partially explained by the presence of peripheral compliance in the overflow reservoirs. The effect of neglecting the curvature of the vessels was not

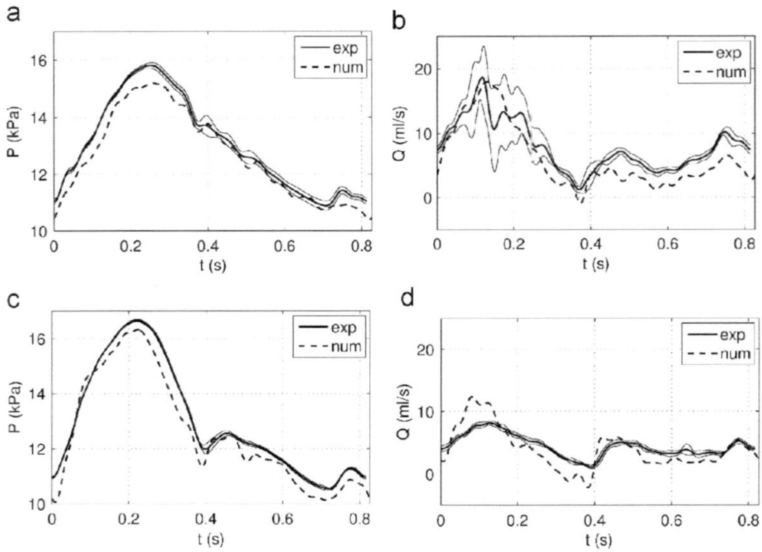

Fig. 12.8. Experimental and theoretical pressure (left) and flow (right) waveforms in typical first-generation vessels: (top) left subclavian I (segment 11), (bottom) right iliac-femoral II (segment 29). The figures also show the standard deviation (thin solid lines) of the ensemble average of each experimental measurement. Taken from [316]

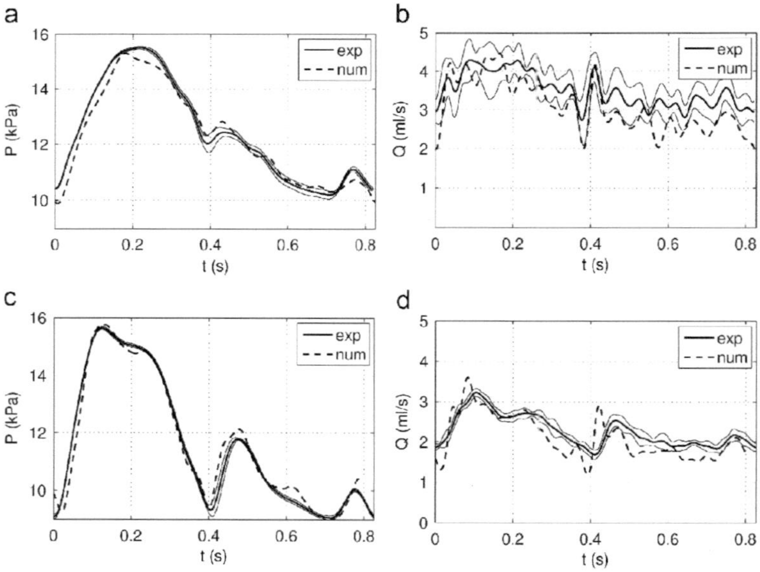

Fig. 12.9. Experimental and theoretical pressure (left) and flow (right) waveforms in typical second-generation vessels: (top) left ulnar (segment 14), (bottom) right anterior tibial (segment 34). The figures also show the standard deviation (thin solid lines) of the ensemble average of each experimental measurement. Taken from [316]

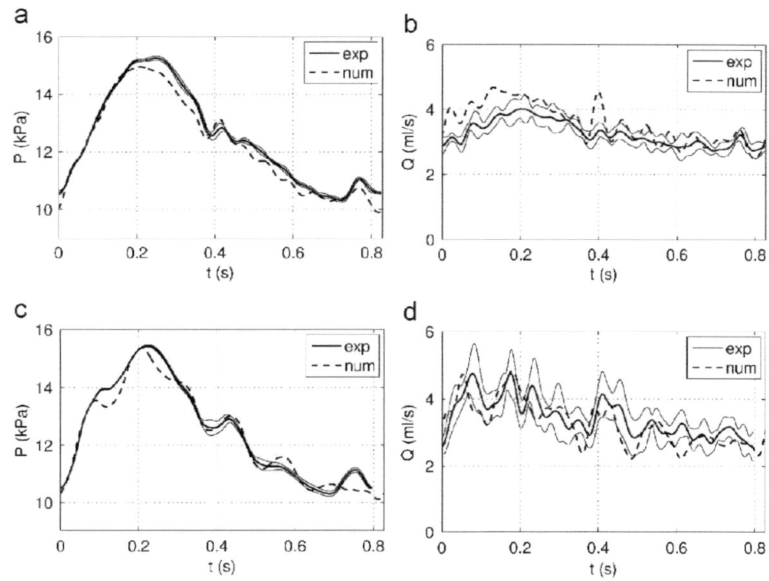

Fig. 12.10. Experimental and theoretical pressure (left) and flow (right) waveforms in typical-third generation vessels: (top) right ulnar (segment 7), (bottom) splenic (segment 20). The figures also show the standard deviation (thin solid lines) of the ensemble average of each experimental measurement. Taken from [316]

analysed, although it should be secondary because of the geometry of the experimental network. Consequently, the viscoelasticity of the silicone wall might have had an important effect on damping peripheral oscillations.

12.2 A FSI benchmark on a straight compliant vessel

Miguel A. Fernández, Jean-Frédéric Gerbeau, and Marina Vidrascu

We consider the academic numerical test, originally proposed in [155], which consists in simulating the pressure wave propagation through a straight compliant vessel. This test case has been extensively used in the literature as a benchmark (see e.g., [55, 146, 150, 188]), in order to illustrate the efficiency of the different fluid-structure coupling algorithms described in Chapter 9.

The fluid domain is a straight cylinder of radius 0.5 cm and length 5 cm. The fluid and solid unknowns are described by the fluid-structure problem (3.106)–(3.108) introduced in Chapter 3, in which the elastodynamics equation (3.107) is replaced by a a non-linear shell model (based on MITC4 shell elements [75]).

The fluid physical parameters are $\mu = 0.03\, poise$ and $\rho_f = 1\,\mathrm{g/cm^3}$, whereas for the solid we have $\hat{\rho}_{s,0} = 1.2\,\mathrm{g/cm^3}$, $E = 3 \times 10^6\,\mathrm{dynes/cm^2}$,

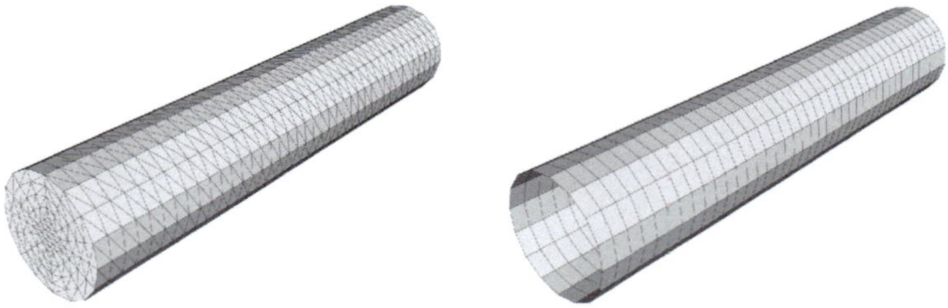

Fig. 12.11. The fluid and solid computational meshes: 21534 tetrahedra for the fluid and 640 quadrilaterals for the solid

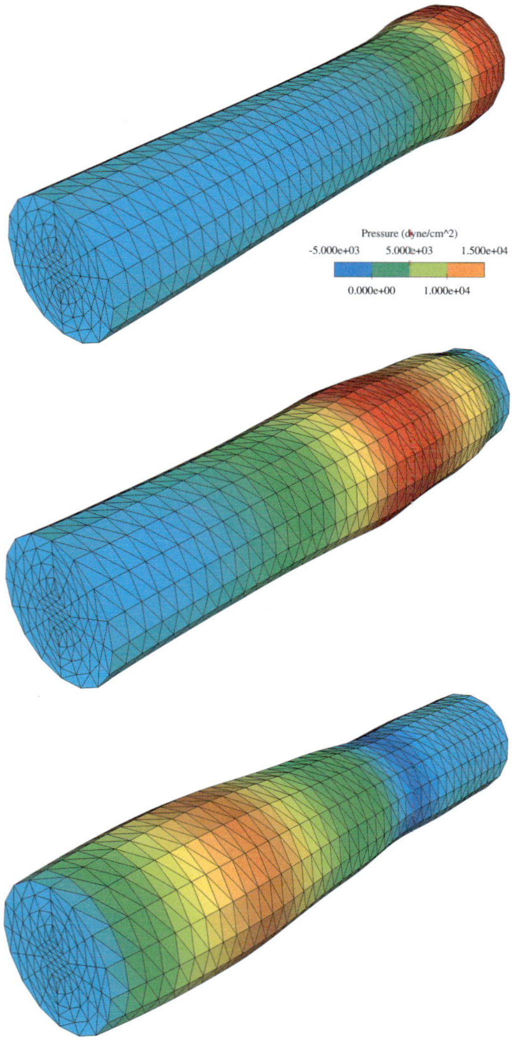

Fig. 12.12. Snapshots of the fluid pressure and fluid domain deformation (magnified by a factor 10) at three different time instants: $t = 0.0025,\ 0.006,\ 0.01\,\mathrm{s}$

$\xi = 0.3$. The thickness of the vessel wall is 0.1 cm. The fluid is initially at rest and a pressure of 1.332×10^4 dynes/cm^2 (10 mmHg) is imposed on the inlet boundary during 0.005 s.

The resulting fluid-structure coupled problem is semi-discretised in time using the implicit coupling framework described in Section 9.3.1, with a time step size of $\delta t = 0.0001$ s. As regards the space discretisation, a $\mathbb{P}_1/\mathbb{P}_1$ stabilised finite element discretisation is considered for the fluid, and the MITC4 shell finite element for the solid. The fluid and solid computational meshes are depicted in Fig. 12.11. At each time step, the resulting non-linear problem is solved using Newton's method (with exact Jacobian evaluations, see e.g., [150]) applied to the Dirichlet-to-Neumann formulation, as described in Section 9.3.3.

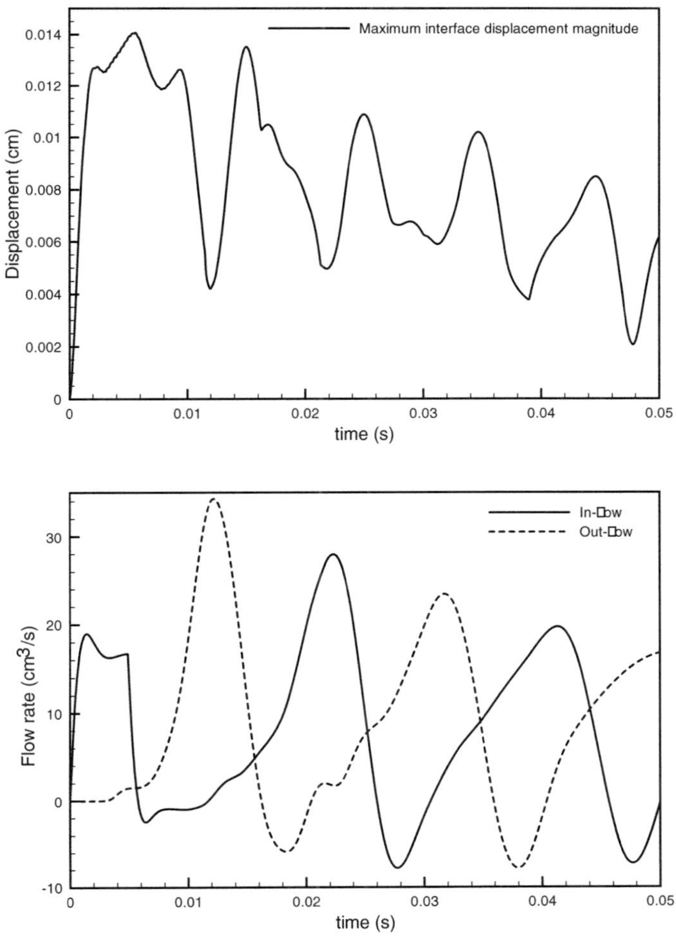

Fig. 12.13. Maximum displacement magnitude of the fluid-structure interface (top), in- and out-flow rates (bottom)

A pressure wave propagation is observed during the simulation (see Fig. 12.12). These results are similar to those obtained in the literature, see e.g. [55, 146, 150, 155, 188]. We conclude this test case by providing, in Fig. 12.13, a few quantitative outputs: the maximum interface displacement and the inlet and outlet flow-rates. In particular, we can clearly observe the expected phase shift between the in- and out-flow rates due to the compliance of the vessel wall.

12.3 Mass transfer phenomena. A case study: drug-eluting stents[1]

Paolo Zunino, Carlo D'Angelo, Christian Vergara, and Martin Prosi

A stent is a small mesh tube that is inserted permanently into a stenotic artery. The stent restores the original value of the arterial section to ensure the physiological flow rate. One of the problems caused by stent insertion is re-narrowing of the treated vessel. To overcome this phenomenon drug-eluting stents (DES) have recently been introduced. Referred to as a *coated* or *medicated* stent, a DES is a normal metal stent that has been coated with a pharmacologic agent (drug) that is known to interfere with the process of restenosis (reblocking). However, the design of such devices is a very complex task because their performance in widening the arterial lumen and preventing further restenosis is influenced by many factors such as the geometrical design of the stent, the mechanical properties of the materials and the chemical properties of the drug that is released. Mathematical models and numerical simulation techniques are appropriate to study such phenomena, aiming for use as predictive tools for the effective design of drug-eluting stents.

We present in this section a brief review of fluid dynamics and drug release models developed by the authors for the numerical simulation of drug-eluting coronary stents.

12.3.1 A mathematical model for drug release

We assume that the drug released by the stent behaves as a passive scalar. This statement holds true under the assumption that the drug does not react with the arterial walls. This is a zero-level simplification of a number of chemical phenomena that involve the drug as a ligand and suitable sites of the extra-cellular matrix as receptors, as discussed in [444]. As a consequence, our drug release model features just one chemical species, the drug, that is governed

[1] This work has been developed in collaboration with the Laboratory of Biological Structure Mechanics (LaBS), Department of Structural Engineering, Politecnico di Milano.

by standard advection-diffusion equations. Thanks to the assumption that coronary arteries treated with cardiovascular stents are large enough to apply a Newtonian model for blood rheology, we consider the Navier-Stokes equations for fluid dynamics in the arterial lumen. Furthermore, the drug we will consider in the numerical experiments is heparin, a relatively small molecule with non-negligible diffusive properties. Then, the advective phenomena in the arterial walls can be neglected. In other words, we address the interaction of the mass transfer in the lumen and in the arterial walls as the fluid-wall model, already *fluid-wall* mentioned in the introduction of Chapter 7 and analysed in [411] for the transport of oxygen. Concerning the coronary artery, here we simplify the complex multilayered structure of the wall; more precisely we assume that the arterial wall is a homogeneous medium, whose physical properties are, for simplicity, the ones corresponding to the intermediate layer, the *media*.

Under these assumptions, the geometrical setting of our reference problem is the following. We denote with Ω_l the lumen of a coronary artery where we set up our analysis. This is the cylindric channel deformed by the introduction and the expansion of a stent. We denote with Γ_{in} and Γ_{out} the proximal and distal sections since they coincide with the inflow and outflow sections of the domain Ω_l. The remaining part of the boundary of Ω_l can be subdivided into two parts: the interface with the arterial wall and the stent. The former is denoted with Γ and the latter with $\Gamma_{s,l}$. In conclusion we obtain $\partial\Omega_f = \Gamma_{in} \cup \Gamma_{out} \cup \Gamma_{s,l} \cup \Gamma$, as shown in Fig. 12.14. Finally, we denote with $\boldsymbol{n}_l$ the outward unit normal vector on $\partial\Omega_l$. Let Ω_w be the truncated portion of the arterial walls corresponding to the lumen Ω_l. We denote with Γ_a the interface of the arterial wall with the outer tissue, with $\Gamma_{n,w}$ the artificial sections originated by the truncation of the artery and with $\Gamma_{s,w}$ the interface of the stent with the arterial wall. Moreover, let $\boldsymbol{n}_w$ be the outward unit normal vector relative to Ω_w. These sections are also shown in Fig. 12.14.

The governing equations for drug release are time dependent, because the drug release process is intrinsically transient and it dies out in a long but finite time. Then, our model for drug concentrations, namely $c_l(t, \mathbf{x})$ and $c_w(t, \mathbf{x})$, read as follows,

$$\partial_t c_* + \nabla \cdot (-D_* \nabla c_* + \boldsymbol{u}_* c_*) = 0 \text{ in } \Omega_*, \text{ with } * = l, w, \tag{12.3}$$

together with a condition prescribing the initial state of the concentration into blood stream and arterial walls, $c_*(t = 0) = 0$ in Ω_* and suitable boundary conditions. For the arterial lumen, Ω_l, on the inflow boundary we prescribe $c_l = 0$ on Γ_{in} since the blood does not contain drug proximally to the stent. Assuming that the outflow boundary is far enough from the stent, we can neglect any diffusive effects across this section and set $\nabla c_l \cdot \boldsymbol{n}_l = 0$ on Γ_{out}. Also, for the arterial wall we prescribe $\nabla c_w \cdot \boldsymbol{n}_l = 0$ on $\Gamma_a \cup \Gamma_{n,w}$.

According to Chapter 7, for the transmission conditions between Ω_l and Ω_w we take into account the endothelium, which is modelled as a membrane at the interface between the lumen and the arterial walls, corresponding to

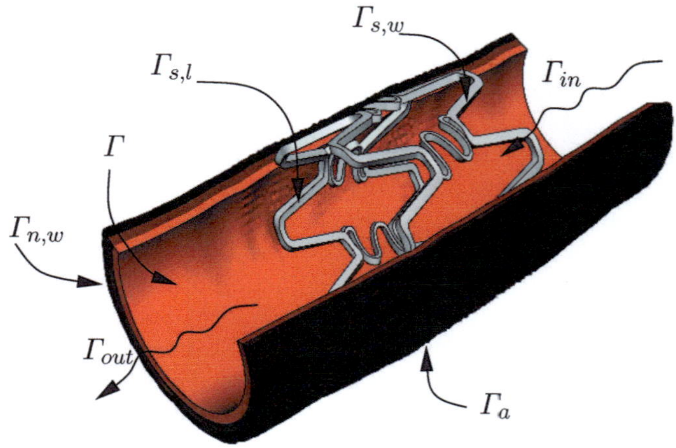

Fig. 12.14. The lumen, the arterial wall and the stent with the partition of their boundaries for the set up of fluid dynamics and drug release models

Γ, having a permeability $\mathcal{P}$ with respect to the transfer of drug. Then, the coupling between equations (12.3) is provided by the following conditions,

$$-D_l \nabla c_l \cdot \boldsymbol{n}_l = \mathcal{P}(c_l - c_w) \text{ and } - D_w \nabla c_w \cdot \boldsymbol{n}_w = \mathcal{P}(c_w - c_l), \text{ on } \Gamma, \quad (12.4)$$

which are symmetric with respect to the lumen and the arterial walls. As shown in [411] this represents an advantage both for the analysis and the numerical approximation of the coupled problem.

Finally, particular attention should be dedicated to the boundary condition at the interface between the stent and the lumen, because this is primarily responsible for determining the drug release rate. We remember that DES for cardiovascular applications are miniaturised metal structures that are coated with a micro-film containing the drug that will be locally released into the arterial walls for healing purposes. The thickness of this film generally lays within the range of microns. Owing to the fact that stent coating is extremely thin, we apply the model proposed in [529] consisting in the following formula for the release rate,

$$J(t,x) = \varphi(t)(c_s^0 - c_*) \quad \text{on} \quad \Gamma_{s,*} \text{ with } * = l, w, \quad (12.5)$$

$J(t,x)$ being the flux that is released from the stent and c_s^0 the initial drug charge of the stent that is equal to unity in the undimensional setting for the concentration. Given the thickness of the stent coating, Δl, and its diffusion parameter, D_s, the scaling function $\varphi(t)$ is defined as follows,

$$\varphi(t) = \frac{2D_s}{\Delta l} \sum_{n=0}^{\infty} e^{-(n+1/2)^2 kt} \quad \text{with} \quad k = \pi^2 D_s / \Delta l^2. \quad (12.6)$$

Owing to (12.5), the boundary condition on $\Gamma_{s,l}$ and $\Gamma_{s,w}$ for equation (12.3) turns out to be the following Robin-type condition,

$$-D_* \nabla c_* \cdot \boldsymbol{n}_* + \varphi(t)(c_s^0 - c_*) = 0 \text{ on } \Gamma_{s,*} \text{ with } * = l, w.$$

The initial/boundary value problem relative to equation (12.3) is now ready to be approximated by means of the numerical discretisation methods addressed in Section 7.3.

12.3.2 Numerical simulation data

The stent used in this study resembles the coronary Cordis BX-Velocity (Johnson & Johnson, Interventional System, Warren, NJ, USA). The stent geometry is created using Rhinoceros 3.0 Evaluation CAD program (McNeel & Associates, Indianapolis, IN, USA), after an acquisition of the Cordis dimensions by the use of a Nikon SMZ800 stereo microscope (Nikon Corporation, Tokyo, Japan). The length of the unit of the stent considered in the analysis is 3.62 mm, the inner radius 0.6 mm and the thickness 0.14 mm. The simulation of the expansion of the folded stent into the coronary artery is achieved by means of the commercial code ABAQUS/Explicit v. 6.4 (see [330]) and references therein.

The lumen and the wall of the artery are subdivided with Gambit (ANSYS Inc., Canonsburg, PA, USA) into 1,637,336 and 1,118,420 tetrahedra respectively. In order to obtain an accurate resolution with a reasonable computational cost and memory storage, we have applied a non-uniform spacing for the mesh generation. In particular, the central part of the domain has been subdivided by means of variable size elements, particularly refined around the stent.

Concerning the blood physiological data, the fluid density is $\rho = 1\,\mathrm{mg/mm^3}$ and the viscosity is $\mu = 3\,\mathrm{mg\,s^{-1}\,mm^{-1}}$. Moreover, at the inflow of the artery we have imposed a parabolic velocity profile with a peak of 270 mm/s. As regards the drug release, we adopt the parameters determined by the experimental investigations presented in [300] for heparin. This corresponds to set $D_l = 1.5 \times 10^{-4}\,\mathrm{mm^2/s}$, $D_w = 7.7 \times 10^{-6}\,\mathrm{mm^2/s}$ and $\mathcal{P} = 4 \times 10^{-4}\,\mathrm{mm/s}$. The diffusivity of the drug into the stent coating typically ranges from 10^{-8} to $10^{-12}\,\mathrm{mm^2/s}$, depending on the mechanical properties of the polymeric substrate. To avoid too stiff parameters we set $D_s = 10^{-8}\,\mathrm{mm^2/s}$.

12.3.3 Analysis of fluid dynamics around the stent

Looking at the Cordis BX-Velocity stent, it is possible to identify two kinds of structures: the struts and the links. The former are twisted rings that provide the circumferential strength of the stent, while the latter are tiny connections along the longitudinal axis between subsequent struts.

An important feature of the struts is that they are twisted in the circumferential direction. For this reason, the blood flow hits the struts at different angles. Consequently, the flow pattern downstream from the struts may be substantially different from the well known flow after a backward facing step that corresponds to the ideal case of a perfectly circular ring that is orthogonal to the flow. This conjecture is confirmed by the fluid dynamics simulations.

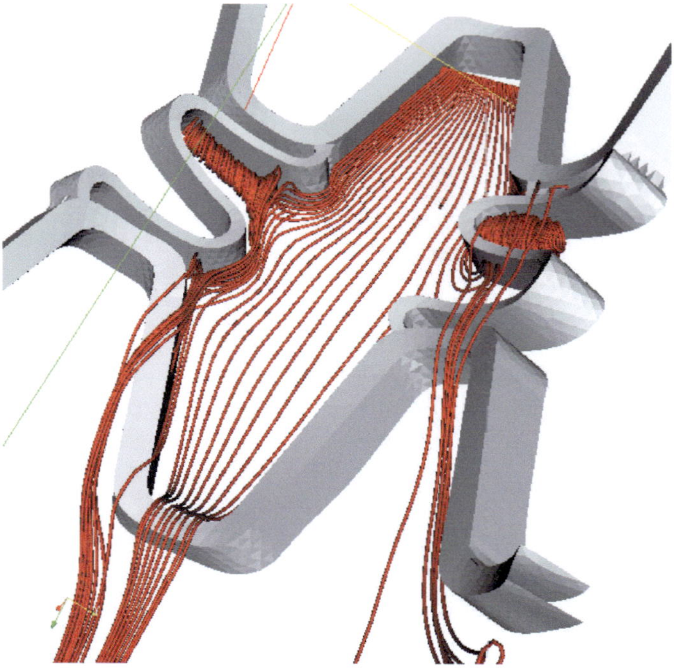

Fig. 12.15. The interaction between the stent and the blood flow visualised by means of streamlines. The proximal section is located on the top while the distal section is on the bottom

Indeed, in Fig. 12.15 we visualise the streamlines of the blood flow around the stent. This picture shows that we are dealing with a fully three-dimensional flow with recirculations, vortexes and secondary motions. For instance, we observe that the vortex induced by the presence of the link on the top left corner is stretched and absorbed in the main stream on its right side. This confirms that the vortex is not only characterised by a planar rotating flow but an out-of-plane motion is present. This secondary motion generates the displacement of the fluid from the centre of the vortex to the extrema and the fluid is thus cast out of the vortex into the main stream.

12.3.4 Analysis of drug release

The numerical simulation based on equation (12.3) shows that the drug released into the lumen is very quickly washed out by the blood flow. Indeed, the peaks of drug concentration into the lumen are reached about 40 seconds after the beginning of the release process. Conversely, the drug dynamics into the arterial walls is much slower, but after 1 hour the drug has reached the outer boundary of the arterial walls, as can be seen in Fig. 12.17 (bottom).

The drug concentration on the surface of the lumen is reported in Fig. 12.16. The highest peaks of drug concentration appear in the neighbourhood of the

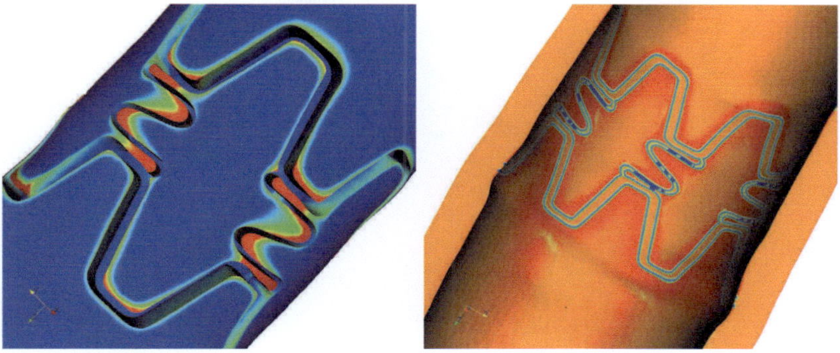

Fig. 12.16. The contour plots of the concentration on the surface of the arterial lumen at 40 seconds after the beginning of the process are shown on the left. The colour scale ranges linearly from 0 (blue) to $10^{-3}c_s^0$ (red). The mass flux exchanged between the lumen and the arterial wall is shown on the right. The red colour denotes a positive flux from the lumen to the wall, while the blue colour refers to the opposite case

links. In these regions, the concentration contours suggest that the recirculation of the blood flow interacts with the drug accumulation. In particular, the smooth and concave shape of the contours suggests that part of the drug released and accumulated in the neighbourhood of the links is transported away and may affect the arterial walls located downstream. Indeed, regions related to non-negligible concentration levels are clearly visible downstream from the stent in Fig. 12.17 (top), where the presence of the drug in the lumen is visualised by means of the iso-surface of the concentration. This means that a wide portion of the endothelium, which is often severely injured during the stent implantation, is exposed to a non-negligible drug concentration. When the drug has anti-proliferative properties, the re-endothelialisation process may be slowed down. This seems to be one of the major drawbacks of DES, and it should be further investigated.

Concerning the struts, the accumulation of drug is unexpectedly prominent upstream with respect to the blood flow. High concentration levels take place where the struts are highly curved and their curvature is convex with respect to the blood flow. This can be explained observing that blood transports the drug downstream to the location where it has been released. The accumulation of the drug takes place where this effect is hindered by the convex stent pattern with respect to the blood flow.

This balance can be analysed by means of more quantitative results. One hour after the stent implantation, almost all the drug has been released. The contact interface between the stent and the walls ensures that 15 % of the total amount of drug is released into the walls. However, more than a half of this fraction is simultaneously transferred into the lumen because of the negative concentration gradient between the lumen and the walls.

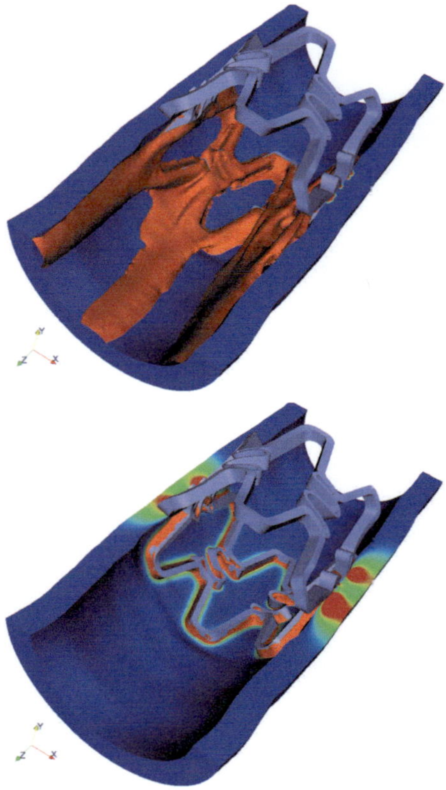

Fig. 12.17. The iso-surface corresponding to the value $10^{-5}c_s^0$ for the drug concentration in the arterial lumen and contour plots into the arterial walls, at 40 seconds (top) and 1 hour (bottom) after the beginning of the process. The colour scale ranges linearly from 0 (blue) to $10^{-3}c_s^0$ (red). The blood flow is directed from top to bottom, as depicted in Fig. 12.14

12.4 Multiscale modelling applied to surgery for the treatment of congenital heart diseases[2]

Francesco Migliavacca, Giancarlo Pennati, Rossella Balossino, and Gabriele Dubini

In this paragraph a test case is presented where the multiscale methodology (see Chapter 11) is applied to paediatric cardiac surgery. The objective is to show its efficacy in surgical planning, side by side with cardiology and cardiac

[2] This work was made possible by the far-sighted and strongly supportive cooperation with Professors Marc R. de Leval and Edward L. Bove. Financial support from the British Heart Foundation and the University of Michigan is also acknowledged.

surgery evaluations, to select the best surgical procedure to treat a complex congenital heart defect. In particular, the treatment of hypoplastic left heart syndrome (HLHS) is hereinafter considered.

12.4.1 The clinical problem

In the HLHS the left side of the heart (including the aorta, the aortic valve, the left ventricle and the mitral valve) is either underdeveloped when compared with the normal heart or absent. Blood returning from the lungs must flow through an opening in the wall between the atria (atrial septal defect). The right ventricle pumps blood into the pulmonary artery and blood reaches the aorta through a patent *ductus arteriosus*. The baby often seems normal at birth, but will come to medical attention within a few days of birth as the ductus closes. This heart defect is usually fatal within the first days or months of life unless it is treated surgically. The anatomical outcome of this surgical operation is briefly described hereinafter.

In the presence of a hypoplastic left heart the palliative procedure usually undertaken up until a few years ago was the *Norwood stage I* [354]. Figure 12.18 depicts a possible solution for the reconstructed anatomy following this operation. The basic idea of this operation is the connection of part of the systemic circulation directly with the pulmonary one after the reconstruction of a new aorta incorporating the original main pulmonary artery. Indeed, the pulmonary artery is detached from the heart above the valve and the end is oversewn. The gap between the valve and the aorta is then bridged by a homograft allowing blood to pump from the right ventricle into the aorta. To get blood into the lungs a systemic-to-pulmonary shunt is performed between the innominate artery and the right pulmonary artery.

In the recent years a new procedure [242, 447], referred to as the *Sano operation* (SO), has been proposed to treat the hypoplastic left heart. It consists mainly in the connection of the systemic circulation to the pulmonary one by means of a synthetic conduit connecting the right ventricle and the pulmonary arteries (Fig. 12.18). It seems that there may be many potential advantages to the placement of a right ventricle to pulmonary artery shunt. Diastolic coronary perfusion may be more stable and shunt thrombosis may be less likely in the perioperative period. Babies treated with a SO shunt seem better able to tolerate temporary low cardiac output and hypotension than if they had had a conventional Norwood procedure. Many questions remain regarding optimal size, location and material of the shunt, growth and distortion of the pulmonary arteries, and possible ventricular volume overload due to shunt backward flow.

12.4.2 The multiscale model

Two different 3-D detailed models of Norwood stage I procedure (Figs. 12.18a and 12.18b) have been developed: a Sano shunt operation (SO) and a systemic-to-pulmonary shunt (the modified Blalock-Taussig shunt, NO). The size of

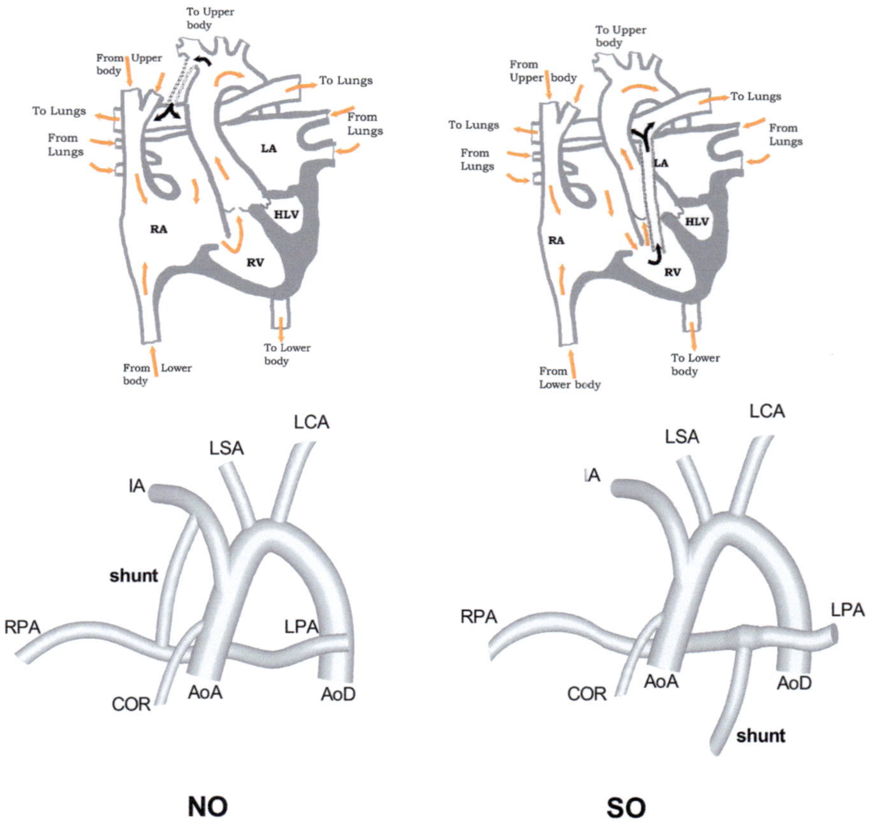

Fig. 12.18. Anatomic skemes (top) and 3-D models (bottom) of the two operations. Left: Modified Blalock-Taussig Shunt (NO) showing the reconstructed neo-aorta and the conduit between the innominate and the right pulmonary artery; right: Sano Operation (SO) showing the conduit between the right ventricle and the pulmonary arteries. Arrows indicate blood flow directions. Dark arrows indicate the blood flow through the shunt. AoA: ascending aorta; AoD: descending aorta; COR: coronary artery; HLV: hypoplstic left ventricle; LA: left atrium; IA: innominate artery; LCA: left carotid artery; LSA: left subclavian artery; LPA: left pulmonary artery; RPA: right pulmonary artery; RA: right atrium; RV: right ventricle (Modified from [328])

the conduits were 4, 5 and 6 mm for the SO model and 3, 3.5 and 4 mm for NO model. The geometric dimensions of the blood vessel were taken from angiograms of a group of patients with a modified Blalock-Taussig shunt performed during catheterisation prior to the second-stage operation. The Finite Volume Method (FVM) was adopted to solve the mass and momentum conservation equations for an incompressible, Newtonian fluid (blood density and viscosity equal to 1,060 kg m^{-3} and 0.005 kg m^{-1} s^{-1}, respectively).

The `Fluent` general-purpose fluid dynamic code (Fluent Inc., Lebanon, NH, USA) was utilised for calculations. Meshes were developed (Fig. 12.19)

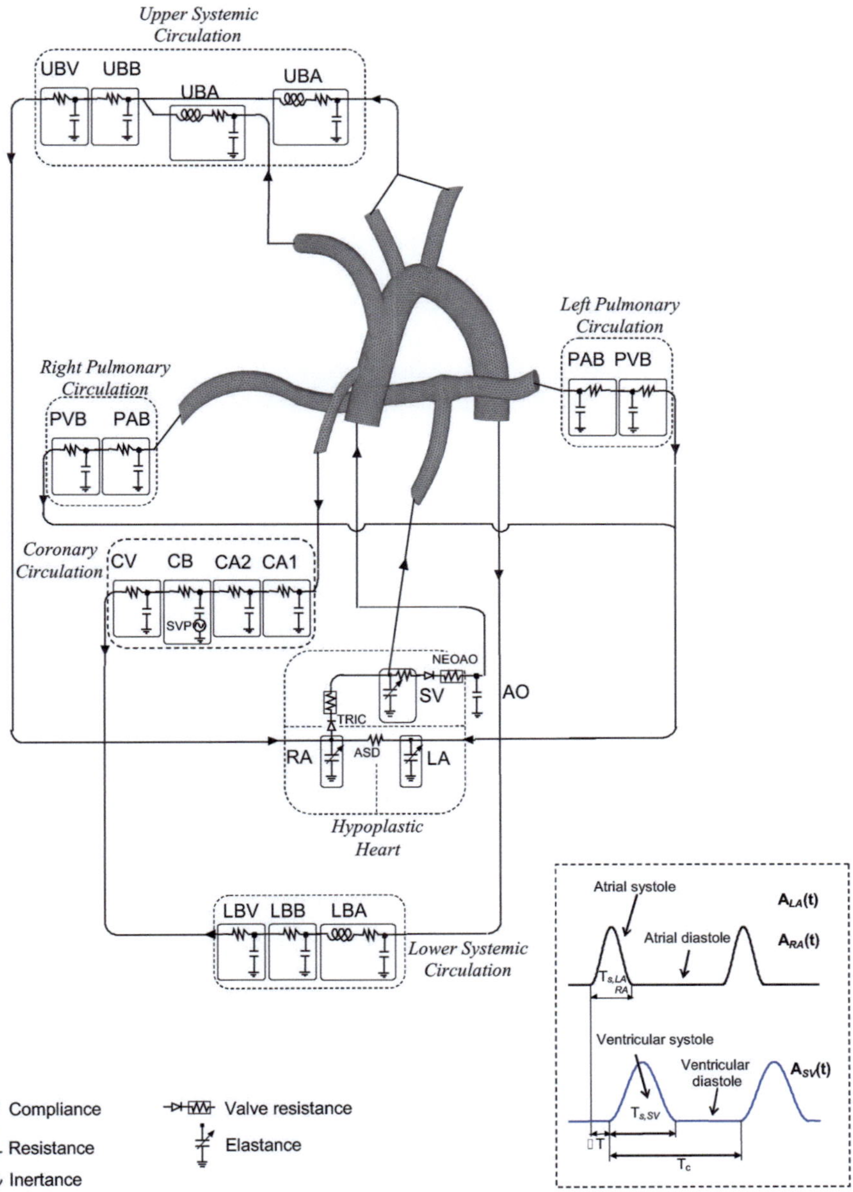

Fig. 12.19. Coupled 3-D and lumped parameter models for the Sano operation. AO: aorta; ASD: atrial septal defect; CA: coronary arteries; CB: coronary bed; CV: coronary veins; LA: left atrium; LBA: lower body arteries; LBB: lower body bed; LBV: lower body veins; NEOAO: aortic valve; PAB: pulmonary arterial bed; PVB: pulmonary venous bed; RA: right atrium; UBA: upper body arteries; UBB: upper body bed; UBV: upper body veins; SVB: systemic venous bed; SV: single ventricle; SVP: single ventricle pressure; SLV: systemic large veins; TRIC: tricuspid valve (Modified from [328])

including about 130,000 4-node tetrahedral cells. The implicit backward Euler method was utilised to as time integration technique, implementing a fixed time increment equal to $\Delta t = 10^{-4}$s. A segregated solver was chosen. Four cardiac cycles were simulated for each model to guarantee a periodic solution.

The circulatory network and the cardiac function were taken into account by means of a lumped parameter model (Fig. 12.19). This model is made of four subsystems: heart, systemic, pulmonary and coronary circulations; it was built following the methodology previously adopted to model the foetal [376] and neonatal circulations [332, 378]. As regards the heart, the pressure within any cardiac chamber (P_{cc}) varies throughout the cardiac cycle due to changes of volume within the chamber (V_{cc}) and to contractile activity of the sarcomeres. Active (systolic) and passive (diastolic) properties of the myocardium account for the total chamber pressure. This can be expressed mathematically as [467]:

$$P_{cc}(t) = P_{cc,active}(t, V_{cc}) + P_{cc,passive}(t, V_{cc}), \quad cc = \{\mathrm{SV}, \mathrm{RA}, \mathrm{LA}\}. \qquad (12.7)$$

Both active and passive pressure-volume relationships are non-linear [488], despite the usual practice of approximating the active curve as a straight line [515]. The active relationship changes during systole as contractile activity of the cardiac chamber changes. Furthermore, the slope (i.e., the elastance) of the active curve decreases with increasing volume. This behaviour was mimicked with a time-varying elastance $E_{cc}(V_{cc}, t)$, which depends also on chamber volume. This elastance, which accounts for the isometric pressure-volume function, was coupled with a constant viscous term R_{wall}, which is related to the dissipative properties of the myocardium:

$$P_{cc,active}(t, V_{cc}) = E_{cc}(t, V_{cc})\,(V_{cc} - V_{u,cc}) + R_{wall,cc}\frac{dV_{cc}}{dt} \qquad (12.8)$$

where $V_{u,cc}$ is the unstressed volume of the cardiac chamber (i.e., the volume at zero pressure). The viscous term was considered only for the ventricle [17].

Elastance can be expressed as a product of a pulsatile activation time-function Acc(t) and a purely volume elastance term E^*_{cc}:

$$E_{cc}(t, V_{cc}) = A_{cc}(t)E^*_{cc}(V_{cc}). \qquad (12.9)$$

Ranging between 0 during the diastole and 1 at the end of systole as a squared sinusoidal function, $A_{cc}(t)$ describes the excitation–relaxation pattern of the myocardial sarcomeres (i.e., the muscle basic contractile units) [17, 515]. Activation function has the same form for the single ventricle and the atria, but has different initiation (ΔT) and temporal lapse. The expression of $E^*_{cc}(V_{cc})$ depends on the pressure-volume relationship during systole of the cardiac chamber. For both atria, a linear pressure-volume function was assumed so that $E^*_{RA}(V_{RA})$ and $E^*_{LA}(V_{LA})$ are constant. For the single ventricle, a second-order polynomial function was adopted where the elastance decreases linearly with increasing volume:

$$E^*_{SV}(V_{SV}) = E^*_{1,SV} + E^*_{2,SV}\,(V_{SV} - V_{u,SV})\,. \qquad (12.10)$$

At diastole, when muscle fibres are relaxed, both the single ventricle and the atria fill through an exponential pressure-volume function [486,515], reflecting the non-linear elasticity of the relaxed muscle and pericardium:

$$P_{cc,passive}(t, V_{cc}) = P_{0,cc}\left(e^{K_{E,cc}(V_{cc}-V_{u,cc})} - 1\right) \qquad (12.11)$$

where $P_{0,cc}$ and $K_{E,cc}$ are constant parameters. Atrio-ventricular (tricuspid) and ventriculo-arterial (neoaorta) valves were mimicked as a series of an ideal unidirectional valve and resistance. Flows through these valves were described by a non-linear relationship between the pressure drop $\Delta P(t)$ and the volume flow rate $Q(t)$ across them:

$$\Delta P_{valv} = K_{valv} Q^2 \qquad valv = \{\mathrm{TRIC}, \mathrm{NEOAO}\}\,. \qquad (12.12)$$

Finally, the non-restrictive atrial septal defect (ASD), which allows flow from the left into the right atrium, was simulated as a constant resistance (R_{ASD}). The systemic circulation was divided into seven compartments, describing the arterial and venous districts located in the upper and lower body. The left and right pulmonary arterial and venous beds were defined by four compartments. The parameter values for the systemic and pulmonary circulations were obtained from previous studies of ours [332, 378], while those for the coronary circulation were scaled from the adult model [311] according to the criteria reported in Pennati and Fumero [377]. Tables 12.2 and 12.3 list the values adopted for this study with the nomenclature as in Fig. 12.19, which depicts the SO coupled to the whole circulatory network. For the whole simulation the heart rate (HR) was 120 beats per minute. HR and duration of the cardiac cycle ($T_c = 1/HR$) were derived from a clinical data set. The duration of ventricular systole ($T_{s,SV} = 0.16 + 0.3T_c$), which increases linearly with the duration of cycle [17], and duration ($T_{s,LA} = T_{s,RA} = 0.3T_c$ and time advance ($\Delta T = 0.02T_c$) of atrial systole were calculated as fractions of the cycle duration [472]. The resulting ordinary differential equation system arising from the lumped parameter model was solved with an explicit Euler method implemented in the `Fluent` package by means of a purposely developed user-defined function. This allowed us to obtain a fully coupled solution at each time-step without stopping the `Fluent` execution. In particular, uniform, time-dependent normal stresses were derived from pressure values calculated in the lumped parameter model and imposed at the boundaries of the 3-D model, while the local velocity profiles were not forced but calculated at each time instant by `Fluent`. After spatial averaging they were fed back to the lumped parameter model. All simulations were carried out on a Pentium IV Personal Computer.

12.4.3 The results

Comparing the cardiac output (CO) in the SO model with the NO models when the same shunt size is used (4 mm), a higher value was found for the

Table 12.2. Values of the parameters describing the circulation. (AO: aorta; CA: coronary arteries; CB: coronary bed; CV: coronary veins; LBA: arterial lower body, LBB: bed lower body; LBV: venous lower body; LPA: left pulmonary artery; RPA: right pulmonary artery; UBA: arterial upper body, UBB: bed upper body; UBV: venous upper body)

R	*mmHg s/ml*	L	*mmHg s²/ml*	C	*ml/mmHg*
		Pulmonary circulation			
R_{RPA1}	0.83376			C_{RPA1}	0.02039
R_{RPA2}	0.02194			C_{RPA2}	0.44375
R_{LPA1}	0.83376			C_{LPA1}	0.02039
R_{LPA2}	0.02194			C_{LPA2}	0.44375
		Upper body circulation			
R_{UBL}	14.04478	L_{UBL}	0.02138	C_{UBL}	0.088592
R_{UBR}	14.04478	L_{UBR}	0.02138	C_{UBR}	0.088592
R_{UBB}	0.64510			C_{UBB}	0.15515
R_{UBV}	0.16529			C_{UBV}	2.03945
		Lower body circulation			
R_{LBA}	7.02239	L_{LBA}	0.01069	C_{LBA}	0.077575
R_{LBB}	0.64510			C_{LBB}	0.077575
R_{LBV}	0.16529			C_{LBC}	2.03945
		Coronary circulation			
R_{CA1}	10.6739			C_{CA1}	1.94351×10^{-3}
R_{CA2}	10.6739			C_{CA2}	5.18269×10^{-3}
R_{CB}	21.3477			C_{CB}	7.77404×10^{-3}
R_{CV}	10.6739			C_{CV}	0.5×10^{-4}
		Aorta			
				C_{AO}	0.0415548

NO model (2.38–2.43 *vs.* 2.09 l min^{-1}). This observation led to the conclusion that the shunt to be adopted in the SO should be bigger than that selected for the NO. This was already known in clinical practice as reported also by clinical studies. Thus results of this mathematical study are consistent with this practice. The comparison between the two technical procedures in terms of hemodynamics outcomes should hence be done comparing small NO shunts with greater SO shunts (for example, 3 mm NO *vs.* 4 mm SO, 3.5 mm NO *vs.* 5 mm SO, 4 mm NO *vs.* 6 mm SO). From volume flow rate values it is possible to calculate also the oxygen saturations. Similar arterial saturations were obtained with greater SO shunts and smaller NO shunts [328].

Keeping in mind this observation, the results showed that the SO models exhibit, when compared with the NO models with similar CO and aortic pressure, lower pulmonary-to-systemic flow ratio, lower arterial pulse pressure (difference between the maximum and minimum pressures in a cardiac cycle)

Table 12.3. Values of the parameters describing the heart

Compartment	*Parameter*	*Value*	*Units*
Single ventricle	$E^*_{1,SV}$	8.5	mmHg/ml
Right atrium	$E^*_{2,SV}$	-0.042	mmHg/ml^2
	$R_{\text{wall},SV}$	0.09	mmHg s/ml
	$P_{0,SV}$	0.9	mmHg
	$K_{E,SV}$	0.062	ml^{-1}
	$V_{u,SV}$	4	ml
Left atrium	E^*_{RA}	7.35	mmHg/ml
	$P_{0,RA}$	0.17	mmHg
	$K_{E,RA}$	0.484	ml^{-1}
	$V_{u,RA}$	1	ml
ASD	R_{ASD}	0.001	mmHg s/ml
Tricuspid	K_{TRIC}	0.00004	mmHg s^2/ml^2
Neoaorta	K_{NEOAO}	0.0004	mmHg s^2/ml^2

and lower pulmonary arterial pressure, higher coronary perfusion pressure (difference between the diastolic aortic and the diastolic right atrial pressure), which are consistent with literature measurements [307, 308]. Figure 12.20 reports some of those data in a graphical and more readable form. Interestingly, mathematical models also predicted behaviours which are not confirmed at the moment by clinical evidence, except for a work by Ohye et al. [356]. Shunt Doppler analysis performed in one SO and one NO patient demonstrated continuous anterograde flow (i.e., from heart to periphery) through both systole and diastole in the NO patient and anterograde flow through the conduit only during systole for the SO patient.

Figure 12.21 reports the time tracing of the maximum velocity (corresponding to the velocity usually recorded by a Doppler analysis) in the NO model with 4 mm shunt and SO with 6 mm. An almost stable velocity occurred in the NO model while reversal flow during diastole was observed in the SO model. The same figure also shows the axial velocity profiles at different cross-sections along the two shunts at four instants of the cardiac cycle.

12.4.4 Conclusions

Many computationally challenging problems that arise in science and engineering exhibit multi-scale behaviour. In this test case the multiscale simulation methodology has been applied to a surgical procedure whose haemodynamic outcomes are still difficult to foresee in the clinical practice. The presented test case still suffers from limitations such as the assumption of a rigid arterial wall in the 3-D model and the absence of any feed back control (except for the Starling law of the heart). For instance, changes in the

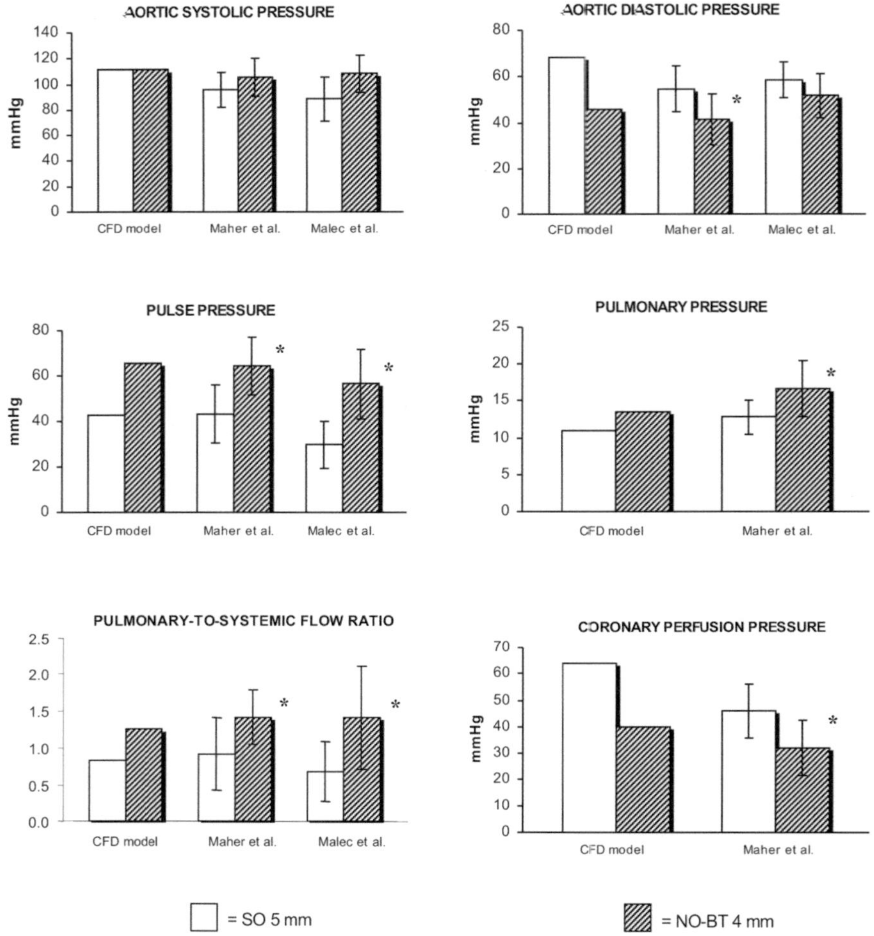

Fig. 12.20. Comparison between CFD simulation and clinical observed data in terms of arterial and coronary perfusion pressure and pulmonary-to-systemic flow ratio. Computational data refer to the 5 mm SO and the 4 mm NO models. Clinical data are from Maher et al., 2003 [307] and Malec et al., 2003 [308]. * Statistically significant differences (Modified from [328])

coronary perfusion do not affect the cardiac contractility. On the other hand, use of simpler, stand-alone 3-D or lumped parameter models would not yield results as meaningful as those obtained here. Indeed, the adopted approach allows one to quantitatively evaluate the postoperative situation, thus suggesting its use as a tool for preoperative surgical planning. In conclusion, this case study illustrates a very successful application of the methodology in the research about paediatric cardiovascular diseases wherein patient-specific anatomy and physiology are used in an engineering model to predict surgical outcome and to guide patient management.

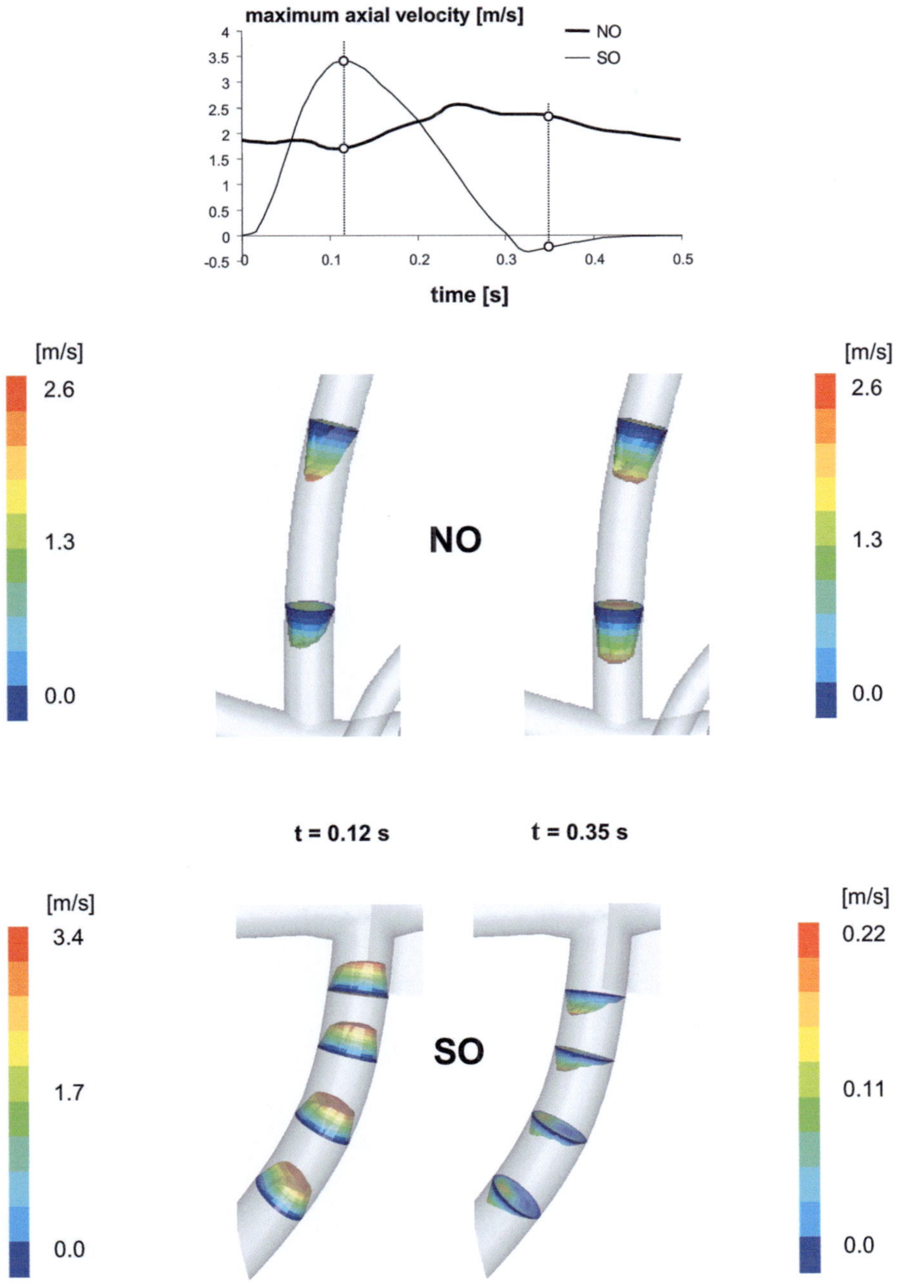

Fig. 12.21. Shunt flow tracings in the 4 mm NO and 6 mm SO models. Velocity profiles along the two shunt models at two different instants of the cardiac cycle

Glossary of medical terms

Name	Explanation
Actin	A fibrous protein which together with myosin provides the contractile force of muscles
Action potential	A wave of electrical discharge that travels along the membrane of a cell
Aerobic	Involving oxygen (opp. anaerobic)
Afferent	toward (opp. efferent)
Anaerobic	Not involving oxygen (opp. aerobic)
Anastomosis	A direct connection between arteries or veins.
Aneurysm	A localised dilation or ballooning of a blood vessel by more than 50 % of the diameter of the vessel. If broken can lead to severe haemorrhage and rapid death. Aneurysms most commonly occur in arteries at the base of the brain (cerebral aneurysm) and in the aorta (aortic aneurysm). The understanding of the basic mechanisms of the genesis and progression of an aneurysms is still matter of active medical research
Anterior	Towards the front (opp. posterior)
Atheroma	Abnormal lesions in the artery walls causing atherosclerosis (also called arteriosclerosis)
Autonomic nervous system	The part of the nervous system not under conscious control
Bilipid membrane	A membrane composed of two layers of lipids arranged so that their hydrophilic head groups are facing outward and their hydrophobic tails are facing each other, the fundamental component of all cell membranes
Cardiac	Pertaining to the heart
Catabolism	The metabolic breakdown of complex molecules into simpler ones, often resulting in a release of energy
Catabolites	The products of catabolism
Coagulate	To transform from a liquid to a solid form, generally applied to the clotting of blood
Cytoskeleton	The fibrous proteins within a cell which provide mechanical integrity to the cell

Depolarise	The decrease, or eliminate, the electric potential across a membrane
Diastole	The period of cardiac relaxation (opp. diastole).
Distal	Further away (opp. proximal)
Efferent	away from (opp. afferent)
Electrocardiogram	The electrical signal caused by the depolarisation of the myocardium during the cardiac cycle
Embolus	An air bubble, fat globule or blood clot drifting in the blood
Endocrine	Pertaining to the glands that excrete hormones.
Endothelium	The monolayer of cells lining blood vessels
Erythrocytes	Also known as "red blood cells", they are the most common type of blood cell and are the vertebrate body principal means of delivering oxygen from the lungs or gills to body tissues via the blood (see also haemoglobin)
Extravasation	Leaving a blood vessel
Fascia	Sheets of connective tissue, largely collegen, that surround or separate muscle fibres
Focal	occurring at specific locations
Gene expression	The process by which a gene DNA sequence is converted into the structures and functions of a cell
Glycocalyx	The polysaccharide or glycoprotein covering on a cell surface
Haemoglobin	The iron-containing oxygen-transport protein in the red cells of the blood in mammals and other animals. Haemoglobin in vertebrates transports oxygen from the lungs to the rest of the body. Haemoglobin also has a variety of other gas-transport and effect-modulation duties, which vary from species to species
Haemorrhage	Haemorrhage is the medical term for bleeding. In common usage, a haemorrhage means a particularly severe bleeding; although technically it just means any escape of blood to extravascular space. The complete loss of blood is referred to as exsanguination
Hematocrit	The hematocrit is the percent of whole blood that is composed of red blood cells. The hematocrit is a measure of the number and the size of red blood cells
Humoral	Relating to bodily fluids, particularly serum.
Hyperplasia	An abnormal increase in the as cells composing a tissue

Inflammation	The first response of the immune system to infection or irritation which triggers the immune cascade
Lesion	A localised abnormality in tissue organisation.
Leukocytes	Also known as "white cells", they form a component of the blood. They are produced in the bone marrow and help to defend the body against infectious disease and foreign materials as part of the immune system. There are normally between 4×10^9 and 11×10^9 white blood cells in a litre of healthy adult blood
Matrix	The ground substance of connective tissue
Metabolism	The chemical processes occurring within a cell that are necessary for the maintenance of life
Metabolites	The products of metabolism
Mitochondria	An organelle in the cytoplasm of cells containing genetic material and many enzymes important for cell metabolism, including those responsible for the conversion of food to usable energy
Mucosa	A mucous membrane containing an epithelium and excretory cells
Myocardium	The cardiac muscle tissue of the heart
Myofiber	A muscle fibre composed of myocytes
Myosin	A protein which, together with actin, is responsible for the generation of contractile force in muscles
Neural	Pertaining to nerves
Ostium	An opening or passage
Pacemaker	The collection of specialist myocytes in the sinoatrial node which oscillate electrically to initiate the cardiac cycle
Parasympathetic	The part of the autonomic nervous system that is generally responsible for conserving energy and reducing metabolism. (opp. sympathetic)
Plaque	a localised abnormal patch on a body part
Posterior	toward the back (opp. anterior)
Prolapse	the abnormal protrusion of a part of an organ, in particular the movement of a cardiac valve into its upstream chamber
Proliferate	To grow or multiply rapidly by producing new tissue or cells
Proximal	Closer (opp. distal)
Pulmonary	Pertaining to the lung
Red blood cells	See erythrocytes

Remodelling	The change of tissue morphology due to external or internal stimulus
Renal	Pertaining to the kidney
Sarcoplasm	The cytoplasm of the muscle cell
Septum	A partition that divides an organ; specifically in the heart it is the layer of myocardium that divides the left chambers from the right
Serous membrane	The membrane composed of epithelium and underlying loose connective tissue; particularly the lining of the pericardial, pleural and peritoneal cavities
Smooth muscle cells	Non-striated, involuntary muscle found in vessel walls
Stasis	An unchanging state
Stenosis	A constriction or narrowing of a passageway
Stent	A short narrow tube, often in the form of a mesh, that is inserted into the lumen of a vessel such as an artery or bile duct to keep a previously blocked passageway open
Sympathetic	The part of the autonomic nervous system that is generally responsible for elevating metabolism and increasing alertness (opp. parasympathetic).
Systemic	pertaining to the cardiovascular system with the exception of vessels perfusing the lungs (opp. pulmonary)
Systole	The period of cardiac contraction (opp. diastole).
Thrombus	a blood clot
Vasoactive	Stimuli that affect the cardiovascular system, particularly vasoconstriction and vasodilation
Vasoconstriction	A reduction of the diameter of blood vessels, particularly the arterioles that control the distribution of blood in the body (opp. vasodilation)
Vasodilation	An increase of the diameter of blood vessels, particularly the arterioles (opp. vasoconstriction)
White blood cells	See leukocytes
Windkessel	The mechanism by which the elastic arteries smooth out the cardiac pulse by expanding during systole and contracting during diastole, the principle was used in early fire engine pumps by including an air chamber (Windkessel in German) downstream of the pump

Symbol explanation

div	The divergence of a vector field
div	The divergence of a tensor field
$\dfrac{Dv}{Dt}$	The material derivative of the field v
$\Omega(t)$	The domain at a given time t
$\boldsymbol{\nabla} v$	The gradient operator
$\boldsymbol{\nabla}\mathbf{v}^T$	Transpose gradient operator $\boldsymbol{\nabla}\mathbf{v}^T = (\boldsymbol{\nabla}\mathbf{v})^T$
$\widehat{\boldsymbol{F}}$	The deformation gradient at time t
J	The Jacobian of the deformation at time t, $J = \lvert\widehat{\boldsymbol{F}}\rvert$
$\mathcal{L}_t$	The Lagrangian Mapping at time t
Δ	The Lapace operator
P	The pressure
$\mathbb{R}$	The set of real numbers
$\boldsymbol{\sigma}$	The Cauchy stress tensor
$(\boldsymbol{u} \cdot \boldsymbol{\nabla})$	The convective operator associated with the velocity field $\boldsymbol{u}$
$\widehat{\Omega}$	The reference domain
$\mathrm{d}\gamma$	The surface measure
ρ	The density
$\underset{\sim}{\eta}$	The displacement vector
$\boldsymbol{E}$	The Green-Lagrange tensor
$\widehat{\boldsymbol{x}}$	The Lagrangian space coordinate
$\widehat{\boldsymbol{\varphi}}$	The motion map
$\boldsymbol{n}$	The normal to a domain boundary (outward oriented)
$\frac{\partial u}{\partial n}$	The normal derivative: $\frac{\partial u}{\partial n} = \boldsymbol{\nabla} u \cdot \boldsymbol{n}$
$\mathcal{P}$	The permeability
$\widehat{\boldsymbol{\Pi}}$	The Piola-Kirchhoff 1st tensor
p	The Scaled pressure $P = P/\rho$
$\widehat{\boldsymbol{\Sigma}}$	The Piola-Kirchhoff 2d tensor
$\boldsymbol{s}$	Extra diagonal part of the rate of deformation tensor
ε	The strain tensor
$\boldsymbol{D}$	The rate of deformation tensor
$\boldsymbol{u}$	The velocity
μ	The dynamic viscosity
ν	The kinematic viscosity $\nu = \mu/\rho$

References

1. V. Agoshkov, A. Quarteroni, and G. Rozza. Shape design in aorto-coronaric bypass anastomoses using perturbation theory. *SIAM J. Numer. Anal.*, 44(1):367–384, 2006
2. J. Alastruey, S.M. Moore, K.H. Parker, T. David, J. Peiró, and S.J. Sherwin. Reduced modelling of blood flow in the cerebral circulation: Coupling 1-D, 0-D and cerebral auto-regulation models. *Int. J. Num. Meth. Fluids*, 56(8):1061–1067, 2008
3. J. Alastruey, K.H. Parker, J. Peiró, S.M. Byrd, and S.J. Sherwin. Modelling the circle of Willis to assess the effects of anatomic variations and occlusions on cerebral flows. *J. Biomech.*, 40(8):1794–1805, 2007
4. J. Alastruey, K.H. Parker, J. Peiró, and S.J. Sherwin. Can the modified Allen's test always detect sufficient collateral flow in the hand? A computational study. *Comp. Meth. Biomech. Biomed. Engng.*, 9(6):353–361, Dec 2006
5. J. Alastruey, K.H. Parker, J. Peiró, and S.J. Sherwin. Lumped parameter outflow models for 1-D blood flow simulations: Effect on pulse waves and parameter estimation. *Comm. Comp. Phys.*, 4(2):317–336, 2008
6. G. Ali, A. Bartel, and M. Gunther. Parabolic differential-algebraic models in electrical network design. *Multiscale Model. Simul.*, 4:813–838, 2005
7. D. Amadori, F. Ferrari, and L. Formaggia. Derivation and analysis of a fluid-dynamical model in thin and long elastic vessels. *Networks and ether. media*, 2(1):99–125, 2007
8. N. Amenta and M. Bern. Surface reconstruction by Voronoi filtering. *Discrete and Computational Geometry*, 22:481–504, 1999
9. N. Amenta, S. Choi, and R.K. Kolluri. The power crust. In *Proceedings of Solid Modeling '01*, pp. 249–260, 2001
10. M. Anand and K.R. Rajagopal. A shear-thinning viscoelastic fluid model for describing the flow of blood. *Int. J. Cardiovasc. Med. and Science*, 4:59–68, 2004
11. J.L. Anderson and D.M. Malone. Mechanism of osmotic flow in porous membranes. *Biophys. J.*, 14:957–982, 1974
12. L. Antiga, B. Ene-Iordache, and A. Remuzzi. Computational geometry for patient-specific reconstruction and meshing of blood vessels from MR and CT angiography. *IEEE T. Med. Imaging.*, 22(5):674–684, May 2003

13. C.H. Arthur Chang, D. Coutand, and S. Shkoller. Navier-stokes equations interacting with a nonlinear elastic fluid shell. http://arxiv.org/abs/math.AP/0611670, 2006
14. U.M. Ascher and L.R. Petzold. *Computer methods for ordinary differential equations and differential-algebraic equations.* Society for Industrial and Applied Mathematics, Philadelphia, 1998. U.M. Ascher, L.R. Petzold. ill.
15. G. Astarita and G. Marrucci. *Principles of Non-Newtonian Fluid Mechanics.* McGraw Hill, London, 1974
16. M. Astorino, J.-F. Gerbeau, O. Pantz, and K. Traoré. Fluid-structure interaction and multi-body contact. Application to aortic valves. *Comp. Meth. Appl. Mech. Eng.*, 2009 (electronic version)
17. G. Avanzolini, P. Barbini, A. Cappello, and A. Cevese. Time-varying mechanical properties of the left ventricle. a computer simulation. *IEEE Trans. Biomed. Engng.*, 32:756–763, 1985
18. F. Avnaim, J.-D. Boissonnat, O. Devillers, F.P. Preparata, and M. Yvinec. Evaluating signs of determinants using single-precision arithmetic. *Algorithmica*, 17:111–132, 1997
19. F. Baaijens. A fictitious domain/mortar element method for fluid-structure interaction. *Int. J. Numer. Meth. Fluids*, 35:743–761, 2001
20. L. Back, J. Radbill, and D. Crawford. Analysis of oxygen transport from pulsatile, viscous blood flow to diseased coronary artery of man. *J. Biomech.*, 10:763–774, 1977
21. S. Badia, F. Nobile, and C. Vergara. Fluid-structure partitioned procedures based on robin transmission conditions. *J. Comput. Phys.*, 227(14):7027–7051, 2008
22. S. Badia, A. Quaini, and A. Quarteroni. Splitting methods based on algebraic factorization for fluid-structure interaction. *SIAM J. Scient. Comp.*, 30(4):1778–1805, 2008
23. R.L. Baek, S. Gleason, and K.R. Rajagopal, and J.D. Humphrey. Theory of small on large: Potential utility in computations of fluid-solid interactions in arteries. *Comp. Meth. Appl. Mech. Eng.*, 196(31):3070–3078, 2007
24. J.M. Ball. Remarks on blow up and non existence theorems in nonlinear evolution equations. *Quart. J. Math. Oxford*, 28(2):473–486, 1977
25. A.C.L. Barnard, W.A. Hunt, W.P. Timlake, and E. Varley. A theory of fluid flow in compliant tubes. *Biophys. J.*, 6:717–724, 1966
26. H.A. Barnes. Thixotropy – a review. *J. Non-Newtonian Fluid Mech.*, 70:1–33, 1997
27. H.A. Barnes. The yield stress – a review of $\pi\alpha\nu\tau\alpha\rho\epsilon\iota$ – everything flows? *J. Non-Newtonian Fluid Mech.*, 81:133–178, 1999
28. H.A. Barnes, J.F. Hutton, and K. Walters. *An Introduction to Rheology.* Elsevier, Amsterdam, 1989
29. H.A. Barnes and K. Walters. The yield stress myth? *Rheol. Acta*, 24:323–326, 1985
30. K.J. Bathe and H. Zhang. Finite element developments for general fluid flows with structural interactions. *Int. J. Numer. Meth. Engng.*, 60(1):213–232, 2004
31. W.H. Bauer and E.A. Collins. Thixotropy and dilatancy. In F.R. Eirich (ed.), *Rheology: Theory and Applications*, volume 4. Academic Press, New York, 1967

32. C. Begue, C. Conca, F. Murat, and O. Pironneau. *Les equations de Stokes et de Navier-Stokes avec condtions aux limites sur la pression*, pp. 179–264. Pittman, RNM Longman, 1988. In H. Brezis, J. Lions (eds): Nonlinear Partial Differential Equations and their applications, College de France, Vol. IX. Pitman, Boston
33. H. Beirão da Veiga. On the existence of strong solutions to a coupled fluid-structure evolution problem. *J. Math. Fluid. Mech.*, 6:21–52, 2004
34. J.L. Bentley and J.H. Friedman. Data structures for range searching. *ACM Comput. Surv.*, 11(4):397–409, 1979
35. S. Berger, L. Talbot, and L.-S. Yao. Flow in curved pipes. *Ann. Rev. Fluid Mech.*, 15:461–512, 1983
36. P. Bergeron. Radiation doses to patients in neurointerventional procedures. *American J. of Neuroradiology*, 15(10):1809–1812, 1994
37. C. Bernardi, Y. Maday, and A.T. Patera. Domain decomposition by the mortar element method. In *Asymptotic and numerical methods for partial differential equations with critical parameters (Beaune, 1992)*, volume 384 of *NATO Adv. Sci. Inst. Ser. C Math. Phys. Sci.*, pages 269–286. Kluwer Acad. Publ., Dordrecht, 1993
38. C. Bernardi, Y. Maday, and A.T. Patera. A new nonconforming approach to domain decomposition: the mortar element method. In *Nonlinear partial differential equations and their applications. Collge de France Seminar, Vol. XI (Paris, 1989–1991)*, volume 299 of *Pitman Res. Notes Math. Ser.*, pp. 13–51. Longman Sci. Tech., 1994
39. H.M. Blackburn and S.J. Sherwin. Instability modes and transition of pulsatile flow: pulse-period dependence. *J. Fluid Mech.*, 573:57–88, 2007
40. T.D. Blacker and M. Stephenson. Paving: A new approach to automated quadrilateral mesh generation. *Int. J. Numer. Meth. Engng.*, 32:811–847, 1991
41. T.D. Blaker and R.J. Meyers. Seams and wedges in plastering: A 3D hexahedral mesh generation algorithm. *Engng. with Computers*, 2(9):83–93, 1993
42. J. Bloomenthal. Polygonization of implicit surfaces. *Comp. Aided Geom. Design*, 5:341–355, 1988
43. H.G. Bogren and M.H. Buonocore. 4D magnetic resonance velocity mapping of blood flow patterns in the aorta in young vs. elderly normal subjects. *J. of Magnetic Resonance Imaging*, 10(5):861–869, 1999
44. J.D. Boissonnat and F. Cazals. Smooth surface reconstruction via natural neighbour interpolation of distance functions. *Comp. Geometry. Theory and Appl.*, 22(1-3):185–203, 2002
45. N. Bom, W. Li, A.F. van der Steen, C.T. Lancee, E.I. Cespedes, C.J. Slager, and C.L. de Korte. New developments in intravascular ultrasound imaging. *Eur. J. Ultrasound*, 7(1):9–14, 1998
46. R.M. Bookchin and V.L. Lew. Pathophysiology of sickle cell anemia [review]. *Hematology /Oncology Clinics of North America*, 10:1241–1253, 1996
47. A.I. Borisenko and I.E. Tarapov. *Vector and tensor analysis with applications.* Dover Inc., New York, 1979
48. K. Boukir, Y. Maday, B. Métivet, and E. Razafindrakoto. A high-order characteristics/finite element method for the incompressible Navier-Stokes equations. *Int. J. Num. Meth. Fluids*, 25(12):1421–1454, 1997
49. R.L. Bratzler, G.M. Chisolm, C.K. Colton, K.A. Smith, and R.S. Lees. The distribution of labeled low-density lipoproteins across the rabbit thoracic aorta in vivo. *Atherosclerosis*, 28:289–307, 1977

50. E. Braunwald. *Braunwald's Heart Disease: A Textbook of Cardiovascular Medicine*, 7th ed. Saunders, Philadephia, 2005
51. H. Brezis. *Analyse fonctionnelle, Thorie et applications.* Masson, Paris, 1983
52. A. Bugalho de Moura. *The geometrical multiscale modelling of the cardiovascular system: coupling 3D FSI and 1D models.* PhD thesis, Politecnico di Milano, 2007
53. R. Burattini and G. Gnudi. Computer identification of models for the arterial tree input impedance: comparison between two simple models and first experimental results. *Med. Biol. Eng. Comp.*, 20:134–144, 1982
54. M. Bureau, J.C. Healy, D. Bourgoin, and M. Joly. Rheological hysteresis of blood at low shear rate. *Biorheol.*, 17:191–203, 1980
55. E. Burman and M.A. Fernández. Stabilization of explicit coupling in fluid-structure interaction involving fluid incompressibility. Submitted. Available as INRIA Research Report, RR-6455, Feb 2008
56. E. Burman and M.A. Fernández. Stabilized explicit coupling for fluid-structure interaction using Nitsche's method. *C. R. Acad. Sci. Paris Sr. I Math.*, 345(8):467–472, 2007
57. A.C. Burton. *Physiology and the Biophysics of the Circulation.* Year Book Medical Publishers Inc., Chicago, 1972
58. F. Calabrò and P. Zunino. Analysis of parabolic problems on partitioned domains with nonlinear conditions at the interface: application to mass transfer through semi-permeable membranes. *Math. Mod. Meth. Appl. Sciences*, 16(4):479–501, 2006
59. S.A. Canann, S. Saigal, and S.J. Owen (eds.). *Special issue of the International J. for Numerical Methods in Fluids on 'Unstructured Mesh Generation'*, volume 49. Wiley, New York, 2000
60. C. Canuto, M.Y. Hussaini, A. Quarteroni, and T.A. Zang. *Spectral methods in fluid dynamics.* Springer-Verlag, New York, 1988
61. C.G. Caro, N.J. Cheshire, and N.J. Watkins. Preliminary comparative study of small amplitude helical and conventional eptfe arteriovenous shunts in pigs. *J. Roy. Soc. Interface*, 2:261–266, 2005
62. C.G. Caro, T.J. Pedley, R.C. Schroter, and W.A. Seed. *The Mechanics of the Circulation.* Oxford University Press, Oxford, 1978
63. C.G. Caro, D.J. Doorly, M. Tarnawaski, K.T. Scott, Q. Long, and C.L. Dumoulin. Non-planar curvature and branching of arteries and non-planar type flow. *Proc. Roy. Soc. London, Ser. A*, 452:185–197, 1996
64. C.G. Caro, J.M. Fitz-Gerald, and R.C. Schroter. Atheroma and arterial wall shear stress. observations, correlation and proposal of a shear dependent mass transfer mechanism for atherogenesis. *Proc. Roy. Soc. London, Ser. B*, 177:109–159, 1971
65. C.G. Caro and R.M. Nerem. Transport of 14c-4-cholesterol between serum and wall in the perfused dog common carotid artery. *Circ. Res.*, 32:187–205, 1973
66. C.G. Caro, T.J. Pedley, R.C. Schroter, and W.A. Seed. *The mechanics of the circulation.* Oxford University Press, Oxford, 1978
67. J. Carr, W. Fright, and R. Beatson. Surface interpolation with radial basis functions for medical imaging. *IEEE T. Med. Imaging.*, 16(1):96–107, February 1997
68. P.J. Carreau. Rheological equations from network theories. *J. of Rheology*, 16:99–127, 1972

69. N. Casson. A flow equation for pigment-oil suspensions of printing ink type. In *Rheology of Disperse Systems*, pages 84–102. Pergamon, London, 1959
70. P. Causin, J.-F. Gerbeau, and F. Nobile. Added-mass effect in the design of partitioned algorithms for fluid-structure problems. *Comp. Meth. Appl. Mech. Eng.*, 194(42–44):4506–4527, 2005
71. J.R. Cebral, R. Löhner, P.L. Choyke, and P.J. Yim. Merging of intersecting triangulations for finite element modeling. *J. Biomech.*, 34(6):815–819, Jun 2001
72. J.R. Cebral, M.A. Castro, O. Soto, R. Löhner, and N. Alperin. Blood flow models of the circle of Willis from magnetic resonance data. *J. Eng. Math.*, 47(3-4):369–386, 2003
73. A. Chambolle, B. Desjardins, M. Esteban, and C. Grandmont. Existence of weak solutions for an unsteady fluid–plate interaction problem. *J. Math. Fluid. Mech.*, 7(3):368–404, 2004
74. K.L. Chan and W.Y. Chau. Mathematical theory of reduction of physical parameters and similarity analysis. *Int. J. Theoretical Physics*, 18:835–844, 1979
75. D. Chapelle and K.J. Bathe. *The Finite Element Analysis of Shells-Fundamentals.* Springer-Verlag, New York, 2003
76. S.E. Charm and G.S. Kurland. *Blood Flow and Microcirculation.* John Wiley & Sons, New York, 1974
77. S.E. Charm, W. McComis, and G. Kurland. Rheology and structure of blood suspension. *J. Appl. Physiol.*, 19:127–133, 1964
78. S.E. Charm and G. Kurland. Viscometry of human blood for shear rates 0–100,000 $\sec^{-1}$. *Nature*, 206:617–618, 1965
79. G. Chavent and J.E. Roberts. A unified physical presentation of mixed, mixed-hybrid finite elements and standard finite-difference approximations for the determination of velocities in waterflow problems. *Adv. in Water Res.*, 14(6):329–348, 1991
80. D.C.-H. Cheng. Yield stress: A time dependent property and how to measure it. *Rheol. Acta*, 25:524–554, 1986
81. G. Chesshire and W.D. Henshaw. Composite overlapping meshes for the solution of partial differential equations. *J. Comput. Phys.*, 90:1–64, 1990
82. S. Chien. Shear dependence of effective cell volume as a determinant of blood viscosity. *Science*, 168:977–979, 1970
83. S. Chien, S. Feng, M. Vayo, L.A. Sung, S. Usami, and R. Shalak. The dynamics of shear disaggregation of red blood cells in a flow channel. *Biorheol.*, 27:135–147, 1990
84. S. Chien, R.G. King, R. Skalak, S. Usami, and A.L. Copley. Viscoelastic properties of human blood and red cell suspensions. *Biorheol.*, 12:341–346, 1975
85. S. Chien, S. Usami, and J.F. Bertler. Abnormal rheology of oxygenated blood in sickle cell anemia. *J. Clin. Invest.*, 49:623–634, 1970
86. S. Chien. Shear-dependent deformation of erythrocytes in rheology of human blood. *Am. J. Physiol.*, 219:136–142, 1970
87. M. Chipot. *Elements of Nonlinear Analysis.* Birkhäuser Verlag, Basel 2000
88. Y.I. Cho and K.R. Kensey. Effects of the non-Newtonian viscosity of blood on flows in a diseased arterial vessel. part I: Steady flows. *Biorheol.*, 28:241–262, 1991
89. A.J. Chorin. Numerical solution of the Navier-Stokes equations. *Math. Comput.*, 22:745–762, 1968

90. A.J. Chorin and J.E. Marsden. *A Mathematical Introduction to Fluid Mechanics*, volume 4 of *Texts in Applied Mathematics*, 3rd ed. Springer-Verlag, New York, 1990
91. U.J. Christensen, S.F. Andersen, J. Jacobsen, P.F. Jensen, and H. Ording. The Sophus anaesthesia simulator v. 2.0. *International Journal of Clinical Monitoring and Computing*, 614(1):11–16, 1997
92. P.G. Ciarlet. *Mathematical elasticity. Vol. I*, volume 20 of *Studies in Mathematics and its Applications*. North-Holland Publishing Co., Amsterdam, 1988
93. P.G. Ciarlet. *Introduction to Linear Shell Theory*. Gauthiers-Villars, 1998
94. P.G. Ciarlet. *Mathematical Elasticity. Vol. III. Theory of shells*. North-Holland, Amsterdam, 2000
95. P.G. Ciarlet. *An Introduction to Differential Geometry with Applications to Elasticity*. Springer, Dordrecht, 2005. Reprinted from J. Elasticity **78/79** (2005), no. 1–3
96. B. Cockburn and C.W. Shu. TVB Runge-Kutta projection discontinous Galerkin finite element methods for conservation laws II. general framework. *Math. Comm.*, 52:411–435, 1989
97. L.D. Cohen and I. Cohen. Finite-element methods for active contour models and balloons for 2-d and 3-d images. *IEEE Trans. on Patt. Analysis and Mach. Intell.*, 15(11):1131–1147, Nov 1993
98. G.R. Cokelet. Viscometric, in vitro and in vivo blood viscosity relationships: how are they related? *Biorheol.*, 36:343–358, 1999
99. G.R. Cokelet, E.W. Merrill, E.R. Gilliland, H. Shin, A. Britten, and R. E. Wells, Jr. The rheology of human blood – Measurement near and at zero shear rate. *Trans. Soc. Rheol.*, 7:303–317, 1963
100. B.D. Coleman, H. Markovitz, and W. Noll. *Viscometric Flows of Non-Newtonian Fluids*. Springer-Verlag, New York, 1966
101. A.L. Copley, C.R. Huang, and R.G. King. Rheogoniometric studies of whole human blood at shear rates from 1000 to 0.0009 sec^{-1} Part I – Experimental findings. *Biorheol.*, 10:17–22, 1973
102. A.L. Copley, R.G. King, S. Chien, S. Usami, R. Skalak, and C.R. Huang. Microscopic observations of viscoelasticity of human blood in steady and oscillatory shear. *Biorheol.*, 12:257–263, 1975
103. D. Coutand and S. Shkoller. Motion of an elastic solid inside of an incompressible viscous fluid. *Arch. Rational Mech. Anal.*, 176:25–102, 2005
104. D. Coutand and S. Shkoller. Interaction between quasilinear elasticity and the Navier-Stokes equations. *Arch. Rational Mech. Anal.*, 179:303–352, 2006
105. C. Crone and D.G. Levitt. Capillary permeability to small solutes. In E. Renkin and C. Michel (eds.), *Handbook of Physiology, Section 2: Microcirculation. The Cardiovascular System*, volume IV, Part1, Chapt. 10, pp. 411–466. Bethesda, MD: Am. Physiol. Soc., 1984
106. F.R.E. Curry. Mechanics and thermodynamics of transcapillary exchange. In E. Renkin and C. Michel (eds.), *Handbook of Physiology: The Cardiovascular System. Microcirculation.*, volume 4, Part 1, pp. 309–374. American Physiological Society, Bethesda, MD, 1984
107. R. Dáger and E. Zuazua. Controllability of tree-shaped networks of vibrating strings. *C. R. Acad. Sci. Paris*, 332(12):1087–1092, 2001
108. C. D'Angelo. Mathematical modelling of the cardiovascular system and skeletal muscle interaction during exercice. In Eric Cancès and J.-F. Gerbeau (eds.), *ESAIM-Proceedings*, volume 14, pp. 72–88, 2005

109. L. Davis. *Handbook of genetic algorithms.* Van Nostrand Reinhold, New York, 1991
110. J. De Hart. Evaluation of a fictitious domain method for predicting dynamic response of mechanical heart valves. *Journal of Fluids and Structures*, 19:835–850, 2004
111. D. De Kee and P.J. Carreau. A constitutive equation derived from Lodge's network theory. *J. Non-Newtonian Fluid Mech.*, 6:127–143, 1979
112. D. De Kee and C.F. Chan Man Fong. Rheological properties of structured fluids. *Polym. Eng. Sci.*, 34:438–445, 1994
113. W.R. Dean. Fluid motion in a curved channel. *P. R. Soc. A*, 121:402–420, 1928
114. A. Delfino, N. Stergiopulos, J.E. Moore, and J.J. Meister. Residual strain effects on the stress field in a thick wall finite element model of the human carotid bifurcation. *J. Biomech.*, 30(8):777–786, Aug 1997
115. H. Demiray and N. Antar. Nonlinear waves in an inviscid fluid contained in a prestressed viscoelastic thin tube. *Z. Angew. Math. Phys.*, 48(2):325–340, 1997
116. G. D'Enrico, A. Onorati, and G. Ferrari. An integrated 1D-2D fluid dyanamic model for the simulation of wave action in I.C. engine manifolds. In *Proceedings of ICE99*, International Conference on Internal Combustion Engines, Capri, Sep 1999
117. S. Deparis. *Numerical Analysis of Axisymmetric Flows and Methods for Fluid-Structure Interaction Arising in Blood Flow Simulation.* PhD thesis, EPFL, 2004
118. S. Deparis, M. Discacciati, G. Fourestey, and A. Quarteroni. Fluid-structure algorithms based on Steklov-Poincaré operators. *Comp. Meth. Appl. Mech. Eng.*, 195(41-43):5797–5812, 2006
119. T. Deschamps. *Curve and shape extraction with minimal path and level sets techniques. Applications to 3D medical imaging.* PhD thesis, Université Paris-IX Dauphine, France, Dec 2001
120. B. Desjardins and M.J. Esteban. Existence of weak solutions for the motion of rigid bodies in a viscous fluid. *Arch. Rational Mech. Anal.*, 146:59–71, 1999
121. C.A. Desoer and E.S. Kuh. *Basic circuit theory.* McGraw-Hill, New York, 1969
122. W. Dettmer and D. Perić. A computational framework for fluid-structure interaction: Finite element formulation and applications. *Comp. Meth. Appl. Mech. Engrg.*, 195(41-43):5754–5779, 2006
123. P. Deuflhard and R. Hochmuth. Multiscale analysis of thermoregulation in the human microvascular system. *Math.Meth. Appl. Sci.*, 27:971–989, 2004
124. S. Dey, R.M. O'Bara, and M.S. Shephard. Curvilinear mesh generation in 3D. *Computer-Aided Design*, 33:199–209, 1999
125. T.K. Dey and W. Zhao. Approximate medial axis as a Voronoi subcomplex. In *Proceedings of the 7th ACM Symposium of Solid Modeling Applications*, pp. 356–366, 2002
126. N.M. Diniz Dos Santos, J.-F. Gerbeau, and J.-F. Bourgat. A partitioned fluid-structure algorithm for elastic thin valves with contact. *Comp. Meth. Appl. Mech. Eng.*, 197:1750–1761, 2008
127. L. Dintenfass. *Blood Microrheology-Viscosity Factors in Blood Flow, Ischaemia and Thrombosis.* Butterworth, London, 1971
128. D.J. Doorly, S.J. Sherwin, P.T. Franke, and J. Peiro. Vortical flow structure identification and flow transport in arteries. *Comp. Meth. Biomech. Biomed. Engng.*, 5:261–275, 2002

129. R.O. Dull, H. Jo, H. Still, T.M. Hollis, and J.M. Tarbell. The effect of varying albumin concentration and hydrostatic pressure on hydraulic conductivity and albumin permeability of cultured endotheloal monolayers. *Microvasc. Res.*, 41:390–407, 1991
130. P.L. Easthope and D.E. Brooks. A comparison of rheological constitutive functions for whole human blood. *Biorheol.*, 17:235–247, 1980
131. H. Edelsbrunner and E.P. Mücke. *Three-dimensional alpha shapes.* ACM Press New York, 1992
132. L.W. Ehrlich and M.H. Friedman. Steady convective diffusion in a bifurcation. *IEEE T. Bio-Med. Eng.*, BME-24(1):12–18, 1977
133. S.H. Embury, R.P. Hebbel, N. Mohandas, and M.H. Steinberg (eds.). *Sickle Cell Disease: Basic Principles and Clinical Practice.* Raven Press, 1994
134. L.E. Eriksson. Practical three-dimensional mesh generation using transfinite interpolation. *SIAM J. Scient. Stat. Comput.*, 6(3):712–741, 1985
135. D. Errate, M. Esteban, and Y. Maday. Couplage fluide-structure. un modèle simplifié en dimension un. *Note aux Comptes rendus de l'Academie des Sciences de Paris*, 318:275–281, 1994
136. C.R. Ethier. Computational modeling of mass transfer and links to atherosclerosis. *Ann. Biomed. Eng.*, 30:461–71, 2002
137. C.R. Ethier and J.A. Moore. Oxygen mass transfer calculations in large arteries. *ASME J. Biomech. Eng.*, 119:469–475, 1997
138. C.R. Ethier and D.K. Stangeby. Computational analysis of coupled blood-wall LDL transport. *ASME J. Biomech. Eng.*, 124:1–8, 2002
139. L. Euler. Principia pro motu sanguinis per arterias determinando. In *Leonhard Euler, Opera Omnia*, volume 16(2), pp. 178–196. Birkhäuser Verlag, Basel, 1989
140. R. Fåhraeus and T. Lindqvist. The viscosity of the blood in narrow capillary tubes. *Am. J. Physiol.*, 96:562–568, 1931
141. J. Fang and R.G. Owens. Numerical simulations of pulsatile blood flow using a new constitutive model. *Biorheol.*, 43:637–668, 2006
142. C. Farhat, M. Lesoinne, and P. Le Tallec. Load and motion transfer algorithms for fluid/structure interaction problems with non-matching discrete interfaces: Momentum and energy conservation, optimal discretization and application to aeroelasticity. *Comp. Meth. Appl. Mech. Eng.*, 157:95–114, 1998
143. W.J. Federspiel and G.R. Cokelet. Blood viscoelasticity for conditions of physiological flow in small arteries. *Chem. Eng. Commun.*, 30:275–284, 1984
144. A. Fenster, D.B. Downey, and H.N. Cardinal. Three-dimensional ultrasound imaging. *Phys Med Biol*, 46(5):67–99, 2001
145. M.A. Fernández, J.-F. Gerbeau, A. Gloria, and M. Vidrascu. Domain decomposition based Newton methods for fluid-structure interaction problems. In G. Galoz and M. Dauge, editors, *ESAIM Proceedings*, volume 22, pp. 67–82, 2007
146. M.A. Fernández, J.-F. Gerbeau, and C. Grandmont. A projection semi-implicit scheme for the coupling of an elastic structure with an incompressible fluid. *Int. J. Numer. Meth. Engng.*, 69(4):794–821, 2007
147. M.A. Fernández, V. Milisic, and A. Quarteroni. Analysis of a geometrical multiscale blood flow model based on the coupling of ODE's and hyperbolic PDE's. *Multiscale Model. Simul.*, 4(1):215–236, 2005
148. M.A. Fernández and M. Moubachir. An exact block-newton algorithm for the solution of implicit time discretized coupled systems involved in fluid-structure

interaction problems. In K.J. Bathe (ed.), *Second M.I.T. Conference on Computational Fluid and Solid Mechanics*, pp. 1337–1341. Elsevier, Amsterdam, 2003

149. M.A. Fernández and M. Moubachir. Numerical simulation of fluid-structure systems via Newton's method with exact Jacobians. In P. Neittaanmki, T. Rossi, K. Majava, and O. Pironneau (eds.), *Fourth European Congress on Computational Methods in Applied Sciences and Engineering*, vol 1, Jyvskyl, Finland, Jul 2004
150. M.A. Fernández and M. Moubachir. A Newton method using exact Jacobians for solving fluid-structure coupling. *Comp. Struct.*, 83:127–142, 2005
151. I.E. Figueroa, C.A. Vignon-Clementel, K.E. Jansen, T.J.R. Hughes, and C.A. Taylor. A coupled momentum method for modeling blood flow in three-dimensional deformable arteries. *Comp. Meth. Appl. Mech. Eng.*, 195(41–43):5685–5706, 2006
152. M. Fila. Boundedness of global solutions for the heat equation with nonlinear boundary conditions. *Comm. Math. Univ. Carol.*, 30:479–484, 1989
153. M. Fila. The blow up rate for the heat equation with a nonlinear boundary condition. *Math. Methods Appl. Sci.*, 14:197–205, 1991
154. T.M. Fisher, M. Stöehr-Lissen, and H. Schmid-Schönbein. The red cell as a fluid droplet: Tank tread-like motion of the human erythrocyte membrane in shear flow. *Science*, 202:894–896, 1978
155. L. Formaggia, J.-F. Gerbeau, F. Nobile, and A. Quarteroni. On the coupling of 3D and 1D Navier-Stokes equations for flow problems in compliant vessels. *Comp. Meth. Appl. Mech. Eng.*, 191:561–582, 2001
156. L. Formaggia, J.-F. Gerbeau, F. Nobile, and A. Quarteroni. Numerical treatment of defective boundary conditions for the Navier–Stokes equations. *SIAM J. Numer. Anal.*, 40(1):376–401, 2002
157. L. Formaggia, D. Lamponi, A. Quarteroni. One dimensional models for blood flow in arteries. *J. Eng. Math.*, 47:251–276, 2003
158. L. Formaggia, D. Lamponi, M. Tuveri, and A. Veneziani. Numerical modeling of 1D arterial networks coupled with a lumped parameters description of the heart. *Comp. Meth. Biomech. Biomed. Engng.*, 9(5):273–288, 2006
159. L. Formaggia, A. Moura, and F. Nobile. On the stability of the coupling of 3D and 1D fluid-structure interaction models for blood flow simulations. *Math. Model. Num. Anal.*, 41:743–769, 2007
160. L. Formaggia, F. Nobile, and A. Quarteroni. A one dimensional model for blood flow: application to vascular prosthesis. In I. Babuška, T. Miyoshi, and P.G. Ciarlet (eds.), *Mathematical Modeling and Numerical Simulation in Continuum Mechanics*, volume 19 of *Lecture Notes in Computational Science and Engineering*, pp. 137–153, Springer-Verlag, Berlin, 2002
161. L. Formaggia, S. Perotto, and P. Zunino. An anisotropic a-posteriori error estimate for a convection-diffusion problem. *Comp. Visual. Science*, 4(2):105–109, 2001
162. L. Formaggia and A. Veneziani. Reduced and multiscale models for the human cardiovascular system. Technical report, PoliMI, Jun 2003
163. L. Formaggia, A. Veneziani, and C. Vergara. A new approach to the numerical solution of defective boundary problems in incompressible fluid dynamics. *SIAM J. Numer. Anal.*, 0:0, 2006

164. C. Förster, W.A. Wall, and E. Ramm. Artificial added mass instabilities in sequential staggered coupling of nonlinear structures and incompressible viscous flows. *Comp. Meth. Appl. Mech. Eng.*, 196(7):1278–1293, 2007
165. S. Fortune. Voronoi diagrams and Delaunay triangulations. *Algorithmica*, 2:153–174, 1992
166. D.H. Frakes, C.P. Conrad, T.M. Healy, J.W. Monaco, M. Fogel, S. Sharma, M.J.T. Smith, and A.P. Yoganathan. Application of an adaptive control grid interpolation technique to morphological vascular reconstruction. *IEEE T. Bio-Med. Eng.*, 50(2):197–206, Feb 2003
167. A.F. Frangi, W.J. Niessen, R.M. Hoogeveen, T. van Walsum, and M.A. Viergever. Model-based quantitation of 3-D magnetic resonance angiographic images. *IEEE T. Med. Imaging.*, 18(10):946–956, Oct 1999
168. A.F. Frangi, W.J. Niessen, P.J. Nederkoorn, J. Bakker, W.P. Mali, and M.A. Viergever. Quantitative analysis of vascular morphology from 3D MR angiograms: In vitro and in vivo results. *Magn. Reson. Medic.*, 45(2):311–322, Feb 2001
169. J.A. Frangos, T.Y. Huang, and C.B. Clark. Steady shear and step changes in shear stimulate endothelium via independent mechanisms-superposition of transient and sustained nitric oxide production. *Biochem. Biophys. Res. Comm.*, 224(3):660–665, 1996
170. O. Franke. Die Grundform des arteriellen Pulses. *Zeitung fur Biologie*, 37:483–586, 1899
171. P. Franke. *Blood Flow and Transport in Artifical Devices.* PhD thesis, Imperial College London, University of London, 2002
172. P.J. Frey and P.L. George. *Mesh generation. Application to finite elements.* Herms Science Publ., Paris, Oxford, 2000
173. M.H. Friedman. *Principles and Models of Biological Transport.* Springer-Verlag, New York, 1986
174. M.H. Friedman and D. Fry. Arterial permeability dynamics and vascular disease. *Atherosclerosis*, 104:189–194, 1993
175. D. Fry. Mass transport, atherogenesis, and risk. *Arteriosclerosis*, 7(1):88–100, 1987
176. D.L. Fry. Mathematical models of arterial transmural transport. *Am. J. Physiol.*, 248(2):H240–H263, 1985
177. Y.C. Fung. What are the residual stresses doing in our blood vessels? *Ann. Biomed. Eng.*, 19(3):237–249, 1991
178. Y.C. Fung. *Biomechanics: Mechanical Properties of Living Tissues.* Springer-Verlag, New York, 1993
179. Y.C. Fung. *Biomechanics: Mechanical Properties of Living Tissues.* Springer-Verlag, New York, 1993
180. Y.C. Fung, K. Fronek, and P. Patitucci. Pseudoelasticity of arteries and the choice of its mathematical expression. *Am. J. Physiol.*, 237(5):H620–H631, Nov 1979
181. G.P. Galdi, R. Rannacher, A.M. Robertson, and S. Turek. *Hemodynamical Flow: Modeling, Analysis and Simulation.* Birkhäuser, Basel, 2008
182. A. Gaspar-Rosas and G.B. Thurston. Erythrocyte aggregate rheology by transmitted and reflected light. *Biorheol.*, 25:471–487, 1988
183. T.C. Gasser and G.A. Holzapfel. A rate-independent elastoplastic constitutive model for biological fiber-reinforced composites at finite strains: continuum

basis, algorithmic formulation and finite element implementation. *Comput. Mech.*, 29(4-5):340–360, Oct 2002

184. C.W. Gear. Differential algebraic equations, indexes, and integral algebraic equations. *SIAM J. Numer. Anal.*, 27(6):1527–1534, 1990
185. B. Geiger. Three-dimensional modeling of human organs and its application to diagnosis and surgical planning. Technical Report 2105, Institut National de Recherche en Informatique et Automatique, 06902 Sophia Antipolis, France, Dec 1993
186. P.-L. George, F. Hecht, and E. Saltel. Automatic mesh generator with specified boundary. *Comp. Meth. Appl. Mech. Eng.*, 92:269–288, 1991
187. J.-F. Gerbeau and D. Chapelle. Numerical simulation of the cardiovascular system. *Med Sci (Paris)*, 21(5):530–534, May 2005
188. J.-F. Gerbeau and M. Vidrascu. A quasi-Newton algorithm based on a reduced model for fluid-structure interactions problems in blood flows. *Math. Model. Num. Anal.*, 37(4):631–648, 2003
189. J.-F. Gerbeau, M. Vidrascu, and P. Frey. Fluid-structure interaction in blood flows on geometries coming from medical imaging. *Comp. Struct.*, 83:155–165, 2005
190. M. Germano. The Dean equations extended to a helical pipe flow. *J. Fluid Mech.*, 203:289–305, 1989
191. M. Gharib, E. Rambod, and K. Shariff. A universal time scale for vortex ring formation. *J. Fluid. Mech.*, 360:121–140, 1998
192. D. Gilbarg and N. Trudinger. *Elliptic Partial Differential Equations of Second Order.* Springer-Verlag, Berlin, 1998
193. S. Giordana, S.J. Sherwin, D.J. Doorly, J.S. Crane, K.E. Lee, N.J.W. Cheshire, and C.G. Caro. Local and global geometric influence on steady flow in distal anastomoses of peripheral by-pass grafts. *ASME. J. Biomech. Engrg.*, 127:1087–1098, 2005
194. S. Giordana, S.J. Sherwin, J. Peiró, D.J. Doorly, Y. Papaharilaou, C.G. Caro, N. Watkins, N.J.W. Cheshire, M. Jackson, C. Bicknall, and V. Zervas. Automated classification of peripheral distal by-pass geometries reconstructed from medical data. *J. Biomech.*, 38(1):47–62, 2005
195. V. Girault and P.-A. Raviart. *Finite element methods for Navier-Stokes equations.* Springer-Verlag, Berlin, 1986
196. R. Glowinski, T.W. Pan, T.I. Hesla, D.D. Joseph, and J. Périaux. A fictitious domain approach for the direct simulation of incompressible fluid flow past moving rigid bodies: Application to particulate flow. *J. Comput. Phys.*, 169:363–426, 2001
197. R. Glowinski, T.W. Pan, T.I. Hesla, and J. Périaux. A fictitious domain method for Dirichlet problem and applications. *Comp. Meth. Appl. Mech. Eng.*, 111:283–303, 1994
198. R. Glowinski, T.W. Pan, T.I. Hesla, and D.D. Joseph. A distributed Lagrange mutiplier/fictitious domain method for particulate flows. *Int. J. of Multiphase Flow*, 25:755–794, 1999
199. E. Godlewski and P.-A. Raviart. *Numerical Approximation of Hyperbolic Systems of Conservation Laws*, volume 118 of *Applied Mathematical Sciences.* Springer, New York, 1996
200. J. Goldstone, H. Schmid-Schönbein, and R. E. Wells. The rheology of red blood cell aggregates. *Microvas. Res.*, 2:273–286, 1970

201. C. Grandmont. Existence for a three-dimensional steady state fluid-structure interaction problem. *J. Math. Fluid Mech.*, 4(1):659–694, 2002
202. C. Grandmont and Y. Maday. Existence for an unsteady fluid-structure interaction problem. *Math. Model. Num. Anal.*, 34(3):609–636, 2000
203. M.J. Graves. Magnetic resonance angiography. *Br. J. Radiol.*, 70(829):6–28, 1997
204. A.E. Green and P.M. Naghdi. A direct theory of viscous fluid flow in pipes. I. Basic general developments. *Phil. Trans. R. Soc. Lond., Ser. A*, 342:525–542, 1993
205. A.E. Green, P.M. Naghdi, and M.J. Stallard. A direct theory of viscous fluid flow in pipes. II. Flow of incompressible viscous fluid in curved pipes. *Phil. Trans. R. Soc. Lond., Ser. A*, 342:543–572, 1993
206. N.E. Green, S.Y.J. Chen, J.C. Messenger, B.M. Groves, and J.D. Carroll. Three-dimensional vascular angiography. *Current Problems in Cardiology*, 29(3):104–142, 2004
207. J.-L. Guermond, P. Minev, and J. Shen. An overview of projection methods for incompressible flows. *Comp. Meth. Appl. Mech. Engng.*, 195:44–47 (2006). 6011–6045
208. J.-L. Guermond and J. Shen. Velocity-correction projection methods for incompressible flows. *SIAM J. Numer. Anal.*, 41:112–134, 2003
209. H. Guillard and C. Farhat. On the significance of the geometric conservation law for flow computations on moving meshes. *Comp. Meth. Appl. Mech. Eng.*, 190(11-12):1467–1482, 2000
210. M. Gunzburger. *Perspectives in flow optimization.* SIAM, Philadelphia, 2003
211. M.E. Gurtin. *An introduction to continuum mechanics*, volume 158 of *Mathematics in Science and Engineering.* Academic Press Inc., New York, 1981
212. A.C. Guyton. *Circulatory Physiology: Cardiac Output and its Regulation.* Saunders (2nd ed.), Philadelphia, 1973
213. A.C. Guyton. *Textbook of Medical Physiology.* Elsevier Saunders (11th ed.), Philadelphia, 2005
214. P. Hartman. *Ordinary differential equations.* Wiley, New York, 1964
215. J.C. Healy and M. Joly. Rheological behavior of blood in transient flow. *Biorheol.*, 12:335–340, 1975
216. G.W. Hedstrom. Nonreflecting boundary conditions for nonlinear hyperbolic systems. *J. Comput. Phys.*, 30:222–237, 1979
217. M. Heil. An efficient solver for the fully coupled solution of large displacement fluid-structure interaction problems. *Comp. Meth. Appl. Mech. Eng.*, 193(1-2):1–23, 2004
218. J.G. Heywood, R. Rannacher, and S. Turek. Artificial boundaries and flux and pressure conditions for the incompressible Navier–Stokes equations. *Int. J. Numer. Meth. Fluids*, 22:325–352, 1996
219. R. Hochmuth and P. Deuflhard. Multiscale analysis for the bio-heat-transfer equation: The nonisolated case. *Math. Mod. Meth. Appl. Sciences*, 14(11):1621–1634, 2004
220. M.H. Holmes. A spectral problem in hydroelasticity. *J. Differential Equations*, 32(3):388–397, 1979
221. G.A. Holzapfel. *Non linear solid mechanics. A continuum approach for engineering.* John Wiley & Sons, Chichester, 2000

222. G.A. Holzapfel. Determination of material models for arterial walls from uniaxial extension tests and histological structure. *J. Theor. Biol.*, 238(2):290–302, 2006
223. G.A. Holzapfel, T.C. Gasser, and R.W. Ogden. A new constitutive framework for arterial wall mechanics and a comparative study of material models. *J. Elasticity*, 61(1-3):1–48, 2000. Soft tissue mechanics
224. G.A. Holzapfel, T.C. Gasser, and M. Stadler. A structural model for the viscoelastic behavior of arterial walls: Continuum formulation and finite element analysis. *European J. of Mechanics. A/Solids*, 21(3):441–463, May–June 2002
225. R.M. Hoogeveen, C.J. Bakker, and M.A. Viergever. Limits to the accuracy of vessel diameter measurement in Mr angiography. *J. Magn. Reson. Imaging*, 8(6):1228–1235, 1998
226. H. Hoppe, T. DeRose, T. Duchamp, J. McDonald, and W. Stuetzle. Surface reconstruction from unorganized points. In *Siggraph '92 Proceedings*, pp. 71–78, 1992
227. F.H. Hoppensteadt and C. Peskin. *Mathematics in Life Sciences and Medicine.* Springer, New York, 1992
228. P.R. Hoskins. Ultrasound techniques for measurement of blood flow and tissue motion. *Biorheol.*, 39(3):451–459, 2002
229. http://www.nlm.nih.gov/medlineplus. A service of the U.S. National Library of medicine and the National Institutes of Health. Statistics on the incidence of cardiovascular disease in the U.S.
230. C.R. Huang and S.S. Horng. Viscoelastic-thixotropy of blood. *Clinic. Hemorheol.*, 15:25–36, 1995
231. C.R. Huang, N. Siskovic, R.W. Robertson, W. Fabisiak, E.H. Smith-Berg, and A.L. Copley. Quantitative characterization of thixotropy of whole human blood. *Biorheol.*, 12:279–282, 1975
232. Y. Huang, D. Rumschitzki, D. Chien, and S. Weinbaum. A fiber matrix model for the growth of macromolecular leakage spots in the arterial intima. In *Advances in Biological Heat and Mass Transfer*, volume 231 of *HTD*, pp. 81–92. ASME, 1992
233. Y. Huang, Y. Rumschizki, D. Chien, and S. Weinbaum. A fiber matrix model for the filtration through fenestral pores in a compressible arterial intima. *Am. J. Physiol.*, 272:H2023–H2039, 1997
234. Y. Huang, S. Weinbaum, S. Rumschitzki, and D. Chien. A fiber matrix model for the growth of macromolecular leakage spots in the arterial intima. *ASME Adv. Biol. Heat Mass Trans.*, HTD-231:81–92, 1992
235. Z.J. Huang and J.M. Tarbell. Numerical simulation of mass transfer in porous media of bloob vessel walls. *Am. J. Physiol.*, 273:H464–H477, 1997
236. J.R. Hughes and M. Mallet. A new finite element formulation for computational fluid dynamics: III. The generalized streamline operator for multidimensional advective-diffusive systems. *Comp. Meth. Appl. Mech. Eng.*, 58:305–328, 1986
237. J.M.B. Hughes and N.W. Morrell. *Pulmonary Circulation: Basic Mechanisms to Clinical Practice.* Imperial College Press, London, 2001
238. T.J.R. Hughes. A study of the one-dimensional theory of arterial pulse propagation. Report 74-13, University of California Berkeley, Structural Engineering Laboratory, Dec 1974
239. T.J.R. Hughes and J. Lubliner. On the one-dimensional theory of blood flow in the larger vessels. *Math. Biosci.*, 18:161–170, 1973

240. T.J. Huttl, C. Wagner, and R. Friedrich. Navier Stokes solutions of laminar flows based on orthogonal helical co-ordinates. *Int. J. Numer. Meth. Fluids*, 29:749–763, 1999
241. L. Ibanez, W. Schroeder, L. Ng, and J. Cates. *The ITK Software Guide.* Kitware, Inc. ISBN 1-930934-15-7, http://www.itk.org/ItkSoftwareGuide.pdf, (2nd ed.), 2005
242. Y. Imoto, H. Kado, Y. Shiokawa, K. Minami, and H. Yasui. Experience with the Norwood procedure without circulatory arrest. *J. Thor. Cardiov. Surg.*, 122:879–882, 2001
243. M. Itskov and N. Aksel. Elastic constants and their admissible values for incompressible and slightly compressible anisotropic materials. *Acta Mech.*, 157(1):81–96, Mar 2002
244. G.N. Jager, N. Westerhof, and A. Noordergraaf. Oscillatory flow impedance in electrical analog of arterial system: Representation of sleeve effect and non-newtonian properties of blood. *Circ. Res.*, 16:121–33, 1965
245. J. Jeong and F. Hussain. On the identification of a vortex. *J. Fluid Mech.*, 285:69–94, 1995
246. Z. Jianhai, C. Dapeng, and Z. Shengquan. ALE finite element analysis of the opening and closing process of the artificial mechanical valve. *Appl. Math. Mech.*, 17(5):403–412, 1996
247. M. Joly, C. Lacombe, and D. Quemada. Application of the transient flow rheology to the study of abnormal human bloods. *Biorheol.*, 18:445–452, 1981
248. M.R. Kaazempur-Mofrad, A.G. Isasi, H.F. Younis, R.C. Chan, D.P. Hinton, G. Sukhova, G.M. LaMuraglia, R.T. Lee, and R.D. Kamm. Characterization of the atherosclerotic carotid bifurcation using MRI, finite element modeling, and histology. *Ann. Biomed. Eng.*, 32(7):932–946, 2004
249. G. Karner and K. Perktold. Effect of endothelial injury and increased blood pressure on albumin accumulation in the arterial wall: a numerical study. *J. Biomech.*, 33:709–715, 2000
250. G. Karner, K. Perktold, M. Hofer, and D. Liepsch. Flow characteristics in an anatomically realistic compliant carotid artery bifurcation model. *Comp. Meth. Biomech. Biomed. Engng.*, 2(3):171–185, 1999
251. G. Karner, K. Perktold, H.P. Zehentner, and M. Prosi. Intra and extracorporeal cardiovascular fluid dynamics. In P. Verdonck and K. Perktold (eds.), *Fluid Structure Interaction*, volume 2 (23), chapter Intra and Extracorporeal Cardiovascular Fluid Dynamics, pp. 209–247. WIT-Press, Southampton, Boston, 2000
252. G.E. Karniadakis, M. Israeli, and S.A. Orszag. High-order splitting methods for the incompressible Navier-Stokes equations. *J. Comput. Phys.*, 97(2):414–443, 1991
253. G.E. Karniadakis and S.J. Sherwin. *Spectral/hp element methods for CFD.* Oxford University Press, Oxford, 1999
254. A. Katchalsky and P.F. Curran. *Nonequilibrium Thermodynamics in Biophysics.* Harvard University Press, Cambridge, 1981
255. O. Kedem and A. Katchalsky. Thermodynamic analysis of the permeability of biological membranes to non-electrolytes. *Biochim. Biophys. Acta*, 27:229–246, 1958
256. J. Keener and J. Sneyd. *Mathematical Physiology.* Interdisciplinary Applied Mathematics. Springer, New York, 1998

257. C.T. Kelley. *Solving nonlinear equations with Newton's method.* SIAM, Philadelphia, 2003
258. S. Kim, Y.I. Cho, A.H. Jeon, B. Hogenauer, and K.R. Kensey. A new method for blood viscosity measurement. *J. Non-Newtonian Fluid Mech.*, 94:47–56, 2000
259. O. Kitoh. Swirling flow through a bend. *J. Fluid Mech.*, 175:429–446, 1987
260. P. Knupp and S. Steinberg. *Fundamentals of Grid Generation.* CRC Press, Boca Raton, 1993
261. R. Krams, J.J. Wentzel, J.A. Oomen, R. Vinke, J.C. Schuurbiers, P.J. de Feyter, P.W. Serruys, and C.J. Slager. Evaluation of endothelial shear stress and 3D geometry as factors determining the development of atherosclerosis and remodeling in human coronary arteries in vivo. combining 3D reconstruction from angiography and IVUS (ANGUS) with computational fluid dynamics. *Arterioscl., Thromb. Vascul. Biol.*, 17(10):2061–2065, Oct 1997
262. E. Krause. Modeling of the circulatory system. Lecture Notes of the VKI Course on Fluid Dynamics and Biological Flow. 04-1998, 1998
263. D.N. Ku. Blood flow in arteries. *Annu. Rev. Fluid Mech.*, 29:399–434, 1997
264. D.N. Ku, D.P. Giddens, C.K. Zarins, and S. Glagov. Pulsatile flow and atherosclerosis in the human carotid bifurcation. *Arteriosclerosis*, 5:293–302, 1985
265. H.M. Ladak, J.S. Milner, and D.A. Steinman. Rapid three-dimensional segmentation of the carotid bifurcation from serial MR images. *J. Biomech. Engng.*, 122(1):96–99, Feb 2000
266. H.M. Ladak, J.B. Thomas, J.R. Mitchell, B.K. Rutt, and D.A. Steinman. A semi-automatic technique for measurement of arterial wall from black blood MRI. *Med. Phys.*, 28(6):1098–1107, Jun 2001
267. B. Lakshminarayana and J.H. Horlock. Generalized expressions for secondary vorticity using intrinsic co-ordinates. *J. Fluid. Mech.*, 59:97–115, 1973
268. J. Lambert. *Numerical Methods for Ordinary Differential Systems: The Initial Value Problem.* John Wiley & Sons, New York, 2001
269. D. Lamponi. *One dimensional and multiscale models for blood flow circulation.* PhD thesis, EPFL, Lausanne, Thesis n. 3006, 2004
270. E.M. Landis and J.R. Pappenheimer. Exchange of substances through the capillary walls. In W.F. Hamilton, editor, *Handbook of Physiology, Section 2: Circulation*, volume II, Chap. 29, pp. 961–1034. Washington, DC: Am. Physiol. Soc., 1963
271. P. Le Tallec. *Introduction la dynamique des structures.* Ellipses, Paris, 2000
272. P. Le Tallec and J. Mouro. Fluid structure interaction with large structural displacements. *Comp. Meth. Appl. Mech. Eng.*, 190:3039–3067, 2001
273. K.L. Lee. *Coronary Flow: Magnetic Resonance Measurement and Computational Prediction.* PhD thesis, Imperial College London, University of London, 2006
274. K.Y. Lee. *The study of flows in idealised double curved non-branching vessels and realistic distal anastomosis geometries.* PhD thesis, Imperial College London, University of London, 2006
275. K.Y. Lee, K. Parker, C. Caro, and S.J. Sherwin. Spectral/hp element modelling of steady flow in non-planar double bends. *Int. J. Num. Meth. Fluids*, 57(5):519–529, 2008
276. S. Lehoux and A. Tedgui. Cellular mechanics and gene expression in blood vessels. *J. Biomech.*, 36(5):631–643, May 2003

277. R.J. LeVeque. *Numerical Methods for Conservation Laws.* Birkhäuser, Basel, 1990
278. M.J. Lever. Mass transport through the walls of arteries and veins. In M.Y. Jaffrin and C.G. Caro (eds.), *Biological Flow*, pp. 177–197. Plenum Press, New York, 1995
279. J.R. Levick. *An Introduction to Cardiovascular Physiology.* Arnold (4th ed.), London, 2003
280. H.A. Levine and L.E. Payne. Nonexistence theorems for the heat equation with nonlinear boundary conditions and for the porous medium equation backward in time. *J. Diff. Equations*, 16:319–334, 1974
281. H.A. Levine and R.A. Smith. A potential well theory for the heat equation with a nonlinear boundary condition. *Math. Methods Appl. Sci.*, 9:127–136, 1987
282. M.N. Levy and R.M Berne. *Cardiovascular Physiology.* Mosby Elsevier (9th ed.), Philadelphia, 2007
283. T. Lévy. Fluid flow through an array of fixed particles. *Int. J. Engng. Sci.*, 21(1):11–23, 1983
284. M.A. Lewis. Multislice CT: opportunities and challenges. *Br. J. Radiol.*, 74(885):779–781, 2001
285. Z. Li and C. Kleinstreuer. Fluid-structure interaction effects on sac-blood pressure and wall stress in a stented aneurysm. *J. Biomech. Engng.*, 127(4):662–671, Aug 2005
286. A. Libai and J.G. Simmonds. *The Nonlinear Theory of Elastic Shells.* Cambridge University Press, Cambridge, 1998
287. P. Libby. Atherosclerosis: the new view. *Scientific American*, 286(5):46–55, may 2002
288. D. Liepsch and St. Moravec. Pulsatile flow of non-Newtonian fluid in distensible models of human arteries. *Biorheol.*, 21:571–586, 1984
289. D.W. Liepsch. Flow in tubes and arteries – A comparison. *Biorheol.*, 23:395–433, 1986
290. M.J. Lighthill. *Waves in fluids.* Cambridge University Press, Cambridge, New York, 1978
291. J.-L. Lions. *Quelques mèthodes de rèsolution des problèmes aux limites non linèaires.* Dunod, Paris, 1969
292. J.-L. Lions and Zuazua E. Approximate controllability of a hydroelastic coupled system. *ESAIM: Contr.Optim.Calc.*, 1:1–15, 1995
293. J.-L. Lions and E. Magenes. *Problèmes aux limites non homogènes et applications.* Dunod, Paris, 1968
294. J.-L. Lions and E. Magenes. *Non-homogeneous boundary value problems and applications. Vol. I.* Springer-Verlag, New York, 1972
295. S. Liu and J.H. Masliyah. Axially invariant laminar flow in helical pipes with a finite pitch. *J. Fluid Mech.*, 251:315–353, 1993
296. I. Lomtev, C.W. Quillen, and G. Karniadakis. Spectral/*hp* methods for viscous compressible flows on unstructured 2D meshes. *J. Comput. Phys.*, 144:325–357, 1998
297. Q. Long, X.Y. Xu, M.W. Collins, M. Bourne, and T.M. Griffith. Magnetic resonance image processing and structured grid generation of a human abdominal bifurcation. *Comp. Meth. Progr. Biomed.*, 56:249–259, 1998

298. R. Loon, P.D. Anderson, J. De Hart, and F.P.T. Baaijens. A combined fictitious domain/adaptative meshing method for fluid-structure interaction in heart valves. *Int. J. Numer. Meth. Fluids*, 46:533–544, 2004
299. W.E. Lorensen and H.E. Cline. Marching cubes: a high resolution 3D surface construction algorithm. *Computer Graphics*, 21:163–169, 1987
300. M.A. Lovich and E.R. Edelman. Mechanisms of transmural heparin transport in the rat abdominal aorta after local vascular delivery. *Circ. Res.*, 77:1143–1150, 1995
301. A.F. Low, G.J. Tearney, B.E. Bouma, I.K. Jang. Technology insight: optical coherence tomography – current status and future development. *Nature Clinical Practice Cardiovascular Medicine*, 3:154–162, 2006
302. D.O. Lowe. *Clinical Blood Rheology, Vol.I, II.* CRC Press, Boca Raton, 1998
303. M. Lucius and J. F. Stolz. Importance of erythrocyte aggregation on the viscoelastic and thixotropic properties of blood. *Clinic. Hemorheol.*, 7:63–70, 1987
304. P.P. Lunkenheimer et al. The myocardium and its fibrous matrix working in concert as a spatially netted mesh: a critical review of the purported tertiary structure of the ventricular mass. *European Journal of Cardio-thoracic Surgery* 295:41–49, 2006
305. E.M. Lutostansky, G. Karner, G. Rappitsch, D.N. Ku, and K. Perktold. Analysis of hemodynamic fluid phase mass transport in a separated flow region. *J. Biomech. Engng.*, 125:189–196, 2003
306. C.W. Macosko. *Rheology: Principles, Measurements and Applications.* VCH Publishers Inc., New York, 1994
307. K.O. Maher, C. Pizarro, S.S. Gidding, K. Januszewska, E. Malec, W.I.Jr. Norwood, and J.D. Murphy. Hemodynamic profile after the Norwood procedure with right ventricle to pulmonary artery conduit. *Circulation*, 108:782–784, 2003
308. E. Malec, K. Januszewska, J. Kolcz, and T. Mroczek. Right ventricle-to-pulmonary artery shunt versus modified Blalock-Taussig shunt in the Norwood procedure for hypoplastic left heart syndrome – influence on early and late haemodynamic status. *Eur. J. Cardiothor. Surg.*, 23:728–733, 2003
309. R. Malladi and J. A. Sethian. A real-time algorithm for medical shape recovery. In *Proceedings of International Conference on Computer Vision*, pp. 304–310, Jan 1998
310. L.E. Malvern. *Introduction to the mechanics of continuous medium.* Prentice-Hall, Englewood Cliffs, 1969
311. S. Mantero, R. Pietrabissa, and R. Fumero. The coronary bed and its role in the cardiovascular system: a review and an introductory single-branch model. *J. Biomed. Engng.*, 14:109–116, 1992
312. M. Mäntylä. *An Introduction to Solid Modeling.* Computer Science Press, College Park, 1988
313. J.E. Marsden and T.J.R. Hughes. *Mathematical Foundations of Elasticity.* Prentice-Hall, Englewood Cliffs, 1983
314. V. Martin, F. Clèment, A. Decoene, and J.-F. Gerbeau. Parameter identification for a one-dimensional blood flow model. In *Proceedings Cemracs 2004, ESAIM*, 2005
315. F.H. Martini. *Fundamentals of Anatomy and Physiology.* Prentice Hall, Englewood Cliffs, 1995
316. K.S. Matthys, J. Alastruey, J. Peiró, A.W. Khir, P. Segers, P.R. Verdonck, K.H. Parker, and S.J. Sherwin. Pulse wave propagation in a model human arterial network: Assessment of 1-D numerical simulations against in vitro measurements. *J. Biomech.*, 40(15):3476–3486, 2007

317. D.A. McDonald. *Blood Flow in Arteries.* Edward Arnold, London, 1960
318. T. McInerney and D. Terzopoulos. A dynamic finite element surface model for segmentation and tracking in multidimensional medical images with application to cardiac 4D image analysis. *Comp. Med. Imag. Graph.*, 19(1):69–83, 1995
319. T. McInerney and D. Terzopoulos. Deformable models in medical image analysis: a survey. *Med. Imag. Anal.*, 1(2):91–108, Jun 1996
320. T. McInerney and D. Terzopoulos. Topology adaptive deformable surfaces for medical image volume segmentation. *IEEE T. Med. Imaging.*, 18(10):840–850, Oct 1999
321. E.W. Merill. Rheology of blood. *Physiol. Rev.*, 49:863–888, 1969
322. E.W. Merill, C.S. Cheng, and G.A. Pelletier. Yield stress of normal human blood as a function of endogeneous fibrinogen. *Journal of Applied Physology*, 26:1–3, 1969
323. E.W. Merrill, A.M. Benis, E.R. Gilliland, T.K. Sherwood, and E.W. Salzman. Pressure-flow relations of human blood in hollow fibers at low flow rates. *Journal of Applied Physology*, 20:954–967, 1965
324. E.W. Merrill, E.R. Gilliland, G. Cokelet, H. Shin, A. Britten, and R.E. Wells, Jr. Rheology of human blood, near and at zero flow. Effects of temperature and hematocrit level. *Biophys. J.*, 3:199–213, 1963
325. J. Mewis. Thixotropy – A general review. *J. Non-Newtonian Fluid Mech.*, 6:1–20, 1979
326. G. Meyer, R. Merval, and A. Tedgui. Effects of pressure stretch and convection on low-density lipoprotein and albumin uptake in the rabbit aortic wall. *Circ. Res.*, 79(3):532–540, 1996
327. H.J. Michaely, O. Dietrich, K. Nael, S. Weckbach, M.F. Reiser, and S.O. Schoenberg. MRA of abdominal vessels: technical advances. *Europ. Radiol.*, 16(8):1637–1650, 2006
328. F. Migliavacca, R. Balossino, G. Pennati, G. Dubini, T-Y. Hsia, M. R. de Leval, and E.L. Bove. Multiscale modelling in biofluidynamics: application to reconstructive paediatric cardiac surgery. *J. Biomech.*, 39(6):1010–20, 2006
329. F. Migliavacca, G. Dubini, E.R. Bove, and M.R. de Leval. Computational fluid dynamics simulations in realistic 3-D geometries of the total cavopulmonary anastomosis: the influence of the inferior caval anastomosis. *J. Biomech. Engng.*, 125(6):805–813, Dec 2003
330. F. Migliavacca, F. Gervaso, M. Prosi, P. Zunino, S. Minisini, L. Formaggia, and G. Dubini. Expansion and drug elution model of a coronary stent. *Comp. Meth. Biomech. Biomed. Engng.*, 10(1):63–73, 2007
331. F. Migliavacca, G. Pennati, G. Dubini, and M.R. de Leval. A study of mathematical modelling of the competitions of flow in the cavopulmonary anastomosis with persistent forward flow. *Card. Young*, 14 Suppl 3:32–37, 2004
332. F. Migliavacca, G. Pennati, G. Dubini, R. Fumero, R. Pietrabissa, G. Urcelay, E.L. Bove, T-Y. Hsia, and M.R. de Leval. Modeling of the Norwood circulation: effects of shunt size, vascular resistances, and heart rate. *Am. J. Physiol. Heart Circ. Physiol.*, 280:H2076–H2086, 2001
333. J.S. Milner, J.A. Moore, B.K. Rutt, and D.A. Steinman. Hemodynamics of human carotid artery bifurcations: computational studies with models reconstructed from magnetic resonance imaging of normal subjects. *J. Vasc. Surg.*, 27(1):143–156, 1998

334. W.R. Milnor. *Hemodynamics*. Williams & Wilkins (2nd ed.), Baltimore, 1989
335. R.D. Mindlin. Influence of rotary inertia and shear on flexural motion of isotropic elastic plates. *J. Appl. Mech.*, 18:31–38, 1951
336. D.P. Mok, W.A. Wall, and E. Ramm. Partitioned analysis approach for the transient, coupled response of viscous fluids and flexible structures. In W. Wunderlich, editor, *Proceedings of the European Conference on Computational Mechanics*. ECCM'99, TU Munich, 1999
337. D.P. Mok, W.A. Wall, and E. Ramm. Accelerated iterative substructuring schemes for instationary fluid-structure interaction. In K.J. Bathe (ed.), *Computational Fluid and Solid Mechanics*, pp. 1325–1328. Elsevier, Amsterdam, 2001
338. P.C.F. Møller, J. Mewis, and D. Bonn. Yield stress and thixotropy: on the difficulty of measuring yield stress in practice. *Soft Matter*, 2:274–288, 2006
339. M. Mooney. Explicit formulas for slip and fluidity. *J. Rheol.*, 2:210–221, 1931
340. J.E. Moore, N. Guggenheim, A. Delfino, P.A. Doriot, P.A. Dorsaz, W. Rutishauser, and J.J. Meister. Preliminary analysis of the effects of blood vessel movement on blood flow patterns in the coronary arteries. *J. Biomech. Engng.*, 116(3):302–306, Aug 1994
341. H. Morand and R. Ohayon. *Fluid-Structure Interaction: Applied Numerical Methods*. John Wiley & Sons, Chichester, 1995
342. L. Morris, P. Delassus, P. Grace, F. Wallis, M. Walsh, and T. McGloughin. Effects of flat, parabolic and realistic steady flow inlet profiles on idealised and realistic stent graft fits through Abdominal Aortic Aneurysms (AAA). *Med. Eng. Phys.*, 28:19–26, 2006
343. K.W. Morton and D.F. Mayers. *Numerical solution of partial differential equations*. Cambridge University Press, Cambridge, 2005
344. J. Mouro. *Interactions fluide structure en grands déplacements. Résolution numérique et application aux composants hydrauliques automobiles*. PhD thesis, Ecole Polytechnique, Paris, 1996
345. C.M. Murea. Optimal control approach for the fluid-structure interaction problems. In J.Bemelmans et al., editor, *Proceedings of the Fourth European Conference on Elliptic and Parabolic Problems*, volume 52 (2), pp. 442–450. World Scientific Publ. Co. Pte., 2001
346. C.M. Murea and C. Vazquez. Sensitivity and approximation of coupled fluid-structure equations by virtual control method. *Appl. Math. Optim.*, 52(2):357–371, 1952
347. D.L. Nelson and M.M. Cox. *Lehninger Principles of Biochemistry*. W.H. Freeman (5th ed.), New York, 2008
348. P. Neofytou. Comparison of blood rheological models for physiological flow simulation. *Biorheol.*, 41(6):693–714, 2004
349. Q.D. Nguyen and D.V. Boger. Measuring the flow properties of yield stress fluids. *Annu. Rev. Fluid Mech.*, 24:47–88, 1992
350. W.W. Nichols and M.F. O'Rourke. *McDonald's Blood Flow in Arteries: Theoretical, Experimental and Clinical Principles*. Hodder Arnold (4th ed.), London, 2005
351. F. Nobile. *Numerical approximation of fluid-structure interaction problems with application to haemodynamics*. PhD thesis, EPFL, 2001
352. F. Nobile and C. Vergara. An effective fluid-structure interaction formulation for vascular dynamics by generalized robin conditions. *SIAM J. Scient. Comp.*, 30(2):731–763, 2008

353. A. Noordergraaf, H.B.K. Boom, and P.D. Verdouw. A human systemic analog computer. In A Noordergraf, editor, *1st Congr. Soc. for Ballistocardiographic Res.*, 1960
354. W.I. Norwood. Hypoplastic left heart syndrome. *Ann. Thor. Surg.*, 52:688–695, 1991
355. O. Ogunrinade, G.T. Kameya, and G.A. Truskey. Effects of fluid shear stress on the permeability of the arterial endothelium. *Ann. Biomed. Eng.*, 30:430–446, 2002
356. R.G. Ohye, A. Ludomirsky, E.J. Devaney, and E.L. Bove. Comparison of right ventricle to pulmonary artery conduit and modified blalock-taussig shunt hemodynamics after the norwood operation. *Ann. Thor. Surg.*, 78(3):1090–1093, 2004
357. M. Olufsen, F. Nielsen, P.F. Jensen, and S.A. Pedersen. The models underlying anaesthesia simulator Sophus. TEKST 278, IMFUFA, Roskilde Universitets-center, Roskilde, 1994
358. M.S. Olufsen. Structured tree ouflow condition for blood flow in larger systemic arteries. *Am. J. Physiol.*, 276:H257–H268, 1999
359. M.S. Olufsen and A. Nadim. On deriving lumped models for blood flow and pressure in the systemic arteries. *Math. Biosci. Engng*, 1:61–80, 2004
360. M.S. Olufsen, C.S. Peskin, W.Y. Kim, E.M. Pedersen, A. Nadim, and J. Larsen. Numerical simulation and experimental validation of blood flow in arteries with structured tree outflow conditions. *Ann. Biomed. Eng.*, 28(11):1281–1299, 2000
361. A. Osses and J.P. Puel. Approximate controllability for a linear model of fluid structure interaction. *ESAIM: Contr. Optim. Calc. Var.*, 4:497–513, 1999
362. N. Otsu. A threshold selection method from gray level histograms. *IEEE Trans. on System, Man and Cybernetics*, 9:62–66, Mar 1979
363. J.T. Ottesen. Modeling the baro-reflex feedback mechanism with time-delay. *J. Math. Biol.*, 36:41–63, 1997
364. J.T. Ottesen, M.S. Olufsen, and J.K. Larsen (eds.). *Mathematical Models in Human Physiology*. SIAM, Philadelphia, 2004
365. S.J. Owen. A survey of unstructured mesh generation technology. In *7th International Meshing Roundtable*, pp. 239–267, 1998
366. S.J. Owen and M. Shephard (eds.). *5th Symposium on Trends in Unstructured Mesh Generation*. Special issue of *Engineering with Computers*, 24:3, 2008
367. R.G. Owens. A new microstructure-based constitutive model for human blood. *J. Non-Newtonian Fluid Mech.*, 140:57–70, 2006
368. R.G. Owens and T.N. Phillips. *Computational Rheology*. Imperial College Press, London, 2005
369. Ö. Özsarlak, J.W. Van Goethem, M. Maes, and P.M. Parizel. MR angiography of the intracranial vessels: technical aspects and clinical applications. *Neuroradiology*, 46(12):955–972, 2004
370. Y. Papaharilaou, D.J. Doorly, S.J. Sherwin, J. Peiro, C. Griffth, N. Cheshire, V. Zervas, J. Anderson, B. Sanghera, N. Watkins, and C.G. Caro. Combined MRI and computational fluid dynamics detailed investigation of flow in idealised and realistic arterial bypass graft models. *Biorheol.*, 39(3/4):525–532, 2002
371. S.V. Patankar. *Numerical Heat Transfer and Fluid Flow*. Computational Methods in Mechanics and Thermal Sciences. Taylor and Francis, London, 1980
372. L. Pauling, H. Itano, S.J. Singer, and I.C. Wells. Sickle cell anemia: A molecular disease. *Science*, 110:543–548, 1949

373. T.J. Pedley. *The Fluid Mechanics of Large Blood Vessels.* Cambridge University Press, Cambridge, 1980
374. J. Peiró. Surface grid generation. In J.F. Thompson, N.P. Weatherill, and B.K. Soni (eds.). *Handbook of Grid Generation,* Chapter 19. CRC Press, Boca Raton, 1999
375. J. Peiró, L. Formaggia, M. Gazzola, A. Radaelli, and V. Rigamonti. Shape reconstruction from medical images and quality mesh generation via implicit surfaces. *Int. J. Numer. Meth. Fluids,* 53:1339–1360, 2007
376. G. Pennati, M. Bellotti, and R. Fumero. Mathematical modelling of the human fetal cardiovascular system based on Doppler ultrasound data. *Med. Eng. Phys.,* 19:327–335, 1997
377. G. Pennati and R. Fumero. Scaling approach to study the changes through the gestation of human fetal cardiac and circulatory behaviors. *Ann. Biomed. Eng.,* 28:442–452, 2000
378. G. Pennati, F. Migliavacca, G. Dubini, R. Pietrabissa, and M.R. de Leval. A mathematical model of circulation in the presence of the bidirectional cavopulmonary anastomosis in children with a univentricular heart. *Med. Eng. Phys.,* 19:223–234, 1997
379. K. Perktold and G. Karner. Computational principles and models of hemodynamics. In M. Hennerici and S. Meairs (eds.), *Cerebral Ultrasound, Theory, practice and future developments,* p. 63. Cambridge University Press, Cambridge, 2001
380. K. Perktold, M. Hofer, G. Rappitsch, M. Loew, B.D. Kuban, and M.H. Friedman. Validated computation of physiologic flow in a realistic coronary artery branch. *J. Biomech.,* 31:217–228, 1998
381. K. Perktold and M. Prosi. Computational models of arterial flow and mass transport. In G. Pedrizzetti and K. Perktold (eds.), *Cardiovascluar fluid mechanics,* number 446 in CISM Courses and lectures, pp. 73–136. Springer-Verlag, Wien, New York, 2003
382. K. Perktold, M. Prosi, and A. Leuprecht. Computer simulation of arterial flow and related transport phenomena. In J. Middleton, N.G. Shrive, and M.L. Jones (eds.), *Computer Methods in Biomechanics and Biomedical Engineering.* University of Wales College of Medicine, Cardiff, 2002. CD Rom, ISBN: 1 903847 09 5
383. K. Perktold, M. Resch, and H. Florian. Pulsatile non-Newtonian flow characteristics in a three-dimensional human carotid bifurcation model. *J. Biomech. Engng.,* 113:464–475, 1991
384. P. Perona and J. Malik. Scale-space and edge detection using anisotropic diffusion. *IEEE T. Pattern. Anal.,* 12(7):629–639, 1990
385. C. Peskin. The immersed boundary method. *Acta Numerica,* 11:479–517, 2002
386. D.L. Pham, C. Xu, and J.L. Prince. Current methods in medical image segmentation. *Annu. Rev. Biomed. Eng.,* 2:315–337, 2000
387. C. Picart, J.-M. Piau, H. Galliard, and P. Carpentier. Blood low shear rate rheometry: influence of fibrinogen level and hematocrit on slip and migrational effects. *Biorheol.,* 35:335–353, 1998
388. C. Picart, J.-M. Piau, H. Galliard, and P. Carpentier. Human blood shear yield stress and its hematocrit dependence. *J. Rheol.,* 42:1–12, 1998
389. G. Pierce. Basics of computed tomography angiography of the lower extremity vessels. *Semin. Vasc. Surg.,* 17(2):102–109, 2004

390. R. Pitt. *Numerical Simulation of Fluid Mechanical Phenomena in Idealised Physiological Geometries: Stenosis and Double Bend.* PhD thesis, Imperial College London, University of London, 2005
391. G. Pontrelli. The role of the arterial prestress in blood flow dynamics. *Med. Eng. Phys.*, 28(1):6–12, Jan 2006
392. R. Ponzini, C. Vergara, A. Redaelli, and A. Veneziani. Reliable CFD based estimation of flow rate in haemodynamics measures. *Ultras. Biol. Med.*, 32(10):1545–1555, 2006
393. A.S. Popel and P.C. Johnson. Microcirculation and hemorheology. *Ann. Rev. Fluid Mech.*, 37:43–69, 2005
394. A.R. Pries and T.W. Secomb. Rheology of the microcirculation. *Clinic. Hemorheol. Microc.*, 29:143–148, 2003
395. M. Prosi. *Computersimulation von Massetransportvorgängen in Arterien.* PhD thesis, TUG, Austria, 2003
396. M. Prosi, K. Perktold, Z. Ding, and M.H. Friedman. Influence of curvature dynamics on pulsatile coronary artery flow in a realistic bifurcation model. *J. Biomech.*, 37:1767–1775, 2003
397. M. Prosi, P. Zunino, K. Perktold, and A. Quarteroni. Mathematical and numerical models for the transfer of low-density lipoproteins through the arterial walls: a new methodology for the model set up with application to the study of disturbed lumenal flow. *J. Biomech.*, 38:903–917, 2005
398. M.H. Protter and H.F.Weinberger. *Maximum Principles in Differential Equations.* Springer-Verlag, New York, 1984
399. Y. Qiu and J.M. Tarbell. Numerical simulation of oxygen mass transfer in a compliant curved tube model of a coronary artery. *Ann. Biomed. Eng.*, 28:26–38, 2000
400. A. Quaini and A. Quarteroni. A semi-implicit approach for fluid-structure interaction based on an algebraic fractional step method. *Math. Mod. Meth. Appl. Sciences*, 17(6):957–983, 2007
401. A. Quarteroni and L. Formaggia. Mathematical modelling and numerical simulation of the cardiovascular system. In N. Ayache, editor, *Computational Models for the Human Body*, Handbook of Numerical Analysis (P.G. Ciarlet ed.), pp. 3–129. Elsevier, Amsterdam, 2004
402. A. Quarteroni, S. Ragni, and A. Veneziani. Coupling between lumped and distributed models for blood problems. *Comp. Visual. Science*, 4:111–124, 2001
403. A. Quarteroni, R. Sacco, and F. Saleri. *Numerical Mathematics.* Springer-Verlag (2nd ed.), Berlin, 2006
404. A. Quarteroni, F. Saleri, and A. Veneziani. Analysis of the Yosida method for the incompressible Navier-Stokes equations. *J. Math. Pures et Appl.*, 78:473–503, 1999
405. A. Quarteroni, F. Saleri, and A. Veneziani. Factorization methods for the numerical approximation of the incompressible Navier-Stokes equations. *Comp. Meth. Appl. Mech. Eng.*, 1998:505–526, 2000
406. A. Quarteroni, M. Tuveri, and A. Veneziani. Computational vascular fluid dynamics: problems, models and methods. *Comp. Visual. Science*, 2:163–197, 2000
407. A. Quarteroni and A. Valli. *Numerical Approximation of Partial Differential Equations.* Number 23 in Springer-Verlag Series in Computational Mathematics. Springer-Verlag, Berlin, 1997

408. A. Quarteroni and A. Valli. *Domain decomposition methods for partial differential equations*. Numerical Mathematics and Scientific Computation. The Clarendon Press and Oxford University Press, Oxford, 1999. Oxford Science Publications
409. A. Quarteroni and A. Veneziani. Analysis of a geometrical multiscale model based on the coupling of PDE's and ODE's for blood flow simulations. *Multiscale Model. Simul.*, 1(2):173–195, 2003
410. A. Quarteroni, A. Veneziani, and P. Zunino. A domain decomposition method for advection-diffusion processes with application to blood solutes. *SIAM J. Scient. Comp.*, 23(6):1959–1980, 2002
411. A. Quarteroni, A. Veneziani, and P. Zunino. Mathematical and numerical modelling of solute dynamics in blood flow and arterial walls. *SIAM J. Numer. Anal.*, 39(5):1488–1511, 2002
412. D. Quemada. Rheology of concentrated disperse systems III. General features of the proposed non-Newtonian model. Comparison with experimental data. *Rheol. Acta*, 17:643–653, 1978
413. D. Quemada. A non-linear Maxwell model of biofluids: Application to normal human blood. *Biorheol.*, 30:253–265, 1993
414. D. Quemada. Rheological modelling of complex fluids. I. The concept of effective volume fraction revisited. *Eur. Phys. J. AP*, 1:119–127, 1998
415. D. Quemada. Rheological modelling of complex fluids. IV. Thixotropic and "thixoelastic" behaviour. Start-up and stress relaxation, creep tests and hysteresis cycles. *Eur. Phys. J. AP*, 5:191–207, 1999
416. B. Rabinowitsch. Über die Viskosität und Elastizität von Solen. *Z. Physik Chem.*, A145:1–26, 1929
417. K.R. Rajagopal and A.R. Srinivasa. A thermodynamic framework for rate-type fluid models. *J. Non-Newtonian Fluid Mech.*, 88:207–227, 2000
418. P.W. Rand, E. Lacombe, H.E. Hunt, and W.H. Austin. Viscosity of normal human blood under normothermic and hypothermic conditions. *J. Appl. Physiol.*, 19:117–122, 1964
419. G. Rappitsch and K. Perktold. Computer simulation of convective diffusion processes in large arteries. *J. Biomech.*, 29:207–216, 1995
420. G. Rappitsch and K. Perktold. Pulsatile albumin transport in large arteries: a numerical simulation study. *ASME J. Biomech. Eng,*, 118:511–519, 1996
421. G. Rappitsch, K. Perktold, and E. Pernkopf. Numerical modelling of shear-dependent mass transfer in large arteries. *Int. J. Numer. Meth. Fluids*, 25:847–857, 1997
422. S.P. Raya and J.K. Udupa. Shape-based interpolation of multidimensional objects. *IEEE T. Med. Imaging.*, 9(1):32–42, 1990
423. A. Redaelli, F. Boschetti, and F. Inzoli. The assignment of velocity profiles in finite element simulations of pulsatile flow in arteries. *Comp. Biol. Med.*, 27(3):233–247, 1997
424. B.D. Reddy. *Introductory Functional Analysis. With applications to boundary value problems and finite elements*. Springer-Verlag, New York, 1998
425. E. Reissner. The effect of transverse shear deformation on the bending of elastic plates. *J. Appl. Mech.*, 67:A69–A77, 1945
426. V.C. Rideout and D.E. Dick. Difference-differential equations for fluid flow in distensible tubes. *IEEE T. Bio-Med. Eng.*, 14(3):171–7, 1967
427. J.M. Rippe. *Heart Disease for Dummies*. Wiley, Indianapolis, 2004

428. A.M. Robertson. Review of Relevant Continuum Mechanics. In G.P. Galdi, R. Rannacher, A.M. Robertson, and S. Turek (eds.), *Hemodynamical Flows: Modeling, Analysis and Simulation*, volume 37, pp. 1–62. Birkhäuser Verlag, Basel, 2008. Oberwolfach Seminars
429. A.M. Robertson, A. Sequeira, and M.V. Kameneva. Hemorheology. In G.P. Galdi, R. Rannacher, A.M. Robertson, and S. Turek (eds.), *Hemodynamical Flows: Modeling, Analysis and Simulation*, vol. 37, pp. 63–120. Birkhäuser Verlag, Basel, 2008. Oberwolfach Seminars
430. C.M. Rodkiewicz, P. Sinha, and J.S. Kennedy. On the application of a constitutive equation for whole human blood. *J. Biomech. Engng.*, 112:198–206, 1990
431. J.S. Rosenblatt, D.S. Soane, and M.C. Williams. A Couette rheometer design for minimizing sedimentation and red-cell aggregation artifacts in low-shear blood rheometry. *Biorheol.*, 24:811–816, 1987
432. M. Rosenfeld, E. Rambod, and M. Gharib. Circulation and formation number of laminar vortex rings. *J. Fluid Mech.*, 376:297–318, 1998
433. M. Rowe. Measurements and computations of flow in pipe bends. *J. Fluid Mech.*, 43:771–783, 1970
434. G. Rozza. On optimization, control and shape design of an arterial bypass. *Int. J. Numer. Meth. Fluids*, 47(10-11):1411–1419, 2005
435. W. Ruan, M.E. Clark, M. Zhao, and A. Curcio. A hyperbolic system of equations of blood flow in an arterial network. *SIAM J. Appl. Math.*, 64(2):637–667, 2004
436. W. Ruan, M.E. Clark, M. Zhao, and A. Curcio. Global solution to a hyperbolic problem arising in the modeling of blood flow in circulatory systems. *J. Math. Anal. Appl.*, 331(2):1068–1092, 2007
437. W. Ruan, M.E. Clark, M. Zhao, and A. Curcio. Initial-boundary-value problem of hyperbolic equations for blood flow in a vessel. *Nonlinear Anal. Real World Appl.*, 9(5):2068–2085, 2008
438. W. Rudin. *Functional Analysis*. McGraw-Hill, New York, 1991
439. Y. Saad. *Iterative Methods for Sparse Linear Systems*. PWS Publishing Company, Boston, 1996
440. Y. Saad and M.H. Schultz. GMRES: a generalized minimal residual algorithm for solving nonsymmetric linear systems. *SIAM J. Scient. Stat. Comput.*, 7(3):856–869, 1986
441. A.H. Sacks, K.R. Raman, J.A. Burnell, and E.G. Tickner. Report no. 119, technical report, vidya, 1963
442. P.G. Saffman. *Vortex Dynamics*. Cambridge University Press, Cambridge, 1992
443. K. Sagawa, H. Suga, and K. Nakayama. Instantaneous pressure-volume ratio of the left ventricle versus instantaneous force-length relation of papillary muscle. In J. Baan, A. Noordergraaf, and J. Raines (eds.), *Cardiovascular System Dynamics*, pp. 99–105, 1999
444. D.V. Sakharov, L.V. Kalachev, and D.C. Rijken. Numerical simulation of local pharmacokinetics of a drug after intravascular delivery with an eluting stent. *J. Drug Targ.*, 10:507–513, 2002
445. A.G. Salinger, R. Aris, and J.J. Derby. Finite element formulations for large-scale coupled flows in adjacent porous and open fluid domains. *Int. J. Numer. Meth. Fluids*, 18:1185–1209, 1994
446. H. Samet. *The Design and Analysis of Spatial Data Structures*. Addison-Wesley, Reading, 1990

447. S. Sano, K. Ishino, M. Kawada, S. Arai, S. Kasahara, T. Asai, Z. Masuda, M. Takeuchi, and S. Ohtsuki. Right ventricle-pulmonary artery shunt in first-stage palliation of hypoplastic left heart syndrome. *J. Thor. Cardiov. Surg.*, 126:504–509, 2003
448. H. Schmid-Schönbein, P. Gaehtgens, and H. Hirsch. On the shear rate dependence of red cell aggregation in vitro. *J. Clin. Invest.*, 47:1447–1454, 1968
449. H. Schmid-Schönbein and R. Wells. Fluid drop-like transition of erythrocytes under shear. *Science*, 165:288–291, 1969
450. H. Schmid-Schönbein and R.E. Wells, Jr. Rheological properties of human erythrocytes and their influence upon the "anomalous" viscosity of blood. *Ergeb. Physiol.*, 63:146–219, 1971
451. H. Schmid-Schönbein, H.G. Gallasch, E. Volger, and H.J. Klose. Microrheology and protein chemistry of pathological red cell aggregation (blood sludge) studies in vitro. *Biorheol.*, 10:213–222, 1973
452. H. Schmid-Schönbein, E. Volger, and H.J. Klose. Microrheology and light transmission of blood, II. the photometric quantification of red cell aggregation formation and dispersion in flow. *Pflüggers Arch.*, 333:140–155, 1972
453. J.A. Sethian. *Level Set Methods and Fast Marching Methods.* Cambridge University Press, Cambridge, 1999
454. T. Sexl. Über den von E.G. Richardson entdeckten 'Annulareffekt'. *Z. Phys.*, 61:349–362, 1930
455. L.F. Shampine and C.W. Gear. User view of solving stiff ordinary differential-equations. *SIAM Review*, 21(1):1–17, 1979
456. S.J. Sherwin and H.M. Blackburn. Three-dimensional instabilities and transition of steady and pulsatile flows in an axisymmetric stenotic tube. *J. Fluid Mech.*, 533:297–327, 2005
457. S.J. Sherwin. Dispersion analysis of the continuous and discontinuous Galerkin formulations. In *Discontinuous Galerkin methods: Theory, computational and applications.* Springer-Verlag, Berlin, 2000
458. S.J. Sherwin and D.J. Doorly. *Flow dynamics within model distal arterial bypass grafts*, volume 34 of *Advance in Fluid Mechanics*, A. Tura (ed.), Chapter 9. WIT Press, Southampton, 2003
459. S.J. Sherwin and J. Peiró. Mesh generation in curvilinear domains using high-order elements. *Int. J. Numer. Meth. Engng.*, 53(1):207–223, 2002
460. S.J. Sherwin, O. Shah, D.J. Doorly, J. Peiró, Y. Papaharilaou, N. Watkins, C.G. Caro, and C.L. Dumoulin. The influence of out-of-plane geometry on the flow within a distal end-to-side anastomosis. *J. Biomech. Engng.*, 122:76–86, 2000
461. J.R. Shewchuk. Adaptive precision floating-point arithmetic and fast robust geometric predicates. *Discr. Comput. Geom.*, 18:305–363, 1997
462. J.R. Shewchuk. What is a good linear element? Interpolation, conditioning, and quality measures. In *Eleventh International Meshing Roundtable*, pp. 115–126, 2002
463. S.D. Shpilfoygel, R.A. Close, D.J. Valentino, and G.R. Duckwiler. X-ray videodensitometric methods for blood flow and velocity measurement: A critical review of literature. *Med. Phys.*, 27:2008–2023, 2000
464. J.H. Siggers and S.L. Waters. Steady flows in pipes with finite curvature. *Phys. Fluids*, 17(7):077102, 2005
465. S. Singhal, R. Henderson, K. Horsfield, K. Harding, and G. Cumming. Morphometry of the human pulmonary arterial tree. *Circ. Res.*, 33(2):190–197, Aug 1973

466. R. Skalak and S. Chien. Theoretical models of rouleaux formation and disaggregation. *Ann. N. Y. Acad. Sci.*, 416:138–148, 1983
467. R. Skalak and S. Chien (eds.). *Handbook of Bioengineering*, Chapter: Cardiovascular Models and Controls, pp. 2386–2403. CRC Press, Boca Raton, 1995
468. R. Skalak and C.Zhu. Rheological aspects of red blood cell aggregation. *Biorheol.*, 27:309–325, 1990
469. F.T. Smith. Fluid flow into a curved pipe. *Proc. Roy. Soc., Ser. A*, 351:71–87, 1968
470. R.E. Smith. Transfinite interpolation (TFI) generation systems. In J.F. Thompson, N.P. Weatherill, and B.K. Soni (eds.), *Handbook of Grid Generation*, Chapter 3. CRC Press, Boca Raton, 1999
471. J. Smoller. *Shock Waves and Reaction-Diffusion Equations.* Springer-Verlag, New York, 1983
472. M.F. Snyder and V.C. Rideout. Computer simulation of the venous circulation. *IEEE Trans. Biomed. Engng.*, 16:325–334, 1969
473. J. Sokołowski and J.-P. Zolsio. *Introduction to shape optimization*, volume 16 of *Springer Series in Computational Mathematics.* Springer-Verlag, Berlin, 1992
474. B.K. Soni. Grid generation: Past, present, and future. *Appl. Numer. Math.*, 32:361–369, 2000
475. H.B. Squire and K.G. Winter. The secondary flow in a cascade of airfoils in a non-uniform stream. *J. Aero. Sci*, 18:271–277, 1951
476. D.K. Stangeby and C.R. Ethier. Computational analysis of coupled blood-wall arterial ldl transport. *J. Biomech. Engng.*, 124:1–8, 2002
477. B.N. Steele, M.S. Olufsen, and C.A. Taylor. Fractal network model for simulating abdominal and lower extremity blood flow during resting and exercise conditions. *Comp. Meth. Biomech. Biomed. Engng.*, 10:39–51, 2007
478. D.A. Steinman, J.S. Milner, C.J. Norley, S.P. Lownie, and D.W. Holdsworth. Image-based computational simulation of flow dynamics in a giant intracranial aneurysm. *AJNR Am. J. Neuroradiol.*, 24(4):559–566, Apr 2003
479. D.A. Steinman and C.A. Taylor. Flow imaging and computing: Large artery hemodynamics. *Ann. Biomed. Eng.*, 33:1704–1709, 2005
480. D.A. Steinman. Image-based computational fluid dynamics modeling in realistic arterial geometries. *Ann. Biomed. Eng.*, 30(4):483–497, Apr 2002
481. D.A. Steinman and C.R. Ethier. The effect of wall distensibility on flow in a two-dimensional end-to-side anastomosis. *J. Biomech. Engng.*, 116(3):294–301, Aug 1994
482. D.A. Steinman, J.B. Thomas, H.M. Ladak, J.S. Milner, B.K. Rutt, and J.D. Spence. Reconstruction of carotid bifurcation hemodynamics and wall thickness using computational fluid dynamics and MRI. *Magn. Reson. Medic.*, 47(1):149–159, 2002
483. N. Stergiopulos, B.E. Westerhof, and N. Westerhof. Total arterial inertance as the fourth element of the windkessel model. *Am. J. Physiol.*, 276:H81–H88, 1999
484. J.F. Stoltz and M. Lucius. Viscoelasticity and thixotropy of human blood. *Biorheol.*, 18:453–473, 1981
485. J.F. Stoltz, M. Singh, and P. Riha. *Hemorheology in Practice.* IOS Press, Amsterdam, 1999
486. H. Suga. Theoretical analysis of a left ventricular pumping model based on the systolic time-varying pressure-volume ratio. *IEEE Trans. Biomed. Engng.*, 18:47–55, 1971

487. H. Suga. Cardiac mechanics and energetics–from Emax to PVA. *Front. Med. Biol. Eng.*, 2(1):3–22, 1990
488. H. Suga and K. Sagawa. Instantaneous pressure-volume relationships and their ratio in the excised, supported canine left ventricle. *Circ. Res.*, 35:117–126, 1974
489. H. Suga, K. Sagawa, and L. Demer. Determinants of instantaneous pressure in canine left ventricle. Time and volume specification. *Circ. Res.*, 46(2):256–263, Feb 1980
490. N. Sun and D. De Kee. Simple shear, hysteresis and yield stress in biofluids. *Can. J. Chem. Eng.*, 79:36–41, 2001
491. J.M. Tarbell. Mass transport in arteries and the localization of atherosclerosis. *Annu. Rev. Biomed. Eng.*, 5:79–118, 2003
492. J.M. Tarbell, M.J. Lever, and C.G. Caro. The effect of varying albumin concentration and hydrostatic pressure on hydraulic conductivity of the rabbit common carotid artery. *Microvasc. Res.*, 35:204–220, 1988
493. C.A. Taylor and M.T. Draney. Experimental and computational methods in cardiovascular fluid mechanics. *Annu. Rev. Fluid Mech.*, 36:197–231, 2004
494. C.A. Taylor, M.T. Draney, J.P. Ku, D. Parker, B.N. Steele, K. Wang, and C.K. Zarins. Predictive medicine: Computational techniques in therapeutic decision-making. *Comp. Aid. Surg.*, 4(5):231–247, 1999
495. R. Temam. Une méthode d'approximation de la solution des équations de Navier-Stokes. *Bull. Soc. Math. France*, 96:115–152, 1968
496. T.E. Tezduyar. Finite element methods for fluid dynamics with moving boundaries and interfaces. *Arch. Comput. Meth. Engrg.*, 8:83–130, 2001
497. M. Thiriet. *Biology and Mechanics of Blood Flows.* CRM Series in Mathematical Physics. Springer-Verlag, New York, 2007
498. J.W. Thomas. *Numerical Partial Differential Equations: Finite Difference Methods.* Texts in Applied Mathematics. Springer-Verlag, New York, 1995
499. J.F. Thompson, B.K. Soni, and N.P. Weatherill (eds.). *Handbook of Grid Generation.* CRC Press, Boca Raton, 1999
500. J.F. Thompson, Z.U.A. Warsi, and C.W. Mastin. *Numerical Grid Generation. Foundations and Applications.* North-Holland, New York, 1985
501. J.F. Thompson and N.P. Weatherill. Aspects of numerical grid generation: Current science and art. In *11th AIAA Applied Aerodynamics Conf. (Amer. Inst. of Aeronautics and Astronautics)*, pp. 1029–1070, Aug 1993. AIAA paper 93-3539
502. K.W. Thompson. Time dependent boundary conditions for hyperbolic systems. *J. Comput. Phys.*, 68:1–24, 1987
503. G.B. Thurston. Frequency and shear rate dependence of viscoelasticity of human blood. *Biorheol.*, 10:375–381, 1973
504. G.B. Thurston. Elastic effects in pulsatile blood flow. *Microvasc. Res.*, 9:145–157, 1975
505. G.B. Thurston. Rheological parameters for the viscosity, viscoelasticity, and thixotropy of blood. *Biorheol.*, 16:149–162, 1979
506. G.B. Thurston. Plasma release-cell layering for blood flow. *Biorheol.*, 26:199–214, 1989
507. G.B. Thurston. Non-Newtonian viscosity of human blood: Flow induced changes in microstructure. *Biorheol.*, 31(2):179–192, 1994
508. G.B. Thurston. Viscoelastic properties of blood and blood analogs. *Adv. Hemodyn. Hemoreol.*, 1:1–30, 1996

509. W.D. Timmons. Cardiovascular models and control. In J. Bronzino (ed.), *The Biomedical Engineering Handbook*, Chapter 158, pp. 2386–2403. CRC Press, Boca Raton, 1999
510. S. Timoshenko. *Vibration Problems in Engineering*. D. van Nostrand, New York, 1955
511. A. Toselli and O. Widlund. *Domain Decomposition Methods – Algorithms and Theory*. Volume Series in Computational Mathematics, Vol. 34. Springer-Verlag, New York, 2005
512. C. Truesdell and W. Noll. *The non-linear field theories of mechanics*. Springer-Verlag (3rd ed.), Berlin, 2004. Edited and with a preface by Stuart S. Antman
513. G.A. Truskey, W.L. Roberts, R.A. Herrmann, and R.A. Malinauskas. Measurement of endothelial permeability to I-low density lipoproteins in rabbit arteries by use of en face preparations. *Circ. Res.*, 7(4):883–897, 1992
514. M. Unser. Splines: A perfect fit for signal and image processing. *IEEE Signal. Proc. Mag.*, 16(6):22–38, Nov 1999
515. M. Ursino. Interaction between carotid baroregulation and the pulsating heart: a mathematical model. *Am. J. Physiol.*, 275:H1733–H1747, 1998
516. M. Ursino and S. Cavalcanti. A mathematical model of the carotid baroreflex control in pulsatile conditions. *Surveys on Mathematics for Industry*, 7:203–220, 1997
517. S. Usami, R.G. King, S. Chien, R. Skalak, C.R. Huang, and A.L. Copley. Microcinephotographic studies of red cell aggregation in steady and oscillatory shear – A note. *Biorheol.*, 12:323–325, 1975
518. C.M. van Bemmel, L. Spreeuwers, M.A. Viergever, and W.J. Niessen. Level-set based carotid artery segmentation for stenosis grading. In *MICCAI*, volume 2489, pp. 36–43. Springer-Verlag, Berlin Heidelberg, 2002
519. C.M. van Bemmel, L.J. Spreeuwers, M.A. Viergever, and W.J. Niessen. Level-set-based artery-vein separation in blood pool agent CE-MR angiograms. *IEEE T. Med. Imaging*, 22(10):1224–1234, Oct 2003
520. C.M. van Bemmel, M.A. Viergever, and W.J. Niessen. Semiautomatic segmentation and stenosis quantification of 3d contrast-enhanced mr angiograms of the internal carotid artery. *Magn. Reson. Med.*, 51(4):753–760, Apr 2004
521. R. van Loon, P.D. Anderson, and F.N. van de Vosse. A fluid-structure interaction method with solid-rigid contact for heart valve dynamics. *J. Comput. Phys.*, 217:806–823, 2006
522. S. Čanić, J. Tambaca, A. Mikelić, C.J. Hartley, D. Mirković, J. Chavez, and D. Rosenstrauch. Blood flow through axially symmetric sections of compliant vessels: new effective closed models. *Conf. Proc. IEEE Eng. Med. Biol. Soc.*, 5:3696–3699, 2004
523. S. Čanić, J. Tambača, G. Guidoboni, A. Mikelić, C.J. Hartley, and D. Rosenstrauch. Modeling viscoelastic behavior of arterial walls and their interaction with pulsatile blood flow. *SIAM J. Appl. Math.*, 67(1):164–193, 2006
524. S. Čanić and E.H. Kim. Mathematical analysis of the quasilinear effects in a hyperbolic model blood flow through compliant axi-symmetric vessels. *Math. Methods Appl. Sci.*, 26(14):1161–1186, 2003
525. A. Veneziani. *Mathematical and Numerical Modeling of Blood Flow Problems*. PhD thesis, University of Milan, 1998
526. A. Veneziani and C. Vergara. Flow rate defective boundary conditions in haemodynamics simulations. *Int. J. Numer. Meth. Fluids*, 47(8-9):803–816, 2005

527. A. Veneziani and C. Vergara. An approximate method for solving incompressible navier-stokes problems with flow rate conditions. *Comp. Meth. Appl. Mech. Eng.*, 196:1685–1700, 2007
528. C. Vergara. *Numerical Modeling of Defective Boundary Problems in Incompressible Fluid-Dynamics – Applications to Computational Haemodynamics.* PhD thesis, Politecnico di Milano, 2006
529. C. Vergara and P. Zunino. Multiscale boundary conditions for drug release from cardiovascular stents. *Multiscale Model. Simul.*, 7:565–588, 2008
530. H. Versteeg and W. Malalasekera. *An Introduction to computational fluid dynamics: the finite volume method.* Prentice Hall (2nd ed.), London, 2007
531. I.E. Vignon-Clementel, C.A. Figueroa, K.E. Jansen, and C.A. Taylor. Outflow boundary conditions for three-dimensional finite element modeling of blood flow and pressure in arteries. *Comp. Meth. Appl. Mech. Eng.*, 195(29–32):3776–3796, 2006
532. G. Vlastos, D. Lerche, and B. Koch. The superposition of steady on oscillatory shear and its effect on the viscoelasticity of human blood and a blood-like model fluid. *Biorheol.*, 34:19–36, 1997
533. S. Wada and T. Karino. Computational study on LDL transfer from flowing blood to arterial walls. In T. Yamaguchi (ed.), *Clinical Application of Computational Mechanics to the Cardiovascular System*, pp. 157–173. Springer-Verlag, New York, 2000
534. F.J. Walburn and D.J. Schneck. A constitutive equation for whole human blood. *Biorheol.*, 13:201–210, 1976
535. J.J. Wang and K.H. Parker. Wave propagation in a model of the arterial circulation. *J. Biomech.*, 37(4):457–470, Apr 2004
536. K.C. Wang, R.W. Dutton, and C.A. Taylor. Improving geometric model reconstruction for blood flow modeling. *IEEE Eng. Med. Biol.*, 18(6):33–39, Nov/Dec 1999
537. D.F. Watson. Computing the n-dimensional Delaunay tessellation with application to Voronoi polytopes. *The Computer Journal*, 24:167–172, 1981
538. N.P. Weatherill and O. Hassan. Efficient three-dimensional delaunay triangulation with automatic point creation and imposed boundary constraints. *Int. J. Numer. Meth. Engng.*, 37:2005–2039, 1994
539. N. Westerhof, F. Bosman, C.J. De Vries, and A. Noordergraaf. Analog studies of the human systemic arterial tree. *J. Biomech.*, 2(2):121–43, 1969
540. R. Whitaker. Algorithms for implicit deformable models. In *Proceedings of the Fifth International Conference on Computer Vision*, pp. 822–827, 1995
541. R.T. Whitaker and X. Xue. Variable-conductance, level-set curvature for image denoising. In *ICIP01*, pp. III: 142–145, 2001
542. S. Whitaker. *Introduction to Fluid Mechanics.* R.E. Krieger, Malabar, 1984
543. R.L. Whitmore. *Rheology of the Circulation.* Pergamon Press, Oxford, 1968
544. S.E. Widnall, D.B. Bliss, and C.-Y. Tsai. The instability of short waves on a vortex ring. *J. Fluid Mech.*, 66(1):35–47, 1974
545. M.C. Williams, J.S. Rosenblatt, and D.S. Soane. Theory of blood rheology based on a statistical mechanics treatment of rouleaux, and comparisons with data. *Intern. J. Polymeric Mater.*, 21:57–63, 1993
546. J.R. Womersley. Method for the calculation of velocity, rate of flow and viscous drag in arteries when the pressure gradient is known. *J. Phys.*, 127:553–563, 1955

547. L.-S. Yao and S. Berger. Entry flow in a curved pipe. *J. Fluid Mech.*, 67:177–196, 1975
548. K.K. Yeleswarapu. *Evaluation of Continuum Models for Characterizing the Constitutive Behavior of Blood.* PhD thesis, University of Pittsburgh, Pittsburgh, 1996
549. K.K. Yeleswarapu, M.V. Kameneva, K.R. Rajagopal, and J.F. Antak. The flow of blood in tubes: Theory and experiment. *Mech. Res. Comm.*, 25:257–262, 1998
550. P.J. Yim, G. Boudewijn, C. Vasbinder, V. B. Ho, and P. L. Choyke. Isosurfaces as deformable models for magnetic resonance angiography. *IEEE T. Med. Imaging.*, 22(7):875–881, Jul 2003
551. P.J. Yim, J.R. Cebral, R. Mullick, and P.J. Choyke. Vessel surface reconstruction with a tubular deformable model. *IEEE T. Med. Imaging.*, 20(12):1411–1421, Dec 2001
552. K. Yosida. *Functional Analysis.* Springer Classics in Mathematics. Springer-Verlag (5th ed.), Berlin, 1980
553. Z. Yu. A DLM/FD method for fluid/flexible-body interactions. *J. Comput. Phys.*, 207(1):1–27, 2005
554. L. Zabielski and A. J. Mestel. Steady flow in a helicaly symmetric pipe. *J. Fluid Mech.*, 370:297–320, 1998
555. M. Zacek and E. Krause. Numerical simulation of the blood flow in the human cardiovascular system. *J. Biomech.*, 29(1):13–20, 1996
556. E. Zeidler. *Applied functional analysis.* Springer-Verlag, New York, 1991
557. H. Zhang, X. Zhang, S. Ji, Y. Guo, G. Ledezma, N. Elabbasi, and H. deCougny. Recent development of fluid-structure interaction capabilities in the ADINA system. *Comp. Struct.*, 81(8–11):1071–1085, 2003
558. Q.S. Zheng. Constitutive relations of linear elastic materials under various internal constraints. *Acta Mech.*, 158(1):97–103, Mar 2002
559. J.Z. Zhu, O.C. Zienkiewicz, E. Hinton, and J. Wu. A new approach to the development of automatic quadrilateral mesh generation. *Int. J. Numer. Meth. Engng.*, 32:849–866, 1991
560. D.P. Zipes. *Cardiac Electrophysiology: from Cell to Bedside.* Saunders (4th ed.), Philadephia, 2004
561. D. Zorin and P. Schröder. *Subdivision for modeling and animation.* Technical report, SIGGRAPH 2000, 2000. Course Notes
562. M.A. Zulliger, P. Fridez, K. Hayashi, and N. Stergiopulos. A strain energy function for arteries accounting for wall composition and structure. *J. Biomech.*, 37(7):989–1000, Jul 2004
563. P. Zunino. *Mathematical and numerical modeling of mass transfer in the vascular system.* PhD thesis, Ecole Polythéchnique Fédérale de Lausanne, 2002

Index

MIX
Papier aus verantwortungsvollen Quellen
Paper from responsible sources
FSC® C105338

If you have any concerns about our products,
you can contact us on
ProductSafety@springernature.com

In case Publisher is established outside the EU,
the EU authorized representative is:
Springer Nature Customer Service Center GmbH
Europaplatz 3, 69115 Heidelberg, Germany

Printed by Libri Plureos GmbH
in Hamburg, Germany